THE DYNAMICS OF HEALTH AND WELLNESS

A BIOPSYCHOSOCIAL APPROACH

THE DYNAMICS OF HEALTH AND WELLNESS

A BIOPSYCHOSOCIAL APPROACH

Judith Green
Aims Community College, Greeley, Colorado
Psychotherapy and Biofeedback Associate

Robert Shellenberger
Aims Community College, Greeley, Colorado
Psychotherapy and Biofeedback Associate

Harcourt Brace College Publishers
Fort Worth   Philadelphia   San Diego
New York   Orlando   Austin   San Antonio
Toronto   Montreal   London   Sydney   Tokyo

Publisher	Ted Buchholz
Acquisitions Editor	Eve Howard
Project Editor	Michele Tomiak/Steve Welch
Production Manager	Tad Gaither
Manager of Art & Design	Guy Jacobs
Text Designer	Rita Naughton
Cover Designer	George Rigg

Library of Congress Cataloging-in-Publication Data

Green, Judith Alyce.
    The dynamics of health and wellness : a biopsychosocial approach /
Judith Green, Robert Shellenberger.
        p.   cm.
    Includes bibliographical references.
    Includes index.
    ISBN 0-03-014583-X
    1. Health.   2. Stress management.   3. Personality—Health aspects.
4. Health behavior.   5. Health promotion.   I. Shellenberger,
Robert.   II. Title.
    [DNLM: 1. Biofeedback (Psychology).   2. Health Promotion.   WL 103
G796d]
RA776.G7887   1991
613—dc20
DNLM/DLC
for Library of Congress   90-5181
                                                                CIP

Requests for permission to make copies of any part of the work should be mailed to: Copyrights and Permissions Department, Holt, Rinehart and Winston, Inc., Orlando, FL 32887

Address Editorial Correspondence To: 301 Commerce Street, Suite 3700, Fort Worth, TX 76102

Address Orders To: 6277 Sea Harbor Drive, Orlando, FL 32887
1-800-782-4479, or 1-800-433-0001 (in Florida)

The paper used in this book was made from recycled paper.

Printed in the United States of America

3 4 016 9 8 7 6 5 4 3

To the Instructor

Throughout many years of teaching, clinical practice, and research, we have been intrigued by the question "Why are healthy people healthy?" To find the answer, we journeyed into many fields—medical sociology, health psychology, developmental psychology, pediatric psychology, personality, health education, community health, behavioral medicine, psychoneuroimmunology, psychophysiology, and research methodology. We have found a diverse and growing body of knowledge that is the foundation for understanding health and wellness, knowledge gained through the study of people who are physically and psychologically healthy, who have survived traumatic experiences in a healthful way, or who have recovered from disease or illness. *The Dynamics of Health and Wellness: A Biopsychosocial Approach* is an introduction to health and wellness based upon

these sources, and it describes health and wellness as complex processes that are the result of the interaction of biological, psychological, and social systems.

The biopsychosocial approach reflects the many forces that contribute to health and wellness, just as the biopsychosocial model of disease and illness reflects the forces that contribute to physical disorders, most obviously the chronic disorders that arise from lifestyle and stress. The biopsychosocial approach to health and wellness provides the framework for bringing together in a single textbook such diverse topics as personality; stress; physiology; psychophysiology and mind/body interaction; relaxation, biofeedback training, and other behavioral techniques; social support; self-responsibility and social responsibility; self regulation and lifestyle; the development of health behaviors; and behavioral medicine.

Behavioral medicine is the application of the dynamics and ingredients of health and wellness in treatment. The dynamics and ingredients of health and wellness help healthy people stay healthy, and the study of health and wellness is an integral part of the health sciences. At the same time, knowledge of health and wellness is rapidly becoming an integral part of the treatment of disease and illness. For this reason we look closely at clinical applications of the dynamics and ingredients of health and wellness in the unit on behavioral medicine. The chapters on behavioral medicine will be of particular interest to students who plan a career in a health field, but they are likely to be of personal interest to all students. The incidence of stress-related disorders is high among college students, and these chapters will be helpful.

We have drawn upon the experience and research of many leaders in the health sciences and upon our own work as clinicians and teachers. Our clinical orientation, research interests, and experience in teaching psychology and health classes enables us to weave together a research orientation, an applied clinical orientation, and a personal experiential orientation. These three orientations are woven into an integrated whole, moving easily among research and models, clinical applications, and the use of the dynamics and ingredients of health and wellness in daily life. We believe that the academic study of health and wellness is complete when augmented by personal experience and a focus on personal health and wellness.

These orientations are woven together through case reports, stories, and self-evaluation inventories; through the presentation and analysis of research and constructs; and through the classroom assignments described in the instructor's manual. We begin with the puzzling case of Mr. Wright to intrigue and motivate the student, as we introduce the content of this text.

We hope that the style and presentation bring to life these central themes: (1) research, research evaluation, and critical thinking are essential in the health sciences to the student, health professional and consumer; (2) self-responsibility and self regulation are the cornerstones of health and wellness; (3) understanding stress and developing cognitive and behavioral stress-management skills are important dynamics in health and wellness; (4) knowledge is power, including the knowledge of one's physiological response to stress; (5) health and wellness are not merely the result of good luck but can be studied, cultivated, and taught to others; (6) knowledge of the dynamics and ingredients of health and wellness is the foundation of prevention and treatment of illness and disease; (7) health and wellness are complex processes arising from the interaction of biological, psychological, and social systems.

The Dynamics of Health and Wellness: A Biopsychosocial Approach has many features not found in other textbooks:

- A biopsychosocial systems approach.
- A focus on health, while also emphasizing personal and societal forces that jeopardize health and wellness.
- An examination of the personality characteristics of healthy people, such as hardiness and learned resourcefulness, and the development of these characteristics.
- An introduction to psychoneuroimmunology.
- Separate chapters on the history, principles, and applications of relaxation and biofeedback training, and visualization and imagery. In conjunction with cognitive and behavioral techniques, these procedures form a solid foundation for development of personal stress-management and self regulation skills. This combination is also the basic structure for the skills-oriented

treatment protocols described in the behavioral medicine chapters.

- A detailed analysis of the ingredients of self regulation.
- A discussion of three healthy lifestyle ingredients not normally included in lifestyle—nonviolence, assertiveness, and play.
- A chapter on treatment of children, including behavioral techniques for helping children cope with traumatic and painful medical procedures.
- A detailed examination of innovative programs in health education and behavioral treatment.
- Critical analysis of cultural and societal forces against health and wellness, appropriate to the biopsychosocial approach, counterbalanced by discussion of forces for health and wellness.
- A self-knowledge, self-help theme appropriate to the academic study of the dynamics and ingredients of health and wellness.
- A writing style that is easy to read and personal, without sacrificing clarity or content.

The study of the dynamics of health and wellness from a biopsychosocial perspective is interdisciplinary and is not limited to one speciality. Therefore, *The Dynamics of Health and Wellness: A Biopsychosocial Approach*, with its particular themes and unique features, is appropriate for classes in several disciplines, such as health psychology, stress management, health, and counseling. The instructor's manual, written by us, provides course outlines and supporting material for classes in these areas. The manual also includes diagrams and topics not included in the text.

Our study of the dynamics and ingredients of health and wellness has been a challenging journey. We expect that a course based on this text will also be challenging, if not provocative, from the first chapter to the last.

Much is known about health and wellness and why healthy people are healthy. Yet there are many mysteries, and there are vast frontiers for research, for promoting health and wellness, for preventing and treating disease and illness, and for overcoming the biological, psychological, and social forces that impede health and wellness. This text lays a foundation for understanding and achieving health and wellness.

To the Student

The title *The Dynamics of Health and Wellness: A Biopsychosocial Approach* must suggest to you that health and wellness are more complicated than simple, static conditions that can easily be defined and studied. You can guess that health and wellness have to do with an interaction—a dynamic interaction—of biological, psychological, and social variables. You might also guess that human beings are not "slated" at birth to be healthy and well or sick and poorly. While the genetic and environmental cards may be stacked either for us or against us, the fact that psychological and social factors interact with biological factors gives humans an opportunity to maximize health and wellness when healthy and to recover when sick. This textbook describes the biological, psychological, and social forces, and the resources, that underlie health and wellness.

The study of the dynamics of health and wellness is in its infancy, but it is a robust and rapidly growing infant no longer overshadowed by the study of illness and disease. Today we recognize that knowledge of the dynamics of health and wellness is vital to enhancing health and wellness, and is vital to overcoming illness and disease. Knowledge of those dynamics promotes health in healthy people, and when incorporated in treatment, promotes health in sick people. This is a new concept.

Health as a process—as a state of being that is maintained, created, and enhanced—is also a new concept. Today we recognize that health and wellness are not just a lucky chance. They are the result of conscious effort and knowledge.

Given this sense of health and wellness, as dynamic and under personal control, we write about health and wellness in a particular way.

We write about them as academic subjects that you can study and pass exams on, and we write about them as processes that you "do." To be truly knowledgeable in this field, you do more than study from a textbook. You take action, participate, get involved.

We hope to engage you in this book in three ways: as a person who is interested in maximizing health and wellness; as a student who must know certain facts and concepts and learn how to evaluate research; and as a future health professional who will use both personal and academic knowledge of the dynamics of health and wellness in helping others. As a result of this perspective, we have three writing styles. One style speaks to you personally, one is a reporting style, and one is an academic style appropriate to the content of theories and models. When we speak to you personally, the tone is direct and easy, but do not be deceived by this writing style. The content is as important academically as it is to you personally. We trust that the change in styles will be interesting and easy to read.

Our writing also reflects who we are. We are personally involved in health and wellness, and we attempt to "practice what we preach"; we are students, continually learning; and we are health professionals in three areas—we teach college- and graduate-level classes, we have been involved in a variety of research projects, and we are therapists in private practice. Throughout this book we share these "selves" with you, describing our personal experiences and knowledge of the dynamics of health and wellness.

We dedicate this book to the goal of the World Health Organization:

HEALTH FOR ALL BY THE YEAR 2000

Contents

Acknowledgments

We are pleased to acknowledge the needed encouragement and support of our colleagues at Aims Community College and the help of Kim Shellenberger, who conducted library searches, and Mike Shellenberger, who willingly aided in tedious computer tasks and provided several photographs. We are also grateful for the encouragement and sound advice of our many reviewers:

Aian Ackerman—Aims Community College

Lewis Barker—Baylor University

Alan Benedict—Mesa Community College, Arizona

Jon Carlson—Lake Geneva Wellness Center Clinic

James Clopton—Texas Tech University

Brian Cooke—University of Northern Colorado

James B. Cooney—University of Northern Colorado

David Danskin—Kansas State University

Tom Dietvorst—University of Denver

George Fuller von Bozzay—City College of San Francisco

Bob Gatchel—University of Texas Southwestern Medical Center

Eugene Gilden—Linfield College, Oregon

Alan Glaros—University of Missouri–Kansas City

Sandy Gramling—Virginia Commonwealth University

Mariellen Griffith—Butler University

Bob Hoyt—University of Wisconsin–Stout

Jim King—Chemeketa Community College, Oregon

Ed Krupat—Boston University

Janet Lapp

Tyler Long—Yale University

Majel Martin—University of Northern Colorado

Doug Matheson—University of the Pacific, California

Robert McCaffrey—State University of New York–Albany

David Mostofsky—Boston University

Carol Schneider—University of Colorado

John Sesney—Lewis & Clark State College, Idaho

Frederic Shaffer—Northeast Missouri State University

Ed Wilson—Colorado Center for Biobehavioral Health

Greg Wilson—Washington State University

Brian Yates—The American University, Washington, D.C.

Photographers: Robert Waltman, Aims Community College Media. Services; and Gordon Stewart, Denver.

Line graphs and bar graphs by Bob Shelalenberger.

THE DYNAMICS OF HEALTH AND WELLNESS

A BIOPSYCHOSOCIAL APPROACH

PART ONE

The Dynamics of Health and Wellness

It is customary to begin a textbook with an overview of the subject matter, and this text is no exception. In Chapter 1, The Dynamics of Health and Wellness, the purpose and scope of this textbook are described, terms are defined, concepts are outlined, and each chapter is briefly described.

The dynamics of health and wellness enable healthy people to stay healthy, they are the basis of prevention of disease and illness, and they are the foundation of treatment for regaining health when sick. Because health and wellness are complex biopsychosocial processes, the study of the dynamics of health and wellness is interdisciplinary, meaning that knowledge about health comes from many disciplines—physiology, medicine, psychology, health education, nursing, sociology, anthropology—and contributes to many disciplines—health psychology, behavioral medicine, health education, medical sociology, nursing, behavioral health, psychology, psychotherapy, medicine.

In Chapter 2, Mind and Body Dynamics, we focus on two fundamental, innate dynamics that are the basis of health and wellness: the influence of mind on body and homeostasis, the ability of the body to maintain a steady internal state. That mind influences health has probably been known for as long as humans have been observing their own behavior. Only in the last half century, however, has the importance of mind-body relationships in health and illness been recognized. Today we are experiencing a rebirth of the study and use of the mind in all health fields.

CHAPTER 1

Introduction

IIII▶

SECTION ONE: THE CASE OF MR. WRIGHT

The *Journal of Projective Techniques* reported the following case in 1957. The case was described to the author of the article by the patient's physician, Dr. West.

Mr. Wright had a generalized far advanced malignancy involving the lymph nodes. Eventually the day came when he developed resistance to all known treatments. Also, his increasing anemia precluded any intensive efforts with X-rays or nitrogen mustard, which otherwise might have been attempted. Huge tumor masses, the size of oranges, were in the neck, groin, chest, and abdomen. The spleen and liver were enormous. He was taking oxygen by mask frequently, and our impression was that he was in a terminal state, untreatable, other than to give sedatives to ease him on his way. In spite of all this, Mr. Wright was not without hope, even though his doctors most certainly were. The reason for this was that the new drug that he had expected to come along and save the day had already been reported in the newspapers! Its name was Krebiozen.

Then he heard in some way that our clinic was to be one of a hundred places chosen by the Medical Association for evaluation of this treatment. We were allotted supplies of the drug sufficient for treating twelve selected cases. Mr. Wright was not considered eligible, since one stipulation was that the patient must not only be beyond the point where standard therapies could benefit, but also must have a life expectancy of at least three, and preferably six months. He certainly didn't qualify on the latter point, and to give him a prognosis of more than two weeks seemed to be stretching things.

However, a few days later, the drug arrived, and we began setting up our testing program, which, of course, did not include Mr. Wright. When he heard we were going to begin treatment with Krebiozen, his enthusiasm knew no bounds, and as much as I tried to dissuade him, he begged so hard for this "golden opportunity," that against my better judgment, and against the rules of the Krebiozen committee, I decided I would have to include him.

Injections were to be given three times weekly, and I remember he received his first one on a Friday. I didn't see him again until Monday and thought as I came to the hospital he might be moribund or dead by that time, and his supply of the drug could then be transferred to another case.

What a surprise was in store for me! I left him in fever, gasping for air, completely bedridden. Now, here he was, walking around the ward, chatting happily with the nurses, and spreading his message of good cheer to any who would listen. Immediately I hastened to see the others who had received their first injection at the same time. No change, or change for the worse was noted. Only in Mr. Wright was there brilliant improvement. The tumor masses had melted like snowballs on a hot stove, and in only these few days, they were half their original size!

Within 10 days he was able to be discharged from his "death-bed," practically all signs of his disease having vanished in this short time. Incredible as it sounds, this "terminal" patient, gasping his last breath through an oxygen mask, was not only breathing normally, and fully active, he took off in his plane and flew at 12,000 feet, with no discomfort!

This unbelievable situation occurred at the beginning of the Krebiozen evaluations, but within two months, conflicting reports began to appear in the news, all of the testing clinics reporting no results.

This disturbed our Mr. Wright considerably as the weeks wore on. He began to lose faith in his last hope, which so far had been life-saving and left nothing to be desired. As the reported results became increasingly dismal, his faith waned, and after two months of practically perfect health, he relapsed to his original state, and became very gloomy and miserable.

Knowing something of my patient's innate optimism by this time, I deliberately took advantage of him. This was for purely scientific reasons, in order to perform the perfect control experiment, which could answer all the perplexing questions he had brought up. Furthermore, this scheme could not harm him in any way, I felt sure, and there was nothing I knew anyway that could help him.

When Mr. Wright had all but given up in despair with the recurrence of his disease, in spite of the "wonder drug" which had worked so well at first, I decided to take a chance. Deliberately lying, I told him not to believe what he read in the papers, the drug was really most promising after all. "What then," he asked, "was the reason for my relapse?" "Just because the substance deteriorates on standing," I replied, "a new super-refined, double-strength product is due to arrive tomorrow which can more than reproduce the great benefits derived from the original injections."

This news came as a great revelation to him, and Mr. Wright, ill as he was, became his optimistic self again, eager to start over. By delaying a couple of days before the "shipment" arrived, his anticipation of salvation had reached a tremendous pitch. When I announced that the new series of injections were about to begin, he was almost ecstatic and his faith was very strong.

With much fanfare, and putting on quite an act, I administered the first injection of the doubly potent fresh preparation, consisting of fresh water and nothing more. The results of this experiment were quite unbelievable. Recovery from his second near-terminal state was even more dramatic than the first. Tumor masses melted, chest fluid vanished, he became ambulatory, and even went back to flying again. At this time he was certainly the picture of health. The water injections were continued, since they worked such wonders. He then

remained symptom-free for over two months. At this time the final AMA announcement appeared in the press: "Nationwide tests show Krebiozen to be a worthless drug in treatment of cancer."

Within a few days of this report Mr. Wright was re-admitted to the hospital in extremis. His faith was now gone, his last hope vanished, and he succumbed in less than two days.

From Klopfer (1957) *Journal of Projective Techniques, Vol. 21*, 331–340. Reprinted by permission of the Society for Personality Assessment.

The title of the article in which this case report appears is "Psychological Variables in Human Cancer," and it was written by Bruno Klopfer, then president of the Society of Projective Techniques. Klopfer was particularly interested because he had given Mr. Wright the Rorschach test (Box 1.1) as part of a study of personality and cancer.

If your reaction is like that of many people, you find the case of Mr. Wright unbelievable and perplexing, yet intriguing because it is true. If your reaction is like many, you are wondering whether Dr. West said to Mr. Wright, "This may surprise you, Mr. Wright, but the fact is that the power was in you all along—it was your belief, not Krebiozen, that melted those tumors like snowballs on a hot stove, so do it again." And if the physician said this, why was Mr. Wright unable to melt the tumors again?

If Dr. West had discussed with Mr. Wright the extraordinary power of belief to heal the body, and if he had encouraged the patient to use this power, he would have been an unusual doctor. In the mid-1950s, at the time of the Krebiozen experiments, most physicians and patients relied on medications, surgery, and other medical interventions. Today, armed with new insights about the dynamics of health and wellness and with new treatment procedures, we can continue this story.

Within a few days of this report, Mr. Wright is re-admitted to the hospital in extremis. His faith is now gone, his last hope vanished . . . .

THE RORSCHACH INKBLOT TEST

Determining a person's "true" and often hidden personality characteristics has been a continuing interest and problem for psychology and psychiatry. Herman Rorschach, a Swiss psychiatrist, created a method—the inkblot—that he thought would reveal the person's true characteristics. The inkblots are amorphous, with no specific content. The patient studies the inkblot and describes what she or he sees. The subject's responses reflect personal interpretations of the designs. The originality of the responses, the content, and many other characteristics of the responses are scored. Trained interpreters of the Rorschach relate scores to personality characteristics such as maturity, emotional control, anxiety, and physical and sexual drives.

Mr. Wright's physician enters the patient's hospital room with an infectious look of encouragement. "Ed, I have startling and encouraging news for you—news so surprising that you might find it hard to believe, just as I did. You remember that I gave you a second, stronger dose of Krebiozen; well, this is what really happened. I gave you a strong dose of water and nothing else! So you see, Ed, you healed yourself. You believed that the drug healed you, but we understand now that it wasn't the drug; it was your own belief. Then, when you believed that Krebiozen had failed, it was your belief and subsequent depression that allowed the tumors to return. Not once did this happen, but twice! We could never have guessed that your beliefs could have such power, but the experiment proves it. Now I realize that we have another

treatment for you. This treatment isn't another drug. This treatment uses your mind to heal your body, which we discovered does work."

Listening intently, Mr. Wright is speechless. Emotions changing as he listens, he feels deceived, disbelieving, and puzzled. "You are wrong, Doctor. You must have given me Krebiozen the second time. It worked just like the first dose; I recovered so quickly."

Dr. West is ready for this response. "Ed, I too have been puzzled by your case, so puzzled that when it was clear to me that more was involved in your recovery than Krebiozen, I began consulting a team of experts from around the country who specialize in the study of mind and body interaction. Because you're so unusual, these experts have agreed to consult with you today. They will help you understand how your healing and regression occurred, and with you, they will create a treatment program to bring you back to health."

Before Mr. Wright can voice another doubt, Dr. West ceremoniously opens the door, admitting nine experts who are introduced as world-famous authorities. Mr. Wright hastily pushes his call button. "Find chairs for my guests!" he shouts with excitement. "They will be staying awhile."

The Experts

Dr. West read the interpretation of the Rorschach test that Ed Wright took before the Krebiozen experiment. The test indicated that he is the type of person who responds well to the power of external authority. This means that the "power of authority" that Mr. Wright gave to Krebiozen must somehow be given back to him. Dr. West knows that because of Mr. Wright's personality type, it would probably not help to simply tell him, "It was your *belief* that made the tumors shrink like snowballs on a hot stove. Now that you know this, you can use that power to make them go away again." It would be the task of the experts and the medical staff who work with Mr. Wright to help him accept the possibility of healing himself and to give himself the power that he had given to Krebiozen. Dr. West has already brought in Mr. Wright's nurse specialist, who is familiar with every member of the team and has worked with many patients. She will coordinate the program and provide constant support for Mr. Wright. Now, with obvious respect, Dr. West introduces the first authority, Dr. Cognitive Psychology.

Dr. Cognitive Psychology

"Mr. Wright, I am sure that you know about psychology, but you might not have heard of cognitive psychology. It is easy to explain—the word *cognitive* refers to thinking. I could say, 'Your child has good cognitive skills.' That would mean that your child knows how to use concepts and thinking processes. My particular interest is in how cognitions influence behavior and in the fact that because people can change their thinking, they can change their behavior. I can give you a quick example—people who think that they will always fail act in ways that cause them to fail. That seems obvious, I know, but the important point is that when people begin to think more positively and gain some hope, they then act in ways that bring about success. Another example is that people can *think* themselves into being stressed—like worrying about something that might not even happen."

"Boy, do I know about that," Ed Wright says. "I've been worried from the beginning of this thing. Now I can't shut my mind off, and I feel depressed all the time." Mr. Wright leans back and shuts his eyes. "It seems so hopeless."

"I know, Ed, it seems hopeless. We'll talk about that, about what you are thinking— thinking about yourself, about the cancer, about the treatment program. You might find ways to think about things a little differently, and that will help—we don't want you to waste energy on worry. I want you to know that *we* don't feel so hopeless. In fact, the team

is feeling pretty encouraged right now. You made a remarkable recovery before; I want to talk about that and tell you about one of my other interests.

"I have worked over 30 years studying the relationships among cancer, personality, beliefs, and emotions. I have found many cases of spontaneous remission such as yours. Spontaneous remission means that the cancer completely disappears without medical treatment. In my research, I have identified certain personality traits of people who had spontaneous remission of cancer. From the description of you by Dr. West and the personality test that you took, you seem to be one of those fortunate people with a personality that can help the body heal.

"You are probably familiar with the miraculous cures that come from the healing waters at the shrine of Lourdes in France. A group of scientists examined the water and discovered that it was no different from any other water. So what caused the cures at Lourdes? One answer is the belief of these people that they will be healed, just as it was your belief in Krebiozen that caused your tumors to melt. I am very interested in the power of beliefs. And where is 'belief,' Mr. Wright—the thinking that I have been talking about? Not outside of you, like water or a drug, but *inside* of you, something that you can control. I see that you are puzzled and are probably wondering how we know for sure that your beliefs healed you and not Krebiozen, or the water for that matter. To explain this, we have on our team an authority on medical research methodology."

Dr. Methodology

"Mr. Wright, as the primary researcher for the Krebiozen study, it is my task to be sure that any benefits of drugs like Krebiozen are caused by the drug alone and not other factors, such as the belief of the patient. Before using a drug, we must know that it can help people and how much it helps.

"To study the effects of a drug, we divide our patients into two groups. One group receives the real drug, and the other group receives what we call a placebo. It is a sugar pill, or a shot of water, or something like that. We always find that some people in both groups improve. If the drug is effective, however, more people in the drug group get better than in the placebo group. This is how Krebiozen was studied. As you know, patients taking the drug showed little improvement, no more than patients taking the placebo, so it was clear that Krebiozen did not reduce cancers. But you were different. Of all the patients in this hospital taking Krebiozen, you alone significantly improved, and dramatically quickly. It seemed obvious to Dr. West that the drug could not have had this special effect on you and on no one else, so he concluded that it must have been your belief in the drug that somehow caused the tumors to shrink. To test this hypothesis, and with the hope of ridding you of cancer once and for all, he decided to do an experiment.

"After giving you the Krebiozen with the amazing result, he then gave you a placebo, the water shot, telling you that it was a new type of Krebiozen. You know what happened: once again you were up and out of here very quickly. Now, we knew for sure that you were cured by your own belief—it had to be your belief, because I can tell you water shots do not melt tumors! But there is even more evidence. When you no longer believed in Krebiozen, the tumors returned. I guess it must work both ways: If your beliefs can help to make you well, they can probably help to make you sick, too.

"I tell you, Mr. Wright, your case has been exciting and perplexing for us all. To help us understand how beliefs can have such power, we have consulted Dr. Psychoneuroimmunology, who has spent years studying the interaction of the mind and the immune system. Dr. Psychoneuroimmunology is here to explain to you the elements of this interaction so that you can understand what happened and why we believe that the new treatment program will work."

Dr. Psychoneuroimmunology

"I can tell by the look on your face that you are wondering what my speciality could possibly be! The best way to tell you is to break the word into its parts: *psycho-*, *neuro-*, and *immunology*. Psycho- refers to mind, neuro- to the nervous system, and immunology to the immune system. Psychoneuroimmunology is the study of how the mind and the nervous system interact and affect the immune system.

"My research investigates the way in which beliefs, expectations, and personality affect natural killer cells. Natural killer cells are aggressive, and they kill tumor cells, so they are an important defense against cancer. I have compared the activity of natural killer cells in individuals with positive personality traits to those in individuals with negative personality traits. The results were very interesting. Natural killer cells were more active in the individuals with positive traits than they were in those with negative traits. My research may explain how you were able to eliminate your tumors when you were excited and hopeful about Krebiozen, and how the tumors returned when you were in a negative, discouraged state. I conclude that your positive expectations heightened the activity of the natural killer cells and other components of the immune system, which eliminated the cancer, and that your negative states lowered the activity of the immune system, allowing the cancer to return.

"That this could happen is not really surprising. We have known for many years that the human brain and body have mechanisms for responding to the mind. There are nerve centers, chemicals, and such, that respond to your fears, to what you imagine, and to your beliefs and emotions, and it makes sense that your immune system would respond to these things as well.

"Ed, you're beginning to get an idea of the new treatment program, aren't you? We will create a program for your mind and body, using the power of the mind to influence the body, and using the natural ability of the body to heal itself. Before you start doubting the power of your mind, let me introduce our expert on mind-body interaction, who, I see, is eager to speak with you."

Dr. Psychophysiology

"Mr. Wright, I want you to imagine the following scene. You are driving home on a rainy night. The street lights are out. You drive up the driveway, turn off the lights and ignition, open the car door, and put your foot down on a long black snake. It squirms under your foot. In an instant you are caught in a stress response. In panic you jump back into the car and slam the door. You barely notice your pounding heart, tight stomach, and rapid breathing. With shaking hands you slip the key into the ignition and turn on the headlights. There it is—the *garden hose*. Laughing with relief, you say to yourself, 'Good grief, the garden hose. Left it there this afternoon.' Now your breathing becomes deeper, your muscles relax, your heart stops pounding, your blood pressure drops, and your physiological responses begin to return to normal.

"Well, what do you think, Mr. Wright? Anything like that ever happen to you? Did you ever stop to think how incredibly powerful the mind is? Garden hoses can't raise blood pressure or increase heart rate. So what really created all those body responses? The mind, and the idea 'Snake!' You know, I have studied the effect of mind on body for many years, and every time I tell this story I am as amazed as ever that the mind has such power over the body. Of course, it has to be this way. If the mind could not direct the body, the human race would have perished long ago. So here we are, with a mind and body that interact 24 hours a day, consciously and

unconsciously, and the question is, how can we use this interaction for health? That is my particular specialty—using the mind for health. I like to think that we have a mind-body team, and that good health comes from training the whole team. So you can see that your treatment program will include both mind and body.

"By the way, *psychophysiological* is a word that you will hear often. It refers to processes, like the stress response, that are related to mind-body interaction. If you think of a snake and your body responds, that is a psychophysiological response. Relaxation is a psychophysiological process, because relaxation involves body and mind.

"But let's get back to the story of the snake and the garden hose. It is clear that what you perceive with your mind gets into your body. In this case we call it the stress response; perhaps you know it as the fight-or-flight response. When you perceive something as stressful, the body responds because of the way that various centers in your brain talk to each other and to glands such as the adrenals, which release adrenaline.

"This is what I think happened to you: You read that Krebiozen does not affect cancer, and you saw a snake, a very frightening, depressing snake, am I right? And of course, your body responded to that snake. Then, when your doctor tried the 'new Krebiozen,' it was like seeing a garden hose on a hot day, and your body responded to that.

"Now we are back with the snake again, and again your immune system is going downhill. But now you understand what has been happening, and now it is time to get your mind geared up again to fight, which it has done twice before. Mr. Wright, an image just came into my mind of a powerful garden hose inside of you. It is spraying poison all over the cancer cells, and they are dying by the thousands. But now I am getting out of my field. We have an expert on our team who specializes in the use of imagery for healing, so let me introduce Dr. Imagery."

Dr. Imagery

"How are you doing so far, Mr. Wright? Does all this make sense? It's no mystery that your mind affects your body. So it's no mystery that what you imagine can affect your body. We don't know exactly how the brain responds to images, but that it happens is certain. The image of a snake is pretty powerful, isn't it! Or try this—imagine that you have a juicy lemon. Take a sharp knife and slice that lemon in half. Now pick up one half and squeeze the juice into your mouth—drink that sour lemon juice. I don't know about you, Ed, but my mouth is watering—you see the power of images! I am going to guess that when you heard that Krebiozen did not work, you had very negative images, maybe seeing the cancer getting worse and yourself dying. And when you were given the 'new Krebiozen,' you had images of the cancer melting again, and you flying again—is that right?"

"Yup, that's right," said Mr. Wright. "I never thought about it. I see what you are saying, and the first guy said that beliefs affect the body, too. That is really something—I just never thought about it before."

"The fact is, Ed, that the mind creates images all the time—that is what it loves to do. So our task is to figure out what images to use to help your body heal. I'll tell you an image that came to my mind while Dr. Psychophysiology was talking to you about the garden hose spraying poison. I suddenly remembered the scene in the *Wizard of Oz* where Dorothy throws water on the Wicked Witch of the East and the witch melts into the floor, and that reminded me that your doctor told us that your tumors melted like snowballs on a hot stove. There are many possibilities for images here, don't you think! The amazing thing about imagery is that even as fanciful and symbolic as it is, your body seems to know what your mind is directing it to do.

"My first assignment for you is to create imagery that directs your immune system to destroy the cancer cells. You will need to experiment with a variety of images until you find the imagery that feels best for you. Tomorrow we will talk about how you use the imagery.

"We have found that when a person uses imagery to direct the body, it is important to have the body quiet and relaxed. I use an analogy to describe this. Imagine a classroom full of children, all out of their seats and running around making a racket. When the teacher speaks, no one hears. Now imagine that all the children are seated, looking forward, and being quiet; now when the teacher speaks, everyone hears. Your body is the classroom and your mind is the teacher. It is important to have your body quiet and paying attention when you speak to it with your mind. Actually, Mr. Wright, I think it is important to have the teacher paying attention too, listening to the classroom. It is important to learn to quiet both body and mind. You are wondering how you can learn to relax your body and your mind. Now I must introduce you to the next member of our team who knows all about this, our relaxation expert."

Dr. Relaxation

"That's right, I am an expert on relaxation. I study the physiology, the neuroanatomy, and the psychology of relaxation, and the methods for relaxing mind and body. This is a new field of study, Mr. Wright. For years scientists and physicians studied stress, but few studied relaxation. After all, you don't get rich from it, and it doesn't make you sick, so why study it? Dr. Imagery gave you part of the answer, but the complete answer takes us back again to the snake and the garden hose. If you have created a snake in your mind, then your body reacts, and we call that reaction the stress response. But what happens when you discover that the snake is really just the garden hose? You begin to relax. You say to yourself, 'It's just the garden hose.' Your breathing is deeper, your muscles relax, your heart rate slows, your blood pressure comes down, and your adrenaline and many other hormonal reactions turn off. It seems to me, Mr. Wright, that just as nature created the stress response to make us ready to fight or flee, so nature created the equally powerful relaxation response to bring the body back to normal. Stress turns on hundreds of responses, and relaxation turns them off and brings body and mind back to a healthy state. So you see, relaxation has a powerful and beneficial effect on the body. We are finding that deep relaxation helps the body heal itself. Sometimes I say to my patients that we have a new medicine called relaxation, and this medicine has no bad side effects.

"The problem is that we have not been taught how to relax. In school we are taught how to worry and work hard. But now we realize how important relaxation is for health. So your treatment program will include extensive relaxation training—which, as I say, will help your body heal—and will aid you in your imagery work as well. When I speak of relaxation, most people think of things like going to a movie or watching television, but I am talking about something quite different. I mean deep relaxation of mind and body. We have many techniques and tools to help patients learn this type of relaxation, and it really does involve learning. I will be teaching you a variety of techniques. Our primary tool for aiding you and for monitoring your response will be biofeedback training. Perhaps you have heard of it. We have on our team a leader in the field of biofeedback training who is here to explain the procedure to you.

Dr. Biofeedback

"You have probably heard about biofeedback training. In fact, this hospital has a biofeedback therapy center. I always describe biofeedback training by defining the two parts of the word, *bio-* and *feedback*. Feedback refers to the feedback of information to you, and *bio-* refers to the body, so biofeedback is the process of feeding back information to you about your own body. Biofeedback training uses sensitive electronic instruments that pick up

signals from your body, such as heart rate, blood pressure, or muscle tension. The biofeedback instrument amplifies the body signal, turns it into useful information, and feeds it back to you; now you have information about what is going on inside your body. Taking your own blood pressure with a blood-pressure cuff is a simple example of biofeedback. We have found that people can regulate many body processes that are normally difficult to control, when they get information about the process that they are trying to regulate.

"If you think about it, you will realize that just about everything you have learned, you learned because you got feedback—from your own body, from teachers, or from parents. We need feedback in order to learn. Take the example of learning to play darts. The first time you play darts, what happens? You just pick up a dart and throw it without knowing exactly what to do, unless, of course, you have a good coach who can help you. You throw the first dart, and then what?"

Ed responds immediately, "I see where it lands."

"Exactly, You see where it lands, and that is what we call the feedback of information. You get information from the dartboard. Now what do you do with that information?"

"Well, I use it. I see where the dart lands, and that gives me information about my shot, so I use the information to make a better second shot."

"Right. So you throw the second shot, see where it lands, and use that information to adjust your behavior—I might say mind-body behavior—and you throw again. You can see that feedback of information is essential for learning. With feedback from the dartboard, you become more conscious of what you are doing, and finally you gain control and hit the bull's-eye. Imagine trying to learn to hit the bull's-eye blindfolded. Do you think you could?"

"No. I would never get any information, so I wouldn't know where my last shot went, so I wouldn't know how to change my aim."

"That's right. You can see that in learning any skill, you have to become conscious of what you are doing to gain control, and to become conscious and learn, you need feedback. Now here is the problem with the body, and why it is hard to control. The body has lots of blindfolds. Let me give you an example. Close your eyes and put your attention into your heart. Can you feel your heart beating?"

Ed nods.

"Good. Now focus within again, and try to feel your blood sugar."

Ed looks puzzled, then smiles.

"Can't feel a thing, can you? But you have blood sugar," says Dr. Biofeedback. "The problem is that it is in the unconscious, blindfolded so to speak. So if I told you to increase your blood sugar, you wouldn't know how to begin, because you are getting no feedback about blood sugar from your body. This is where biofeedback comes in. If I had an instrument that could monitor your blood sugar for you and feed that information back to you, then you could use that information just as you do in learning to play darts. You could use the information to become conscious of your mind and body processes that change blood sugar, and finally you would learn how to increase and decrease blood sugar. The fact is, Ed, we are unable to find a body process that cannot be regulated to some extent, if the person gets feedback about the body process. Now that you have spoken with Drs. Psychophysiology and Psychoneuroimmunology, I know that this is no surprise to you. Your mind affects your body, and you can use this power to make changes in both mind and body. The information from the biofeedback instrument guides you in the same way that information from the dart board guides you. Does all this make sense, Ed?"

"Yes, it does. I wonder if there is an instrument that can give me information about my immune system."

"That's an exciting idea, and people are working on it, but so far we don't have an instrument for that. An instrument that would feed back natural killer-cell activity would be great, but we find that it is not essential. You can enhance the activity of your immune system without direct information. In your treatment program, you will use biofeedback training to learn relaxation skills that will help the body recover. There is just one catch—it isn't magic, and it sure isn't like taking a drug that does the work for you. When you use biofeedback training and the other techniques in this program, you do the work. The benefit is that you gain self regulation skills that you will have for the rest of your life."

"I see what you mean by skills, but self regulation—what does that mean?"

"The simple answer is that self regulation means that you regulate yourself, rather than be controlled by something or someone else. The new therapies, like biofeedback training, are called self regulation therapies. Another team member can explain the concept in greater detail, so let me introduce Dr. Self Regulation."

Dr. Self Regulation

"Ed, the longer I study the dynamics of health and wellness and recovery from disease, the more impressed I am by the importance of self regulation and by the extraordinary ability that people have to regulate themselves. In fact, I think that everyone here would agree that self regulation is the cornerstone of health."

"Sounds like punishment to me."

"Well, it can feel like punishment when you are overcoming a bad habit, like smoking. Did you ever smoke?"

"I started smoking when I was in the Army and I smoked for 30 years. I quit when I found out that I had cancer. Dr. West said that I had to quit, and I did. Before that, I tried to quit but it never worked. That is why I said that it sounds like punishment."

"I am impressed. Then you know a lot about self regulation, and you have to admit that it is healthier for you to be self regulating than to let a nicotine addiction control you. But breaking a bad habit is only one kind of self regulation. When you learn to change negative thinking into positive thinking, that is cognitive self regulation. When you learn to relax and turn off the stress response, that is psychophysiological self regulation, and so is using imagery to create physiological change. When you change your lifestyle habits, as you did with smoking, we might call that behavioral self regulation. When you decide to be hopeful, that is emotional self regulation. We all emphasize self regulation to make it absolutely clear that you are in charge of yourself, and that you have the power to make many changes that may affect your health. We are here to coach you as you learn these skills and make lifestyle changes, but you will find that soon you will not need us. Once you learn a self regulation skill, you have it forever."

"So you are saying that I have more power than I knew to regulate myself, and self regulation is what health is all about. But I have to learn how, and I have to choose to do so."

"Exactly. It is a choice, and this self regulation treatment program involves a lot of time and effort. Do you think you want to do it?"

"I'll tell you one thing, I don't have anything else to do. I can sure give it a try!"

"Great. I hoped that you would say that, because now I want to introduce our last team member, Dr. Lifestyle. That's right, lifestyle, one of the most fundamental elements in health, and one that involves a lot of self regulation as you change your diet and exercise habits and such things. But I will let Dr. Lifestyle explain all this to you."

Dr. Lifestyle

"Last but not least, Ed. I was interested to hear you tell Dr. Self Regulation that you quit smoking. That was an important lifestyle change that, as you said, wasn't all that easy. Some lifestyle changes are not easy, but are very important. *Lifestyle* refers to your daily habits that affect health, like diet and exercise. You and I will take a long, hard look at your habits,

including things that you might not have thought of as lifestyle, like how much fun you have every day and how assertive you are. We will create a diet for you that may be quite different from the one you are used to, and we will start you on an exercise program. Are you married, Ed?"

"I sure am."

"Good. We will ask your wife to take part in the planning. She will be interested in everything you learn and will help you make the necessary changes. We find that a family can be a great help. In fact, I will probably put you in touch with several other cancer patients who have formed a group, because group support really helps, too."

"I like that idea. You know, I have felt pretty isolated, and I think my wife has too. Yes, I'd like to be in the group."

"Well, that's settled. You will find that many people in the group are making lifestyle changes, and it won't be so hard for you. Now I'm going to give you some homework. I have several lifestyle questionnaires that I want you to fill out to help us analyze your habits. Then in a few days, when you have begun the other parts of your treatment program, we will study the questionnaires together. You can think of me as your lifestyle teacher. Like all the members of your team, I will have a great deal to teach you."

Dr. West is smiling broadly. "I sure am pleased, Ed. Well, what are you thinking now?"

Mr. Wright replies, "After Dr. Methodology told me how my beliefs caused the tumors to shrink, I was pretty amazed. It doesn't seem possible, but really, in a way, it does seem possible. I mean, I understand the story about the snake and the garden hose. That happened to me once—my heart really pounded. I never thought about it being the mind that had done that. And I thought that Krebiozen had made me well and then failed, but I did it myself and didn't know it. I really believed it would work, but what really worked was me! I did it twice. What a surprise! And it's not a mystery, is it? Your team of experts has made it clear to me that the mind can change the body. But what do you think, Dr. West? It's exciting, but I'm scared, too. Do you think that I can do it again?"

Without hesitation, Dr. West replies, "Ed, I believe that it is possible. I know something else too. I know that knowledge is therapeutic, and the more you learn about your mind and body and how they interact, the more power you will have.

"Ed, for a long time medicine and psychology used 'either/or' approaches to health and disease—something was either physical or psychological. The physician used therapies like drugs or surgery to treat the body, and there wasn't much understanding of how feelings, beliefs, and even lifestyles produce sickness. On the other hand, the treatment of psychological problems pretty much ignored the body. Fortunately, we have made great progress in recent years. We understand that many physical and mental processes interact to produce disease and health. Your experts represent a team approach to treatment, a very powerful approach. So, Ed, I know that you have a good chance of melting those tumors again!"

Laughing and pretending to hold up a hypodermic needle, Dr. West pushes back Ed's sleeve. "Just to be safe though, I can inject you with water again!"

"No thanks, Doc, that won't be necessary!" Ed's laughter sounds good, but now he is serious again. "I have a choice, don't I. I can give up and die, which is what I was doing, or I can get some energy going for this program and fight for my life." Saying, "I know what I'm going to do," Ed turns to the team. "Let's get started!"

||||➡

SECTION TWO: THE DYNAMICS OF HEALTH AND WELLNESS

Take a minute: Take a minute to answer this question: If you were the head of the team of experts, how would you have treated Mr. Wright?

Do It Now.

You might have included other authorities, such as a family therapist, a minister or spiritual counselor, a specialist on death and dying, an exercise physiologist, or even a laughter therapist. Many people would be involved in Mr. Wright's treatment program, including his family. The professionals on your team would reflect your understanding of the dynamics of health and wellness. Please read Box 1.2 now.

We introduced this textbook with a team to reflect the fact that there are many ingredients in health and wellness, ingredients and underlying dynamics that interact. This textbook is about these ingredients and dynamics—they can be studied, and used. We opened with the case of Mr. Wright to dramatically illustrate this central theme: the ingredients and dynamics of health and wellness are under personal control and therefore can be used to maximize health and to recover from illness and disease. Health and sickness are not just a matter of good or bad luck, nor are they the result of a single variable. Health and wellness are complex, dynamic processes.

BOX 1.2

CONCLUDING THE CASE OF MR. WRIGHT

Although we continued the case of Mr. Wright, we did not create an ending in which he lives. We cannot write an ending because, in spite of justified optimism, we cannot know with certainty that Mr. Wright would be able to eliminate the cancer again, although undoubtedly the quality of his life would improve. Nonetheless, we pose this question for your consideration: Will Mr. Wright live?

Dynamics: Force, Process, Effective Action

Focus on the word **dynamic**. What comes to mind? Consider these examples: "She has a *dynamic* personality." "That is a *dynamic* program." The word *dynamic* comes from the Greek word *dynamis,* meaning "force." In physics, for example, dynamics refers to the forces that govern motion. Dynamic also means "changing," as opposed to "static." This meaning of dynamic refers to processes in which change occurs, such as growth—growth is a dynamic process because continual change is part of the process. Dynamic also means "characterized by effective action" (*Random House Dictionary,* 1980). In this sense of the word, dynamic suggests that the change or process is for the better and involves conscious effort.

You can anticipate the meaning of "the dynamics of health and wellness."

Health

Take a minute: What comes to mind when you think of health? Was Mr. Wright healthy although he had cancer; was he healthy when the cancer melted like snowballs on a hot stove? Answer this question: What is health?

Do It Now.

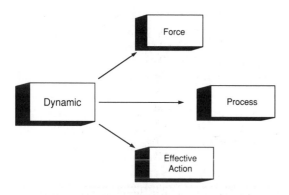

Figure 1.1   The Characteristics of "Dynamic."

Consider this example: "My friend finally regained her health after a traumatic illness." When we say that a friend "regained her health," we usually mean that she became free of injury or disease. "Mr. Wright regained his health" means that Mr. Wright became free of cancer. Freedom from illness and disease has been the most common meaning of health. This is exemplified in terms such as "health center," "health care," and "health insurance," which actually refer to the treatment of disease and financial coverage of medical expenses. The fact that these activities are described as "health" activities, when the emphasis is on treatment of disease and illness, means that health is considered to be recovery from and absence of disease and illness. Please read Box 1.3 now.

Today we are experiencing a significant change in the meaning of "health," a redefinition that was first voiced in 1947 by the World Health Organization (WHO), a branch of the United Nations. WHO defined health as "a state of complete physical, mental, and social well-being and not merely the absence of disease and infirmity" (World Health Organization, 1947). Although this statement does not tell us what "well-being" is, it does say that health is not merely the absence of disease. A person is not healthy simply because he or she is not sick. A heart-attack victim cannot say, "I was healthy until the day I had my heart attack." This would be false because the physiological conditions that led to the heart attack, such as atherosclerosis or hypertension, developed over many years in which the victim was not well, although symptoms were not detected. We suspect that the belief that people are healthy if they are not obviously sick has promoted disease and death over the centuries and particularly in this one, by allowing people to continue destructive habits while believing that they are healthy. Smokers continue to smoke because they feel healthy and not sick; obese people consider themselves healthy because they are not sick. Obviously, a definition of health that promotes sickness is not a good definition.

BOX 1.3

DISEASE AND ILLNESS

Note that we use two words for sickness—"illness" and "disease." Many authors use these terms interchangeably, but increasingly, illness is used to refer to discomfort or to disorders that are not caused by a disease-causing agent, such as a virus or genetic defect. For example, a tension headache could be classified as an illness because tension headaches generally are related to stress, work habits, and poor posture, and are not caused by a pathogen or genetic defect. On the other hand, polio or juvenile-onset diabetes (not related to lifestyle or obesity) are diseases. The distinction between illness and disease is not always clear. For example, clogging of the arteries that supply the heart muscle (atherosclerosis) is referred to as "coronary heart disease" and yet, in most people, atherosclerosis is not related to a disease-causing agent. In most people, coronary heart disease results from many interacting lifestyle factors.

We distinguish between illness and disease to highlight the fact that many physiological disorders are related to lifestyle and health behaviors and to stress. They are fundamentally different from diseases, which result from infectious agents or other environmental factors like carcinogens ("carcino" = cancer, "genic" = generating or causing).

from addictions. Today, most health professionals would not consider you to be healthy just because you are not currently sick; your lifestyle is an integral part of your health. This means that if you have an "unhealthy" lifestyle, you are not healthy, even though you may have no physiological signs of disease.

In addition to freedom from sickness and living a healthy lifestyle, a third element must be included in the definition of health: physiological conditions that add no risk to health, such as low blood pressure and low blood cholesterol (Hamburg, Elliott, & Parron, 1982; Matarazzo, Weiss, Herd, Miller, & Weiss, 1984). Although a healthy lifestyle promotes physiological health, it is no absolute guarantee. A person could have a healthy lifestyle and also have high blood pressure or high blood fats, and therefore would not have a "clean bill of health." For this reason, we include physiological measures within ranges that indicate no risk to health in the definition of health. Please read Box 1.4 now.

In summary, you are healthy when: (1) you are free of illness and disease, (2) your physiological measures indicate no risk to health, and (3) you have a healthy lifestyle.

Because this three-part definition of health incorporates lifestyle, a significant and profound dimension is added—**self-responsibility**. Health is not a matter of chance or good luck, nor simply a matter of good genes. True health includes personal choice—the choice of adopting a lifestyle that promotes health or one that increases risk for sickness. Pro-health choices involve self-responsibility and self regulation, as Mr. Wright learned.

Health is not a simple matter, as you might have thought or hoped.

Recognizing this fact, most health professionals agree that the definition of health must include lifestyle—a good diet, adequate exercise, coping effectively with stress, and freedom

Wellness

The World Health Organization's definition of health states that "health is not merely the absence of disease and infirmity but a state of complete well-being." **Well-being** adds another

MEETING THE NATION'S HEALTH GOALS FOR 1990

In 1976, a select group of health professionals was asked by the United States government to analyze the causes of disease and death of U.S. citizens, based on criteria described in a landmark report by Marc LaLonde, the Canadian Minister of Health and Welfare, published in 1974 (LaLonde). In addition to adequacy of health care, LaLonde emphasized lifestyle, environmental hazards, and biological factors as determinants of sickness and death, and he referred to this broad approach to the study of health as the "health field concept."

The United States team studied the 10 leading causes of death and found that approximately 50 percent of the deaths were because of unhealthy behavior and lifestyle, and approximately 20 percent of the deaths were because of environmental factors. These deaths were preventable. These shocking data were the initiative for establishing national health goals. The goals were published in a document, *Healthy People: The Surgeon General's Report on Health Promotion and Disease Prevention, 1979.* The goals were: reduction of deaths in all age groups; reduction in the number of days of sickness in the elderly; improved health for all. In the introduction to the document, the secretary of the Department of Health, Education and Welfare, Joseph Califano, wrote: "Let us make no mistake about the purpose of this, the first Surgeon General's Report on Health Promotion and Disease Prevention. Its purpose is to encourage a second public health revolution in the history of the United States" (1979, p. vii).

To accomplish these general goals, many task forces were created to establish specific health objectives for the nation, to be achieved by the year 1990. The task forces established 226 objectives in the following areas:

Preventive services
  High blood pressure control
  Family planning
  Pregnancy and infant health
  Immunization
  Sexually transmitted diseases
Health protection
  Toxic agent control
  Occupational safety and health
  Accident prevention and injury control
  Fluoridation and dental health
  Surveillance and control of infectious
    diseases
Health promotion
  Smoking and health
  Misuse of alcohol and drugs
  Nutrition
  Physical fitness and exercise
  Control of stress and violent behavior

A brief look at these areas indicates that the health of the nation is a matter of healthy lifestyle habits, healthy behavior, and a healthful environment.

In 1985 a "midcourse" evaluation was made of progress toward meeting the national objectives. The evaluation team found that progress had been made in several areas, including reducing hypertension, occupational injuries, and smoking, and in improving dental health. No progress had been made in reducing violence and teenage pregnancies, nor in improving nutrition.

The health objectives for the nation cut across all health professions from heads of government departments to community health workers, from private clinics to classrooms, and they apply to all people.

Source: The 1990 Health Objectives for the Nation: A Midcourse Review. Public Health Service, U.S. Department of Health and Human Services (1986).

dimension to the meaning of health, but like the term "health," "well-being," and our term "wellness," are not easily defined. In the 1950s, Halbert Dunn, a physician working for the United States Department of Public Health, was intrigued by the World Health Organization's definition of health, and attempted to clarify the meaning of well-being. Dunn (1961) described well-being as:

1. A joyous existence in which one feels "zest for life,"
2. A way of living that maximizes one's potential,
3. A purposeful direction that gives meaning to life,
4. Adapting to the challenge of a changing environment, and
5. Having a sense of social responsibility.

Dunn coined the term "high level wellness" to describe a person's state of being when these elements are an intrinsic part of life (Dunn, 1961). Key concepts are noteworthy: joy, way of living, maximizing potential, purposeful direction, and social responsibility. Dunn's concept of high level wellness goes beyond the WHO definition of health by adding elements such as maximizing potential and purpose in life. In this textbook, we use the term "wellness" as Dunn used "high level wellness." Wellness then, refers to a quality of being that can be called psychological health or psychological well-being—maximizing one's potential, having direction and purpose in life, meeting the challenges of the environment, looking beyond the needs of the self to the needs of the society, and doing it all with zest.

Health and wellness are not "all-or-none" states. Each dimension of health and wellness is a continuum—from sickness to absence of disease, from unhealthy lifestyle to healthy lifestyle, from despair to wellness. One can be at a different place on each continuum— feeling healthy while having an unhealthy lifestyle, or having goals but little joy in pursing them, or having joy and no goals. With knowledge and self-responsibility, however,

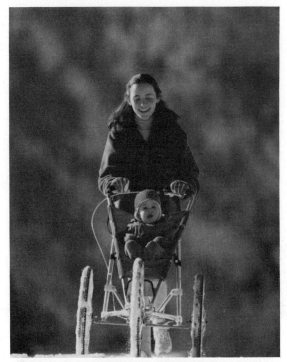

Zest for Life and Healthy Lifestyle Are Dynamics of Health and Wellness.
Source: Carl Yarbrough, Boulder, CO.

it is possible to move toward greater health and wellness, deliberately and wisely. You can think of these dimensions as strands that are intertwined to form a cord. The strength of the cord is determined by the strength of the individual strands.

The Dynamics of Health and Wellness

This book is about the forces, processes, and actions that promote health and wellness, and it describes health and wellness as processes that are changing and that involve effective action.

The forces, processes, and actions that promote health and wellness—the dynamics of health and wellness—apply at all points on the continua of health and wellness. The dynamics operate in health and wellness, and they also operate in recovery from disease and illness. This is an important point. We say to

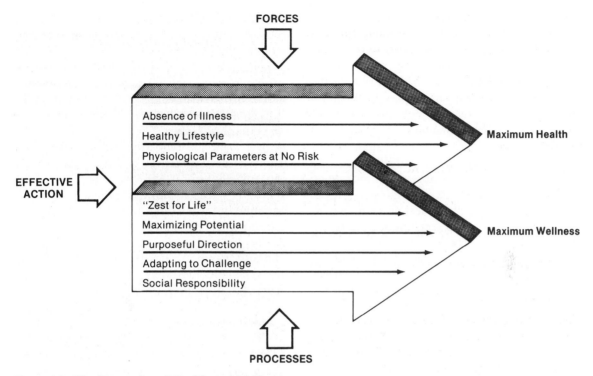

FORCES

EFFECTIVE
ACTION

Absence of Illness

Healthy Lifestyle

Physiological Parameters at No Risk

Maximum Health

"Zest for Life"

Maximizing Potential

Purposeful Direction

Adapting to Challenge

Social Responsibility

Maximum Wellness

PROCESSES

Figure 1.2   The Dynamics of Health and Wellness.

our clients: "We teach about wellness because people get well out of their wellness, not out of their illness." The dynamics that ensure health and wellness are the same dynamics that enable people to recover when sick. The members of Mr. Wright's treatment team understand the dynamics of health and wellness, and they will help Mr. Wright draw upon these dynamics within himself to hasten the process of health through effective action. Figure 1.2 summarizes these concepts. Arrows are used to suggest action and process.

SECTION THREE: THE BIOPSYCHOSOCIAL APPROACH

The title of this textbook indicates that the dynamics of health and wellness are described from a particular perspective, the **biopsychosocial approach**.

When syllables are run together to form a new term, the implication is that the term represents an integration, or interaction, of whatever the syllables represent. The biopyschosocial approach to health and wellness views health and wellness as the result of the interaction of biological, psychological, and social factors. **Biological** factors include "givens," such as genetics; environmental factors that affect physiological functioning, such as pesticides that migrate into the food chain and may cause birth defects and cancer; and behaviors that affect biological functions, such as smoking, diet, and exercise. **Psychological** factors include personality, stress management, life goals, perceptions, feelings, and health and sickness behaviors. **Social** factors include social systems such as the family, work, school, church, and government, and social values, customs, and social support.

Although biological, psychological, and social variables may be studied independently, the importance of the biopsychosocial approach is the recognition that these variables are not independent of each other. Health and wellness result from a complex interaction of biological, psychological and social variables. For example, consider a person who has a long and healthy life. The biological factors might include "good" genes, a wholesome diet, and an unpolluted environment; social factors might include a supportive and loving family, a fulfilling job, and wealth; psychological factors might include an easygoing personality and high self-esteem. Individually, these variables promote health to some degree, but in combination they produce a stronger effect. They interact—the easygoing personality encourages family support and love, which in turn enhances self-esteem, which encourages risk-taking at work, which leads to advancement and wealth; financial security reduces stress, which promotes health, and so on. If these variables were studied independently, the essential interaction would be overlooked.

The importance of the biopsychosocial approach can be illustrated in a simple example—maintaining an exercise program. Suppose that you join a fitness class and faithfully exercise for the duration of the class. The instructor has designed a program for you that fits your schedule and needs, and the group support encourages you. When the class is over, will you continue to exercise? If the instructor has a biopsychosocial perspective, your tendency to relapse into laziness is anticipated, and you are taught skills for coping with social pressure to quit and for coping with stress, and continued social support and follow-up would be arranged. Without the biopsychosocial perspective, the instructor might assume that because you had been faithful to the program you would continue to do so, failing to realize that maintaining an exercise program is a complex process involving psychological and social variables.

Perhaps you have realized that the biopsychosocial perspective can be applied equally well to the dynamics of disease and illness. In fact, one of the first discussions of the biopsychosocial approach was in the context of understanding disease. The biopsychosocial approach was contrasted to the **biomedical model of disease**, which focuses on biological factors, failing to take into account psychological and social factors. Consider a fictional Mr. Wright from the biopsychosocial perspective (fictional because we do not know the details of Mr. Wright's life). Mr. Wright may have had a genetic tendency toward cancer (biological variable); he was a long-time smoker (biological and social variable), who lacked the willpower to quit and convinced himself that smoking was not a health risk (psychological variable); and about one year before the diagnosis of cancer he lost his job and was deeply depressed (social and psychological variables). Independently, these variables may not cause cancer, but as interacting variables they produce the conditions that may promote cancer. The study of these variables as though they were independent would lead to a misunderstanding of Mr. Wright's disease and would lead to inadequate treatment. For example, if Mr. Wright enrolled in a smoking-cessation program that did not understand the interaction of depression and smoking, the smoking program might fail.

Although it is easier to study variables in isolation, the biopsychosocial approach acknowledges the basic reality—biological, psychological, and social variables are involved in health and wellness, and in disease and illness, and together create the total picture.

Figure 1.3 depicts the interaction of many biological, psychological, and social forces both for and against health and wellness. The intersection of the petals depicts this interaction. A description of the interaction of these factors is referred to as the biopsychosocial model of health and wellness.

Although any one of these factors may influence health disproportionately—for example, being born physically handicapped or

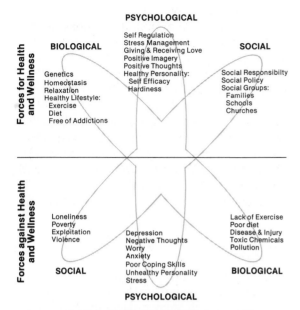

Figure 1.3   Biological, Psychological, and Social Factors That Affect Health and Wellness. The Biopsychosocial Model of Health and Wellness Emphasizes the Interaction of These Factors.

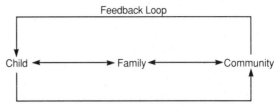

Figure 1.4   A Simple System of Interacting Elements—Individual, Family, and Community. Feedback Is an Important Dynamic in the Way That Subsystems and Systems Interact.

being brought up in a dysfunctional family—the three dimensions are inseparable and are mutually determining. For example, a person born with a physical handicap will have a profoundly different experience in a family and society that easily accommodate handicapped persons than in a family and society that have no resources for helping handicapped persons. As another example, consider drug addiction. To understand drug addiction we study the addictive qualities of a particular drug (biological), the personality characteristics of the addicted person (psychological), and the incentives in the environment, such as peer pressure or earning money by selling a drug (social). The idea that anyone could "just say no" to drugs overlooks the complex influences of social systems such as a high unemployment rate for teenage youths, the lack of psychological skills for coping with the influences of the mass media and peer groups, the lack of job skills, and the network of people who profit from the sale of illegal drugs.

We use the term "biopsychosocial approach" to specify the types of variables that are involved in health and wellness; we could have used the term **systems approach** because biological, psychological, and social variables interact as a system and are systems themselves. A **system** is an organization of interacting parts. Figure 1.4 diagrams a simple system in which a child interacts with the family and with the community, and these elements interact and reflect back to the individual, thus forming a system. Note that each element in the system is itself a system, just as the body can be described as a complex system that is composed of many other systems. Also notice the arrows in the diagram. The arrows indicate an essential element in the way that systems function—**feedback**, sometimes referred to as **feedback loops**. To understand this process, imagine that the child behaves in a way that upsets the family system; social values determine what behaviors the family will tolerate. Immediately the family reacts; the reaction provides feedback to the child, who changes the behavior. The behavior change acts as feedback to the family, which adjusts to the change, and peace is re-established. Feedback is an essential process in living systems, from cellular functioning to social functioning, and we refer to it repeatedly throughout this text in different contexts.

In general, the systems closest to a person have the greatest impact on the person and the greatest feedback. A child is influenced primarily by his family and community and less by elements that are further removed. A challenge for adults is to be involved in feedback loops that may be far removed from the immediate personal system of family and peers. This is a matter of social responsibility, which means interaction with remote systems and assuming responsibility for changing systems in ways that promote health and wellness.

A Systems Approach to Health and Wellness

In modern science, the first description of a systems approach occurred in biology. The functions of the body provide the clearest example of how subsystems interact to produce more complex systems, which interact to produce the whole organism, which can be viewed as a system itself. The German biologist Ludwig von Bertalanffy defined systems as "complexes of elements in interaction" (Bertalanffy, 1968). Bertalanffy emphasized an essential aspect of systems that the body also clearly illustrates: systems function as they do because they continually interact with their environment. For example, the cardiovascular system continually interacts with its environment, the body, and the body continually interacts with its environment, the world outside it. Bertalanffy made the point that to study living organisms, one must study them as they interact with their environment. Consideration of the organism's environment is incorporated in the systems perspective and is referred to as an "ecological" perspective (Boulding, 1978).

The systems approach has been adopted in many sciences in which complex interactions occur, including sociology and economics. In the behavioral sciences, the systems approach has been particularly useful in describing human behavior as the result of many interacting biological, psychological, and social systems. The systems approach to health and wellness (or disease and illness) and the biopsychosocial approach are different ways of describing the same phenomena; the interacting systems of the systems approach are the biological, psychological, and social dimensions of the biopsychosocial approach.

In describing the biopsychosocial approach, we said that biological, psychological, and social variables cannot be studied independently because they interact. The focus on interaction is also the essence of the systems approach, and it describes the nature of living organisms. For example, the functions of the cardiovascular system cannot be fully understood without studying its interaction with the pulmonary system, and vice versa. Their function, delivery of oxygen to body tissue, is the result of interaction.

The biopsychosocial systems approach in the behavioral and medical sciences is relatively new, even though today it seems like an obvious perspective. This is because the essence of science has been to dissect wholes into parts and to study the parts in isolation. Science has made brilliant progress in the physical sciences with this analytic approach. A major proponent of the systems approach in the behavioral sciences, Yale University professor Gary Schwartz writes, "Science has historically overemphasized the analytic approach at the expense of the systemic approach" (Schwartz, 1984, p. 157). However, the biopsychosocial systems approach to understanding the dynamics of health and wellness, and illness and disease, is not easy; it is far easier to study isolated variables than it is to study the interaction of many variables. The complexity of the biopsychosocial systems approach, however, correctly reflects the complexity of human nature.

The idea that the whole is greater than the sum of the parts is embodied in a systems approach and is true of the biopsychosocial approach to health and wellness. Although we might study biological, psychological, and social factors separately and attempt to create a whole picture based on the findings, the biopsychosocial approach suggests that the picture would not be complete because the total picture is a composite of those variables interacting. Having said this, we must tell you that the biopsychosocial picture of health and wellness is so complex that, as yet, we have no way of creating a whole picture. The biopsychosocial approach is still as much a concept, or way of thinking, as it is a field of study. The concept is valid; the picture is still unfolding. For this reason, much of the research that we present focuses on only one or two dimensions of health and wellness. For example, Chapter 6 contains a discussion of social support and health. Social support, a social variable, has psychological effects that in turn affect physiological functioning; but in general, social support researchers do not study the psychological variables that mediate the effects of social support on health.

In other words, there is no field of biopsychosociology that studies the whole picture. The picture that we have is the work of many people in many disciplines who contribute to our knowledge of the biological, psychological, and social dimensions of health and wellness.

The Study of the Dynamics of Health and Wellness: An Interdisciplinary Approach

The studies of biology, physiology, psychology, and sociology have traditionally been individual disciplines. Knowledge from these disciplines is brought together in the biopsychosocial approach to health and wellness, and thus the study of health and wellness from the biopsychosocial perspective is interdisciplinary.

If you ask, "What dynamics of health are operating in Mr. Wright?" the answer will depend in part on one's discipline. A cognitive psychologist might focus on the fact that the Rorschach test shows that Mr. Wright is a highly suggestible person, and highly suggestible persons are good hypnotic subjects who can do amazing things with their bodies. A cognitive psychologist might also focus on the placebo

effect and Mr. Wright's belief that he was receiving injections of Krebiozen when in fact he was receiving water. A psychoneuroimmunologist might focus on the mechanisms of the immune system to explain the rapid changes in tumors. A psychophysiologist might focus on the mechanisms of mind-body interaction that translate hope into physiological change. The physician might focus primarily on the physical disease and on physical treatment. The team approach to the treatment of Mr. Wright says that his disease, treatment, and health are biopsychosocial processes, and no part can be ignored. The team is also a metaphor for the interdisciplinary nature of the study of health and wellness and of treatment.

As the case of Mr. Wright illustrates, the study of health is a complex and intriguing subject. Insights from biological, psychological, and social sciences and related health professions are combined in one picture, to use the previous metaphor—an interdisciplinary approach. Figure 1.5 lists the many academic disciplines and professions that contribute to the biopsychosocial approach to health and wellness and to treatment.

The interdisciplinary approach to health and wellness is reflected in developments in disciplines such as psychology, medicine, and nursing, and in the evolution of such fields as health psychology, behavioral health, and behavioral medicine.

College and university departments of health use an interdisciplinary approach in training specialists in health education, exercise physiology, coaching, community health, and public health. Principles and methods from psychology, sociology, medicine, and education are taught. A psychologist and the first president of the Health Psychology division of the American Psychological Association, Joseph Matarazzo (1984), believes that professionals in the academic disciplines of health—such as health education, nursing, medicine, behavioral medicine, and health psychology—should cooperate in teaching

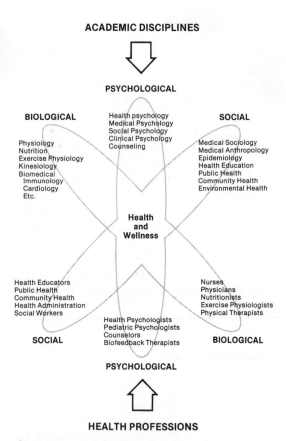

ACADEMIC DISCIPLINES

PSYCHOLOGICAL

BIOLOGICAL

Health psychology
Medical Psychology
Social Psychology
Clinical Psychology
Counseling

SOCIAL

Physiology
Nutrition
Exercise Physiology
Kinesiology
Biomedical
Immunology
Cardiology
Etc.

Medical Sociology
Medical Anthropology
Epidemiology
Health Education
Public Health
Community Health
Environmental Health

Health
and
Wellness

Health Educators
Public Health
Community Health
Health Administration
Social Workers

Nurses
Physicians
Nutritionists
Exercise Physiologists
Physical Therapists

Health Psychologists
Pediatric Psychologists
Counselors
Biofeedback Therapists

SOCIAL

BIOLOGICAL

PSYCHOLOGICAL

HEALTH PROFESSIONS

Figure 1.5 Knowledge of the Biological, Psychological, and Social Factors in Health and Wellness Comes from Many Disciplines and Contributes to Many Disciplines.

health classes, in research, in faculty exchanges, and in community-action projects.

Schools of nursing include professionals in their faculty from a variety of disciplines, and some provide training in behavioral therapies such as biofeedback and stress management (Nakagawa-Kogan, Betrus, Beaton, Burr, Larson, Mitchell, & Wolf-Wilets, 1984). "Nurses, as a group, are experts at working in interdisciplinary environments. In their work environment, nurses interact regularly with physicians, dieticians, physical therapists, psychologists, speech pathologists, and other health care professionals. In fact, at times one of the nurse's major roles is to be the liaison between these

specialities and to coordinate and implement the therapies they recommend" (O'Connell, 1988, p. 15).

Specialities within medicine, such as cardiology and family practice, are becoming more interdisciplinary, in both faculty and in treatment, by emphasizing the roles of nutrition, exercise, personality, and stress management in health. Medical sociologists have an interdisciplinary focus, collaborating with psychologists and physiologists in research and in publications. Henry and Stephens' (1977) classic book, *Stress, Health, and the Social Environment: A Sociobiologic Approach to Medicine,* integrates data from research in personality psychology, sociology, anthropology, and animal studies in an effort to identify the ingredients of health.

In the past two decades, great strides have been made in understanding the multidimensional dynamics of health and wellness, as illustrated by the biopsychosocial approach, and in the development of nonmedical therapeutic techniques for treating sickness, particularly the behavioral aspects. We used the team of health professionals working with Mr. Wright to introduce several dynamics, such as mind-body interaction, and several therapeutic techniques, such as biofeedback training, that are building blocks in the biopsychosocial approach to health and treatment. The team also illustrates the interdisciplinary nature of the new approaches. To bring health professionals together "under one roof" as we did with Mr. Wright's team, and to establish and formalize conceptual foundations, several disciplines and organizations were created in the late 1970s.

Health Psychology

A discipline is formally created when a name is chosen, a society is formed, a journal for professional publication is created, and a definition is given for the new discipline. In 1978, the American Psychological Association, an association of more than 70,000 psychologists, formed the division of Health Psychology, "dedicated to the promotion and maintenance of health" (Matarazzo, 1980). The journal *Health Psychology* began publication in 1981. Health psychology is rapidly becoming an academic field, as textbooks are written that define the field and describe its content. The first health psychology college textbook was written in 1983 (Gatchel and Baum, 1983). In her health psychology textbook, Shelley Taylor writes: "Health psychology is the field within psychology devoted to understanding psychological influences on how people stay healthy, why they become ill, and how they respond when they do get ill. Health psychologists both study such issues and promote interventions to help people stay well and get over illness" (Taylor, 1986, p. 5).

The name "health psychology" and the stated purpose of the field emphasize health as one focus. In addition, health psychology is concerned with issues of disease and illness, with treatment, and with the modification of risk behaviors such as smoking.

Joseph Matarazzo advocates the collaboration of researchers from various fields in tackling such problems as cigarette consumption among young people. Because smoking is a biopsychosocial problem, specialists in these three domains would pool their knowledge and resources. Matarazzo also advocates integrating the disciplines that train health professionals, suggesting that health psychologists team up with schools of nursing, medicine, health education, dentistry, and public health to integrate knowledge and develop methods for enhancing health.

Behavioral Medicine

Behavioral medicine was formally created in 1977 at a conference sponsored by Yale University and the National Heart Lung and Blood Foundation, and in 1980 the *Journal of Behavioral Medicine* began publication. The definition of behavioral medicine most often cited emerged from a second conference in 1978. Behavioral medicine is defined as "the interdisciplinary field concerned with the development and integration of behavioral and biomedical science, knowledge and techniques relevant to health and illness and the application of this knowledge and these techniques to prevention, diagnosis, treatment and rehabilitation" (Schwartz & Weiss, 1978, p. 250). This definition emphasizes the interdisciplinary nature of the field, in keeping with the biopsychosocial approach to health and illness (Schwartz & Weiss, 1977). In Chapters 14, 15, and 16, we describe behavioral medicine and the application of behavioral techniques in treatment of adults and children.

Behavioral Health

Behavioral medicine, as the term suggests, is concerned primarily with treatment of disease and illness. Thus, according to Matarazzo, behavioral medicine needs a sister field that emphasizes the maintenance and promotion of health. Matarazzo calls this field "behavioral health," which he describes as an interdisciplinary field that emphasizes the responsibility of the individual for maintaining health and preventing disease through lifestyle. The challenge for students of the health sciences, says Matarazzo, is to "map some of the important landmarks in this beckoning and relatively unexplored frontier—the health-maintaining, health-enhancing, and illness-preventing behaviors of currently healthy people" (Matarazzo, 1984, p. 29).

These new disciplines clearly overlap in purpose and content. At the same time, they provide a common focus for many health-related disciplines. The focus is the biopsychosocial approach to the dynamics of health and wellness, to disease and illness, and to treatment.

IIII▶

SECTION FOUR: AN OVERVIEW

This book takes up Matarazzo's challenge—to chart the frontier of health-maintaining, health-enhancing, and illness-preventing behaviors in currently healthy people. Matarazzo referred to the study of health (and we would include the study of wellness) as a frontier because health and wellness, as more than the absence of disease, have received little attention until recently.

Israeli sociologist Aaron Antonovsky (1987) coined the word *salutogenesis* from the Greek *saluto* meaning health and *genesis* meaning origins, to describe a new approach. Salutogenesis means the study of the origins of health. Antonovsky believes that health research has been concerned with pathogenesis, namely, the origins of pathology or disease, to the exclusion of salutogenesis. For example, when an epidemic occurs, health professionals are concerned with the disease and with treatment of the sick. The people who stay healthy are not studied. Similarly, much is known about alcoholism, but little is known about people who do not become alcoholics in spite of conditions that promote alcoholism. The salutogenic approach asks, "Who stays well and why?"

One approach to understanding the dynamics of health and wellness, then, is the study of healthy people. This text brings together the main lines of research on healthy people, distilling from the research the forces, processes and effective actions—the dynamics—that promote health and wellness. This includes personality, social, lifestyle, and cognitive variables.

It would be excellent if we could write about the dynamics of health and wellness based entirely on the study of health and wellness, without mentioning disease, treatment, stress, violence, pollution, and other antihealth conditions. But the reality is that healthy people do become sick, everyone experiences stress, pollution threatens everyone's health, and unhealthy relationships can happen to healthy people. The dynamics of health and wellness include meeting the challenges of life in a healthy way. To meet the challenges of life in a healthy way, one must understand what the challenges are and be able to deal with them.

Another approach to the dynamics of health and wellness is to study the forces that undermine health and wellness—stress and its physiological counterpart, the stress response; maladaptive personality styles such as Type A behavior; and lifestyle habits that are health risks. Because health and wellness are not merely the result of good luck, but are also the result of knowledge and effective action, we benefit from understanding risk factors and the dynamics of disease and illness. That way, these factors can be avoided. To promote health, we must know what not to do, as well as what to do. Therefore, although it is not the focus of this text, we do present the downside, the conditions under which health and wellness are in jeopardy. We assume that the readers of this text are fairly representative of the general population. This means that some of you are not in perfect health and wellness: some of you have stress-related illnesses, are involved in destructive relationships, are not maintaining a healthy lifestyle, and are not engaged in life with the zest of wellness. And, sadly, some of you carry the scars of physical and sexual abuse in childhood. Knowing that health and wellness are in jeopardy is an important dynamic that cannot be ignored, and it precedes effective action.

Knowing how to maintain health and wellness and using that knowledge are the focus of this book. These are the dynamics that take health and wellness beyond "just good luck, nothing I did" to health and wellness as dynamic processes under personal control, and these are the cornerstones in the prevention of sickness, another central dynamic. Importantly, these are also the dynamics that take sickness beyond "just bad luck, nothing I can do" to sickness as a process that can be changed through personal control. For these reasons we focus on what to do—how to reduce stress through cognitive and behavioral techniques, how to counteract anger, how to regulate yourself, how to reduce performance anxiety, how to have a healthy lifestyle. We said in the Preface that it would be of little value to write a book "about" the dynamics of health and wellness and not engage the reader in "doing" the dynamics of health and wellness. Take seriously the "how to and now do" theme.

This book is packed with ideas, information, and techniques for health and wellness. You use this knowledge because you want to be healthy. We noted, however, that some of you are not healthy or well today. As we said, an important dynamic in health and wellness is recovery from disease and illness, and disability, and living a healthy and well life in spite of handicaps. The knowledge and skills that you gain from this text will help you recover and maximize health and wellness in spite of sickness. And some of you will become health professionals. You may work in prevention or treatment programs; you may work in a medical setting or in private practice; you may be involved in community health; or you may become an educator. Whatever your health-care focus, understanding and applying the dynamics of health and wellness will be an integral part of your work, from prevention to treatment. And we add this note: Whatever your focus, you will be a model of the health and wellness dynamics that you teach.

We noted earlier that the dynamics of health and wellness are the cornerstones of treatment and recovery. Therapists help people overcome disease and illness by drawing upon, and enhancing, resources for health and wellness. We include in this textbook three chapters on treatment to share with you the upside of sickness—recovery—to acquaint you with behavioral medicine and treatment procedures, and to excite you about human potential.

Chapter by Chapter

Return to the case of Mr. Wright. What do you think was the principal dynamic that helped Mr. Wright regain his health? His belief in Krebiozen, his suggestible personality, and his hope overcame despair and enhanced his immune system. Underlying these powerful forces, however, is a more fundamental dynamic: the mind-body interaction, and particularly the effect the mind has on physiological functions. The effect of mental processes on physiological processes is the underlying dynamic that makes possible the mind-body techniques described in this book, such as hypnosis and biofeedback training. In Chapter 2, Mind-Body Dynamics, we discuss the mind-body connection in detail, with several common and uncommon examples. We also include a brief history of the demise and rebirth of the mind in science and invite you to consider your view of the mind. The principal body dynamic that underlies health—homeostatis—is the second topic of Chapter 2. Homeostasis refers to the body's tendency to maintain a balanced internal state, and to return to balance when disrupted. Homeostasis is an automatic process that can be disrupted or facilitated. Stress is a key factor in disrupting homeostasis. Finally, we introduce the concept of psychological homeostasis.

The topic of Chapter 3, Stress, is stress. Because stress is a part of everyone's life, understanding stress is important for health and wellness. Chapter 3 discusses the nature and dimensions of stress and includes several stress inventories. We focus on work stress and the effects that stress has on academic performance. Chapter 4, The Stress Response, describes the physiological effects of stress. We emphasize this truism: knowledge is power. The more you know about stress and your body's reaction, the more power you have to maintain health. We describe several physiological systems, the stress response of each system, and the primary stress-related illnesses of each system. Chapter 4 provides the physiological information needed for understanding the disorders and treatment procedures described in the chapters on behavioral medicine in Part Five.

Chapter 5, Evaluating Research, stands alone, and yet, it is an integral part of this text. Much of what we know about health and wellness comes from research, and it is essential that you understand the basics of research evaluation. We need not accept research data as absolutely true, and we need not remain continually skeptical; we provide guidelines for evaluating research. We have placed this chapter early in the text so that as you proceed, you will understand research results and appreciate the difficulties of research on complex human processes. We comment on research throughout this text because good research is fundamental to progress in the health fields.

Chapter 6, The Psychosocial Dynamics of Stress Resistance, is the first of five chapters in Part Three, the core chapters on handling the challenges and stressors of life in a healthy way. In Chapter 6, we introduce the question, "Who stays well?" The characteristics and resources of healthy people are described, beginning with the "hardy" personality. Other characteristics and resources include purpose in life, stoical fortitude, and emotional insulation, social support, and love. We also discuss social skills such as empathy, and we introduce an important concept, "learned resourcefulness."

Chapter 7, Relaxation, describes relaxation as an essential skill and a dynamic in health, because relaxation is the psychophysiological process that brings the body back to healthy homeostasis when body functioning is disrupted. Several relaxation techniques are described, including short exercises that you can practice throughout the day. Chapter 8, Biofeedback Training, is a detailed introduction to biofeedback training, including the underlying dynamics, the rationale, and the history. Biofeedback training began in the laboratory and evolved into a powerful self regulation tool that is used in educational, medical, and business settings. Chapter 9, Imagery for Health and Wellness, introduces another tool for self regulation, health, and healing. Imagery has been used primarily in therapy. Many of these uses are described, including the exciting possibility of helping cancer patients influence the immune system and eliminate cancer. However, imagery is everyone's resource and can be used in self-exploration, to enhance performance and creativity, and to help in relaxation and biofeedback training. Chapter 10, Cognitive and Multicomponent Methods for Stress Resistance, describes methods for becoming hardy and stress-resistant. These techniques, which integrate many skills, include cognitive restructuring and stress inoculation.

Chapter 11, Self Regulation for Health, could have been placed at the beginning of this text, because self regulation is another fundamental dynamic. Without this dynamic, people become victims of circumstances rather than victors. Self regulation has many components and many applications in the physiological, behavioral, and cognitive dimensions of health and wellness. Chapter 12, Lifestyle and Health, is a natural companion to Chapter 11 because, for most people, adopting a healthy lifestyle necessitates self regulation. Chapter 12 is a brief look at the basic elements of a healthy lifestyle—diet, exercise, and freedom from addictions, elements that are commonly included in discussions of lifestyle—and assertiveness, nonviolence, and play, elements that we think are essential but that are not usually included. In Chapter 13, Development of Health Behaviors, we describe a variety of school, community, hospital, and clinical programs for the prevention and modification of problem behaviors and the promotion of healthy behaviors.

Chapter 14, Introduction to Behavioral Medicine: Treatment Protocols, introduces Part

Five, the section of this text that deals with treatment. We begin with an example of a treatment protocol, describing five generic sessions. In this chapter, we also describe the skills of the therapist. Chapter 15, Behavioral Medicine: Applications with Adults, describes the use of behavioral therapy in the treatment of several disorders in adults, including hypertension, tension, and migraine headache, irritable bowel syndrome, and epilepsy. Chapter 16, Behavioral Medicine: Applications with Children, is a continuation of Chapter 15, describing treatment protocols and applications of behavioral techniques with children. Chapter 16 includes two applications for which the need and the benefit are great: helping children cope with painful and traumatic medical procedures and with chronic, crippling, and terminal diseases. These chapters illustrate the ways that behavioral techniques may be applied and the potential that people have for masterful self regulation and recovery. Chapter 17, Coronary Prone Personality: Type A, focuses on the Type A behavior pattern, the way the concept was developed and researched, and the relationship of Type A behavior to heart disease. The discovery of Type A behavior and its link to heart disease played an important role in bringing awareness of biopsychosocial variables into the medical arena. We also describe Type B behavior and how to become a Type B person. Chapter 18, Personality and Cancer, describes research on personality and the development of cancer and other immune system disorders. The study of personality and disease provides insight into mind-body relationships and the psychosocial aspects of treatment. This chapter also includes an in-depth look at cancer survivors, who provide invaluable information on the dynamics of health and wellness. In Chapter 19, The Development of Personality Characteristics of the Healthy Person, we discuss the psychosocial factors that foster healthy, stress-resistant children.

The final part of this text moves the focus to society and to the influence of cultural and social forces. We cannot present the biopsychosocial approach without including social variables, recognizing that the health and wellness of the individual depend upon the health and wellness of the society. Simultaneously, we shift the focus from self-responsibility to social responsibility. In Chapter 20, Societal and Cultural Forces Against Health and Wellness, we examine values and institutions that promote worseness of all types and that work against self-responsibility and social responsibility. We also examine violence, which cuts across all boundaries, and poverty, which affects a growing number of people, especially children, who carry the greatest burden of disease and illness and who have the least opportunity to create change. Some of the forces for worseness in our society are subtle, and some are obvious, but all are worthy of our attention.

From the negative we move to the positive. Chapter 21, Societal and Cultural Forces for Health and Wellness, describes health and wellness programs in a variety of settings, from poverty-stricken families to the boardrooms of industry, from prisons to the halls of state government. These programs, which promote personal, social, and environmental health, are models that can be replicated. We also describe, and applaud, the work of citizens' groups. Finally, we move to a global perspective, with the awareness that planetary health is not separate from our own.

CHAPTER 2

Mind-Body Dynamics

Reviewing the case of Mr. Wright and the experts who visited him, what do you think was the most important dynamic of health and wellness that he learned?

In various ways, the experts told Mr. Wright, *"Your mind affects your body; you have power."* We begin with this dynamic of health and wellness because mind-body interaction is a fundamental dynamic of health and sickness, and therefore it is fundamental to many topics in this textbook.

Mind and body continually interact, and physiological states have powerful effects on psychological states. In this textbook, however, we focus primarily on the effect of mind on body, the topic of Section One. This dynamic empowers people in such ordinary processes as choosing healthy lifestyle habits and in such extraordinary processes as eliminating a cancer. In a study that emphasizes the individual's personal responsibility and personal power for achieving health and wellness, the effect of mind on body is the more important dynamic.

■ **NOTE:** You get tired of reading the same phrase over and over, and writers get tired of trying to find new ways to say the same thing. Therefore, when you see mind ⟶ body, you think: *the mind affects the body* or *the influence of the mind on the body* or *the impact of the mind on the body.* ■

Mind ⟶ body has probably been true for as long as bodies have had minds and minds have had bodies. Yet the significance of this dynamic eluded modern science, and the *application* of mind ⟶ body for the prevention and treatment of physical disease and illness has only recently become an important addition in medicine and psychology. In Section Two, we discuss issues and problems involved in the study of the mind, and we describe several factors that contribute to neglect of the mind as an agent in disease and health. We encourage you to consider your beliefs about mind ⟶ body as you read.

In Section Three we describe a second fundamental dynamic of health and wellness— **homeostasis**, the innate ability of the body to maintain physiological health. Homeostasis is a body dynamic of which we are scarcely aware, and yet it is the basis of physiological health. We extend the concept of homeostasis to include psychological health as well.

These two dynamics, mind ⟶ body and homeostasis, are the natural heritage of human beings who are born healthy. Illness and disease may develop when the mind disrupts homeostasis, as with chronic worry, or when the body is thrown off balance with poor lifestyle habits, such as smoking or poor nutrition. By virtue of the fact that mind ⟶ body and homeostasis are the foundations of health, however, they are also the dynamics that allow recovery. Most importantly, health and wellness are maintained and enhanced and sickness is prevented when the mind is used to influence the body in positive ways and when healthy lifestyle habits and a healthy environment are part of everyday living.

SECTION ONE: THE MIND-BODY HYPHEN

Mind-body. There is always a hyphen. The hyphen says: connected, interacting, one system, distinctly different but related.

You have a mind, and you have a body. Subjectively, you experience them as distinctly different but interacting. Without the connection of mind and body, and the ability of mind to influence body, phenomena as simple as reading this book or as complex as Mr. Wright's saga could not occur, nor would we be writing about the disciplines that investigate and apply mind $\longrightarrow$ body for treatment of disease and illness, such as health psychology and behavioral medicine.

The dynamics of health and wellness include many forces and underlying processes. Of these, mind $\longrightarrow$ body is fundamental. In every context in which psychological variables are related to physical health—whether we are discussing social support, cognitions, perceptions and beliefs, images, relaxation, or stress—the underlying mechanism is mind-body interaction, specifically mind $\longrightarrow$ body.

Definitions

Body

Body is relatively easy to define because the body has physical existence. So by body we mean the obvious—your physical being, the vehicle that you cart around and live through.

Through the ages, elements of both Eastern and Western cultures have treated the body either as a source of sin, the seat of appetites that distract the mind from God, or as the source of all pleasure, to be adored and idolized. One view led to a depreciation of the body, the other to its glorification. We accept the Greek ideal: *a healthy mind in a healthy body.* In another framework, it is said that "the body is the temple of the soul." We appreciate the concept that the body is the vehicle for the mind, and as such, deserves first-rate treatment.

We also like this concept: The body is a metaphor of the mind. In other words, the body reflects the mind and in many ways it is a representation of it. Think of posture. Our physical stance can be a reflection of the mind, that is,

our psychological state. Shy people have shy posture; depressed people have depressed posture. The body therapies developed in the past two decades recognize the connection, and therapists may work on the body as a way of working on the mind. The body is also the "servant" of the mind, but it has its kingdoms and hierarchies of structure and function that at times seem to have a life of their own.

Mind

How shall we define the **mind**? What do we mean when we say "my mind?" Psychologists usually define the mind by what it does and by its characteristics. One use of the word "mind" refers to the uniquely human complex of thoughts, emotions, expectations, self-talk, images and visualizations, goals, volition, private agendas, perceptions, beliefs, attitudes, language and memory, attention, and consciousness. These functions, characteristics, and attributes of the mind may be referred to as "mental behavior."

Some psychologists who have a behavioristic orientation are reluctant to use the word "mind." They refer to the activities of the mind in behavioral terms such as "goal-seeking behavior." This stems from the dictates of behaviorism described in Section Two, and from the need to avoid the use of a word that for many centuries referred to a "disembodied spirit" or soul, concepts that are thought to have no place in modern science. In this text we use language for the mind that matches our common experience, such as saying, "I focused my mind on the task" or "I made up my mind." In discussing the influence of mind on body, we might say, "You can talk to your body with your mind" or "The body listens to the mind." This is what we would have said to Mr. Wright, had he been our patient.

But what else is the mind? In describing mental activity, have we defined the mind? When we say "my mind" as we might say "my body," we use language that implies that the mind is a "thing." Is it? The mind seems to have no "thingness"—it is insubstantial, it does not occupy space or have shape, size, or weight. It is **no-thing**. It does not have the properties of things, as does the body. And yet, this "no-thing" influences the physical body. How can "no-thing" influence "some-thing"? This paradoxical nature of mind creates considerable difficulty for science, as discussed later. The mysteries of the structure and functions of the body are slowly being solved, but the greatest mystery of all—the connection of mind and body—remains unsolved. We say that mind and body are connected and we can prove it easily enough. The hyphen exists, but what is the hyphen, and what is the mechanism by which the mind influences the body? How does the image of drinking lemon juice make your mouth water, and how did you create the image in the first place?

There have been many theories about "mind," ranging from mind as a nonphysical entity that interacts with the brain to produce mental phenomena to merely a word for describing certain experiences related to neuronal activity in the brain. Although the nature of mind is a fascinating topic, this textbook is not about the nature of mind. This text concerns the use of the mind and its special connection with the body, for health and wellness.

The Mind-Body Hyphen: Why?

Why did nature create such a powerful mind-body connection? Why did evolution give mental events the power to trigger, and modify, physiological events? Certainly one answer is for survival. If the connection of mind and body did not exist, or existed erratically, we could not have survived over the millennia. Could any species have survived?

In the wild, the natural order in the kingdoms of the carnivores is survival by killing prey and by escaping predators. For many species, killing and escaping demand extraordinary bursts of physical activity. In nonhuman animals, the triggers for physiological responses are external stimuli such as smells, sounds, and visual patterns (for example, the pattern of a hawk overhead, to a rabbit). The response to these triggers is innate, does not have to be learned, and does not seem to involve higher mental processes such as interpretation or anticipation.

In humans, the mechanisms of mind-body interaction for survival have evolved from external triggers to complicated mental processes that involve **interpretation of events**. These interpretations are based on many personal and cultural influences. But we need not complicate the matter with these considerations just yet. We can simply review the snake story told to Mr. Wright.

Imagine: You are driving home at night through a heavy rain. As you approach your house in the foothills, the street lights flash and go out. The headlights illuminate a swirl of shriveled leaves dashing through the light like a thousand miniature ghosts. You turn into the driveway and park in the usual place—it's a quick dash to the front door. You grab your books, open the car door, and step down on a long black snake. It squirms under your foot. In a flash of fear you drop your books on the wet concrete and jump back into the car, slamming the door. You barely notice your pounding heart and rapid breathing. With shaking hands you turn on the lights. There it is, coiled right under the door, ready to strike—the garden hose. Garden hose! Laughing with relief, you think, "Just the garden hose, left it there this afternoon." For a moment you relax. "Good grief, the garden hose." Your breathing returns to normal, heart decelerates, muscles relax. Then you remember the books.

Now, if you had stepped on a snake but had no way of informing your brain of the interpretation "snake" before the snake sank its fangs into your leg, the tardiness of the response would be deadly. Or if you came to the spot in the jungle where a snake had nearly killed you, but there was no way of connecting the memory to the appropriate brain areas to trigger the fight-or-flight response, you would have no way of preparing to fight or flee until you felt the sting of the bite, a bit late. The mind-body connection makes it possible to "get the jump" in threatening situations. The mind activates the appropriate brain areas, which in turn activate the physiological responses needed to fight or flee—it is fast, predictable, and life-saving. Please read Box 2.1 now.

Mr. Wright was asked to imagine drinking the juice of a ripe, sour lemon, and his mouth watered. Where is the lemon? The lemon is in the mind. Is the lemon real? Some people say "No, it isn't a real lemon; it's only in the mind." Wrong. The lemon is real—real in the mind. And here is the important mind ⟶ body dynamic: **What is "real" in the mind is "real" to the body**.

Emotional and mental processes, particularly images, are real in the mind. And because mind and body are connected, they are real to the body, and the body responds.

Attending to and regulating emotional and mental processes are important dynamics in

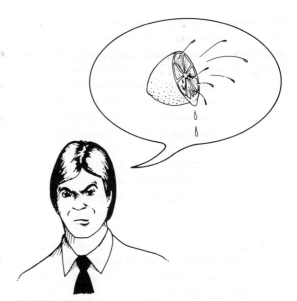

Figure 2.1 The Lemon Is Real in the Mind, and the Body Responds.

health and wellness; several chapters address this topic.

Perceptions, images, self-talk, and other mental processes are messages to the body. We do not necessarily intend to give messages to the body 24 hours a day, but it happens automatically, even during sleep. The hyphen is always there.

Take a minute: Ask yourself: What messages am I giving my body? How many times a day do I see snakes when there are only garden hoses?

Do It Now.

Now imagine that you are driving home on a rainy night, totally exhausted—wiped out. You get out of your car and step on a real snake. In your foggy state, you have the vague thought, "The garden hose; I'll put it away tomorrow." Now what happens? Nothing. No mental/emotional reaction, no physiological reaction. Why? Because you **perceived** the situation as harmless.

The power of perceptions in health and in illness cannot be underestimated. The role of perceptions is discussed throughout this book.

BOX 2.1

Think about this: The body relies on the mind for information about the world. In most cases, the body believes whatever the mind is telling it. Your toes cannot say, "Hey, dummy, this is the garden hose." Fortunately, the body has retained a few triggered responses, the reflexes. For example, the body is good at responding to such things as stepping on a nail and touching a hot stove. By virtue of its reflexes, the body can respond to these stimuli without consulting the mind. Otherwise, the body relies on the mind to tell it about the "outside" world.

"Perception" refers to the cognitive interpretation of events, as in "I perceived him to be angry." Related words are "interpretation," "belief," and "appraisal." Perceptions are a central dynamic in health and wellness because the way in which we "view" ourselves and events affects both behavior and physiological functioning. The dramatic result of perceiving a garden hose as a snake illustrates this point.

You are probably aware that your perceptions, your interpretations of events, and the images in your mind do affect your body, although you might not have considered the significance of this. But when you read the case of Mr. Wright, perhaps you thought, "Mr. Wright's case is too weird . . . that's impossible . . . his mind couldn't do that." The effect of perceptions, beliefs, and images on physiology exemplify mind ⟶ body beyond a shadow of a doubt. In the next subsection we present several illustrations.

Mind ⟶ Body Illustrated

The Placebo Effect

Mr. Wright is perhaps the most extraordinary example of the placebo effect ever recorded. Experts cannot explain the mechanisms of his cure and death, but no one disputes the fact that it happened.

The **placebo effect** is the elimination or reduction of a symptom after the patient receives a sugar pill or other type of placebo, believing that it is a real medicine. Mr. Wright believed that the shot that Dr. West gave him was Krebiozen, and because mind ⟶ body, his body responded. As Dr. Methodology explained, placebos cannot affect symptoms, so the only explanation for the effect is the power of the patient's mind. Please read Box 2.2 now.

The power of belief has undoubtedly been known for as long as the art of healing has been practiced. From the flamboyant shaman to the august physician, healers have understood that

what the patient believes about the treatment affects the outcome of the treatment.

In modern medicine and pharmaceutical research, the placebo effect is used as a scale against which the effectiveness of a drug or procedure is measured. Occasionally the effect of the placebo, which is really the effect of expectation, is equally as impressive as the treatment to which it is compared. For example, the following research abstract reports a British study:

> Sixty-eight women with proved premenstrual syndrome were treated under placebo-controlled conditions for up to ten months in a longitudinal study. Symptoms were monitored with daily menstrual distress questionnaires, visual analogue scales, and the 60-item general health questionnaire. Of the 35 women treated with placebo, 33 improved, giving an initial placebo response rate of 94%. The placebo effect gradually waned, but the response to the [drug] was maintained for the duration of the study.
>
> Magos, et al., 1986,
> *British Medical Journal*

■ **NOTE:** Do not get the idea that the excellent results of the placebo group prove that PMS is "all in the mind." These results prove that the mind is powerful enough to reduce symptoms. ■

Pharmaceutical companies compare every new drug with a placebo to determine the effectiveness of the drug. If the drug is not significantly more effective than the placebo in relieving symptoms, then the drug is assumed to be chemically ineffective, and it cannot be marketed. There is always a placebo effect. Current research on the placebo effect shows that in drug studies and in other types of therapy, the placebo effect may account for as much as 50 percent of the symptom reduction (Evans, 1985).

But how can a medical procedure, other than giving a drug, be faked? Not easily, and probably not ethically today. However, two daring placebo control studies were conducted in 1958 and 1959 to determine the effectiveness

BOX 2.2

RESEARCH METHODOLOGY

As Dr. Methodology explained, in drug studies the placebo effect is determined by comparing symptom reduction in a group of patients given the drug, called the "treatment group," with a group of patients who are given the placebo, called "the control group." The same "dose" and the same instructions and suggestions for improvement are given to the two groups. Ideally, the groups are "matched," meaning that patients in both groups have identical symptoms, are similar in age, have similar prognoses, and have similar beliefs about the "drug" they are taking. When the treatment and the control groups are well matched, it is assumed that the only major difference between the groups that could account for differences in symptom change, is that one group receives the drug and one group receives the placebo.

To increase the ability of the study to isolate the effect of the drug, another element is added: the person giving the "drug" is "blind" and does not know whether it is the medication or the placebo. Because the patient is also blind and does not know whether the drug is a placebo, this research paradigm is called **double-blind**. Why is it important for the person giving the "drug" to be ignorant? If the person giving the drug knows that it is a placebo, this fact might be revealed accidentally to the subjects in the control group. The influence of the experimenter on results is called the "experimenter effect," or "experimenter bias," and is a concern in all research. If subjects find out that the drug is not real, then the study is invalid because the control group no longer has the same beliefs as the treatment group. Dr. West was very persuasive, and Mr. Wright was convinced that he was receiving Krebiozen.

The placebo effect has always been considered a nuisance, but it can't be eliminated because humans are believing and hopeful creatures. Instead, placebo control groups are used. There are many complications with the use of placebo control groups and the double-blind design, and the research is time-consuming and expensive. Yet this type of design is mandatory for drug research. Certainly this is a testimonial to the fact that the pharmaceutical branch of medical science acknowledges the power of beliefs on physiology.

of a surgical procedure for the treatment of angina pectoris. Angina pectoris is pain in the chest that occurs usually with exercise, because of insufficient blood flow to the heart muscle. In the mid-1950s a surgical procedure called mammary artery ligation was developed for the treatment of angina. An incision was made in the chest and an artery was tied. The idea was that due to the blockage, more blood would flow in the collateral arteries, thus increasing flow to the heart muscle. The procedure was quite successful. The treatment was abandoned, however, after two surgeons in separate clinics tested the procedure against a placebo control. In the two studies, involving a total of 35 patients, the patients were randomly assigned to either the treatment or the control group. The treatment group patients received the ligation. The control group patients had the surgery, but no ligation; the chest was opened and closed again. One study had nine patients in each group. All of the control subjects, and six of the treatment subjects, reported a decreased need for medication and an increased tolerance of exercise. When the two studies were combined, the results on all measures—including degree of relief of angina and length of improvement—showed an average improvement in the control group of 37 percent. Two of the untreated patients had total relief of angina, and one had an improved electrocardiogram (Benson & McCallie, Jr., 1979).

The placebo effect is an excellent example of the power of the mind to affect physiology and behavior. It should not be called the "placebo effect," however. To be accurate, the term should be "positive expectation effect" or "positive belief effect." Positive expectations and belief in the treatment—and their counterparts, such as positive imagery—create the effect. The rubric "placebo effect" detracts from its true nature. Please read Box 2.3 now.

The power of hope and positive expectations, faith, and another important ingredient—personal investment—has also been dramatically demonstrated in the healings that have occurred in places such as Lourdes Cathedral in France, as described to Mr. Wright.

We learn from studying the placebo effect, the healings at Lourdes, and similar phenomena, that variables such as hope, positive expectations, and personal investment play a role in overcoming disease and illness and maintaining health, and must be included in theories of health and wellness and in therapies.

Spontaneous Remission

Spontaneous remission is the term given to the remission of a disease and the recovery of the patient when there is no known mechanism for the recovery. Mr. Wright's unexpected

---

BOX 2.3

THE PROBLEM WITH THE PLACEBO EFFECT

The placebo effect is a clear example of the power of the mind to affect the body. In our work with patients, we try to enhance the effect, because symptom reduction that results from positive expectations and belief in the therapy is a boost to the patient. However, the placebo effect is rarely enough. To sustain the change, and to maintain health under all circumstances, patients need **skills and knowledge.**

We wonder how often a drug that seems to work for a time loses its effect because, in fact, what worked was the power of belief. We wonder how often the physician then increases the dosage, or prescribes a new drug that seems to work as the first drug did, but sooner or later seems to work no longer. Patients who experience this phenomenon may do so partly because the placebo effect works until taking the drug becomes routine and enthusiasm for the drug wanes.

---

recovery is an example of spontaneous remission. The literature on spontaneous remission is surprisingly large in comparison to our understanding of how spontaneous remissions occur. The oncologist and pioneer of self-help therapy for cancer patients, Carl Simonton, found that in many cases of spontaneous remission, the patient absolutely believed in recovery and maintained an *image* of being well (Simonton, Matthews-Simonton, & Creighton, 1978).

Mr. Wright is a case of spontaneous remission in the sense that he was not cured by a treatment. We suspect that if physicians and health-care professionals were more inclined to share unusual and inexplicable cases, more Mr. Wrights would be found.

Hypnosis

When I (JG) was young, a hypnotist came to town. Everyone gathered in the town theater to see him. His show was probably like that of many traveling hypnotists. He did an hypnotic induction and suggested that our right arm was becoming as light as air. The right arm of a few people began rising, as if filled with helium. These hypnotized people were invited up to the stage. With eyes wide open, smiling and having a good time, they ate huge white onions because they were told that they were eating delicious red apples. I was too far from the stage to see whether their eyes watered, but I was curious. The hypnotist told the group on the stage that he had a hot rod, and when he touched their arm with it, they would feel pain. They all acted as if they felt the heat of the *pencil*. Then he told them that the theater was becoming cold, freezing cold. Soon they were all shivering. The skeptics in the audience went away saying that it was all fake and that the people had been planted in the audience.

Today traveling hypnotists are rare, but hypnotism survives as a powerful therapeutic technique, in this "classical" form of trance induction and as self-hypnosis. The use of hypnosis for pain and bleeding control in dentistry and surgery is well known, although not commonly used. We discuss hypnosis further in Chapter 9 on imagery and in Chapters 15 and 16 on behavioral medicine; here we use hypnosis as an example of mind ⟶ body. Please read Box 2.4 now.

Hypnosis works. But how? The hypnotist does not touch the person, does not use chemicals, does not alter the person's physiology directly. The hypnotist merely suggests images and feelings; somehow, conditions are created that enhance mind ⟶ body, and the body

follows the suggestion of the mind. How this happens is not understood, but that it happens is clear.

Chemotherapy, Vomiting, and Conditioning

Some cancer patients receiving chemotherapy develop adverse reactions to the drugs, including severe nausea and vomiting. As treatment continues, the nausea and vomiting worsen. Then an interesting process begins. The patients begin to feel nauseated *before* the chemotherapy is started, when they are just sitting in the reclining chair waiting for the treatment. Then nausea may begin in the parking lot, outside the clinic; then it may start while driving to the clinic; and finally nausea begins at home, anticipating chemotherapy. We have worked with patients who began to feel nauseated by simply thinking about chemotherapy. It's not a pleasant example of mind ⟶ body, but one that everyone can understand. Perhaps you became violently sick after eating a particular food, say caramel corn. The next time someone even hints of eating caramel corn, you feel nauseated. The body responds because **what is real in the mind is real to the body**. Please read Box 2.5 now.

Images influence physiology. This aspect of mind ⟶ body may have evolved purely for survival, but today the impact of imagery on physiology is a powerful tool in behavioral medicine, described in detail in Chapter 9.

Data from India

The science of yoga has given the East an ancient and enduring interest in mind ⟶ body. The many systems of yoga are based upon the knowledge that discipline of mind (concentration and meditation) and discipline of body (Hatha yoga, vegetarianism, and so on) bring harmony of mind and body. One dramatic but minor branch of mind-body discipline is the practice and demonstration of feats of

---

BOX 2.4

HYPNOSIS CASE HISTORY

A 40-year-old woman weighing 575 pounds was scheduled for surgical removal of a huge, tumorous mass on her right thigh. Because of her obesity, neither local nor general anesthesia could be attempted. The patient's physician contacted "our colleagues in psychology" to evaluate the patient for possible use of hypnosis.

The patient was seen for four sessions of clinical hypnosis. The authors of the report write: "The patient was very cooperative and responded well to both single and dual inductions. The focal image used involved numbing her body by allowing her to become 'lazy, dull, insensitive, and asleep, like a piece of wood.'" In the fourth session, a metal clip was placed through the web of skin at the base of the thumb to determine the patient's ability to achieve anesthesia. Because the pain test was successful, the two psychologists asked the anesthesiologist to rehearse with the patient the entire surgical procedure, while she was still in trance. The anesthesiologist described the entire procedure and outlined the cut around the tumor with a pencil eraser. One week later the patient was taken to surgery.

In surgery, hypnosis was induced; no premedication was given. The authors report:

"The surgery proceeded smoothly until the surgeon determined that he was unable to lift and hold the massive tumor off the back of the patient's thigh because of its extreme size and its very wide base. A decision was then made to drive a metal spike through the tumor, attach this rod to a hydraulic bed-scale lift, and lift the tumor from the patient."

This procedure was not part of the plan and was not rehearsed. When the spike was driven through the tumor, the patient immediately used a predetermined hand signal indicating that she was in distress. The surgeon halted the procedure, the anesthesiologist immediately gave the patient small doses of fentanyl citrate and diazepam, and the surgery continued. The entire operation lasted two and a half hours; the tumor weighed 55 pounds.

In the postoperative interview, the patient explained that she had felt no pain, but when the spike was driven through the tumor she felt a very hot sensation and was surprised.

The patient recovered uneventfully.

From Morris, Nathan, Goebel, & Blass, 1985

---

psychophysiologic self regulation. These feats include stopping the heart, drying wet sheets wrapped around the body in freezing weather, and being buried underground for days. These demonstrations are rarely studied by

Westerners. Several problems account for this. Unusual feats of physiological control have been inexplicable to traditional Western science and are dismissed by skeptics as fake. Even when there is an opportunity to study

---

BOX 2.5

CONDITIONING

The Russian physiologist Ivan Pavlov first described an element of this process, called classical conditioning, in which physiological responses become conditioned to an external stimulus. Pavlov's basic procedure was to repeatedly place meat powder in the mouth of a hungry dog and simultaneously ring a bell, while measuring salivary gland output via a tube in the dog's mouth. After pairing the meat powder and the bell many times, he rang the bell in the absence of the meat. As all psychology students know, the sound elicited the salivary response; Pavlov called the sound the *conditioned stimulus.* Undoubtedly, the same thing happens to the house pet when we call it to dinner by rattling the food dish. Pavlov was amazed to find that after conditioning, a variety of auditory frequencies would trigger the response. But how? Sounds don't normally trigger the salivary response. It seemed like a momentous discovery.

Pavlov was determined to rid physiology of any hints of psychology because he thought that the study of subjective things muddied science; he thought that studying animals was perfect because the scientist need not worry about emotional or mental responses. In explaining this type of conditioning, in which the body reacts to stimuli that would not elicit the reaction before conditioning, Pavlov stated that the nervous system learns, rather than the dog anticipates the food. This language would have been too mentalistic. However, we can ask: Does the dog imagine the meat at the sound of the bell, and is it the image that triggers salivation? With dogs it is difficult to know.

With human beings it is not so hard to know. Patients who are classically conditioned and experience nausea before chemotherapy, for example, do imagine the experience, and it is the image of chemotherapy that triggers the physiological response of nausea and vomiting.

---

yogis and swamis scientifically, such phenomena are difficult to study because they cannot easily be brought into a laboratory or replicated. It is also undoubtedly true that demonstrations for Westerners is not a priority for yogis and swamis.

Intriguing accounts of unusual phenomena have been written by Westerners living in India and in Tibet (Brunton, 1972; David-Neel, 1971), but personal accounts can be dismissed as anecdotal and fanciful. Fortunately, several investigations of yogis and swamis have been

conducted by Indian scientists (Wenger, Bagchi & Anand, 1961), and in the last two decades several studies have been conducted by Western scientists, including the psychophysiological research team of Green, Green, and Green. In 1973, at the suggestion of Swami Rama (who was participating in research at The Menninger Foundation with Elmer and Alyce Green, pioneers in biofeedback training, whom you will meet in Chapter 8), we traveled to India with a portable laboratory to undertake research with yogis and swamis who were willing to

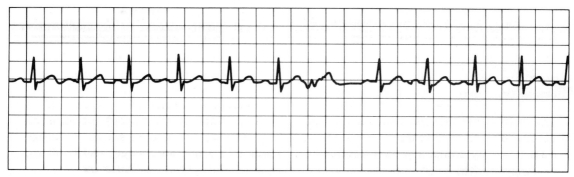

Figure 2.2   The Electrocardiogram of Shri Ramanda Yogi Shows That He Was Able to Cause His Heart to Skip a Beat on Command.

demonstrate physiological control. This research, and the research with Swami Rama, is described in detail elsewhere (Green & Green, 1976). Figure 2.2 shows the heart-rate data of Shri Ramananda Yogi, who made his heart skip a beat on command. During the heartbeat experiment, the yogi sat perfectly still, changing neither his breathing nor his posture.

This demonstration represents a high degree of physiological self regulation.

Summary

We have looked at a variety of mind ⟶ body phenomena, from the common experience of the snake and the garden hose; to the placebo effect; to the unusual, such as spontaneous remission and yogic feats of physiological control. The more usual phenomena remind us of the everyday nature of the mind-body link, and the more unusual show us the possibilities. If you were skeptical when you read the case of Mr. Wright, you now have more supporting data with which to evaluate his case and to understand this fundamental dynamic of health and wellness.

The challenge is to consciously and willfully mobilize the mind side of the mind-body team, bringing both mind and body under personal control. This was the challenge that faced Mr. Wright, and this is the essential dynamic of health and wellness for everyone.

SECTION TWO: THE DEMISE AND REBIRTH OF THE MIND

If the influence of mental processes on physiological functioning is so obvious and powerful, why is there no well established science of mind ⟶ body today? The development of disciplines such as health psychology and of therapeutic techniques such as biofeedback training and imagery, which employ mind ⟶ body, are recent additions in psychology and medical treatment. In fact, the recognition of mind ⟶ body as a fundamental dynamic in health and wellness can be called a renaissance, a rebirth of interest in the mind and its influence on health.

The answer to our question is complex. In this section we present several issues and problems inherent in the study of mind and mental processes. We take a brief excursion through the history of science and psychology, arriving at what seems today an unlikely place: the rejection of mental phenomena as legitimate topics of scientific study and the relegation of mind to the status of a philosophical concept. We end on a more positive note, highlighting changes in psychology—such as the advent of cognitive psychology—that give mental processes a primary role in behavior, changes that pave the way for a broader acceptance of the biopsychosocial approach to health and wellness and of mind ⟶ body.

If you are not familiar with the demise of the mind in the disciplines in which the mind would seem to be most pertinent—the medical sciences, medical practice, and psychology—you may think, "Why should I study this? Everyone knows that the mind affects the body." The answer is that history brings meaning to the present and gains meaning in the present; most importantly, the issues and problems inherent in the study of the mind are relevant today.

The disregard for the mind as a dynamic in health came about partly from neglect; partly because other ingredients in health and disease are easier to study and seem more impressive, such as viruses and other physical causes of disease; partly because medicine developed the biomedical model of disease; and partly because the study of the mind, and even talk about subjective mental phenomena, came to be censored as unscientific in professional circles.

Science and the Mind

The scientific revolution and science as we think of it today have had a profound effect on the way that knowledge is acquired and legitimized in society. Western society is science-oriented, meaning that only data, theories, concepts, and beliefs that can be claimed to be scientific are accepted. You can discredit ideas or arguments by calling them unscientific. To understand how this came about and how this orientation is related to our topic, we begin with the fascinating tale of the birth of modern science, presented in a nutshell.

From our time-condensing 20th-century viewpoint, the gestation and birth of science from the womb of philosophy happened in an instant. We have chosen two illustrious examples of this process. These examples illustrate the power of the experimental approach to knowledge, and they forecast the eventual role of science in the demise of the mind. Both

examples begin in 1543, an easy date to remember—the publication date of both the theory of Copernicus and the first "modern" textbook of human anatomy. In the history of science these are landmarks, not so much for the information that they imparted but for the process of science that they initiated.

The "Copernican revolution," which overcame religious dogma and common sense by putting the sun at the center of the solar system and giving the earth motion, must have the record for being the slowest revolution in history with the greatest impact. The work of the Polish mathematician, physician, and monk Nicolaus Copernicus was published a few months before his death. The heliocentric hypothesis had little impact, however, until a Dutchman, Johannes Kepler, understood its significance and incorporated the idea into his first manuscript, *Mysterium Cosmographicum*, in 1596. Using geometry, mathematics, and celestial observations, Kepler improved on the Copernican system by calculating that the orbits of the planets are elipses, not the perfect circles that Copernicus thought God had intended.

While Kepler was working out his laws of planetary motion, the Italian mathematician and instrument maker Galileo Galilei was teaching the geocentric system and making telescopes for military and commercial use. Kepler could not convince Galileo to adopt the Copernican system, but the evidence that Galileo saw through his telescope in 1610 did—the moons of Jupiter, the phases of Venus, the clouds of stars that form the Milky Way, the rough surface of the moon. Galileo became a scientific hero. The Church of Rome, however, saw heresy and forbade Galileo from teaching the heliocentric system. In 1633 the church banned Galileo's books and forced him to recant. As we know, the church was not converted in Galileo's lifetime.

But science cannot be silenced. By 1705 the English mathematician Issac Newton was honored with knighthood for his scientific achievements, the greatest being his mathematical deduction of universal gravity, which put the final touches on the heliocentric system.

The Copernican revolution was a revolution of knowledge; greater still, it was a revolution in the methods of gaining knowledge. It was a revolution of the power of observation, instrumentation, experimentation, and mathematics over the power of ignorance, "common sense," and dogma—a scientific revolution.

Now we turn from the orbits of heavenly bodies to the structure of the human body. In 1543 the Dutch physician and teacher, Andreas Vesalius, published his great textbook of anatomy, *De Humani Corporis Fabrica*. The *Fabrica* is based upon the dissection of the human body, unlike the hallowed writing of the third-century Roman physician Galen, which had been the anatomy gospel before the *Fabrica*. The boldness of Vesalius in dissection and experimentation is considered the origin of the science of anatomy.

The new experimental approach to anatomy and physiology paved the way for many advances, such as the work of the English physician William Harvey, who used experimentation as the basis of his monumental deduction that blood circulates in the body, propelled by the heart. Harvey published his findings in 1628. This discovery, important in its own right, was of fundamental significance because it replaced the theory of the humors and vital spirits, which was based on conjecture and not on experimentation. At the same time, as the science of anatomy progressed, it became clear that the body can be explained by its own mechanics. Concepts such as "vital spirits" were not needed to explain the functions of the body. Eventually, the mind was given the status of a concept and was not needed to explain physiological functioning or human behavior.

Like the Copernican revolution, the "Vesalius revolution" was a revolution of knowledge and science. Other sciences—physics, physiology, anatomy, and botany—evolved simultaneously, all based on the principles of scientific investigation.

Eventually, science itself became a dogma. Truth would be revealed through science, and science would be truthful. No assumptions about the world would be made. Value judgments were forbidden. Phenomena that could not be subjected to the scrutiny of scientific experimentation could not be studied. Science demonstrated that natural processes are governed by "laws," and science would be the discoverer of these laws.

In the scientific arena, anatomy and physiology fare well because the body can be measured, observed, and experimented upon, and the physiological and mechanical puzzles of the body can be solved. But how does the mind fare in the face of science? The mind fares not well. The motto of the venerable scientific organization, the Royal Society of London, founded in 1662, forecasts the problem: "Take nobody's word for it; see for yourself." Of the mind and the body, which is the easier to see, to measure, to submit to experimentation, and to describe by laws?

Naturally, the study of the mind and mental processes poses a serious problem for the science-minded. The nonphysical nature of the mind, whether defined as subjective experience or as a hypothetical force that influences the brain, excludes mental phenomena from investigation using the methods that have worked so brilliantly in understanding the physical world. The mind was relegated to the mystical, the philosophical, and the unscientific, and thus it could not be the subject of any self-respecting science or scientist.

Behaviorism

Behaviorism played a significant role in the demise in the study of the mind and mental phenomena in psychology, permeating as it did nearly the entire discipline and affecting particularly experimental psychology. We refer to experimental psychology because it was primarily that branch that eliminated mental phenomena as a topic of study. Because we are interested in

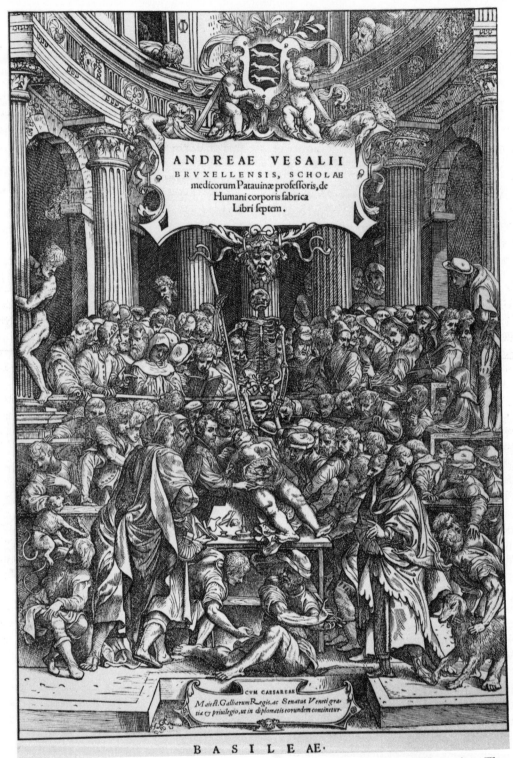

ANDREAE VESALII
BRVXELLENSIS, SCHOLAE
medicorum Patauinæ professoris, de
Humani corporis fabrica
Libri septem.

CVM CAESAREAE
Maiest. Galliarum Regis, ac Senatus Veneti gra-
tia & priuilegio, ut in diplomatis eorundem continetur.

BASILEAE.

Title Page of *De Humani Corporis Fabrica*, Published in 1543, Showing a Dissection. The Engraving Illustrates the Importance Given to the Dissection, to Understanding the Human Body, and to Science.
Source: Yale Historical Medical Library, New Haven, CT.

the mind and its relationship to the body, we do not consider in this book developments in Gestalt, counseling, educational, personality, or developmental psychologies. These are all rich areas in psychology, but they are not directly concerned with mind ⟶ body. We focus on behaviorism because it dominated psychology for several decades, and even today psychology carries the heritage of behaviorism. Psychology came to be defined as the science of behavior. This would have been no problem, except that "behavior" did not include mental behavior such as cognitions or attention or any subjective experience such as hope or fear. Behavior could be studied, but subjective experience itself could not be studied. In his famous paper of 1913, "Psychology as the Behaviorist Views It," John B. Watson eliminated consciousness and all mental concepts from psychology, proclaiming that the study of overt behavior would constitute the true scientific psychology. The pressure to make psychology a science like physics was Watson's primary motive for rejecting the introspectionist methods of Wilhelm Wundt and promoting behaviorism.

The study of overt behavior is appealing because it is a public, measurable event, and laws based on experimentation can be created to describe it. Of all human attributes, however, overt behavior is the aspect of human functioning furthest removed from the mind—it is the end product. So behaviorism took psychology away from the study of the mind and mental phenomena, and led it into areas in which overt behavior was the primary focus of research.

The attention of psychology turned away from the inner world of the person to the outer world of stimuli and reinforcers that were thought to control behavior, and stimulus ⟶ response became the general law of all behavior. A kind of behavioristic reductionism developed in which human behavior was described as response to stimuli, behavior that was strengthened by reinforcers or punishment, and that would stop if reinforcers were absent.

Thus, early behaviorism attempted to bring science to psychology by eliminating the mind. It studied behavior as a response to stimuli and not as the result of a person's internal mental processes. At its worst, behaviorism described human beings as conditioned animals, and quintessential human experiences such as volition or attention became mere hypothetical constructs and were of little interest. As we will see, behaviorism has significantly changed.

The Neurosciences

In the seventeenth century, a French philosopher, René Descartes, thought that he had explained mind-body interaction by arguing that the mind exists as a nonphysical entity, independent of the body, and influences the body through the pineal gland of the brain. The idea that both mind and body exist and are independent is called **dualism**.

It is commonly said that dualism separated mind and body, and that is why we do not have a science of mind ⟶ body today. The issue is much more complicated—arising from the dictates of science, as we noted, and from the compelling data of the neurosciences that can be interpreted as evidence for disputing Descartes' idea of mind as a nonphysical entity. The data suggest that what we call "mind" and "mental phenomena" are actually neuronal and chemical activity in the brain. This theory is called **reductionism** because it reduces the mind to brain activity.

Evidence for reduction of the mind to neuronal activity in the brain is based on instances in which a condition in the brain has clear impact on behavior and mental functioning. When certain parts of the brain are damaged by stroke, injury, surgery, disease, or experimentation, particular mental functions are lost or impaired. Speech, memory, organized thought, emotional control, and purposive behavior can be altered by altering the brain. When drugs are used, mental changes such as euphoria or calm, decreased depression, hallucinations, or arousal occur. In short, behavior, including mental behavior, can be manipulated by manipulating the brain. These data led to the conclusion that the mind is a product of brain activity.

The more precise the analysis of brain structures and neurotransmitters and other chemicals, the more links are found between brain states and mind states. So convincing is the evidence that the brain accounts for the mind that in 1950 the noted Canadian neurologist and neurosurgeon Wilder Penfield stated:

> Everyone knows that the mind of a man is something that depends upon the action of the brain. Everyone knows, too, that a blow on the head may put an end of feeling, action, thought. The man, upon whose unlucky shoulders that head was resting, becomes unconscious. The action of the brain is arrested by the blow, and so the mind does not exist for the time being.
>
> Penfield, 1950

This is the traditional view of the neurosciences, a view that has influenced medicine, psychology, and psychophysiology:

> Mind does not appear to be something separate and apart from the neurons and chemicals that make up our brains. When a person's brain is damaged, his or her mind will be altered, even if ever so slightly. . . . It is humbling to think of the billions of neurons and chemicals in our brains—and then to realize that *they* are doing the thinking.
>
> Wallace, Goldstein, & Nathan, 1985; pp. 66–67

It is expected that when brain mechanisms are understood, right down to the molecular level—when all the neuronal and hormonal interactions in the brain are known—then human behavior will be understood and controllable. While this is a fascinating task, understanding the structure and function of a thing does not necessarily give insight into its owner, just as studying a television does not necessarily give insight into the television station. Today, Descartes might argue that the

twentieth-century study of brain and mental phenomena has no bearing on his notion of an independent mind that interacts with brain, because the mind and the mental phenomena that the brain produces are different from the brain, just as the television station and the picture that the television produces are different. Following this metaphor, Descartes might point out that we do not suppose that the television station is in the television, and if the television is damaged and will not produce a picture, we neither suppose that the television station does not exist nor use this as evidence for the "reduction" of the station to the television. Descartes might argue that just as the signals from the station are converted by the television into a picture and sound, so the mind influences the brain to produce mental phenomena and physiological change. The television station is not the television, however, and the mind is not the brain, although the brain is necessary for mental processes such as sensation, imagining, and thinking.

The reductionist theory that describes all human behavior as the product of neuronal activity raises two issues that are important to all fields of study—**generalization** and **causality versus correlation**.

Generalization is the process of using data about particular events to describe all such events. In logic this process is called inductive reasoning. In the case of reductionism, instances in which the brain clearly causes mental and behavioral change are the basis for generalization about all behavior, including mental behavior and the subjective experience that is called the mind.

The second issue that is of concern to all sciences is correlation versus causality. A fundamental task of science is to distinguish between events or conditions that are correlated—meaning that they occur together—and events that are causally related—meaning that one causes the other. A correlation between events does not mean that the events are causally related. For example, a nobleman died when Halley's comet was overhead. People thought that the comet caused his death. The two events were correlated because they occurred together, but they were not causally related. The comet did not cause the death. The assumption of causality, when only correlation exists, can be the basis of superstition. One reason for confusion between correlation and causality is that events that are causally related are *always* correlated; events that are correlated are not always causally related. Science makes a great effort to separate the two.

In investigating mind-body interaction, the issue is not simple. Do brain events cause mental events, or do mental events cause brain events? Or is it sometimes one and sometimes the other? Are they sometimes correlated and sometimes causally related? For example, data show that a low serotonin level (serotonin is a neurotransmitter) in the brain and major depression may co-exist. But does the low serotonin level cause depression, or does the depression cause the low serotonin level? Or is it different in each individual case? Or are depression and low serotonin level merely correlated, with a third factor—such as psychological or physical abuse in childhood—causing both depression and a low serotonin level?

In a little-known but fascinating study conducted by Dr. Robert Post at the National Institutes of Mental Health, actors simulated the manic behavior of patients with manic-depressive disorder. Post found that after acting out the manic behavior, the actors had increases in certain substances, measured in urine and cerebral spinal fluid. The urine and cerebral spinal fluid samples matched those of patients with known psychiatric illness. These findings led Post to conclude:

> It appears that the behavioral-biological equation often functions in a behavior-determines-biological-change direction rather than the converse, as implied in many of the biological hypotheses of psychiatric illness. Models

emphasizing the rich interaction and bidirectional flow of biological and behavioral influences may be more accurate.

Frontier of Psychiatry, 1973

Please read Box 2.6 now.

The reductionist view of the mind is compelling because the evidence for the mind as a product of brain activity is compelling. We have a basic problem that also lends support to this view—it is difficult to imagine how something that is nonphysical and "no-thing" can interact with the brain, which is matter. It is easier to believe that brain interacts with brain, although we may call it the mind, than to believe that a nonphysical essence called mind exists independently and can influence the brain.

Combined with the scientific orientation, reductionism has led to a narrow focus on brain structure and function. Medicine took a similar path. The scientific revolution swept medicine into the modern era with the biomedical model of disease. Chapter 1 noted that the biomedical model excludes a consideration of psychological and social variables in disease and treatment. Thus, the medical sciences were not concerned with the role of mind and mental processes in disease and illness or in recovery.

Impressed by the neurosciences and by the links between brain chemistry and behavior, many psychologists and psychophysiologists accepted reductionism. Psychology was defined as the science of behavior, and general psychology texts usually began with a chapter on the brain, implying that the brain is the source of behavior and should be studied first.

The Rebirth of the Mind

We have described powerful forces in Western society that combined to exclude the mind and mental processes from scientific study. It is no mystery that the science of mind ⟶ body is only in its infancy. But it is born, or reborn, as

BOX 2.6

CAUSALITY AND THE BIOPSYCHOSOCIAL APPROACH

Do brain events cause mental events, or do mental events cause brain events, or is it sometimes one and sometimes the other, or both simultaneously?

The determination of causality is important because the solution to a problem is usually based on what the cause of the problem is thought to be. For this reason, the evidence for a causal relationship must be examined carefully. For example, we worked with a ten-year-old hyperactive boy who had been taking Ritalin since kindergarten. His kindergarten teacher was certain that the child's hyperactivity was a "brain problem." Her evidence was that as soon as he began taking Ritalin, he calmed down. Does the fact that drugs affect behavior by changing brain chemistry prove that the behavior being changed was caused by brain chemistry? In this case, there was evidence that the hyperactivity was caused by his poor family environment.

The cause of behavior, and of illness and disease, is obviously complex. The biopsychosocial approach suggests that biological, psychological, and social factors may all be involved in the development of disorders. When this is the case, the disorder has many causes. For example, evidence indicates that a tendency for major depressive disorder may be inherited, and yet this tendency may be manifested only in the presence of certain psychological or social conditions, such as abuse in childhood or chronic stress (Gold, Goodwin, & Chrousos, 1988). In this case, what is the cause of the depression? Neither the biological factors nor the psychosocial factors are the sole cause of the depressive disorder; the interaction of these factors caused the manifestation of the disorder.

The multicausal nature of many disorders leads to another question: What type of treatment is best? In the case of depressive disorder, should the patient be treated with drugs that change the biochemical imbalance in the brain, should family therapy be the primary treatment, should the treatment focus on coping skills, or would the best treatment be a combination of approaches? In future chapters, we discuss disorders that have many causes and that are appropriately treated with a variety of methods.

---

stated at the beginning of this chapter, and it is reborn with science.

The optimistic continuation of the case of Mr. Wright was not fantasy. The experts on the team represent important areas of mind ⟶ body exploration, such as psychoneuroimmunology, the use of imagery in healing, and biofeedback training. Cognitive psychology moved beyond the narrow confines of stimulus-response behaviorism and behavior modification, bringing to psychology and psychotherapy knowledge of cognitions, beliefs, expectations, and all manner of mental processes as the basis of behavior. Cognitive psychology also opened the door to the relationship of cognitions and physiological functioning, and quite suddenly phenomena such as the placebo effect became of interest.

One of the most important contributions to the study of mind ⟶ body, and to the

BOX 2.7

COMMENT

Francis Bacon noted that a little philosophy could lead a man to atheism, while study in depth could lead to understanding. Perhaps this was the case for Penfield. At the end of his career Penfield wrote:

"Throughout my own scientific career, I, like other scientists, have struggled to prove that the brain accounts for the mind. But now, perhaps, the time has come when we may profitably consider the evidence as it stands, and ask the question: *Do brain-mechanisms account for the mind?* Can the mind be explained by what is now known about the brain? If not, which is the more reasonable of the two possible hypotheses: that man's being is based on one element, or on two? . . . If one chooses the second, the dualistic alternative, the mind must be viewed as a basic *element* in itself. One might, then, call it a *medium,* an *essence,* a *soma.* That is to say, it has a *continuing existence.* On this basis, one must assume that although the mind is silent when it no longer has its special connection to the brain, it exists in the silent intervals and takes over control when the highest brain-mechanism does go into action" (Penfield, 1975).

development of the biopsychosocial approach, is the increasing awareness of stress and the effect of stress on the body. The effect was illustrated by the snake and garden hose story. This story is an excellent illustration of the power of cognitions and images on physiology, and we use it to illustrate mind ⟶ body. Stress and its effects have become headline topics in

psychology, medicine, sociology, industrial psychology, health psychology, behavioral medicine, pharmacology, and other fields that are concerned with health and wellness. Stress, as defined in the next chapter, is an emotional/mental response that has physiological effects. The advent of stress research, and the widespread recognition of the role of stress in disease and illness, have led to a recognition of the importance of mental processes and their effect on the body. This has opened a door for a study of mind ⟶ body.

We describe mind ⟶ body as a fundamental dynamic of health and wellness, and through the team of experts and in Section One of this chapter, examples of this dynamic are presented. We have come no closer, however, to understanding the fundamental nature of mind. The dualism of Descartes, in which mind and body are independent entities that interact, remains unproven; it is unacceptable in today's science because it suggests the disembodied-spirit concept of mind. Reductionism, also unproven, appears to many to be too narrowly focused on the brain. It runs against the common experience of a "self" that influences the brain, rather than of a brain that creates the self.

Today, philosophers who want to avoid both the disembodied-spirit concept and reductionism have created a third alternative, called the **identity model** of mind and body (Churchland, 1984). The identity model suggests that mind and body exist and are manifestations of a common substance, just as ice and water vapor are manifestations of one substance but are distinctly different. The advantage of the identity model is that it gives to mental processes a life of their own, even though it does not necessarily escape reductionism when the common substance is thought to be brain substance.

Cognitive psychologist Albert Bandura developed an identity model of mind and body that he calls "reciprocal determinism," meaning that the mind and the body act upon, or determine, each other (Bandura, 1986). Bandura argues that mental processes will never

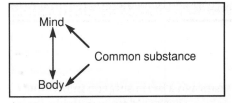

Figure 2.3   In the Identity Model, Mind and Body Interact and Are Separate Manifestations of a Common Substance.

be understood by studying neuronal processes and that understanding the mind and its manifestation, human behavior, will not be achieved by understanding the atomic and molecular structure and processes of brain and their manifestation, brain behavior. Mind and brain, Bandura suggests, are different processes with different laws, requiring different concepts and different sciences.

Summary

The scientific method that so brilliantly advanced knowledge in the physical sciences gradually eroded the study of mind, so that even experimental psychology abandoned it. Hand in hand with scientific experimentation as the royal road to knowledge came the mechanistic view of the body and the reduction of the mind to brain activity. Stimulus-response conditioning became the theme of psychology, and animal laboratories were prominent in every psychology department. Human beings, like their nonhuman laboratory prototypes, were studied as responding mechanisms, rather than as people with perceptions and cognitions and with the power to change behavior and physiological functioning.

The reductionist position prevented the development of mind-body theory and research. The ability of humans to voluntarily control psychological and physiological behavior for health was neglected. The belief that the mysteries of the mind are hidden in the brain created a research bias in the neurosciences and medicine. Research has focused almost exclusively on how the brain affects human functioning, rather than on how the human affects the functioning brain.

Today the mind is reborn as cognitions, perceptions, beliefs, and images. Mental processes are recognized both as the basis of behavior and as factors that affect physiology. Mind $\longrightarrow$ body is increasingly recognized as a fundamental dynamic in health and wellness. Please read Box 2.8 now.

SECTION THREE: HOMEOSTASIS

If at this moment you got up and jogged in place for a few minutes, your body would handle all the necessary physiological changes, such as increases in breathing and pulse rates and in blood sugar and adrenaline levels, and the vasodilation in the large muscles of the legs. When you sit down to read again, these processes would automatically return to "prejog" levels. Your only effort would be to keep moving—at no point would you need to consciously force your body to change physiological functioning to adapt to the exercise and the cessation of exercise. The body orchestrates these changes without the mind.

If you step on a garden hose and think that it is a snake, the same thing happens. You have an immediate stress response—heart rate and blood pressure increase, muscles tense, breathing becomes shallow, adrenaline is released, and the stomach stops digesting—but as soon as you discover the mistake and laugh about it, the body automatically reverses the stress response.

Eat a candy bar, fast for a day, sit in a hot sauna, walk in a chilly rain, eat salty anchovies, drink a quart of tea, expose yourself to a virus, get a sunburn—in other words, put a strain on your body—and your body will automatically attempt to adjust. It will try to keep your "internal environment" fairly constant. This remarkable ability probably has been noted by

---

BOX 2.8

MIND TEASERS

- Yoga says: All of the body is in the mind, but not all of the mind is in the body.

- After general anesthesia, some patients have reported "hearing" the surgeon's comments or bits of conversation. Usually these memories are unconscious, but they can be reached through hypnosis.

- A few people who have had the extraordinary experience of coming very close to death report "withdrawing" from the body. From a distance they watch as the medical team tends the body. It seems to these people that life is in the balance, that they have a choice—they can return to the body and live, or let go of the body and die; they choose to return and live. In my clinical practice, I (JG) have had one patient who had this experience several hours after surgery. In her case, she experienced a surprising dispassion as she watched the activities around her body. She became aware of the choice, and she also became aware of two beings near her conscious self. It seemed that these beings were there to help, should she choose not to return to her body.

- Many years ago a brain surgeon in London devised a shunt that could be inserted in the brain of children born with hydrocephalus. Hydrocephalus is the swelling of the brain because of the blockage of cerebral spinal fluid inside the brain. As the fluid accumulates, the pressure on the brain damages brain tissue and prevents normal development. The shunt allows the fluid to flow normally. In the 1940s, many hydrocephalic children were operated upon successfully. Several of these children became professionals in adulthood. The surgeon who invented the shunt decided to study these people, using the CAT scan that allows computer imaging of brain structures. To his amazement, several of these people had extremely malformed brains, with little cerebral cortex. From the scans he would have guessed that they were severely handicapped and retarded. Is this evidence for the extraordinary power of the brain tissue, or is this evidence for the extraordinary power of the mind and its independence from brain tissue? (*Science Digest,* May, 1981, p. 110.)

---

anyone who pays attention to body processes. Anyone who has observed the tendency to urinate abundantly after drinking abundantly, or who has noticed the reduction in urine and increase of thirst with lack of water, or sweating and a red face with strenuous exercise, undoubtedly realizes that the body has ways of reversing conditions that would normally cause damage. If urination did not increase after one drank more than necessary, body fluid would increase, blood volume would increase, and blood pressure would rise dangerously.

The body's ability to maintain internal constancy was first described in modern times by the French physiologist Claude Bernard in the late nineteenth century. In this century, Walter Cannon, the American physiologist who named the physiological response to stress the fight-or-flight response, investigated this process extensively and called it **homeostasis**. Cannon and other physiologists made great strides in understanding the physiological mechanisms of homeostasis, an exciting field of exploration that continues today.

In Chapter 4, The Stress Response, we describe in detail the effects of stress on physiology, effects that over time can throw the body off balance and produce symptoms and disease. Here we describe the innate ability to maintain physiological homeostasis: the natural tendency of the body to be healthy. Finally, the concept of psychological homeostasis is discussed.

By the end of this section, you will have an increased appreciation of the body's ability to maintain health and of your special responsibility in helping mind and body maintain healthy homeostasis.

Maintaining Homeostasis

Homeostasis means "same state" and describes the body's ability to maintain a steady state. Healthy homeostasis refers to maintaining a healthy state in all body processes—blood pressure, heart rate, blood sugar, hormone levels, stomach secretions, muscle tension, neurotransmitters, components of the immune system, blood components, mineral, vitamin and ion levels, oxygen, and carbon dioxide—in other words, keeping all body processes within a normal healthy range and meeting the needs of the body at every moment. Please read Box 2.9 now.

The regulation of blood sugar is an excellent example of a homeostatic mechanism. Blood sugar is regulated by the pancreas through the release of insulin and glucagon. When blood sugar is higher than normal, the pancreas releases insulin, which stimulates cells to take up sugar from the blood, thus reducing blood sugar. When blood sugar is normal, insulin release is "turned off." When blood sugar is below normal, the pancreas releases glucagon, which stimulates the liver to release glucose into

---

BOX 2.9

HEALTHY HOMEOSTASIS

We preface "homeostasis" with "healthy" to be completely accurate. As a response to stress or unhealthy conditions within it, the body may achieve homeostasis in one process while creating an imbalance in another. For example, if the kidneys do not have enough pressure or blood flow, they release renin, which is converted into angiotensin II, which raises blood pressure by causing vasoconstriction in the periphery. The increase in blood pressure allows the kidneys to function normally, but the result is high blood pressure. The kidneys have achieved homeostasis, but blood pressure is off balance. We refer to this process as unhealthy homeostasis. The body is attempting to maintain homeostasis, but it becomes sick by doing so.

---

the blood, and blood sugar increases. When blood sugar is again normal, glucagon release is turned off.

Any process that turns "on" and "off," such as insulin and glucagon release, has a mechanism that gives the instruction to turn on or off, just as a furnace has a thermostat. The thermostat continually monitors and regulates room temperature. Cells in the pancreas that continually monitor blood sugar give the instruction to release or turn off insulin or glucagon. Information about a process that is used to make a change in the process is called **feedback**. In a loose sense of the word, we can say that the pancreas uses information feedback about blood sugar to regulate blood sugar. Balancing on a tightrope involves feedback from many sources—the balance mechanisms in the ears give information about the body's position in space, muscles give constant feedback, and watching the rope gives visual feedback. With all this feedback, it is possible to learn to walk on a tightrope.

When the body is unable to maintain homeostasis, illness or death may result. Homeostasis is vital to life and is the foundation of health. This is why we refer to homeostasis as a dynamic of health and wellness. We call homeostasis a dynamic because it is a force for health. Homeostasis also underlies the therapeutic techniques that are described in this book. Relaxation techniques, biofeedback training, imagery, and hypnosis would not be effective in the treatment of illness and disease if the body were unable to correct itself. These techniques help the body correct itself through its own homeostatic mechanisms; we describe this process further in Part Three.

Homeostatic mechanisms can function into old age—decade after decade the body will maintain healthy homeostasis. Walter Cannon expressed this in the title of his book *The Wisdom of the Body*. The body knows how to stay healthy; the body is equipped with hundreds of homeostatic mechanisms. And it is natural for the body to return to health if disease does occur. Of this Cannon wrote:

> In the facts which we have surveyed we have become acquainted with good reasons for extending hope and cheer to the sick, reasons based on the ample evidence that in the body there are admirable devices for maintaining its stability against disturbing internal and external conditions, marvelous provisions for protecting its integrity against foes, both wild beasts and microscopic germs, and very liberal margins of structural strength and functional capacity beyond the ordinary requirements. When we are afflicted and our bodily resources seem low, we should think of these powers of protection and healing which are ready to work for the bodily welfare.
>
> Cannon, 1932, pp. 228-229

It is natural for the body to stay healthy—with one giant "if": *if* the right conditions are met, mainly adequate nurturing of our emotional and mental life, adequate nutrition, exercise, and sanitation, and adequate genetics.

Unfortunately, humans have an amazing ability to override homeostatic mechanisms and throw the body off balance. The most popular methods are smoking; lack of exercise; overeating; poor diet; use of medications with side effects; use of recreational drugs, including alcohol; environmental pollution; violence; and chronic stress. Our society provides an impressive array of habits that work against homeostasis and health and wellness. Please read Box 2.10 now.

Homeostatic Failure

Once homeostasis was understood, it was reasonable to postulate that disease results from "homeostatic failure," that is, failure to maintain homeostasis or failure to return to homeostasis. Pathogens, genetics, and injury can disrupt homeostasis and cause disease. The study of homeostatic failure and disease resulting from these agents is in the domain of medicine. The study of homeostatic failure and disease resulting from poor lifestyle, from psychological variables, and from stress is in the domain of health psychology, behavioral health, behavioral medicine, and related fields. The influence of poor lifestyle on health and the ways to overcome poor habits are discussed in several chapters.

Stress and the stress response are described in Chapters 3 and 4. Chapter 4 describes the autonomic nervous system that controls the automatic functions of the body through its complementary branches, as well as the sympathetic nervous system and the parasympathetic nervous system that work together to maintain homeostasis. Because the sympathetic and parasympathetic nervous systems are particularly sensitive to the mind and are responsive to

BOX 2.10

CONSCIOUS HOMEOSTASIS

Homeostasis is an unconscious process. We are not aware of the continual activity of feedback mechanisms and homeostatic processes continually operating in the body. However, we cannot claim ignorance and "trash" the body just because we are not conscious of homeostasis in action. Anyone who reads to the end of this text will know that we have the ability to help or hinder homeostasis, as no other people have before us. This knowledge makes us responsible, just as the ability to destroy life on earth with nuclear power makes us responsible for world peace in a way that was never true before.

To capture this concept, we coined the term "conscious homeostasis" to emphasize the fact that we must make conscious decisions about our health. We can help or hinder homeostasis, and we make a conscious choice whichever way we go.

simple techniques like relaxation and proper breathing, human beings have an extraordinary ability to help the body maintain or recover homeostasis.

Psychological Homeostasis

When the principles of physiological homeostasis were understood, psychoanalytic theorists and others applied the concept to human interaction with the environment, pointing out that humans try to maintain homeostasis with the external world, a process called adaptation. Karl Menninger, a world-renowned psychiatrist, objected to this concept in *The Vital Balance* (Menninger, 1963), saying that it implied maintaining a psychological *status quo*, without growth.

Yet the concept of psychological homeostasis is useful, partly because it implies an idea that we like—the natural psychological healthiness of humans—and partly because the concept implies that, like physiological homeostasis, psychological balance is necessary for life. We use the term **psychological homeostasis** to mean psychological balance—the mixture of emotions and cognitions that create a feeling of inner integrity and comfort with one's self and with the environment. Like physiological homeostasis, which enables continuous growth and change in the body, maintaining a flexible but "vital" balance psychologically enables growth and change. When humans are thrown too far off balance psychologically and lose senses of self-esteem and trust, psychological growth is impeded.

Do humans have innate mechanisms that protect psychological well-being and keep us in balance—a kind of psychological homeostasis? We do not know.

We do know that some children seem to be born with a *joi de vivre* and the ability to get their needs met, and and who bounce back from hurts. Other children are more timid and cautious, and seem to be psychologically fragile. Research on temperament indicates that children may be born with these tendencies (Campos, Barrett, Lamb, Goldsmith, & Sternberg, 1983; Hubert & Wachs, 1985). For example, longitudinal studies of children have identified three patterns: easy children who have low emotional intensity and who are positive in approaching new situations, difficult children who have intense emotions and react negatively to new situations, and slow-to-warm-up children who are shy and negative in moods (Thomas, 1980). These tendencies may explain why children are so different from one another, or they may indicate that early experiences, perhaps even prenatal experiences, influence the child's behavior and psychological functions by either overriding or enhancing psychological homeostasis. It is also possible that humans do not have psychological homeostatic mechanisms that keep us healthy in spite of the environment.

We do know that humans have psychological defense mechanisms that are psychological protection, such as anger, denial and withdrawal, grieving, laughter, and a "who-cares" attitude. These responses to stressors are often helpful and healthy, although they can become out of control and harmful.

We do know that psychological growth, like physical growth, progresses through developmental stages. The study of these stages is a speciality, called **developmental psychology**. Erik Erikson, a pioneer in the field and a leading developmental psychologist, suggests that these stages are like challenges or tasks that the child must overcome, or grow through, before moving on to the next developmental stage (Erikson, 1980). When the child has a supportive environment, progression through the stages is natural and easy. We also know that psychological, physical, and sexual abuse can hinder developmental progression, leaving the victim "stuck" at a particular state. Sometimes the lasting damage is hidden until years later, when the challenges of adulthood cannot be met.

We do know that humans seem to have a natural tendency to strive for completion, for a finishing of unfinished business, referred to as **closure**. Humans have a hard time with ambiguity and uncertainty, and they seek the security of the status quo. Humans strive for a kind of psychological tidiness and will create order out of chaos. Are these tendencies inborn mechanisms for maintaining psychological homeostasis?

We do know that there are many ways in which people can be thrown off balance psychologically. Because humans have the ability to disrupt physiological homeostatic mechanisms, we created the concept **conscious homeostasis** to describe the conscious effort needed to keep the body balanced; we cannot rely solely on the body's own mechanisms for recovery. We must be conscious of the body's needs, and we must consciously bring it back to balance. So too, conscious homeostasis applies to our psychological well-being.

Conscious psychological homeostasis involves being conscious of psychological needs, developing the skills for maintaining psychological balance, and using these skills. Conscious psychological homeostasis is as important as conscious physiological homeostasis. Chronic mental and emotional disturbance, like chronic anger or depression or frustration or fear, perpetuate themselves and affect both the external environment of family and society and the internal environment of psychophysiological functioning.

Psychological balance is as precious as physiological balance; in our opinion, psychological homeostasis needs greater attention than physiological homeostasis. The body is able to take years of abuse, but the psyche cannot. The body will recover from near death, and if cared for, will be good as new. Psychological damage is not so repairable.

Because chronic or severe stress threatens psychological homeostasis, stress management is an important dynamic of health and wellness. Perhaps the most important aspect of stress management is learning to take stressors in stride. This resilience is achieved in four ways: maintaining physiological balance through healthy lifestyle and stress management, including relaxation training; developing behavioral and cognitive skills that counteract and prevent such disruptive psychological lifestyle habits as chronic anger; developing the behavioral and cognitive skills for overcoming the effects of extreme stress, such as abuse in childhood; and developing the skills for preventing stress.

||||➡

CONCLUSION

In this chapter we examined two fundamental dynamics of health and wellness: mind-body connectedness, emphasizing particularly mind ⟶ body, and homeostasis. We illustrated mind ⟶ body through common examples such as the snake and garden hose story, and unusual examples, such as the research in India. We gave you a perspective from the past that will give you an appreciation of the renaissance occurring today, a renaissance of the mind, that like the Italian Renaissance will grow far beyond the present horizon.

In studying the dynamics of health and wellness, it is important to be open-minded about the mind and about the capacity of humans for self-directed change. It is important to consider the possibilities, because belief in "the possible" governs action. We act when we expect a positive outcome. When people do not believe that they have the power to change, they will not attempt to change. This refers to lifestyle change and to psychophysiological self regulation.

In our work as teacher, therapist, and consultant to professionals, we emphasize the importance of maintaining an optimism for human potential that encompasses even the seemingly miraculous cures of people such as Mr. Wright. We appreciate the idea that Norman Cousins states so simply. *No one knows enough to be pessimistic.* Cousins, author of *The Anatomy of an Illness as Perceived by the Patient* (1979) and *The Healing Heart* (1983), came to this position after overcoming a life-threatening disease, described in his first book. We like the idea that no one really knows the limits of the human mind and body for healing—we can afford to be optimistic. We share Cousins' statement with many of our clients to begin building the hope and positive expectations necessary for self regulation and healing. Sometimes a client has received the opposite message—it is better to expect the worst than to be too optimistic.

It is essential to have an optimistic view of mind ⟶ body as a health professional because the beliefs of the therapist/teacher influence the learner. In our work, we introduce the concept of mind ⟶ body immediately, using the story of the snake and garden hose because that story clearly shows the power of perceptions (the mind) to influence the body (the stress response). In therapy, we bolster the client's belief with other examples of mind ⟶ body from our own experience and from the experience of other therapists and clients, and we ask clients to read the stories of people who have healed themselves and who have made significant lifestyle changes.

Following these examples, we introduce the concept of homeostasis, the natural tendency of the body to be healthy. These dynamics, mind ⟶ body and homeostasis, make health and wellness possible.

Homeostasis refers to the ability of the body to maintain the same state. We extended this concept to psychological health.

We call homeostasis a dynamic of health because it is the basis of health, and because homeostatic mechanisms can be consciously used to prevent or remedy homeostatic failure. We developed the concept of conscious homeostasis to emphasize the need for conscious guardianship of homeostasis, both physiological and psychological. The need for self-responsibility and self regulation is a recurrent theme in the dynamics of health and wellness. Healthy homeostasis is our natural heritage that, like other natural resources, is taken for granted until it is lost. It makes no sense to wait until the body is off balance to take an interest in health.

What do you know so far? You know that Mr. Wrights exist. You understand the mind-body hyphen, and why mind ⟶ body is a fundamental dynamic of health and wellness. You understand homeostasis, a fundamental body dynamic. You have a strong foundation of data and ideas to support your personal path to health and your continued study of the dynamics of health and wellness.

PART TWO

The Dynamics of Stress

It is estimated that stress causes or contributes to the majority of the disorders and discomforts for which people seek medical attention. For this reason, and because stress is part of everyone's life, understanding and managing stress are important dynamics of health and wellness. In Part Two we focus on stress and its effects on physiological systems. We begin Chapter 3, Stress, with definitions, and then we examine in detail the nature and dimensions of stress and invite you to evaluate your stressors and assess your stress level. The relationship of stress and physical disorders is also discussed. In Chapter 4, The Stress Response, we describe the physiological systems of the body that are affected by stress and the physiological disorders that are most clearly stress-related. In Chapter 5, Evaluating Research and Physiological Data, we introduce you to several research issues and provide guidelines for evaluating research in the health sciences.

Part Two illustrates a familiar truism, "knowledge is power." In this case, power refers to the important dynamic of health, prevention. In the health fields, knowledge is power because it leads to prevention. The greater your knowledge of stress and how your body responds to stress, the greater your ability to cope with stress and counteract its effects. However, your personal health and wellness are not the only concern. Knowledge of stress and of the stress response are essential to all health professionals, working with people of all ages and in all aspects of health care, from education and primary prevention to treatment.

Stress and the stress response exemplify the importance of the biopsychosocial approach in understanding the dynamics of health and wellness and in understanding disease and illness. Stress has biological, psychological, and social roots, and it has biological, psychological, and social effects, and so its pervasiveness in daily life warrants the attention that it receives. Like the study of mind-body interaction, the study of stress and the stress response has expanded into many fields—medicine, psychology, sociology, epidemiology, immunology, and oncology.

Part One emphasized that two dynamics, mind ⟶ body and homeostasis, are fundamental to health and wellness. These dynamics are also a key to understanding stress and the stress response. Understanding stress and the stress response are key to understanding much of the content of this text, including methods for becoming stress-resistant described in Part Three and the treatment protocols described in Part Five.

Although stress and the stress response may threaten health and wellness, the concern of Part Two, you will discover that by under-standing and implementing the dynamics of health and wellness, humans need not be victims of stress. We repeat, however, that to maximize health, you must understand stress and its physiological counterpart, the stress response.

Understanding the complex interplay of biological, psychological, and social factors in health and sickness is not an easy task. Research in the health sciences is correspondingly complex, and yet research is the foundation of progress and affects everyone's life. For these reasons, Part Two concludes with a brief but important chapter on research issues, research evaluation, and understanding physiological measures. The intention is to acquaint you with key concepts and issues, so that you will have a basis for evaluating research. You will not finish Chapter 5, Evaluating Research and Physiological Data, as a researcher or statistician, but we hope that you will find the issues interesting. We know that you will have a greater appreciation of the importance and challenge of research in the health sciences.

CHAPTER *3*

Stress

||||➡

You cannot go to a bookstore without seeing a shelf of books on stress—everything from how to make stress a part of your life to how to eliminate it. And for good reason. Stress is recognized as a factor in illness and disease and as a factor in social disruption, unproductivity at work, absenteeism, failed goals, child abuse, substance abuse, suicide, and aging. Stress can probably be implicated in every other type of human problem.

It is estimated that 50 percent to 70 percent of all physician visits are for stress-related complaints and stress-related illness (Pelletier, 1977). The growing appreciation of the role of stress in illness and disease is a primary factor in bringing psychological phenomena into the realm of medical science and medical practice, and brings to academic and clinical psychology an interest in medical science and treatment of physical disorders. This reciprocal interest arises from the fact that stress is a psychological experience that has physiological consequences, and it is reflected in the creation of disciplines such as health psychology, medical psychology, medical sociology, and behavioral medicine. In the study of stress and in the treatment of stress-related illness, psychology and medicine find a common interest. Today the need to study and reduce stress is universally accepted.

The pervasiveness of stress gives it top priority in the study of the dynamics of health and wellness and automatically gives to stress management the status of a dynamic in health and wellness. The topic of this chapter is stress, but the elements of stress management will be apparent.

Following the introduction, this chapter has five sections, beginning with the definition of stress and related terms, and a closer look at the nature of stress in Section Two. Section Three provides an opportunity to assess your stress load by analyzing personal stressors, using stress inventories, and by determining your stress signs. This section also discusses a common stressor—work. Section Four examines behavioral and cognitive effects of stress, highlighting the effect of stress on performance. In Section Five the early research on stress and physical disease is described. We critique a popular method for assessing health risk, and you have another opportunity to assess your stress level by determining the number and intensity of life events experienced in the past year. This section also introduces the stress response and how it is activated. A conclusion winds up the chapter.

This chapter exemplifies our orientation described in the Preface—learning is doing. Your knowledge of stress comes from studying theories and research on stress and from understanding personal stress. Stress is one topic in which your personal experiences provide a strong foundation for knowledge; you are a legitimate source of information. Do not be deceived by the personal focus of this chapter; every section is important for understanding the dynamics of health and wellness and prepares you for a career in a health profession, if that is your interest.

||||➡

SECTION ONE: STRESS

Thanksgiving holiday.

Reading in bed in the morning makes my day—no rush to create the relish plate for the

Thanksgiving feast that Fran and I are preparing this afternoon at her apartment. Twelve guests—a lot of relish.

At eleven I am up. The first thing is to try to start the car. When it gets cold at night, it won't start. I put on my windbreaker and go out to my old Ford station wagon behind the house, which is now several tiny apartments. I sure hope it will start. I pump the gas pedal and turn the key. The most bloodcurdling sound—not the engine, not like anything I have ever heard. Reflexively, I turn the key off. Now what?

I raise the hood and look around. Nothing. I get down on the pavement to look at the engine from underneath. Hanging down under the radiator are the hind legs and tail of a cat. Oh Lord, I killed a cat. It must have crawled between the radiator and the fan to keep warm. I feel sick. I don't know what to do. I just stare at the half of a long-haired black and white cat hanging down. But I can't leave it there; I reach up and gently pull the legs; it won't budge. I feel sicker. I can't force myself to pull harder. I don't want to see the mangled head. Okay, I'll call the police.

I tell my story and explain that I need someone to come over and get the cat out of the fan. The Cambridge policeman who answers is unmoved.

"We don't have enough people for that. We can't do that."

I explain why someone has to come over and get the cat.

"Okay, okay, okay. But I don't know how soon."

I wait. The image of the lifeless legs and tail hounds my mind. I wait. Maybe I should go out and look again. I wait. Finally I can't stand it—I go out and very slowly creep under the car. It's gone; the cat is gone. Oh, no, it has gone off to die. I have to find it.

The cat has gone only a few feet into the bushes. Its ears are sliced and its face is cut and bloody. My horror turns to pity. I get down on my hands and knees and talk to it. "Oh, you poor cat. I'm so sorry. Don't worry, I'll take care of you. You will be all right, you poor cat." The cat backs a little farther into the bushes.

"Don't move now, just stay right there." I try to keep my voice low and calm. "I'm going to my car to get a box. Just stay here. I'll be right back."

I get a cardboard box out of the car. Will the cat let me pick it up? If I pick it up, will it die? If I don't try to rescue it, it will die anyway. I talk to the cat again. "That's okay, that's okay. I am going to pick you up, very gently . . . see, just like this . . . I am just picking you up, very gently." Smooth voice, shaking hands.

The cat doesn't resist. It is limp and looks as if it is in shock. Its eyes are open, but is it breathing? Yes, it's breathing. I put the box in the car and quietly close the door. Then I run back to my apartment and call Fran.

Fran has been in Boston longer than I, and she knows where the animal hospital is. It's one of the largest in the world. Surely it would be open on a holiday. I call the hospital—it's open. Get the Boston map, tie a scarf over my uncombed hair, grab my purse.

I search for the hospital on the map while I drive—the hospital is actually on the map, in another part of the city. I think I can find it. I talk to the cat while I drive. "Don't worry, cat, you will be all right. We will get you to the hospital and you will get fixed up. Don't worry, your face will be just great; it's amazing what they can do. You'll be a hero cat." I keep looking into the box to see if the cat is dead.

I am in the area, but I can't find the hospital. Why don't they put one-way streets on the map? What a stupid map. What a stupid city. I hate this city. I pull over and study the map. Okay, I see what happened. It's just a couple of blocks.

The animal hospital is immense. I park in front. The street is deserted and the building looks closed. I carry the box through the huge front doors. Several people are standing in a line at a window that looks like a bank teller's stall in an old western. A sign blocking the hallway says, DO NOT GO BEYOND THIS POINT. PAY AT THE CASHIER.

Oh, no. I can't wait. The cat will die. I can't pay. This is horrible.

I wait a minute at the end of the line. This is terrible; I can't wait. Frustration is building. I wait another minute. The cat has its head up. It probably smells the cats and dogs here. That is good. What should I do? The man at the head of the line walks his dog past the sign and down the hall on the right. I don't have any money, I don't have my checkbook. I don't have time to wait. The cat needs help. Total frustration. I am not going to wait.

I follow the man with the dog down the hall. Everything is gray. I pass several examining rooms; people are working with animals on stainless steel examining tables. I have no idea what I will do next. The man and the dog turn left down another hall. I stop. The cat is limp again, and so bloody. Okay, Green, guts up. I know this feeling. I have had this feeling a few times before. Determination and courage are welling up. I walk directly into the nearest examining room and approach the startled vet.

"This cat is dying. Can you look at it now?"

"You can't be in here. Who told you to come in here?"

"I'm sorry, but I couldn't wait. This cat is dying. The other animals out there aren't dying. The cat has a head injury. It's not my cat. I don't know whose it is." I tell him the story. "You must take care of the cat now." I am being brave and forceful, and at that instant my eyes fill with tears.

The vet studies the cat, and then he takes the box. "Okay, we will take care of the cat." He looks very displeased. "But you must pay when you leave. You will have to get the cat within four days. We won't keep it after four days."

"That's great. Oh, great. Thank you. The cat really needs help. I really appreciate your help." I take another look at the cat. "Goodbye, cat. Don't worry, you will be fine. I will find your owners. Don't worry."

"They will charge you eighty dollars."

I am not going to wait. I am not going to pay. I won't take another hassle.

Hiding the guilt inside with my confident look, I make a beeline for the front door.

What a relief. I escaped, and the cat will live. I just have to find its owners. Before I go to Fran's, I'd better put up signs around the neighborhood.

I am beginning to feel really pressured; it is getting late. I fold up the map and start the car. It won't start. Dead. Try again. Nothing. I open the hood and jiggle all the wires. Try again—nothing.

Miles from my apartment, a holiday, no money. Tears again. Okay, I'll call the guy I just broke up with. He lives near here, and he knows cars, and he has battery cables. What a jerk I am for not buying cables. Humiliation plus. I won't call. I don't want him in the rescuer role. I will call—it's getting late, and he owes me.

I cannot remember the number. My mind is blank. Damn damn double damn, triple damn hell. The operator says that the number is unlisted. That's right. That idiot. Why does he have his phone unlisted, anyway? "Okay, may I talk to your supervisor, this is an emergency." I tell the supervisor that I am having a crisis. The supervisor says that she will call the party and if the party agrees, then she will give me the number.

I call. He is just sitting down to dinner. His mother is up from New York. "Don't worry about it. I'll figure out something else." It was really bad of me to call; I shouldn't have done it.

"No no, that's okay. I'll be there in about half an hour."

I call Fran. I can't possibly make it to her place to help. I haven't made the relish plate, I am a wreck, and I have to find the owners of the cat—I have only four days. Fran understands, but she sounds irritated.

My friend arrives. There is a touch of agony in this, working on the car together. We jump the battery and it starts instantly. I thank him and offer to pay. What a cold creep I am.

I rush back. I hit every red light. Storrow Drive is crammed with dumb holiday drivers. As I drive I compose the sign—FOUND, fluffy black and white cat; cute cat FOUND; where is your cat tonight? FOUND. . . . I need something catchy.

I put up lots of signs. It is getting dark. I am exhausted and starving, and I feel sick. This is what shellshock must be like. I call Fran and tell her that I cannot be there. Fran is great. Everything is under control. She says that folks are drinking wine and talking, and the turkey won't be ready for an hour. I should clean up and come over. I say okay.

Instead, I pull out my hide-a-bed and crash. It feels so good. I try to feel my body sinking into the bed, muscles letting go. But my mind won't quit. I see the cat; I see its ripped ears and bloody face. I see the animal hospital and the long line of people. I see the startled vet. I see myself—I look hysterical. The vet must have thought I was hysterical. I can't pay eighty dollars. After saving the cat, they can't kill it. No one will see the signs. What a wretched day. Shut up, mind! I try to relax again. I can't relax. Okay, I'll go to Fran's. I might as well. Being alone is terrible. In ten minutes I will get up.

Twenty minutes later an alarm goes off inside. The energy lasts about two seconds. I am really exhausted. I force myself to hurry. I look terrible—thank heavens for makeup. I grab a can of olives and a package of carrots. Should I drive or walk? I don't even want to think about starting the car. I run.

Fran has set up a long table in the living room. There are candles, and music, and food. I feel a lot better; I can eat. I sit between people I don't know. I tell my story.

After about three hours, people start clearing the table. I stand up—something is wrong with my right leg! From the knee down, my right leg looks like a nylon stocking with a huge balloon in it. My right leg is twice the size of my left, and it feels terrible. I lie down and put my legs up. What on earth could have caused this? Everyone agrees that it must have

been the wicker chair. During dinner I sat on an old wicker chair; the wicker sank beneath the wooden frame and the frame must have pressed against my leg and blocked the circulation. I look at my horribly swollen leg and hold back tears. What next! I'll probably be mugged going home.

Definitions

We hope that you are not saying to yourself, "You think that was bad—well, listen to this!" But everyone has had bad days, and everyone knows what stress is. Or do they? How would you define "stress"?

In this text, the word **stress** is used as it is in everyday language, meaning *emotional and mental reactions* to psychological and physical threats and challenges, including minor hassles, major events, and ongoing conditions. Stress is a global term that is used in place of many other descriptors. When a friend says that she is stressed, you do not know exactly what she feels. You do know that she feels ill at ease in some way—*not* relaxed, *not* calm, *not* peaceful. The feelings that stress comprises include: threatened, anxious, frustrated, impatient, helpless, guilty, embarrassed, pressured, worried, concerned, courageous—wired, frazzled, uptight. Thanksgiving Day had it all. If I had carried a "how do you feel at this moment" questionnaire with me throughout the day, I would have written a word from the list above at each moment. Or I could have simply written "stressed."

We use the term **stress level** to indicate the degree of stress experienced. Stress is not an on-or-off, all-or-none experience. You could ask a friend, "How stressed are you?" The experience of stress is on a continuum from slight irritation to full-blown anxiety.

"Stress level" is a way of talking about the intensity of stress. The cognitive, behavioral, and physiological effects of stress are related to stress level, although, as it is described in later sections of this chapter, the relationship is complex. The psychological effects of stress can be as mild as slight distraction during a task or as severe as inability to function. The delayed stress syndrome experienced by war veterans is a good example of the lasting effect of severe stress (Jones, 1986), as is the clear connection between abuse in childhood and difficulty in functioning as an adult.

Because mind ⟶ body, stress has physiological effects that are also on a continuum from mild to severe. It is difficult to feel stressed without having a physiological response of some kind—higher pulse rate, tense muscles, shallow breathing, and hundreds of other reactions. We use the term **stress response** to refer to physiological reactions to stress. Stress and the stress response feed each other. Sometimes stress includes awareness of the stress response, as indicated in phrases such as "I feel like a bundle of nerves" or "I feel jumpy." Being aware of the body response often escalates the experience of stress.

Stressor refers to an *external* stimulus or an *internal* thought, perception, image, or emotion that creates stress. External stressors can be as obvious as a red traffic light when we are in a hurry, or as subtle as the barely noticeable change in a lover's smile. Internal stressors may be as obvious as negative self-talk about exams—"I know I won't do well"—or as subtle as an unconscious need to please.

Stress is a mental or emotional response to a stressor, and the stress response is the physiological counterpart of stress. Stress level is the degree of stress experienced. There is another element, **stress behavior**. Without knowing the specific feelings or physiological reactions, we can often tell when a person is stressed. We observe a tight face with a frown, or clenched jaw, rigid or jerky movements, staccato speech; we sense tension that is difficult to describe.

Two other concepts are included in discussions of stress—**coping** and **adaptation**. Long-time stress researcher Richard Lazarus and his colleagues at the Berkeley Stress and Coping Project, University of California at Berkeley,

define coping as "the process of managing demands (external or internal) that are appraised as taxing or exceeding the resources of the person" (Lazarus & Folkman, 1984a, p. 283). Lazarus emphasizes the fact that coping demands effort, skills, and resources. Adaptation is a similar concept. As the term suggests, adaptation means changing to reduce stress. Hans Selye, a pioneer in stress research discussed later in this chapter, used the term *adaptation* to mean the physiological response of the body when exposed to a stressor, such as extreme cold or heat. Selye described adaptation as the body's attempt to maintain homeostasis. Adaptation is also a behavioral and psychological process. It is often discussed in connection with change, as in "He adapted well to the change of schools" or "Our rapidly changing society necessitates continual adaptation." Like coping, the concept of adaptation connotes expenditure of energy or effort. Selye investigated the harmful physiological effects of continual stress, necessitating continual physiological adaptation. Other stress researchers have studied behavioral and cognitive effects of stress, discussed later in this chapter.

Like other topics in psychology and sociology that relate to complex human behavior and experience, the study of stress has had a rocky history. It suffers from difficulty in defining

---

PREVIEW

Stress management includes:

1. Changing external and internal stressors
2. Changing emotional and mental reactions to stressors
3. Changing physiological reactions to stress
4. Changing stress behaviors

the term and from the tendency to simplify. Hans Selye's use of "stress" referred only to the physiological response of the body, and this meaning was retained by industrial psychologist Karl Albrecht (1979), who uses the term "pressure" to refer to the emotional/mental experience of threat or challenge. Aaron Antonovsky (1987) distinguishes between tension and stress, while others prefer to use "strain" rather than stress. Philip Rice (1987) uses strain to refer to the physiological and psychological effects of pressure arising from exposure to stressors.

To add to the confusion, stress has been described as an external stimulus or as a measurable response, following the stimulus-response theory of behaviorism. The tendency to discuss stress as a stimulus or as a response, without reference to the person, was supported by the fact that much stress research was conducted in animal laboratories. There, stimuli and responses are controllable and measurable, but variables such as perceptions or cognitive coping strategies are not. Today, stress research and discussions of stress have shifted dramatically to "person" variables such as perceptions, which affect the experience of stress and determine one's appraisal of stressful stimuli and one's coping response (Guidano, 1988; Lazarus & Folkman, 1984a, 1984b; Mahoney, 1988; Meichenbaum, 1985). The salient fact about stress—the fact that what is stressful for one person may not be stressful for another—illustrates the importance of individual variables in stress.

Summary

Stress is notoriously difficult to define, except in global terms as an emotional/mental response to perceived threats and challenges from either external stimuli or internal stimuli such as thoughts. In fact, this global definition is appropriate because stress is personal and can be a response to just about anything.

Stress is an excellent example of mind ⟶ body because stress has physiological effects, the stress response. You will find as you proceed that the biopsychosocial approach to stress is a perfect fit.

ⅠⅠⅠⅠ➡

SECTION TWO: THE NATURE OF STRESS

Just About Anything

If we were to define stress as our "psychological reaction to . . ." and then attempt to list all the psychological and physical events, situations, conditions, and experiences that threaten or challenge people in some way, we could probably list every conceivable human experience—just about anything. And the interesting thing is that, for some people, some of these stressors would be "challenging," "fun," "invigorating," or "relaxing." So the nature of stress is that it is personal.

Stress is personal in the sense that it is impossible to know exactly what a stressed person is feeling, and stress is personal in the sense that what is stressful for one person is not necessarily stressful for another. Hans Selye claimed that for him the greatest torture would be spending a day on the beach, doing nothing!

Except for the stressors that terrify everyone, every stressor is personally evaluated. The evaluation (interpretation or perception or appraisal) of an event or situation determines the level of stress. Hence the familiar idea among stress researchers and therapists: *Events do not stress us; it is our perception or interpretation of events that stresses us.* For example, even in the case of the death of a loved one, interpretation of the event determines the level of stress. Death perceived as part of the natural ebb and flow of life is less stressful than death that is perceived as a tragedy or punishment.

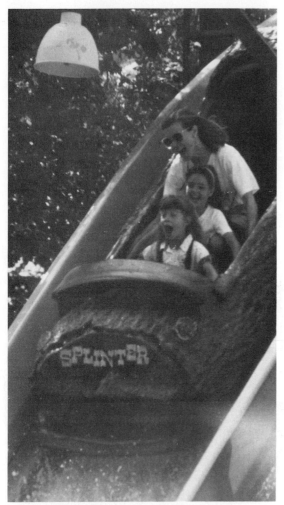

Stress Is the Result of One's Interpretation of an Event, and People Respond Differently to the Same Event, as the Log Ride Illustrates.
Source: Gordon Steward, Denver, CO.

A thorough discussion of the development of perceptions and interpretations is beyond the scope of this chapter but is a recurring topic throughout this text. Suffice it to say that learning is a primary force—learning through role models such as parents and peers, and learning from personal experience. Children learn very early that certain events are threatening when parents model stress reactions.

Negative experiences are powerful teachers. A single failure can turn a neutral task into a stressor. Psychology students are familiar with the experiment by behaviorist John Watson, who taught the young child, Albert, to fear fluffy white objects by frightening the child in the presence of a white rat. This simple example is a prototype for one kind of learned perception, which in its severe form is a phobia. How one reacts to external and internal stressors is also learned, from modeling by parents and peers, from cultural norms, and from experience.

One type of reaction to chronic stress, learned helplessness, is a pattern of giving up and taking no action to escape or change a stressor. This pattern, named by psychologist Martin Seligman, results from repeated failure to change or escape a stressor (Seligman, 1975). For example, a woman who is repeatedly abused by her husband and continually fails to change or escape the situation may eventually give up. And she has learned that she is helpless.

The fact that stress is the result of perceptions and interpretations of events is important in understanding the nature of stress. It is a key to stress management because *stress-producing perceptions and interpretations can be modified.* The power that perceptions have in determining stress automatically makes perceptions and interpretations a key dynamic in health and wellness. Sometimes changing one's perceptions, and thus modifying stress, is easy, and sometimes it is difficult, but the dynamic is always true. This topic is discussed further in Part Three.

A Threat to What?

We defined stress as the mental or emotional response to threat or challenge. A threat to what? One answer: a threat to our needs. What needs do humans have? Abraham Maslow, a psychologist and founder of humanistic psychology, organized human needs into a hierarchy with six

Table 3.1   A Hierarchy of Needs

Needs	Needs Met By	Threats	Challenge Is to
Transcendence	Spiritual orientation	Devastating life experiences; Harm from others	Overcome boundaries of the ego; Gain sense of oneness, unity with all
Self-Actualization	Self-fulfillment; Achieving personal goals; Living by highest ideals	Devastating life experiences; Other-directed demands Self-imposed limitations; Inertia	Overcome limitations; Refuse to take second best; Be true to self; Know self
Esteem	Personal achievement; Satisfying work; Recognition	Devastating life experiences; Dependence on others for self-worth	Learn to be competent; Gain adequate education; Have unconditional positive self-regard
Love, Belongingness	Romance; good marriage, family and friends Team spirit at work Social, political, and religious groups	Psychological or physical abuse as child or adult; Isolation; Inability to give love	Overcome the past; Establish relationships with persons or groups; Learn to be loving
Safety	Personal, family, social, and political security	Abusive family and relationships; Violent environment; Political and social upheaval; War	Change, avoid, or escape abusive relationships; Change the environment; Get help
Physiological Needs	Adequate food, clothing, shelter; Unpolluted environment (including toxins and noise)	Poverty; Extreme handicaps	Get help, find resources; Share resources; Find employment; Postpone gratification of needs; Have hope and courage

levels, with the most basic physiological needs at the bottom of the hierarchy (Maslow, 1970):

Table 3.1 is a brief look at the major issues at each level of Maslow's hierarchy. Several threats and challenges are relevant at each level. For example, devastating life events may hinder progress at every level. At every level, the challenge is to overcome inertia and personal limitations through action. And at every level, the ability to delay gratification is needed. "Delaying gratification" means saving resources today for future needs, or working hard today for rewards in the future. At the most basic level, this might mean storing food in spite of hunger, or saving money instead of buying nonessential items. At the level of Love and Belonging, the ability to delay gratification might mean missing a party in order to study, or refusing to get involved in an unfulfilling relationship despite loneliness and the need for love. To satisfy the needs for esteem and self-actualization, which often depend upon having a job or skill, delaying gratification means effort today for the reward of doing well in the future. Or it might mean turning down a job today to continue school with the hope of a more satisfying job in the future. The ability to delay gratification with ease and equanimity is not a hallmark of our culture, which promotes "instant gratification" and the "quick-fix" approach to solving problems.

Maslow's idea is that the basic needs of each level must be met before the person can move to the challenges of the next level. Needs for food and shelter must be met before the need for a secure environment can be tackled, and the need for love and belongingness cannot be satisfied until a secure environment is obtained, and so on. Each level of the hierarchy represents basic human needs. We all have a need for love and belongingness, esteem, self-actualization and transcendence. When the fulfillment of any of these needs is threatened, we feel stressed.

Today, the majority of people in the United States are not struggling to fulfill physiological and safety needs, and therefore stress does not come from threats to these needs. Yet, if human beings have an inner drive to fulfill the needs of all levels, then we can appreciate the extreme stress of the poor, who cannot satisfy the most basic needs and have little hope of satisfying the needs for esteem and self-actualization, which others take for granted.

Take a minute: Let come into your mind the last time that you were very stressed. Get into the situation, be in it, *relive* it. Feel what your body is doing; feel what your mind is doing.

Do It Now.

What did you think of? Was it the last time you could not find a cave for the night? Was it when there was no food? Was it when the fire in the hearth went out? Probably not. Sometimes people do recall a truly life-threatening event, but in most cases something else is threatened. What is it? If you analyze the stressful event carefully, you might find that your need for love and belongingness, esteem, or self-actualization was threatened, although you might say that the threat was to your plans, expectations, hopes, friendship, ego, the status quo, or peace of mind. As further exploration, consider the stress of final exams (unless this is exactly what came to mind, in which case consider the stress of an important job interview). Why are final exams stressful? What is threatened?

Maslow's hierarchy is a global description of human needs and challenges. It provides a guideline for understanding stressors and stress. Within each level are numerous personal needs that could be threatened and challenges that produce stress when tackled.

One way of understanding stress, then, is as the result of the perception of a threat or challenge to personal needs. Richard Lazarus and his colleagues describe stress from another perspective—as a threat to one's ability to cope. In Lazarus's model of stress, people make two types of appraisal when confronting a potentially stressful situation: the degree of harm that may occur, and their ability to cope with the situation (Lazarus & Folkman, 1984a). A harmful situation will be less stressful when a person feels confident in his or her ability to cope; a less harmful situation will be stressful when the person feels unable to cope. This is undoubtedly verified by everyone's experience, and it points to an important aspect of stress management in general and therapy in particular—the development of positive coping skills. Coping skills include the very practical, such as learning to change a flat tire if getting a flat would be appraised as stressful, to cognitive skills, such as the stress inoculation described in Chapter 10, to simple physiological skills, such as deep breathing to counteract the stress response. Lazarus points out that ability to cope also depends upon coping resources, including social support, financial support, information, and the ability to solve problems. Lazarus's model of stress is referred to as an **interaction** model because it emphasizes the fact that one's experience of stress depends upon a continual process of interaction with the stressor, appraisal and reappraisal, and coping.

In a related model of stress, Irving Janis, professor emeritus of psychology at Yale University emphasized **self-esteem** as a crucial variable in the experience of stress, self-esteem that comes from the ability to make good decisions (Janis, 1982). Numerous studies have shown a relationship between self-esteem and performance on a coping task, in which subjects with low self-esteem perform more poorly than students with higher self-esteem (Rosen, Terry, & Leventhal, 1982). At the same time, successful coping enhances self-esteem. So again, coping techniques are an important aspect of stress management and therapy. Self-esteem and coping are intimately related to another variable that is paramount in determining stress level and that has been extensively researched in laboratory animals and human subjects—**control**. Controllable stressors are less stressful than uncontrollable stressors; control, therefore, reduces negative behavioral and physiological effects of stress. Control is central because it fosters self-esteem and a sense of **self-efficacy**, another important variable (Bandura, 1986), and it fosters the development of successful coping skills and mastery. Lack of control, however, leads to a sense of hopelessness and learned helplessness. Self-esteem, self-efficacy, and control are interacting variables that enhance one another.

Although individual researchers have focused on particular aspects of the experience of stress, most describe a variety of variables that influence a person's experience. Figure 3.1 depicts many variables that are involved in stress. A person hanging on a wire has at least two stressors, the situation itself and that person's perception of the situation. One stressor (hanging on a wire) has many dimensions, not the least of which is duration. In addition to perceptions, the person contributes coping skills and self-efficacy to the situation, determined by experience. Stress level is a result of these variables. If the person were a gymnast, this situation would pose no problem and stress level would be low; if the person were dangling on an electrical wire high above the ground, stress level would be high. The action taken is determined by all the variables in the situation. Positive action enhances self-efficacy and skills, which in turn change the stressor, current and future. Diagrams of subjective experiences, such as stress, are not easy to construct because all of the elements interact in a continuous process. Examine Figure 3.1 now.

This formula for stress suggests several important avenues for intervening in the development of stress and for counteracting the stress response. In teaching stress management, and in working with clients who have stress-related disorders, we attend to each element in the stress formula. We teach coping skills that help the person intervene in the development of stress at several points in the process.

Occasionally, a person's experience of stress does not fit the model of a situation or event as the trigger of stress. People who experience "panic attacks" or "free-floating anxiety" feel extreme stress but are unable to identify a stressor. In our work with these people, we have found that in fact they do have many stressors in life or have experienced extreme stress, such as abuse in childhood. In general,

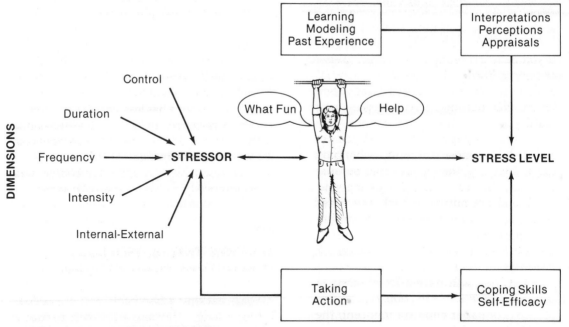

Figure 3.1 Stress Is the Result of Many Variables. The Most Important Variables That Determine Stress Level Are Perception of the Stressor and Coping Skills.

however, people can identify the cause of stress and can learn effective coping skills.

We defined stress as a reaction to threats and challenges. But perhaps you thought, "That is too simple. I can be stressed without being threatened or challenged." This seems true, yet the threat or challenge may be minor. Lazarus and his colleagues at the Berkeley Stress and Coping Project have investigated the effect of the minor irritations of daily life that they call **hassles** (Lazarus & DeLongis, 1981). For an entire year, research subjects recorded and rated daily annoyances. Among all the subjects, three hassles were commonly rated in the top ten: misplacing or losing things, physical appearance, and too many things to do. College students were most hassled by wasting time, trying to meet high standards, and being lonely. Lazarus and his team found that the stress of daily hassles can significantly affect psychological and physiological health. But can something as insignificant as stuck paper clips be a threat or a challenge? Apparently.

To have unmet needs is stressful, meeting the challenge of our needs can be stressful, daily hassles are stressful, and at the wrong moment, stuck paper clips are stressful.

Ask yourself how you create your own stress, how you "do it to yourself." You can create stress with your lifestyle, your personality, your beliefs about the world, your reactions to events, your choices—failure to say "no," failure to be assertive, failure to live up to your own standards, failure to set your own goals. And you can create stress by making all the right choices—the stress of challenge, doing well, succeeding. Hold this question in mind as you read the next section.

Summary

People can be stressed over just about anything; and yet, what stresses one person may not stress another. This is because stress is personal and depends upon one's perceptions,

PAPER-CLIP STRESS

If you have ever fought with stuck paper clips, you know what "paper-clip stress" is all about. Paper-clip stress is about irritation over nothing, sweating the small stuff.

If you are a paper-clip reactor, you get irritated at almost anything—shopping carts stuck together, your child spilling the milk, your roommate borrowing your brush and not putting it back, the pages falling out of your notebook, the vacuum cleaner grabbing a plastic toy, the plastic wrap sticking to itself, and on and on.

When you create a lot of paper clips in your life, you will have a lot of stress, a little at a time. We say "you create" because stuck paper clips are innocent; the child cannot help the spill and can clean up the mess without your anger, and the vacuum cleaner couldn't care less.

Almost everyone turns into a paper-clip reactor when the pressure is on from other stressors. If you are a paper-clip reactor as your *style*, then you probably have something much bigger than the paper clips bothering you, or paper-clip stress is a reaction that you learned, a habit. In any case, you are pushing your body into a stress response and upsetting yourself and people around you. By the time you finish reading this chapter, you will appreciate the need to reduce paper-clip stress, for the sake of mind and body. By the time you finish reading this book, you will have learned techniques for turning off paper-clip stress. In the meantime, when you catch yourself reacting to "paper clips," take an easy, deep breath, let it out slowly, smile, and say to yourself, "Not worth it."

interpretations, and evaluation of events. The experience of stress also depends upon one's resources and ability to cope effectively with the stressor. Self-esteem and sense of self-efficacy interact with ability to cope and determine one's stress level. When needs are threatened, the person who has resources and has learned to cope has less stress than a person who lacks resources and has not learned coping skills. This obvious fact points to an important element in stress management—the development of resources and skills for coping with stressors and stress, even paper-clip stress.

SECTION THREE: THE LOAD— EVALUATING YOUR STRESS

Imagine packing a backpack. You are preparing for a long, strenuous trip, with particular goals. You carefully weigh every item and assess its value. You want to take items that will contribute to the success and fun of the trip, but you know that all the weight adds up, so you are careful.

Life is a long, strenuous trip, with particular goals. Stress adds up psychologically, and the stress response adds up physiologically. It makes sense to know your stress items, their value to you, and how much you are carrying. You would never carry unnecessary weight in a pack, and you would find ways to ease the load that you do carry. You would get in shape, avoid getting lost, share the weight with a partner, and take many breaks. This is what stress management is all about. Take the trip, stick to your goals, and ease the load.

Easing the load is the focus of future chapters. Here we are looking at what the load is.

Personal Stressors

What are your personal "every day" stressors? We do not mean stressors like famine in

Third World countries, or the possibility of nuclear war, or the acute, rare stressors like *nearly* being run over by a car. We mean the stressors that have a continuing effect on health and wellness.

In assessing your stressors, what would you note about them? You would immediately note that stressors are not just events that happen. Stressors have personal meaning, determined by the individual. You would also note that stressors have varying impact and can be evaluated on a continuum from most stressful to least stressful, and you would note that there are many dimensions on which a stressor can be evaluated. Most of your stressors could be evaluated on several dimensions: intensity/frequency, duration, internal/external, psychological/physiological, useful/not useful, short term/long term, chosen/not chosen, controllable/not controllable, fun/not fun, challenging/not challenging, created/I did not create, I can change/I cannot change, I can change and will/I can change but will not, I need support/I do not need support, I have support/I do not have support.

The impact of a stressor depends upon how it stacks up both on your personal hierarchy and on these dimensions. To assess your stressors, you need to create your own list. Rank the stressors according to your personal experience. A format for doing this is presented in Table 3.2.

We encourage you to assess your stressors—the major stressors and the daily hassles. Assessment is important because stressors, stress habits, and the physiological stress response can become unconscious. Consciously or not, stress adds up and becomes a physiological and psychological risk to health and wellness.

If you analyze your five most powerful stressors, you will cover the major sources of stress in your life right now. After ranking your stressors, the next task is to assess each stressor on the dimensions that determine your experience of the stressor and your stress level.

The Dimensions of Stressors and Stress

Intensity

How bad is it? An intense stressor, such as a wounded cat in the radiator fan, a final examination, or a death in the family, cannot be ignored; it becomes the focus of our attention and energy.

Frequency

How often does the stressor occur? By definition, daily hassles are frequent. Final examinations are two or three times a year, the death of a parent occurs twice in life, and a cat in the radiator fan, almost never. Mild stressors that are frequent can add up, as the title of Lazarus's article suggests: "Little Hassles Can Be Hazardous to Health" (Lazarus, 1981).

Duration

How long does each experience of the stressor last? Stuck paper clips last a few seconds; a finger prick for blood is even shorter. Final exams last several days; college may last several years. Daily hassles are short in duration but take their toll because they are frequent.

Short Term/ Long Term

Although daily hassles are of short duration, they will always be with us. Raising children is long-term, the schooling needed for a professional career is long-term, financial responsibilities are long-term, self improvement is long-term. Short-term stressors are over quickly and are not repeated—sewing a wedding dress is short-term, serving dinner for 20 is short-term, learning to drive a car is short-term.

Psychological/Physiological

Almost all stressors are psychological in the sense that they are experienced mentally and

Table 3.2   Personal Stressor Chart

Stressor Characteristics	1	2	3	4	5
List five stressors and check the characteristics that apply to the stressor (1 = most stressful, 5 = least stressful)					
psychological/ physiological					
internal/ external					
useful/ not useful					
short term/ long term					
chosen/ not chosen					
fun/ not fun					
challenging/ not challenging					
I created/ did not create					
I will change/ will not change					
Control/ not control					
I need support/ I do not need support					

emotionally, even though they may be external. These might be final exams, a traffic jam, or a misplaced memo. Physiological stressors have a direct effect on the body, such as physical injury and illness, toxins, extreme cold, hunger, or poor posture.

Useful/Not Useful

This dimension is exactly as the words suggest—useful stressors help us achieve a goal,

useless stressors do not. The usefulness of a stressor is an important dimension because it modifies the level of stress. Stressors that help us achieve a goal, or that support our well-being, are less stressful than stressors that do not.

Chosen/Not Chosen

Stressors that we choose to experience are less stressful than those that are imposed upon us.

Some stressors appear to be "not chosen" when in fact they are chosen, indirectly. A student may say, "I didn't choose to take algebra. I hate algebra," and will feel very stressed. We point out that although algebra may be frustrating, it is a requirement for graduation. And because getting a degree is the student's personal goal, then algebra really was chosen. Sometimes this helps!

Controllable/Not Controllable

As noted in the previous section, one's control of the stressor is the most important factor in determining level of stress. Sense of control over a stressor directly affects stress level, and it changes one's experience of a stressor. The positive effects of control on psychological and physiological well-being have been demonstrated repeatedly in laboratory animal and human studies, as have the negative effects of lack of control.

A sense of control is so powerful that it enabled some prisoners in the German camps of World War II to survive even in the worst conditions. The prisoners forced themselves to maintain mental control, saying inwardly, "They can control my body, but they cannot control my mind." The challenge is to bring a sense of control into all situations.

SERENITY PRAYER

God, give me the serenity to
Accept the things I cannot change,
Courage to change the things I can,
And the wisdom to know the difference.

Allen Grant

I Can Control and Will/I Can Control and Will Not

If you experience a stressor over which you have some control, do you use your control to change the stressor? You may have loud neighbors who disturb your work—you have some power to control that stressor, but do you take action? You may have a boss who gives unreasonable deadlines—you have power to control that stressor, but will you? Your friend is always late, your children are demanding, your spouse will not help with the housework, the landlord overcharges, the traffic light stays red too long—you have power to change these stressors, but will you? You feel stressed a lot—you have power to change, but will you?

Having the potential to control a stressor eases the load somewhat, but *taking* control is the essential variable in easing the load. Humans have a seemingly unlimited ability to "stay stuck." Sometimes a person decides not to rock the boat or decides that changing the stressor is not worth the stress that the effort would bring. Sometimes people fail to take control from pure laziness, but usually people fail to reduce stress by changing the stressor because they do not know how to solve problems or how to be assertive. "I don't have any control over that" is a common explanation for failure to act. Occasionally, people are trapped by a stressor, but often people are trapped by default. They could have control but convince themselves that they do not.

When people fail to use their power to control a stressor, there is usually a "payoff" of some sort, in which inaction seems to be better than action. The most important issue concerning this dimension is the awareness that you are making a choice when you continue to experience a controllable stressor.

Stressors that you choose to hang on to, or cannot change, can have less impact if you use the stress management techniques described in this text. Stressors that you can change will be identified in your list. In the following chapters, you will learn techniques for ridding yourself of unnecessary stressors.

I Need Support/I Do Not Need Support

Like sense of control, having support in handling a stressor is an important dimension that determines how stressful a stressor is. Having the support of a friend, group, organization, or even a pet, is to share the load. Research on social support is discussed in Chapter 6, The Psychosocial Dynamics of Stress Resistance.

Some stressors are purely personal and are easily handled without the support of others. You do not need organizational support to get the paper clips unstuck. On the other hand, the major life stressors, and even many minor stressors, are less stressful when we have support. Study groups reduce the stress of academic work, social groups reduce the stress of loneliness, and citizen action groups reduce the stress of fighting a battle alone. Around the country, support groups are forming to help people cope with stresses, such as alcoholism, abuse as a child, bereavement, or rape. Services, such as crisis and runaway hot lines, offer support to people who feel isolated and unsupported. Society is evolving away from tight families and small communities in which social support in all phases of life was the norm. With the loss of the extended family and the small community, social support must be actively organized and actively sought.

In evaluating your stressors, you have determined whether or not you need support to reduce the stress of the items on your list. One challenge is to seek support from family, friends, and organizations when it is needed; another challenge is to create your own support group.

Challenging/Not Challenging

Stressors that we perceive as challenging are meaningful. They bring out our best, along with a sense of accomplishment and self-worth.

Nonchallenging stressors foster fatigue and denial. When we were little, we could hardly wait to be old enough to do the dishes; the challenge was to finish without breaking anything and without getting water all over the floor. Doing the dishes soon became a very nonchallenging chore that we tried to escape. We have had roommates who were good at escaping the dishes, but they never escaped the challenge of exams in school or a good argument at the dinner table. A stressor can also be nonchallenging because it is overwhelming—there is no hope of overcoming the stressor. Here, too, fatigue, failure, avoidance, and escape are outcomes. The challenge is to create challenge where there is none—to turn a dull, nonchallenging stressor into a challenge, and to bring seemingly overwhelming stressors into the realm of the controllable.

Fun/Not Fun

Is it possible to be stressed and have fun at the same time? Apparently. The obvious example is the roller coaster ride—you scream as if in agony, but you get off saying, "Boy, was that fun!" Most people have a touch of the thrill seeker. Most people can experience stress and fun at the same time. Clearly, stressors that have an element of fun are less stressful than those that do not. The challenge of mundane stressors is to add an element of fun.

I Created/I Did Not Create

We all create more stress for ourselves than we would like to admit. And it is tempting to point a finger elsewhere—"The report that I haven't written makes me worried," "Casper makes me angry," "The boss really stresses me." In reality, we create stress by our interpretations of events, by getting into stressful situations, and by making decisions in life that create stress.

Fortunately, most of the stress that we create is chosen, challenging, and controllable.

BETTER STRESSORS

The better stressors are short-term (the end is in sight), are chosen or consciously created, and are a necessary part of a life plan, and can be terminated if they create more stress than they are worth. In addition, the better stressors are a challenge and are fun.

The worst stressors are those that are not chosen and that cannot be controlled or escaped. Stressors of this type are rare for most people, but they are common for the sick, the undereducated and underskilled, and the poor.

If you noted on the stressor evaluation chart that you have stressors that you did not choose or cannot change, think again.

Changing a career, having children, leaving a relationship, or staying in a bad relationship are conscious choices that create stress. We make choices that create stressors and stress when there is a payoff. Like the issue of choosing or not choosing a stressor, it is less stressful to experience a stressor that was consciously created than to experience one that was not.

If you have seriously attended to the task of evaluating your stressors, you now know much more about them. We direct you through this task because before you can change your stressors and reduce stress, you need to know what your stressors are, how they stack up on these dimensions, and what meaning they have for you.

To identify typical stressors among college students, Bush, Thompson, and Van Tubergen (1985) created a stressor inventory of 100 items, which was given to 1200 students at 23 colleges. Students ranked the stressors from most- to least-stressful on a five-point scale. The ten stressors that were most frequently noted are: (1) final exam week, (2) test anxiety, (3) academic workload, (4) future plans, (5) putting off assignments, (6) financial pressures, (7) grades received, (8) guilt for not performing better, (9) worrying about not exercising, (10) competitiveness for grades.

Women and men scored somewhat differently when stressors were ranked for intensity. Both women and men ranked "death of a parent" as most stressful, and both ranked "final exam week" as the third-most stressful event. Men ranked "loss of intimate relationship" as the second-most stressful event, while the second-most stressful event for women was "involved in pregnancy or abortion." Women ranked "test anxiety" as the tenth-most stressful item, while men ranked it as number 18. Men scored "career opportunities after graduation" as a number eight, while women ranked it as number 21; on the other hand, women ranked "eating habits" as the thirty-eighth-most stressful item of 100, while men scored it as number 74. Both men and women ranked "visiting relatives" as the least stressful event.

If your personal stressor inventory includes items related to school or work, marriage, loneliness, or personal relationships, time pressure, money, or health, then you have stressors in common with almost everyone who reads this textbook.

These classes of stressors are interrelated, and the dimensions discussed above apply to all types of stressors. In all cases, a sense of control and the ability to create change are key factors in reducing stress level.

We hope you took the time to evaluate your stressors. Note that directly or indirectly, your stressors are determined by your socioeconomic status and that of your parents; by your age, sex, race, marital status, neighborhood, and living conditions; by your goals, your education level and that of your parents, and by their goals for you; by your physical and psychological health; and by many other biological, psychological, and social variables. The biopsychosocial approach to stress is a perfect fit because a person's interpretation of and reaction to events is determined by these dimensions, and because

THE STRESS OF POVERTY

Poverty has it all—money problems by definition, insufficient employment, family disruption and disintegration, lack of control, unfulfilled expectations, overcrowding and lack of privacy, and lack of security. Poverty brings hopelessness, uncertainty, poor health, and failure to strive and thrive.

If everyone were poor, the discouragement of poverty might be much less. The stress of poverty in this country is great partly because poverty exists in the midst of plenty. In Chapter 20, Societal and Cultural Forces Against Health and Wellness, we discuss poverty in greater detail.

stressors also have biological, psychological, and social dimensions.

We have stated repeatedly that stress and stressors are personal in the sense that no two people react in the same way to the same stressor.

Personal Stress Signs

You may have several major stressors and many daily hassles, but are you really stressed? This may seem like a nonsensical question because "stressor" is defined as anything that creates stress; by definition, if you have stressors, you must be stressed. But people are not always aware of their own stress levels. Sometimes psychological or physiological stress is so much a part of life that it feels normal, and people no longer notice the subtle signs of stress. Sometimes a painful or frightening symptom is the first clue that alerts a person to stress and its effects. Health and prevention of illness necessitate awareness of stress before it takes its toll.

In this section you may estimate your stress level by assessing your personal stress signs, which indicate how much stress you are carrying. There are three ways to carry stress—in the body, in the mind, and in behavior—and therefore there are three inventories.

These stress-sign questionnaires may bring to your attention a psychological or physiological reaction to stress that you have been ignoring or that has gone unnoticed. If you check an item in the *always* or *often* category, determine whether the behavior is caused by a temporary stressor that you can clearly identify. If you have several stress signs, you may have stressors that need your attention—you may need to change the stressor or your reaction to it. This may be as simple as changing your reading posture when you study or as complex as re-evaluating your goals in life.

We do not include a "key" for scoring your stress-sign inventories *because you are unique.* If the categories had numerical value and your score were low, it would not necessarily mean that you are not stressed or that the items in these categories could be ignored. Or if your score were high, you would not necessarily be overwhelmed by stress. You are the best judge of your stress level and of the importance of your stressors. *The key is self-awareness.*

When you are aware of your stressors, stress habits, and personal stress signs—how you carry stress psychologically, physiologically, and behaviorally—then you are ready to ask yourself: "Am I too stressed? Should I take action to reduce my stress?" How can you tell?

If you have a chronic physical stress sign, such as headache, upset stomach, or chronic fatigue, or if you have several lesser stress signs that add up to feeling "less than perfect" most of the time, then you are probably too stressed, and it is time to begin systematic stress management. If you do have a physical stress sign that persists when you are not stressed or that hinders your daily activity, we recommend that you also see a physician.

If you have psychological stress signs that occur "always" or "often," and you feel less than

Stress Signs	Never	Always/Usually	Often	Seldom
Behavioral				
1. My voice is harsh and high-pitched				
2. I slam doors				
3. I eat quickly				
4. I can't sit still				
5. I drive too fast				
6. I walk quickly				
7. I grimace				
8. I bite my nails				
9. I twitch				
10. I tap my fingers				
11. I chew my pencils or erasers				
Physiological				
1. Tightness or aching in the shoulders				
2. Tightness or aching in the back				
3. Tightness or aching in the jaws				
4. Tightness or aching in the forehead				
5. Clenching teeth				
6. Tightly gripping a chair arm, steering wheel, etc.				
7. Diarrhea				
8. Constipation				
9. Short, irregular, or shallow breathing				
10. Heart racing or pounding				
11. Cold hands or feet				
12. Sweaty palms				
13. Headache				
14. Stomach or gut pain				
15. Sleep problem				
16. Other symptoms				
Emotional				
1. I get upset				
2. I am irritated				

Stress Signs	Never	Always/Usually	Often	Seldom
3. Unimportant things bother me				
4. I feel depressed				
5. I feel angry				
6. I feel "burned out"				
7. I have trouble focusing my mind				
8. I waste time				
9. I am "moody"				
10. I cry inappropriately				
11. I feel anxious				
12. Other				

perfect psychologically even when you have no clear stressors, then you may wish to consult a counselor or someone who can help you determine the cause of your feelings and who can teach you ways of changing your stressors and your reaction to them.

Now we focus on a stressor that is, or will be, a part of everyone's life—work. We highlight work because it is a nearly universal stressor. The stress that evolves from work is a biopsychosocial phenomenon, as is work itself.

Work: Would You Like to Be an Orange Sorter?

Probably everyone you know is working, lives in a family supported by a worker, or is preparing to work. Work is a major source of stress because it has the potential of fulfilling three primary needs—money (which enables fulfillment of other basic needs), self-esteem, and self-actualization. Often these needs cannot all be met through work, or one is sacrificed for another, depending upon a person's priorities (a person might sacrifice salary for a challenging job). The years in education and training for a career are spent in the hope that

work will bring money, self-esteem, and self-actualization. Thus, work has the potential for being the source of great challenge and advancement or a source of continual stress.

In 1978 the National Institute of Occupational Safety and Health (NIOSH) commissioned a group of researchers to determine which occupations are associated with the highest incidence of stress-related disorders, such as ulcer and hypertension (Smith, Collisan, & Hurrell, 1978). The group studied 130 occupations and examined the health records of 22,000 people. Laborers had more stress-related illnesses than other occupations, and secretaries were second. In both situations, the worker has little power or control, and work is governed by "the boss."

Swedish researcher Marianne Frankenhauser (1980) studied two groups of workers in a sawmill. One group graded the quality of timber. The work pace was set by machine, and the judgment of the quality of the wood had to be made in less than five seconds. The graders had little interaction with other workers and had no variation in the task. The second group of workers had jobs that allowed them to move around and socialize.

Frankenhauser found that the graders had higher levels of adrenaline and more stress-related disorders than the second group of workers. In addition, the graders were unable to relax after work and perceived the work as monotonous. Adrenaline level was highest when the job was highly repetitious, when the worker was unable to move about, and when a machine controlled the pace of work (Frankenhauser & Rissler, 1970).

Other investigators have found similar results. Swedish researchers Karasek, Theorell, Schwartz, Pieper, and Alfredsson (1982) studied several thousand workers and found that employees who were under high pressure with little control over the situation had the highest incidence of illness, particularly heart disease. This work situation contributes the same degree of risk for coronary heart disease as do smoking and elevated blood cholesterol.

As we noted earlier, lack of control is a major factor in determining stress load. Research on work stress supports this idea—stressful situations in which the person has no control impair human functioning. Please read Box 3.1 now.

In the 1970s burn-out became a popular word to describe the stress, fatigue, and

---

BOX 3.1

KEYPUNCH OPERATORS AND SENSE OF CONTROL

"East-West Insurance Company employed several dozen keypunch operators. . . . Many of them had begun to show some of the symptoms of job burnout. Work efficiency was at an all-time low. The speed at which the keypunch operators worked had fallen below the accepted industry standard. The number of errors in one group of about 40 keypunch operators had reached an unacceptably high level. Absenteeism, one of the clearest signs of job burnout, had reached the highest level among all departments at East-West.

"Although many of the keypunch operators felt powerless, they were able to use what influence they had. . . . In a group discussion about the problems, they came up with a list of 73 specific suggestions for redesigning their jobs. . . .

"Management at East-West Insurance Company accepted many of the recommendations, particularly the ones that gave greater control over their jobs to the workers. They sought to give each keypunch operator more responsibility, to turn mindless jobs into challenging ones that allowed for personal growth. For instance, under the new design, workers no longer received batches of work that took about an hour to keypunch. Instead, they assumed responsibility for certain 'accounts,' the clients that this department served within the company. Now the keypunch operators each had a personal stake in the job; they could go directly to the user departments to clear up mistakes. A new social network developed within the company, giving the jobs more meaning.

"Under the old job design, keypunch operators felt frustrated because they had to punch the information exactly as it came to them from the service clerk, even when they recognized mistakes! Lack of control also extended to the fact they could not even plan their own work. The new design gave each keypunch operator the power to correct mistakes, schedule his (her) own work, and correct his (her) own mistakes. The keypunch jobs had previously been dead-end positions in the company. The new design tried to remove this stress by providing for advancement within the department and, more important, transfer and promotion to the user departments that send information to the keypunchers.

"In July 1970, a group of keypunchers was selected to institute the changes. Others continued to work at the old jobs to find out which design would enhance the individual worker's life as well as contribute to the overall company goals. East-West Insurance waited one year to see the consequences this redesign would have. The results startled everyone. Absenteeism among the workers in redesigned jobs dropped by 24 percent! A high rate of mistakes in work, a classic symptom of burnout, changed markedly with an improvement of 35 percent. The hourly number of cards that employees punched jumped by nearly 40 percent. In addition, the company could now eliminate supervisory positions, with the result that total savings in one year rose to $64,305!

"But this monetary gain couldn't compare with the savings in human morale, sickness, and the prevention of job burnout. A before-and-after survey of employee attitudes showed an overall improved score of 16.5 percent, while keypunch operators following the old procedures remained at the same levels for the entire year. East-West Insurance Company, while saving money, had improved job satisfaction. The work became more interesting. A much higher percentage now said that 'the job is worth putting effort into.'"

The Work/Stress Connection: How to Cope with Job Burnout, by Robert L. Veninga and James P. Spradley. Copyright © 1981 by Robert L. Veninga and James P. Spradley. Reprinted with permission of Little Brown and Co.

disillusionment that people in the health professions experience. People such as social workers, teachers, and nurses, who have low pay and little control but from whom much is expected, are susceptible to burn-out. Often a person chooses a helping profession with idealistic goals only to discover that the work involves many tasks that are not related to helping. In addition, the work load is heavy, yet many people cannot be helped. Social workers may interview 20 to 30 clients a day, many of whom are poor, depressed, frustrated, and angry. In addition to the client load, many forms must be completed, one of the frustrations of dealing with government bureaucracy. One social worker reported, "I've gone for a year without a period. My doctor said it was stress-related. I broke out in a red rash. My hands broke out in blisters and a couple of layers of skin peeled off. I lost 20 pounds, and I was weighing less than 100 pounds" (Fenly, 1977). Another said, "I seem to have compassion fatigue" (Maslach, 1982).

The most stressful jobs have "high demand" tasks, like sorting oranges, with little relief, power, or pay. Or they involve great responsibility and some control, but they do not meet the esteem and self-actualization needs of the worker. The best jobs have a high salary to compensate for the stress, involve the worker in making decisions, are challenging, and promote growth.

Many other job factors interact with "lack of control" to create job stress. In fact, work stress is an excellent example of the interplay of biological, psychological, and social variables—biological factors such as loud noise, pollution, toxic chemicals, and fatigue interact with social factors such as an insensitive management, interpersonal conflict with bosses or employees, job overload, and racial and sexual discrimination. These factors in turn interact with psychological factors such as low tolerance for monotonous work or being overqualified or un-

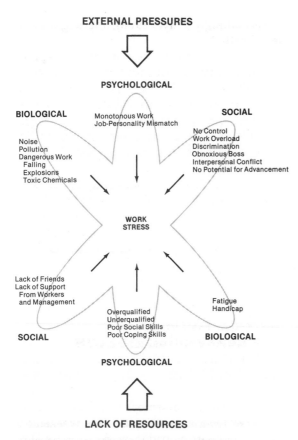

EXTERNAL PRESSURES

PSYCHOLOGICAL

BIOLOGICAL

Monotonous Work
Job-Personality Mismatch

SOCIAL

Noise
Pollution
Dangerous Work
Falling
Explosions
Toxic Chemicals

No Control
Work Overload
Discrimination
Obnoxious Boss
Interpersonal Conflict
No Potential for Advancement

**WORK
STRESS**

Lack of Friends
Lack of Support
From Workers
and Management

Fatigue
Handicap

Overqualified
Underqualified
Poor Social Skills
Poor Coping Skills

SOCIAL

BIOLOGICAL

PSYCHOLOGICAL

LACK OF RESOURCES

Figure 3.2   Work Stress Has Biological, Psychological, and Social Components.

derqualified for a job. Figure 3.2 lists the many biological, psychological, and social factors that contribute to job stress.

Work-related stress is a primary concern of health professionals because it leads to burnout, absenteeism, alcoholism, and physical disorders, and because job stress and its repercussions are preventable. Increasingly, health professionals work with employees and employers in the work environment; they conduct stress-management programs and help the worker and the employer understand and alleviate job stress.

In the past decade, the importance of understanding and reducing stress in the workplace has been given top priority in many industries. From the rank and file, through mid-

dle management, to top-ranking executives, stress takes its toll on health and performance. The incentive for industry to do something about stress grows as industry pays an increasingly larger medical bill and as the cost of replacing disabled or dead executives increases. In Chapter 21, Societal and Cultural Forces for Health and Wellness, we describe steps that industry is taking to reduce workplace stress and improve the health of employees.

Is Stress All That Bad?

Stress has acquired a bad reputation, and rightly so—it plays a central role in many mental and physical disorders. But many people say that they could not live without it.

Could you live without it? "If it weren't for stress, I would be a vegetable." "My stress keeps me going." "If I stopped worrying, I wouldn't do anything." Many stress theorists say that stress is necessary for life. Recently two stress-management experts wrote in a popular magazine for women, "It is the essential ingredient in optimal performance and can be our strongest ally for leading stimulating, healthy, satisfying lifestyles." (Levine, 1987) Really? This upbeat approach to stress is a backlash against the doomsday belief that stress is a killer. It also faces the reality that stress is a part of life and that we may as well use it instead of abuse it. This appreciation of stress is also based on the observation that many people thrive on stress, and stress motivates others to strive for their greatest potential. Here, however, we must distinguish between the two broad categories—stress as a result of perceived threat, and stress as the result of perceived challenge. Common sense and personal experience indicate that the stress of challenge is less harmful than the stress of threat.

Still, we believe that life would be great without stress. Perhaps in a wellness utopia in the future we would say, "Stress is not a fact of life that we should learn to live with, but events that might cause stress are." This approach is stated nicely in the saying, "When life give you lemons, make lemonade."

Do people really need stress as a motivator? Apparently so, but perhaps many people confuse stress with goals. For example, getting through school is stressful, but the stress is not the reason for finishing school. Graduating and reaping the benefits of education are the motivation. This is an important distinction. The stress encountered while pursing a goal, however, does seem to be less destructive when the goal is kept in mind. Stress that drives us seems to be more harmful than stress that results from our own interests. We suspect that the statement, "If it weren't for stress, I would be a vegetable," really means, "If I didn't have goals, I would be a vegetable." Even so, stress is not all bad.

Humans have a wonderful capacity to rebound from stress and to withstand long-term stress, especially when stress-reduction techniques are periodically used. And there is such a thing as "good" stress, which Hans Selye called *eustress. Eu* = good, and eustress refers to the stress of a challenge, for example. Eustress also refers to changing a bad stressor into a good stressor by changing one's attitude. Selye recommended an attitude toward life that helped him through difficult times. "Imitate the sundial's ways, count only the pleasant days" (Selye, 1978). Turning stress into eustress is described in Chapters 6 and 10.

Stress theorists suggest that too little stress is stressful, and too much stress is stressful—people perform poorly with too little stress or with too much, and they perform best with a moderate amount of stress. The relationship between stress level and performance is describe in the next section.

Although the relationship between stress and productivity and well-being is accepted as a general rule, there are individual differences. Our advice is to know yourself and maintain a stress level that is best for your physical and mental health. As Hans Selye put it, know whether you are a racehorse or a turtle, and live accordingly (Selye, 1978). You might even be a "hortle."

Here is another consideration—stress is not all bad, unless your way of coping is self-destructive. How does a person self-destruct while handling stress? Self-destructive behaviors include overeating, smoking, doing drugs, drinking, being reckless, and dropping out. So while stress is not all that bad, it may take work to make it good.

However, in spite of our ability to rebound from stress and live with stress, we return to our major theme: Too much stress is harmful. In the following section, we examine behavioral and cognitive effects of stress, related to academic performance.

||||➡

SECTION FOUR: COGNITIVE AND BEHAVIORAL EFFECTS OF STRESS—ACADEMIC PERFORMANCE

When I (RS) was a senior in college, I dated a woman from a small town. One weekend I went home with her to meet her parents and relatives. A large family picnic was held on Saturday afternoon, and I was asked to give the blessing. I stood up, bowed my head, and began "Dear Lord"—and then my mind went blank. I could not think of another word. After a long silence, I said "Amen." I was startled by this experience, and I was very embarrassed, as was my girlfriend. I could not imagine what had happened. I was a debater with several years' experience, and I had experience in extemporaneous, informative, and oratory speech. I had prayed out loud in front of people many times. Nevertheless, the stress of saying a prayer for my girlfriend's family made my mind go blank for the first time in my life.

Stress can affect thinking and behavior. Some people go blank when taking an exam; others start to shake before giving a speech. Excessive stress impairs thinking, remembering, and physical performance. On the other hand, the right amount of stress can improve performance. For more than 30 years, researchers have studied the harmful and beneficial effects of stress on performance (Hockey, 1983). This section examines the effects of stress on academic performance.

> Brick wrote brilliant essays and was an excellent humanities and social studies student. He spoke intelligently in class and showed mastery of difficult concepts. But Brick did poorly on multiple-choice exams. Whenever it was time to take a multiple-choice exam he became extremely nervous—he had bouts of diarrhea and his mind went blank.

Brick has "test anxiety" and does not function at maximum level. During the exams he "blanks out" and his concentration is impaired.

Irwin Sarason, psychologist at the University of Washington, has studied the relationship between anxiety and academic performance for many years (Sarason, 1975a, 1975b). Sarason finds that the stress of upcoming examinations encourages some students to work harder and improve performance. Many students, however, are debilitated by anxiety and do poorly, like Brick. What is the difference between the students who do well and the students who do poorly?

Sarason found that the key difference between successful test-takers and poor test-takers is **self-preoccupation** (Sarason, 1975b). Poor test-takers focus on their inadequacies and shortcomings, and successful test-takers focus on the task at hand. To fully understand how stress impairs academic performance, it is crucial, says Sarason, to understand how self-preoccupation impairs performance.

Imagine that you stayed up very late last night watching a movie, and you go to your 9:00 A.M. class half asleep. Your professor announces that she will give a test tomorrow instead of next week and will spend the class period reviewing. Immediately you are stressed. Your heart beats faster, your hands begin to perspire, and you feel butterflies in your stomach.

You begin to worry. "When will I have time to study? I feel so tired now I will never have the energy to study tonight." What happens after this initial response will depend on whether you are a "test-anxious student" who becomes debilitated or a "test-hardy student" who can focus on studying and taking the exam.

If you are a test-anxious student, you become self-preoccupied and divert your attention and energy away from task-relevant activities. Your energy and attention go into worrying about your performance instead of learning the material. In addition, your thoughts are negative—"I won't be able to learn enough in one evening," "I will probably panic again," "I'm not smart enough to learn all the material," "What if I get such a low grade that I don't pass the class?" Anxiety may overwhelm you. You may feel panicky and have trouble thinking. Your expectations will be negative—"I will probably forget everything I studied when I take the exam," "My mind will go blank." You may have negative images of going to class and "falling apart." You might see yourself just sitting in class, in a daze. Your body may also overreact. You may have diarrhea or get a headache. You may feel shaky and dizzy. When you finally take the exam you feel drained and incredibly anxious, and you cannot concentrate on the material. Or your mind is unable to mobilize the attention and energy necessary to think efficiently.

If you are a test-hardy student, you stay focused on task-relevant activities. You arrange time to study for the exam. You become absorbed in the material. You memorize, outline, and do what is necessary to learn the material. Your cognitions and expectations are positive—"I have studied hard for the exam and I will do fine." During the test you focus on the questions. Your energy and attention are absorbed by the activity of taking the test.

Another difference emerges between test-anxious and test-hardy people when the result of the examination is returned. The test-hardy student concentrates on wrong answers, examines the mistakes, and determines to avoid mis-

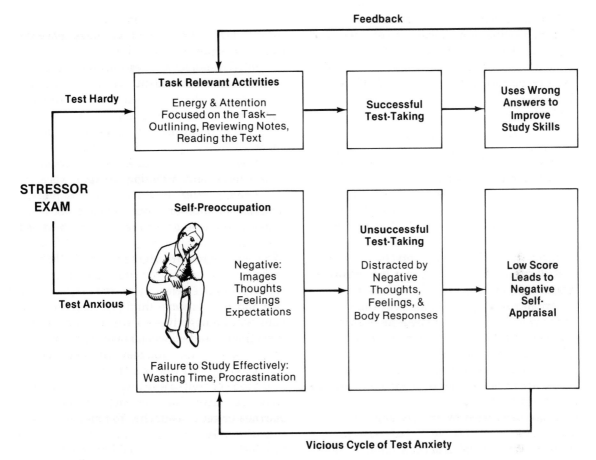

Figure 3.3 Responses of a Test-Hardy and a Test-Anxious Person to Taking an Exam.

takes on the next exam. In other words, the test-hardy person uses wrong answers as feedback to improve performance. In contrast, the text-anxious student becomes preoccupied—"I just can't seem to study," "I just panic when I take tests," "Another bad test."

Figure 3.3 diagrams the test-anxious student's process and the test-hardy student's process. The test-hardy student successfully prepares for the test, takes the test, and learns from mistakes. The test-anxious student has a rigid process of self-preoccupying behaviors that seriously hinder preparing for an exam, taking the exam, and using the results positively.

If you are a test-anxious student, we hope that while reading this section the question

came to mind, "Can I change the habits that foster test-anxiety?" The answer is yes. You can stop the vicious cycle of test anxiety. Part Three provides many ideas for overcoming stress of all types.

Summary

The topic of this section, "The Cognitive and Behavioral Effects of Stress," is worthy of its own textbook. We focused on academic performance. A blank mind and self-preoccupation are cognitive responses to stressors that escalate stress and lead to poor performance, discouragement, and despair. Many other topics are of interest, such as procrastination, underachievement, irrational thinking—cognitive effects of stress that affect behavior. The good news is that the spiral of negative cognitions and behavior can be stopped; this is the subject of Part Three of this text.

IIII➡

SECTION FIVE: STRESS AND PHYSICAL DISORDERS

We noted in the introduction to this chapter that the increasing awareness of the affect of stress on health is a primary factor in bringing the mind back into medicine and psychology. Stress contributes to illness and disease in three ways: as a primary factor, as in tension headache; as a factor that exacerbates an existing disease, such as asthma or epilepsy; or as a factor that increases the likelihood of becoming sick.

Stress and sickness have been partners for as long as minds and bodies have been stressed, but the relationship has been studied scientifically only in this century and has been accepted only recently in medicine. The biomedical model of disease excluded stress as a factor in illness and disease, in spite of the extensive research of the pioneers.

Pioneers: A Brief History

Walter Cannon, a physiologist, discovered that noxious stimuli trigger adrenaline release by studying the physiological response of a cat being frightened by a barking dog; Cannon referred to the reaction as the fight-or-flight response. Cannon used the word *stress* to describe this response in his classic book, *The Wisdom of the Body*, published in 1932.

Hans Selye, physician turned endocrinologist, discovered another branch of the stress response, the pituitary-adrenal cortex system described in Chapter 4, while he was studying the effects of noxious stimuli on rats in the late 1930s and 1940s. Selye's first paper, "A Syndrome Produced by Diverse Noxious Agents," published in 1936, describes the physiological effects of exposure to such stimuli; Selye used the term *stress* to refer to the physiological response of the organism (described below). Selye devoted the rest of his life to the study of stress and its causes; his classic book, *The Stress of Life*, was published in 1956 and revised in 1976.

Working with humans in a laboratory setting, psychiatrist Harold Wolff and his associates accumulated 30 years of data on physiological responses to social stressors. The primary laboratory tool was a stress-inducing interview. Working with patients, Wolff found that it was possible to induce a variety of symptoms such as migraine headache, increased blood pressure, hives, increased wheezing in asthma, and stomach pain by stimulating feelings of anger, bitterness, and helplessness through the interview technique. The original description of this work, *Stress and Disease*, was published in 1952 and was revised by Wolff's colleagues in 1968 (Wolf & Goodell, 1968).

In a larger sphere, Wolff's associate, Lawrence Hinkle, studied the effect of social milieu and interpersonal relationships on health over time. Hinkle, a staff physician for the New York Telephone Company, conducted a 20-year study of telephone workers that is discussed in Chapter 6, The Psychosocial Dynamics of Stress Resistance. The report of this work, "The Effect of Exposure to Culture Change, Social Change, and Changes in Interpersonal Relationships on Health," was published in 1974 (Hinkle, 1974). This was the same year that physicians Friedman and Rosenman published *Type A Behavior and Your Heart*, the culmination of many years of research on a behavior pattern called Type A and heart disease (Friedman & Rosenman, 1974). It is described in Chapter 17, Coronary Prone Personality: Type A.

Another major effort to demonstrate a relationship between stress and sickness was launched by Thomas Holmes, also an associate of Wolff's. Holmes noted that onset or recurrence of tuberculosis often followed a clustering of life events that occurred within a year of the development of symptoms. The original report of this relationship was published in 1957, "Evidence of Psychosocial Factors in the Development of Pulmonary Tuberculosis" (Hawkins, Davies, & Holmes, 1957). After several years of studying life events and illness, Holmes teamed up with psychiatrist Richard Rahe and created the Schedule of Recent Experience. The schedule gives a numerical value to life events, in an attempt to quantify their stress. The original schedule was published in 1967; it is now called the Social Readjustment Rating Scale. This work is described below.

In summary, a wealth of data has been laboriously accumulated over the past few decades, showing that stress affects physiology and health, or, in the larger framework of the dynamics of health and wellness, that mind affects body. The basic physiological mechanisms of the stress response pioneered by Cannon and Selye have become common knowledge. The fact that a psychological variable, stress, can cause or promote disease and illness is also common knowledge today.

For health professionals and for the general public, two areas of stress research have been particularly important in increasing awareness of the relationship between stress and sickness—the effect of Type A behavior on coronary heart disease and the association of life events and sickness.

Life Events and Sickness

The fact that change is stressful is news to no one. Changing jobs, or changing partners, or something as minor as changing the dinner menu because someone ate the pasta can be stressful. A life event as joyous as marriage may be a stressor when it involves change and readjustment.

The relationship between life change and sickness was first noticed by Dr. Thomas Holmes when he was working as the intake physician in a tuberculosis sanitarium. Holmes interviewed new patients, taking a thorough history. Over time, Holmes noticed that new patients, or patients returning to the sanatorium after a relapse, were likely to have a history of several stressful life events before the onset of the disease. This observation stimulated the curiosity of the young physician and led him to a lifelong investigation of the relationship between life events and sickness.

Holmes and Rahe created the inventory of life events, the Social Readjustment Rating Scale, by asking people to rank 43 life events on a scale from those that demanded the most adjustment to the least adjustment, with marriage as a reference point in the middle of the scale. Participants ranked death of spouse as most demanding and minor violations of the law as least. To quantify these events, a number was given to each event; death of spouse was given 100 points, and violations, 11 points. The points indicate the amount of adjustment needed to cope with the stressor. Holmes and Rahe found that there is a relationship between the number of points, or clustering of life changes, and health in the year following the changes.

Holmes wrote:

> What's your own risk? Take a moment and add up the score for all the items that applied to you in the last year.
>
> If you scored below 150 points, you are on pretty safe ground—about a one in three chance of serious health change in the next two years. Remember, you already have a 10 percent chance of winding up in the hospital sometime during the year. If you scored between 150 and 300 points, your chances rise to about 50-50. The odds on Russian roulette are better than that. If you scored over 300 points, be sure your health insurance is paid up—your chances are almost 90 percent.
>
> Blue Cross/Blue Shield, 1978

In fact, the correlation between life events and disease and illness is not as strong as indicated by Holmes's statement or the popularity of the inventory. The grim prognosis is not true for many people who experience an accumulation of life changes. As you take the inventory (Box 3.2), ask yourself why it is not an accurate predictor of illness and disease, and what variables might contribute to its inaccuracy. Please read Boxes 3.2 and 3.3 now.

Although the Social Readjustment Rating Scale does not accurately predict sickness in many individuals, we all know that the change necessitates adjustment and can be stressful. Therefore, life change is one way of estimating stress level. The types of life events experienced depend somewhat on age and status.

BOX 3.2

LIFE EVENTS AND RELATIVE STRESS VALUES

Life Event	Stress Values
Death of spouse	100
Divorce	73
Marital separation	65
Jail term	63
Death of close family member	63
Personal injury or illness	53
Marriage	50
Fired at work	49
Marital reconciliation	45
Retirement	45
Change in health of family member	44
Pregnancy	40
Sex difficulties	39
Gain of new family member	39
Business readjustment	39
Change in financial state	38
Death of a close friend	37
Change to different line of work	36
Change in number of arguments with spouse	35
Mortgage over $10,000	31
Foreclosure of mortgage or loan	30
Change in responsibilities at work	29
Son or daughter leaving home	29
Trouble with in-laws	29
Outstanding personal achievement	28
Spouse begins or stops work	26
Begin or end school	26
Change in living conditions	25
Revision of personal habits	24
Trouble with boss	23
Change in work hours or conditions	20
Change in residence	20
Change in schools	20

Life Event	Stress Values
Change in recreation	19
Change in church activities	19
Change in social activities	18
Mortgage or loan less than $10,000	17
Change in sleeping habits	16
Change in number of family get-togethers	15
Change in eating habits	15
Vacation	13
Christmas	12
Minor violations of the law	11

Source: Adapted from "The Social Adjustment Rating Scale" by T.H. Holmes and R.H. Rahe, 1967, *Journal of Psychosomatic Research,* 11, 213–218. Copyright 1967 by Pergamon Press, Ltd. Reprinted by permission.

BOX 3.3

NOTE ON STRESS EVALUATION AND STRESS RESEARCH

To evaluate the relationship between stress and sickness, it is necessary to have a way of numerically quantifying stressors and stress. Numerical quantification is important because statistical analyses are needed to determine the relationship between stress and sickness. In addition, large groups of people must be studied.

Quantifying stressors and the experience of stress is a difficult problem because stress is a personal experience, and what is stressful for one person may not be stressful for another. Some people are risk-takers who seem to thrive on the experience of stress, and they seek certain types of stressors. Consequently, a numerical score given to a stressor may not accurately reflect the individual's stress level when experiencing the stressor. To add a personal appraisal dimension to the life events inventory, Sarason, Johnson, and Siegel (1978) eliminated the number scale of the Schedule of Life Events

of Holmes and Rahe and added a rating scale. The scale allows a person to evaluate each event from − 3 (extremely negative) to +3 (extremely positive).

This new scale, called the Life Experiences Survey, has 47 general items and 10 additional items for students. Items for students include:

1. Beginning a new school experience at a higher academic level (college, graduate school, professional school, etc.)
2. Dropping a course
3. Financial problems concerning school (in danger of not having sufficient money to continue)
4. Failing an important exam
5. Changing a major

Among college students, negative change was associated with anxiety and depression and poor grades, while positive change was not associated with these variables. Johnson and Sarason (1979) found that negative change was associated with self-report of physical symptoms seven months after students evaluated life change.

The study of large populations presents another problem in research—loss of individual differences that might provide valuable information. For example, a researcher might be interested in the health effect of the stress of final exams in a large university. The researcher could examine the use of the student health services before, during, and after final exams. The data would show trends, but the response of individual students would not be seen. The researcher could also use a questionnaire asking students to rate the stress of exams. The researcher could then examine the health records of students who rated exams as very stressful and students who were not stressed. The data would yield a more precise analysis of stress and health, but the individual response would not be studied.

While studies of stress and sickness are useful and indicate trends, it is always one's personal response to stressors that determines stress level.

The College Schedule of Recent Life Experience was created in 1972 by Anderson, and revised in 1975 by Marx, Garrity, and Bowers. The college scale has values from one to 100. It includes the following items and values:

Event	Values
Entered college	50
Major conflict or change in values	50
Major change in amount of independence and responsibility	49
Major change in use of alcohol	46
Held job while attending school	43
Change in or choice of major field of study	41
Major change in participation in school activities	38

Marx found that college freshmen who had many recent life changes had many more sick days compared with students who had few life changes: 41 days versus 19 days (Marx, Garrity, & Bowers, 1975).

If you are a student, you may have experienced several of these stressors recently. The amount of change during college can be greater than at any other time in life, but only you can judge your stress level; a numerical score cannot tell you how stressed you are, and life change cannot magically create illness and disease. Life changes have the same dimensions as other stressors that contribute to stress level, described earlier. For example, the stress of life events can be significantly modified by a sense of personal control and support. These dimensions are not taken into account on the numerical scale but are taken into account on the Life Experience Survey discussed in Box 3.3.

As we said, the relationship between stress and sickness is not magical. Physiological mechanisms operate over time to create physical symptoms. The physiology of the stress response was the primary focus of the research of Hans Selye, discussed next.

The Stress Response

In the 1930s Selye began his lifelong career by studying the physiological effects of physical stressors on rats. Selye defined stress as the body's physiological response to any stimulus that activates an adaptive response in the organism. A common theme in all theories of stress, regardless of how stress is defined, is that stress occurs when the organism must adapt to a new challenge or a noxious stimulus.

Adaptive response is the organism's physiological change to meet the challenge of the stressor. In this model of stress, a stressor can be anything that activates an adaptive response, either pleasant or unpleasant. To Selye, a passionate kiss and the lash of a whip, while not equally pleasant, are both stressors.

To study stress, Selye and his colleagues subjected rats and other animals to a variety of unpleasant physical stressors, such as immobilization, electric shock, and injection of toxic material. The animals were subjected to these stressors over time; that is, the stressors were chronic. The animal's physical reaction to these chronic stressors was determined by measuring hormone levels, including adrenaline and steroids, and by examining the internal organs. This early work did not contribute to knowledge about the psychological dimensions of stress, but it laid the foundation for the acceptance of the role of nonbiological factors in physical illness and disease. In the 1930s it must have seemed remarkable and puzzling that something as physically innocuous as immobilization could create the variety of physical responses that Selye found. Please read Box 3.4 now.

The stress response can take its toll on the body, as subtly as elevated blood pressure or as obviously as a pounding heart, whether stress is brief or chronic. A body that is already compromised by illness or poor lifestyle becomes a candidate for more illness and disease when the owner of the body continually triggers the stress response.

How to Activate the Stress Response

Imagine that you are driving to the airport. . . . Everything is fine, plenty of time. . . . The city traffic is moving fast. You pass the one-mile sign to the airport and move into the exit lane. Traffic in the exit lane is slowing, really slowing, slowing to a standstill. Traffic jam! Cars and trucks are backed up as far as you can see. You can see the airport. Planes are landing and taking off. You will never make it. You are going to miss your plane. It's terrible!

Let's look at this scene from the body's perspective, as if it were not connected to the mind. "Nice, comfortable, warm." The body does not know anything about airports and traffic jams. But it finds out because mind and body are connected—the fundamental dynamic. Because the situation is interpreted as threatening, the stress response is triggered: pulse rate up, blood pressure up, hands sweaty, breathing shallow, shoulders tight, stomach stops digesting. You have triggered the stress response while sitting comfortably, securely, and passively in your car.

Or review the snake-and-garden hose story about coming home on a rainy night, stepping on the garden hose, and perceiving it as a snake. Let's review what happened. A squishy sensation underfoot creates an instant interpretation, "snake." In this story, snakes are *fearsome*. The interpretation "snake" triggers the familiar flood of physiological responses—pounding heart, trembling hands, tight muscles, shallow breathing. Instantly you take action—hop off the snake, jump into the car. In this case, your interpretation is the stressor, and the physiological reaction is the stress response.

Snake story continues: You pick up your books and run through the rain into the house. Immediately you begin telling your story to whomever is there. "The scariest thing happened. I stepped on the garden hose and I thought it was a snake! It was horrible; I've never felt anything so slimy. It felt just like a snake. It was the garden hose, but it felt just like a snake. I was so scared. You should have seen me shaking. See, I'm still shaking. It was awful, just like a snake."

Now what is happening? You are reliving the event. There is no snake for miles, but to the body there is a snake nearby. And the stress response is maintained—although not to the extent of the initial fright—because what is real in the mind is real to the body.

BOX 3.4

HANS SELYE

Imagine the young medical student witnessing his mentor describe the minute but observable clues that distinguish one disease from another in several patients. While listening to the elaborate descriptions, the student noticed that the patients had something in common—they all looked alike, *sick.* Selye's mentor did not find this unusual because the patients were sick. What caught Selye's attention was the fact that, although the patients had different diseases, they all had a response in common. Years later, Selye remembered this observation when he discovered that, regardless of the stressor, his laboratory rats had a common response. This is what happened.

In the early 1930s Hans Selye began work as an endocrinologist at McGill University in Montreal, Canada. Selye was interested in sex hormones and was hoping to find a new one. Selye did not find a new hormone; instead he discovered that regardless of the hormone injected into the animal, the rats had a similar response—enlarged adrenal glands, shrunken lymph nodes and thymus glands, and bleeding ulcers. Being a good scientist, Selye knew that before conclusions could be made about the effects of the sex hormones he had injected, he needed to test a "control group" with nonhormone substances. That is when he found the surprising common response. No matter what substance was injected, the response was always the same—enlarged adrenals, shrunken immune system glands, and bleeding ulcers. Selye realized that this was a general response, not related to a specific substance. The general nature of the response was confirmed after many experiments, using a variety of stressors including exposure to cold, immobilization, and electric shock. Selye called the physiological reaction *stress* and called the development of the triad of responses the General Adaptation Syndrome.

Selye used the word *adaptation* because he reasoned that the physiology of the animal was trying to adapt to the challenge of the noxious stimulus. The process of adaptation to chronic and severe stressors, however, is harmful in the long run. Selye observed that there are three phases to the response: *alarm, adaptation,* and *exhaustion.*

Selye named these phases of the stress response for a sequence of physical events in the stressed animal. The alarm phase is the characteristic fight-or-flight response. If the animal does not die in this phase, and the stressor continues, the animal appears to adapt. In the adaptation phase, the physiological responses are less extreme, but the animal eventually becomes exhausted. In the exhaustion phase, the animal's adaptation energy is spent, symptoms occur, and the animal dies. Selye thought that animals, including humans, have finite reserves of energy for adaptation to stressors, and that humans should not squander adaptation energy on unimportant stressors.

The evolution of the mind-body connection has brought us into modern life with a stress response that can be activated in an instant. It can be triggered by a thought ("Uh oh, this is where the snake was"), by a misinterpretation of an event (snake for garden hose), by an actual threatening event (stepping on a snake), and even by pure fantasy ("The snake is waiting for me and wants to bite me"). The stress response is a two-edged sword. On one hand, the stress response is needed in situations that threaten survival; on the other hand, it is triggered by anything that a human thinks is threatening, and that can be just about anything. The body does not interpret, it just responds. Fortunately, the body has amazing powers of recovery, and humans have the power to consciously modify the body's reaction to stress.

||||➡

CONCLUSION

The biopsychosocial approach to stress is a perfect fit because humans have biological, psychological, and social stressors that interact to produce stress, and stress has biological, psychological, and social consequences. The common experience of test anxiety exemplifies the biopsychosocial nature of stress. The anxiety is a psychological experience that is intensified by self-preoccupation and negative thinking, but the driving force behind the anxiety is social—social values, social pressure, and expectations. The stress response becomes part of the experience, escalating the stress. Figure 3.4 summarizes many biological, psychological, and social variables involved in stress, including lack of resources. Some variables, like poor self-concept, are both a stressor and a "lack of resource."

We have included a lengthy chapter on stress in this text because stress is a fact of life that can have devastating effects, and yet stress is clearly controllable. Understanding stress and learning to handle it in a healthy way are dynamics in health and wellness.

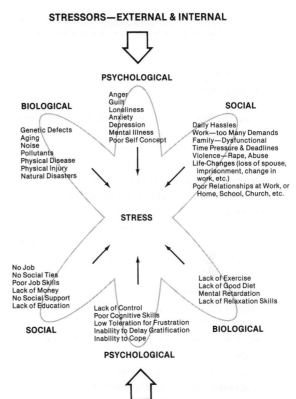

Figure 3.4   The Biopsychosocial Model of Stress.

We conclude this chapter with a return to Thanksgiving Day. The impact of a stressful event is determined and modified by our personal perceptions and needs and by the many dimensions of the stressor. Discovering a cat in the radiator fan is a frightening event. But the extreme stress that was felt came from my intense concern for the cat and from the conflict between caring for the wounded animal and my needs for the day, including my sense of responsibility to my friend.

We know that:

1. Stress is personal, resulting primarily from one's perceptions and interpretations, and
2. Stress escalates when stressors are compounded. When stress escalates,

3. People behave in extreme ways. On Thanksgiving Day I thought I hated the city, and I did a thing that I would not normally do—leave the hospital without paying.
4. When people are stressed, small events are blown out of proportion—forgetting the phone number was a catastrophe, and every red light was a disaster. But,
5. Stress can activate our inner resources—I mustered courage and became assertive; I followed through with signs around the neighborhood; I kept in touch with Fran. Yet,
6. Too much stress can have the opposite effect—apathy, pessimism, helplessness—"I'll probably be mugged going home."
7. Stress has physical effects—fatigue and a leg the size of a large balloon.
8. The impact of stressors is modified by many variables, such as duration, personal choice, and control. The stress of Thanksgiving Day was short, but intense. Of course, rescuing the cat was a choice that I made, and I gained a sense of control by being assertive in the hospital.

At this moment, focus within and determine your stress level.

You have a stressor—you do not know how the cat story ends. If you want to know what happened to the cat, you might describe your feeling as anticipation, curiosity, or "unfinished business." Unfinished business is a stressor.

This is how the story ends:

I stay home to answer the phone. No one calls. The hospital says four days, that is the policy.

On the morning of the fourth day I call the hospital. I will pick up the cat after work. I plan my strategy for not paying. I don't have eighty dollars.

The phone rings. "You must have our cat. We'll come right over and get her." It is the people just across the alley—I have never met them. I explain what happened. These people are so relived to find their pet that eighty dollars is nothing. I say, "Call the hospital immediately." I describe what happened again. I explain three times how to get to the hospital.

I go to work, and after a couple hours I call the animal hospital. The cat was picked up. They really did it! Now, at last, I can relax.

Shortly after I get home, the neighbors call. "You must come over for a drink. We know that you want to see Fluffy. The fluffy black and white cat is really called Fluffy.

I walk across the alley and up to the second-floor apartment. Champagne! They toast me as the rescuer of Fluffy. Fluffy is perfect, just as I told her she would be, and she is totally nonchalant, as only a cat can be.

End of story, almost. For many years after Thanksgiving Day, my right leg swelled whenever I was stressed.

CHAPTER *4*

The Stress Response

In Chapter 2, Mind and Body Dynamics, we discussed mind-body interaction in terms of the stress response and survival. The mind must be able to influence the body for survival, and it must do so before the body is damaged. A rapid and robust stress response, triggered by the perception of threat or challenge, is necessary. Chapter 3 noted that "stress" and "stressor" are broadly defined, only because to define stress by listing stressors would comprise an encyclopedia of human concerns.

Now we can move to the question of how the stress response occurs—how it is that you can step on the garden hose and think that it is a snake, and suddenly have the hundreds of physiological responses that are the stress response.

In Chapter 3, we defined stress as an emotional/mental reaction to a threat or challenge, experienced as anxiety, frustration, fear, edginess, excitement, anticipation, and many other feelings. We defined the stress response as the body's natural reaction to stress. The stress response would not be harmful if humans kept stress short and simple, and kept the body physically fit. Unfortunately, many people do neither. A chronic stress response means trouble—in the form of ulcers, hypertension, headache, low back pain, irritable bowel, heart attack, asthma, gastritis, colitis, arthritis. The medical and the "personal discomfort" bills for stress-related illness are staggering.

To understand the stress response, you need a brief overview of the nervous system. This is because the nervous system is the "go-between," the mediator between mind and physiological responses—it initiates and modifies the stress response. The Appendix at the end of this chapter provides an overview of the nervous system. If you are not familiar with the basics of the nervous system and its functions, please read the Appendix immediately. If you have avoided the study of physiology, we recommend a new perception: Knowledge is power. The more you know about your body, the more power you have to keep it in good health, and the better you will be as a teacher, therapist, or parent. In addition, this chapter provides the basic information for understanding the treatment of stress-related disorders, which are described in the chapters on behavioral medicine in Part Five.

In Section One we discuss the "generic stress response," which initiates physiological responses to stress. Section Two describes four major systems of the body that respond to stress—cardiovascular, gastrointestinal, immune, and skeletal muscles. In each case we describe (1) basic physiology of the system, (2) how the stress response occurs in the system, and (3) the disorders that may develop in each system as a result of the stress response or that may be aggravated by stress.

Although stress is not the sole cause of many disorders, it can contribute to their development or exacerbate them, even clearly organic diseases like epilepsy and multiple sclerosis.

||||➡

SECTION ONE: THE PHYSIOLOGY OF STRESS—THE STRESS RESPONSE

The stress response is actually a **psychophysiological response**. Psychological factors trigger and modulate the physiological response, and the stress response can influence our psychological state. In this chapter, we focus on the physiology of the stress response.

As you read this chapter, remember that we are putting together the pieces of a puzzle—the puzzle of how stress, a mental and emotional experience, affects the physical body—how one can step on a garden hose, *think* that it is a snake, and suddenly experience a cascade of physiological responses. Please read Box 4.1 now.

■ **REMINDER:** The Appendix at the end of this chapter describes the basic terms for the nervous system and explains basic principles. ■

The Generic Stress Response

How does the perception "snake" trigger the stress response? The complete answer is still a mystery, but a partial answer begins with the brain and its ability to initiate the stress response.

If you needed to fight or flee, what would you want your body to do? You immediately think of the obvious: adrenaline available,

---

BOX 4.1

KEY CONCEPTS

• The stress response occurs because mental processes affect the brain, and the brain, via the nervous system, affects the entire body. The brain is always the mediator between the mind and the body. For example, the mind has no way of directly stimulating the heart to increase heart rate when a frightful event is anticipated. Anticipation triggers particular brain centers that in turn affect the heart through nerve connections.

• The brain has two primary pathways for the stress response, **neuronal** and **hormonal**. The brain can affect the body through the intricate systems of nerves and through the release of hormones from glands. These pathways overlap in producing a response.

• **Neuroendocrine** is the term used to describe the connection between nerves and the endocrine glands, which secrete hormones. For example, the release of adrenaline from the adrenal glands is called a neuroendocrine response because the release is initiated by the hypothalamus in the brain, part of the nervous system.

• Any system or process that is influenced by neuronal or hormonal activity is potentially susceptible to stress. Consequently, the entire body is potentially susceptible to stress.

heart rate increase, blood pressure increase, increased blood flow to the large muscles of the legs, and increased depth and rate of breathing. You would also need a supply of fuel, plenty of blood to carry oxygen and fuel, and an increase in metabolism for converting fuel into energy. The body does all this and more when you confront a significant stressor. The stressor could be the type studied by Selye, such as blood loss and exposure to cold, or it could be a psychological stressor that results in fear, anxiety, or frustration; in both cases the body responds.

The body has three ways to initiate the stress response: (1) through sympathetic nerves that terminate on target organs, such as the heart and blood vessels; (2) through the release of adrenaline and noradrenaline (epinephrine and norepinephrine) from the medullae of the adrenal glands; and (3) through the release of other hormones that have a variety of effects.

Before studying these pathways of the stress response, remember that this description is simplified. The brain and nervous system are complex, and as techniques for analyzing brain function improve, knowledge of the complexity grows. Brain processes that seemed simple in one decade are shown to be complex in the next. Our impression is that directly or indirectly, every part of the brain acts in concert with every other part. It is not necessary to know the complexities and intricacies of brain functions to understand the basics of the stress response and to appreciate the significance of the fact that the body reacts to the garden hose that was mistaken for a snake.

Sympathetic Nervous System Arousal

The sympathetic division of the nervous system is the arousal system that gets the body geared up for fight or flight. The stressor could be the snake in the garden hose story, in which

an external stimulus sends sensory signals to the brain. It could also begin with a mental process, such as remembering that you left the airplane tickets at home, or left the keys in your locked car.

Figure 4.1 follows the course of events when you remember that you have locked the keys in the car and your date is waiting for you on the library lawn.

The sequence of events is:

1. Memory-image-thought: Keys are in the locked car. This is interpreted as "disaster," and the **cortex** of the brain responds.

2. The cortex sends signals to the **limbic system**, a complex of nerve centers deep in the brain, sometimes referred to as the "emotional brain" that adds emotional tone to the experience.

3. The limbic system sends signals to the **hypothalamus**, the main center in the brain that regulates the autonomic nervous system.

4. The hypothalamus has three main functions in initiating the stress response: (a) It sends signals to the anterior and posterior lobes of the **pituitary gland**, the "master" gland in the brain that regulates hormones throughout the body; (b) it sends signals to the medullae (inner portion) of the **adrenal glands**, initiating the release of adrenaline and noradrenaline; and (c) it relays "disaster" information to the centers in the lower brain, called the **pons**, that regulate such processes as heart rate and respiration. From there, signals are relayed to the rest of the body via the sympathetic nervous system. The hypothalamus is the hub of the stress response, the mediator between the cortex and lower centers of the brain, and a link between the brain and the endocrine (hormonal) system. The hypothalamus also stores the morphine-like neuropeptides, called enkephalins, which are important in pain reduction. The hypothalamus may also trigger the release of endorphins stored in the pituitary, another neuropeptide involved in

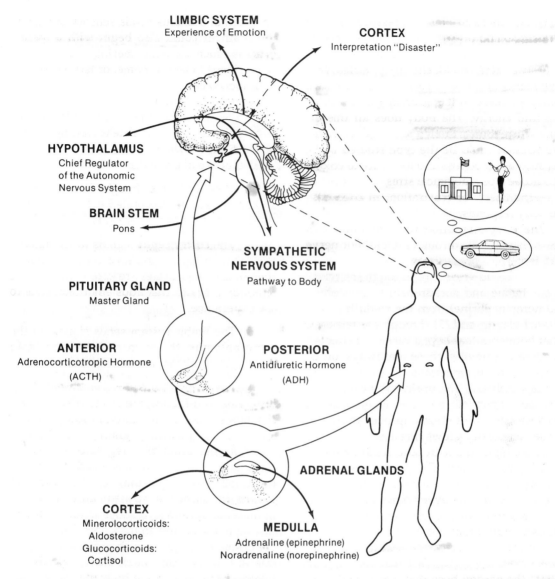

Figure 4.1 Sequence of Events in the Stress Response.

pain control. Recent evidence indicates that the hypothalamus can also affect the immune system.

5. The **anterior lobe** of the pituitary gland releases **adrenocorticotropic hormone** (ACTH). The nature and destination of ACTH can be learned from the initials: a hormone (H) that seeks (*tropic* = T) the cortex

(*cortico* = C) of the adrenal (*adreno* = A) glands. ACTH travels through blood to the **cortex** (outer portion) of the adrenal glands. The **posterior lobe** of the pituitary gland releases **antidiuretic hormone** (ADH), which causes the kidneys to retain water, thus increasing blood volume and blood pressure. Antidiuretic hormone is also called vasopressin and causes the constriction of arterioles, another mechanism for raising blood pressure.

6. The cortex of the adrenals release **corticosteroids** into circulation. There are two main types of cortico (*cortico* = cortex) steroids, **mineralocorticoids** and **glucocorticoids**. Mineralocorticoids have that name because they influence electrolyte balance, mainly sodium and potassium. **Aldosterone** is the primary mineralocorticoid. Aldosterone causes the kidneys to bring sodium and water back into blood circulation (decreasing urine formation). Increased fluid retention increases blood volume, which increases blood pressure. The glucocorticoids are so named because one function is to increase blood sugar. The main glucocorticoid is **cortisol**. In addition to increasing blood sugar, the glucocorticoids increase fat in the blood, increase protein metabolism, reduce inflammation, and reduce immune system responsivity.

Again, this is a simplified description of the stress response, focusing on the short-term response. In fact, the pituitary gland releases many hormones—including growth hormone, thyroid stimulating hormone, and reproductive hormones—that may also be affected by chronic stress. It has been reported that during the bombing of London during World War II, a severe chronic stressor, 40 percent of menstruating women missed their cycles—a sensible physiological response!

As noted above, the stress response is triggered by the sympathetic nervous system and by the release of hormones. If we had only the sympathetic nervous system to activate the body, the body would be packed solid with nerve fibers going to their many destinations. The freeways of blood and the ability of molecules to pass through blood vessels into tissue, however, enable the mechanisms of the stress response to affect the entire body without being cumbersome.

Stress has such immediate and extensive physiological effects because, through nerve pathways and substances in blood circulation, the stress response can occur throughout the body. The neuronal and hormonal mechanisms that respond to stress affect all the organs, tissues, and systems of the body.

IIII➡

SECTION TWO: STRESS AND SICKNESS

Physiology of the Stress Response

The body has many systems: nervous, cardiovascular, respiratory, gastrointestinal, endocrine, immune, and reproductive. These systems have different functions, but they are not separate; they continuously interact to maintain the functions and health of the body. For example, a primary function of the heart is to deliver oxygenated blood from the lungs to the entire body. The cardiovascular and respiratory systems continually interact; what affects one affects the other.

The systems of the body are complex, but for the purposes of this textbook we examine only basic functions that are related to the stress response and to the development of stress-related disorders. If you are planning to enter a health profession such as biofeedback therapy, you will need a thorough understanding of human anatomy and physiology. This section will prepare you for the chapters on biofeedback training and behavior medicine, and you will understand the role of stress management and relaxation in health and wellness.

The Cardiovascular System

The heart and blood vessels have many functions that are vital to life. These tasks are (1) to transport oxygen and nutrients to all tissues; (2) to transport carbon dioxide and waste products of metabolism to the lungs and kidneys;

(3) to transport hormones to target organs; (4) to maintain blood pressure; (5) to regulate body temperature by controlling blood flow to the skin; and (6) to transport the components of the immune system. The cardiovascular system must perform these tasks optimally during conditions of extreme stress or rest and when handicapped by mechanical failure or conditions such as coronary heart disease. In this subsection, we describe the heart and the vascular system separately.

The Heart

The heart has three variables that affect the circulation of blood and blood pressure: rate; force of contraction; and amount of blood pumped by each contraction, called stroke volume.

When the body is at rest, heart rate is maintained at a resting level by the dominant influence of the **parasympathetic** system, via the **vagus nerves** that originate in the brain stem. The vagus nerves carry impulses to the pacemaker in the right atrium (the SA node) at a pace that allows the heart to beat at a rate that meets the oxygen need of the body. The cardiac center in the brain stem "knows" what the oxygen demand is because it receives signals from specialized cells in the aorta and carotid arteries called chemoreceptors and baroreceptors. The heart is controlled so well by these circuits that the heartbeat is maintained even when the connections from the brain stem to the rest of the brain are severed.

The ability of the heart to effectively pump blood depends upon the strength of contraction of the heart muscle. Strength of contraction can be governed by the nervous system or by the heart itself, independently of the nervous system. As the heart fills, atrial and ventricular muscles stretch in direct proportion to the volume of blood filling the chambers. The greater the volume of blood, the greater the stretch, and the greater the force of contraction. The ability of the heart to regulate the force of contraction is called **autoregulation**.

Neuronal Control of the Heart

The heart is innervated by more sympathetic and parasympathetic nerves than any other organ. The parasympathetic fibers terminate near the pacemaker nodes and can decrease heart rate to as low as twenty to thirty beats per minute. The neurotransmitter released by parasympathetic nerve fibers is acetylcholine. The sympathetic fibers are more numerous and are more widely distributed than the parasympathetic fibers. Under maximum sympathetic stimulation, the heart rate may surpass 250 beats per minute, depending upon body weight and a person's age. The neurotransmitter released by sympathetic nerve fibers is primarily norepinephrine; at high concentrations, epinephrine from the adrenal glands can also stimulate the heart.

The contraction strength of the heart is controlled primarily by increases or decreases in sympathetic stimulation of cardiac muscle. Maximum sympathetic stimulation can increase ventricle contraction strength by approximately 100 percent above resting strength. Heart rate and contraction strength can be reduced by increasing parasympathetic stimulation and by reducing sympathetic stimulation or both. Thus a dynamic balance of forces control the heart rate, stroke volume, and blood pressure.

The Stress Response of the Heart

If you have ever waited for your turn to speak in public or to play a great poker hand, or if you have ever heard your bedroom door creak slowly open in the middle of the night, then you know how rapidly the heart responds to anticipation and fear. When you are perfectly still, with no increase in the immediate demand for oxygen, your heart prepares for action that may be no more than putting your cards on the table in triumph.

The increase in heart rate is mediated by the sympathetic nervous system. Your interpretation of the stressor—"Oh no, what if Jack has a royal flush!" or "I might win!"—triggers cortical responses that relay signals to the limbic/hypothalamic system, enabling the emotional experience and the activation of the sympathetic nervous system. The hypothalamus relays information to the cardiac accelerator center in the brain stem, which activates the sympathetic peripheral nerves that synapse near the pacemaker node and at various places along the heart muscle. This response takes about $1/100$ millisecond. Simultaneously, the hypothalamus sends signals to the adrenal medullae, which release epinephrine and norepinephrine. These chemicals stimulate the pacemaker and cardiac muscle receptors; heart rate and force of contraction increase. This response takes a few seconds, and you didn't move a muscle.

When perfectly still, you may feel your heart pounding, but you probably do not feel the automatic rise in blood pressure that occurs with increased heart rate and changes in the vascular system.

Stress-Related Disorders of the Heart

Sudden Cardiac Death. Being "scared to death" is not impossible. **Sudden cardiac death**, a dramatic result of stress, is apparently due to an excessive rush of epinephrine and

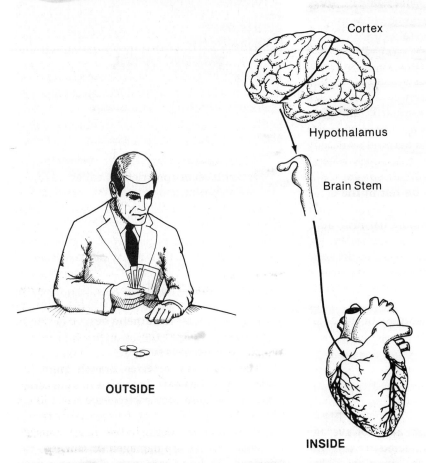

OUTSIDE

Cortex

Hypothalamus

Brain Stem

INSIDE

Figure 4.2 Although the Player Appears to Be Calm and Does Not Move, Heart Rate Will Increase with the Excitement of a Card Game.

norepinephrine that upsets the electrical conduction system of the heart. It may cause spasm of the coronary arteries and destruction of heart muscle fibers or both. Usually, this rare cause of death affects a heart that is already compromised by coronary artery disease and hypertension. In less than 10 percent of deaths, no coronary artery disease is found. Studies with laboratory animals show that large amounts of adrenaline destroy the heart muscle. Robert Eliot, a cardiologist and pioneer of the "hot reactor" personality style, suggests that people who react to life with the stressful "hot reactor" response may slowly erode the heart muscle with noradrenaline and adrenaline, making the heart increasingly more vulnerable to stress (Eliot & Breo, 1984).

Heart Arrhythmias. **Arrhythmia** refers to a disruption of the normal rhythm of the heart. Sympathetic nervous system arousal or increases of adrenaline and noradrenaline can cause the heart to beat irregularly. The most common arrhythmia is premature ventricular contraction (PVC), which is harmless when no other heart problem exists. It is clearly related to stress. PVCs are a double beat followed by a pause that can often be felt in the chest or neck.

Some arrhythmias are more harmful, such as a "fluttering" of the atria or ventricles that make it impossible for the heart to fill and pump blood properly. Although arrhythmia may not be caused by stress alone, stress can often trigger it.

Other stress-related disorders of the heart are actually problems of the vascular system and are described below.

The Vascular System

If all the blood vessels in an adult of average height and weight were connected in a line, the resulting tube could circle the globe three times. The major arteries and veins would be the first 20 feet, and the remaining 75,000 miles would be the arterioles, capillaries, and venules.

Every cell in the body depends upon an unending flow of blood, so naturally the vascular system is efficient. For our discussion of the stress response, the thousands of circular muscles that are wrapped around arteries, arterioles, and veins are the most interesting feature of the vascular system. Like all muscles, the circular muscles of the vascular system contract when activated. They decrease the diameter of the vessel when they contract; this is called **vasoconstriction**. During vasoconstriction, blood flow through vessels is reduced.

The circular muscles respond to tissue injury by constricting, and they respond to the needs of the tissues that they nourish without input from the nervous system. More importantly, however, the circular muscles are activated by the sympathetic nervous system and are therefore responsive to stress. Vasoconstriction plays a significant role in the stress response and in several physical disorders.

The sympathetic nervous system maintains a constant level of constriction, called vasomotor tone, in peripheral vessels. Vasoconstriction occurs when sympathetic impulses increase above this level, and **vasodilation** occurs when sympathetic impulses to the circular muscles decrease and the vessels dilate. Nervous system control of vasoconstriction and vasodilation is primarily through the sympathetic system; most of the vasculature of the body is not innervated by the parasympathetic nervous system. Consequently, blood flow is controlled by the sympathetic nervous system.

The **coronary arteries** branch from the aorta back to the heart. These arteries are called coronary because they encircle the heart like a crown. The importance of the coronary arteries is obvious—they nourish the heart muscle. If the coronaries are damaged or clogged, the heart muscle does not receive sufficient oxygen and cannot function. The coronary arteries have

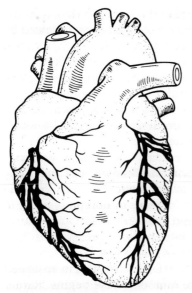

Figure 4.3 The Coronary Arteries Carry Blood to the Heart Muscle. The Circular Muscles in These Arteries Can Constrict, Reducing Blood Flow to the Heart.

circular muscles that can constrict, like the other arteries of the body.

The Stress Response of the Vascular System

The principle goal of the stress response is to prepare you to fight or flee. Both actions involve the large muscles of the body, primarily the legs. To ensure sufficient blood flow to the fight-or-flight muscles, the vascular stress response combines vasoconstriction in the extremities with vasodilation in the deep muscles. The hands, feet, and gastrointestinal tract in particular are deprived of blood; the vessels supplying other organs such as the kidneys may also constrict. When the stressor is very sudden and frightful, the face may "turn white" with vasoconstriction.

Vasoconstriction occurs when signals are relayed from the cortex to the hypothalamus to the vasomotor center in the lower brain, to the peripheral sympathetic nerves that synapse on the circular muscles. You do not need a lot of blood in your paws to escape from a bear. Vasoconstriction in the periphery makes more blood available for the muscles, heart, and brain. All of the arterioles in the periphery can constrict. Vasoconstriction of the arteries that supply the kidneys, liver, and gastrointestinal tract may cause or exacerbate hypertension, ulcers, and colitis, and it may increase blood cholesterol. Reduced blood flow to the liver decreases the removal and metabolism of cholesterol and fat in the blood, and therefore cholesterol and fatty acids in the blood increase. This increase may also be due to long-term elevation of cortisol and adrenaline, which mobilize fatty acids (such as cholesterol) from the fat deposits in the body.

Vasoconstriction reduces blood flow in hands and feet, and they decrease in temperature. If you respond to stress with vasoconstriction, you will notice that your hands and feet are cold when you are stressed, especially when you are in a cold environment. Little did we know as children that when we teased someone for being afraid by saying So-and-so "has cold feet" that we were physiologically correct! Because vasoconstriction is highly responsive to stress and plays a role in several disorders, and because vasodilation is highly responsive to relaxation, blood flow is an ideal indicator of the stress and relaxation responses. Therefore, blood flow, measured as skin temperature, is an ideal modality for biofeedback therapy, described in Chapter 8.

Together, the heart and vascular system manage the complicated tasks listed above. In addition to continuous help from the nervous system, the cardiovascular system has a partner, the kidneys. The kidneys regulate the volume of blood in the system. To understand this, remember that every drop of urine was previously blood fluid. The kidneys continually filter blood and remove fluid and waste products that will be eliminated from the body. Most of the fluid that is removed in the billion nephron units of each kidney is returned to blood a few seconds later as it passes through the tubules and the narrow loop of Henle at the end of each unit. The fluid that remains in the collecting tubule becomes urine.

If the kidneys did not return most of the fluid back into circulation, blood volume would decrease rapidly. Death from dehydration and insufficient blood pressure would occur in a few days. Anything that causes the kidneys to increase the return of fluid into circulation increases blood volume, and anything that causes the kidneys to increase urine production decreases blood volume.

Would there be an advantage to increased blood volume during stress? Yes, as a hedge against blood loss and as a mechanism for maintaining blood pressure.

During stress of the fight-or-flight type, the coronary arteries dilate to allow more blood flow to the heart muscle. In some people, however, when vigorous activity does not occur, stress has the opposite effect. The coronary arteries constrict, causing a condition called coronary artery spasm, which is one cause of angina pectoris (chest pain). When the coronary arteries constrict, blood flow to the heart muscle decreases, and the muscle is deprived of oxygen.

Stress-Related Disorders of the Vascular System

Migraine Headache. People who have **migraine headaches** describe the pain as "excruciating, piercing, throbbing, unbearable." For some patients, the headache can be stopped by drugs and bedrest within hours of onset; in others, the headache may last two or three days. Occasionally the headache is stopped only after a large dose of analgesic is given in the doctor's office or emergency room. The pain of a migraine can be unilateral, meaning in one side of the head only, or bilateral.

Migraine headaches are included under vascular disorders because in many people the headache has a clearly vascular nature. The headache begins with vasoconstriction in the extracranial and cerebral arteries, followed by "rebound" vasodilation, which is the painful phase. Some headache specialists think that migraine is neuronal, not vascular, in origin. They argue that the vascular response and the pain are secondary to a neurotransmitter disturbance in the brain, possibly in the hypothalamus or brain stem.

The mechanisms that initiate vasoconstriction are not fully known, but they may begin with sympathetic nervous system arousal and an increase in norepinephrine in extracranial and cerebral blood. The norepinephrine causes platelet aggregation, and platelets release serotonin, which simulates vasoconstriction. When serotonin in absorbed into tissue, the dilation phase begins. Rather than returning to normal, the vessels become overdilated, perhaps from fatigue of the circular muscles or perhaps to compensate for vasoconstriction. During the dilation phase, several vascular and chemical changes contribute to pain. When vessels expand, blood flow slows down (just as the current does when a river widens), and the vessels become "leaky," causing swelling in surrounding tissues. The hyperdilation, inflammation, and associated chemicals produce pain.

Migraine headaches are referred to as either **classical** or **common**. The sufferer of a classical migraine experiences warning signs such as visual disturbances, or symptoms that mimic a stroke, before the onset of pain; this phenomenon is called the "aura" and is thought to result from lack of blood flow to brain tissue during the vasoconstriction phase. The aura may precede the headache by minutes or days. In common migraine, the patient does not have a warning before headache onset.

Migraine headaches appear to have a genetic component in some people, and may have a definite trigger, especially foods that contain tyramine, such as wine and cheese. Often a migraine headache occurs simultaneously with a muscle tension headache, or it may be triggered by a muscle tension headache. Most migraine patients are aware that stress can also trigger a headache. Although there may not be a clear "migraine personality," people who have chronic migraine headaches are often stressed by a self-imposed sense of duty, perfectionism, and compulsivity.

Raynauds Disease.   Raynaud's disease is extreme vasospasm in the arteries of hands and feet. The spasm, often a reaction to cold or stress, may last a few minutes or several hours. In long-term cases, the tips of the fingers may become tender from poor blood flow. During the spasm, the skin temperature of the affected area may become very cold from lack of blood flow. Often people with Raynaud's have chronic low hand or foot temperature, indicating chronic vasoconstriction. **Raynaud's phenomenon** is a similar condition, but it results from one of the diseases that affect the peripheral vascular system.

Blood Pressure

Although blood pressure is the result of the dynamics of the cardiovascular system and the renal (kidney) system, we discuss blood pressure as though it were a system in itself. As measured with a blood-pressure cuff, blood pressure has two values: the **systolic** pressure, which is the maximum pressure in the arteries at the moment that the heart beats and forces blood into the arterial vessels, and the **diastolic** pressure, or minimum pressure in the arteries, which occurs when the heart is filling. Blood pressure is recorded as systolic "over" diastolic—for example, 120/80 mmHg.

How high is "high?" 140/90 is considered to be "borderline" high. At 140/90 and higher, some physicians recommend drug treatment and others recommend "behavioral" treatment such as exercise, weight loss, stress reduction, and biofeedback therapy. Pressure consistently above 140/90 is considered high, and drug treatment is usually recommended.

120/80 is normal. Data from life insurance companies indicate that at this level, blood pressure does not contribute to mortality. 110/70 is excellent, and as long as you have lots of energy and feel terrific, 100/60 or lower is fine. It is not surprising to find blood pressure as low as 95/60 in young college students.

Blood pressure is the result of three main variables—heart rate, stroke volume, and peripheral resistance, that are themselves influenced by many variables. Figure 4.4 illustrates the major factors involved in blood pressure regulation. Blood pressure is vital to life, and the body has many ways of maintaining adequate blood pressure and raising it in times of stress, including physical stress such as blood loss.

Heart rate is the familiar measure of the number of times that the heart beats in one minute.

Stroke volume is the amount of blood pumped from the left ventricle with each beat (stroke) of the heart. That amount is determined by (1) total volume of blood in the body, (2) total blood volume returned to the heart from the lungs to be pumped to the body, and (3) strength of contraction. Increased blood volume increases stroke volume. Consequently, blood pressure rises, if other factors do not change.

Blood volume is precisely regulated by mechanisms that control kidney function, such as blood pressure, and by stretch receptors in the heart that respond to increasing volume by sending signals to the brain to reduce sympathetic nervous system activity to the kidneys. Reduced sympathetic activity causes vasodilation, and vasodilation in the kidneys increases blood flow through the kidneys, which increases urine production, thus decreasing blood volume, which reduces stroke volume, and blood pressure decreases: ↑ blood volume → ↑ stretch response → ↑ signals to the brain → ↓ sympathetic outflow to kidneys → vasodilation → ↑ blood flow to kidneys → ↑ urine formation → ↓ blood volume → ↓ stroke volume → ↓ blood pressure.

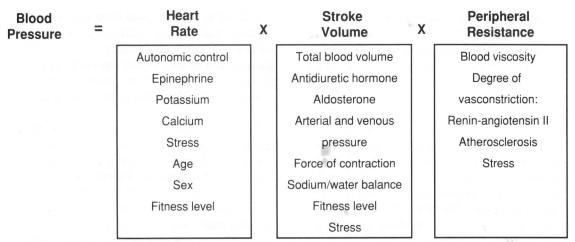

Blood Pressure =	Heart Rate X	Stroke Volume X	Peripheral Resistance
	Autonomic control	Total blood volume	Blood viscosity
	Epinephrine	Antidiuretic hormone	Degree of
	Potassium	Aldosterone	vasconstriction:
	Calcium	Arterial and venous	Renin-angiotensin II
	Stress	pressure	Atherosclerosis
	Age	Force of contraction	Stress
	Sex	Sodium/water balance	
	Fitness level	Fitness level	
		Stress	

Figure 4.4 The Main Variables That Affect Blood Pressure. Note That Stress Affects Heart Rate, Stroke Volume, and Peripheral Resistance.

Blood volume is also decreased by a recently discovered chemical, called atrial natriuretic factor (natri = sodium, uretic = makes water), which is released from the atria of the heart as a response to stretch when blood volume increases. Atrial natriuretic factor increases kidney excretion of sodium, which increases urine output, reducing blood volume and blood pressure. Two hormones cause the kidneys to form less urine, returning more fluid into blood circulation and increasing blood volume. These hormones are **aldosterone**, released by the cortex of the adrenal glands, and **antidiuretic hormone** (ADH, also called vasopressin), released by the posterior pituitary. (These hormones were discussed in the previous chapter because they are involved in the stress response.)

Peripheral resistance is the resistance to the flow of blood in the periphery, meaning all of the body outside the brain and spinal cord. Peripheral resistance is affected primarily by the diameter of the arterioles through which blood flows. When the diameter of the vessels decreases, blood pressure increases.

A garden hose is a commonly used analogy to explain the variables involved in blood pressure.

Imagine a garden hose (vascular system) with a nozzle (circular muscles) for regulating the flow of water (blood) through the hose; the knob controls the flow of water (heart rate); and the pressure and flow can also be regulated by the size and force of the pump in the pumping station (stroke volume). If any variable changes while others remain constant, pressure in the hose will increase (increased blood pressure). For example, as the nozzle is closed (vasoconstriction), there is greater resistance to the flow (increased peripheral resistance), and pressure in the hose increases (increased blood pressure). As the nozzle is opened (vasodilation), there is less resistance (decreased peripheral resistance), and pressure in the hose goes down (decreased blood pressure). If the nozzle and faucet are unchanged but the pump is replaced with a bigger one, pressure in the system increases. If the hose is old and filled with deposits (atherosclerosis) or with icy slush (high blood viscosity), pressure increases. However, if the hose is very elastic and expands easily, then when flow or pressure increases (heart rate or stroke volume increases) or when the nozzle is tightened (vasoconstriction) pressure does not greatly increase

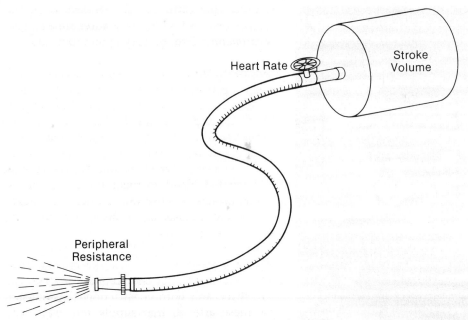

Figure 4.5   The Garden Hose Analogy for the Three Main Factors That Affect Blood Pressure.

because the hose expands (elastic blood vessels).

If a single variable changes while the others remain constant, then blood pressure will change. However, if one of the variables begins to change, the body can automatically change another variable to compensate. For example, if stroke volume and blood pressure drop because of blood loss, vasoconstriction will increase peripheral resistance and blood pressure will increase. The body makes continual adjustments in the system to ensure sufficient blood flow and pressure so that tissues can be nourished and the kidneys can function.

The kidneys can play an active role in the regulation of peripheral resistance. The kidneys are very sensitive to low pressure and have a mechanism for raising it because they cannot function unless blood pressure is high enough for filtration of fluid and wastes. Of all the organs, only the kidneys work on pressure; if pressure is not high enough in the nephron

unit to allow removal of wastes, death follows. Every nephron unit contains cells that release the hormone **renin** when pressure is too low. Renin in the blood is quickly converted into Angiotensin I, which is converted by an enzyme into Angiotensin II. **Angiotensin II** is a powerful vasoconstrictor that increases peripheral resistance. Angiotensin II also interacts with aldosterone, causing an increase in fluid retention and increased stroke volume. As you see, the body has many ways to increase blood pressure.

Heart rate and peripheral resistance respond rapidly to stress via sympathetic nervous system activation of the heart and vasoconstriction. That is why blood pressure can increase in seconds with stress. The stress of having blood pressure taken in the doctor's office can raise blood pressure considerably, a phenomenon called "white coat hypertension" (Pickering, James, Boddie, Harshfield, Blank, & Laragh, 1988).

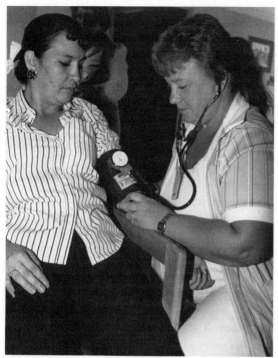

The Stress of Having Blood Pressure Taken in the Doctor's Office Can Raise Blood Pressure. *Source:* Gordon Steward, Denver, CO.

Stress-Related Disorders of the Cardiovascular System

The cardiovascular system has a central role in fight-or-flight response because heightened cardiovascular functioning is crucial for survival. However, as tiger-type threats to survival have decreased, two aspects of cardiovascular functioning have become hazardous to health: the ability of the system to respond to anticipated stress, and the ability of the system to respond to any stressor that the human responds to, even when fight or flight are not required. The emotions that the cardiovascular system responds to most readily are anticipation, fear, anxiety and the Type A personality characteristics of anger, hostility, and competitiveness. When these emotional responses become

chronic, the cardiovascular system is chronically stimulated with jabs of adrenaline and noradrenaline. Over time, symptoms develop.

Angina Pectoris. Angina pectoris refers to feelings of pressure and pain in the chest that may radiate to the neck and jaw, left shoulder and left arm, and occasionally the right arm. The pain usually occurs with exercise, but it can also result from stress. Angina occurs when the coronary arteries cannot deliver enough oxygenated blood to meet the needs of the heart muscle because the arteries are clogged by atherosclerosis or because of a coronary artery spasm, or both.

Coronary Artery Spasm. Like all circular muscles, the muscles of the coronary arteries can constrict, and with constriction, the diameter of these arteries that supply the heart with blood decreases, decreasing blood flow to the heart muscle. Excessive adrenaline and noradrenaline levels resulting from stress may trigger the spasm.

Atherosclerosis. Atherosclerosis results from the formation of fatty plaques on the inner lining of arteries. One cause of plaque formation is injury to the vessel and the consequent build-up of connective tissue and platelets as part of the repair. The injury may be caused by high blood pressure. Fats adhere to the injured area, a process that is worsened by high blood cholesterol and fats in blood. The plaques cause hardening, clogging, and weakening of the artery. The build-up of fatty, cholesterol-containing plaques occurs most frequently in the arteries of the heart, brain, and kidneys, leading to complications that account for the majority of all deaths in the United States. Stress hormones (adrenaline, noradrenaline, and corticosteroids) elevate blood cholesterol and fat and may play a role in atherosclerosis. Stress plays another role when overeating and obesity are stress-related.

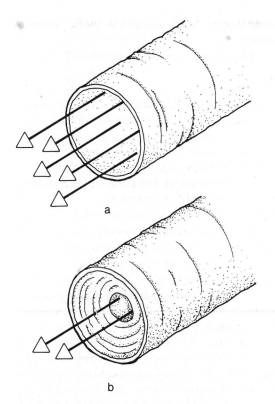

a

b

Figure 4.6   A Normal Artery and an Atherosclerotic Artery. The Atherosclerotic Artery Is Clogged with Fats and Scar Tissue and Can Reduce Blood Flow to the Brain, Heart, Kidneys, or Other Areas of the Body.

Essential Hypertension. Essential hypertension refers to high blood pressure that is not caused by an organic problem, such as kidney failure. High blood pressure is commonly defined as systolic pressure greater than 140 mmHg and diastolic pressure greater than 90 mmHg, but data indicate that pressures higher than 120/80 contribute a degree of risk for coronary heart disease. The relationship between risk and blood pressure is linear, so the higher the blood pressure, the higher the risk. Stress contributes to hypertension by increasing resistance to blood flow with vasoconstriction, by increasing heart rate and stroke volume through increased blood volume that results from the release of aldosterone from the

adrenal glands, and by releasing antidiuretic hormone from the pituitary. In addition, atherosclerosis contributes to hypertension by narrowing arteries and thereby increasing peripheral resistance.

Hypertension is a major risk factor in many types of cardiovascular disease, including coronary artery disease and heart attack; cerebral vascular accidents such as stroke; kidney failure; and the destruction of the tiny arteries in the eyes. Hypertension is also a cause of **left ventricular hypertrophy**, which contributes to **congestive heart failure**. When the heart must pump blood against high resistance in the body, the left ventricle enlarges in the effort. Congestive heart failure results when the heart becomes an ineffective pump and blood flow becomes congested. Back pressure resulting from insufficient blood flow causes fluid to seep from vessels into body tissue. The resulting swelling is called edema. Edema in the lungs results in difficulty in breathing and can cause death.

Platelet Aggregation. Platelets are much smaller than red and white blood cells. They have the ability to stick together and to adhere to the injury site in blood vessels, which enables them to form blood clots to prevent bleeding. Platelet aggregation increases the formation of plaques and emboli, which are clots that travel through the vascular system. When a clot is caught in a narrowed artery in the lungs, brain, or heart, it obstructs blood flow and causes tissue damage. Elevated levels of noradrenaline and adrenaline may increase platelet aggregation; therefore, stress may be a factor in platelet aggregation.

The cardiovascular system is affected by many factors in addition to stress. Lifestyle factors such as obesity, smoking, high blood cholesterol, high triglyceride levels, and inadequate exercise all contribute to cardiovascular disease. It is clear, however, that stress does more damage to a system compromised by other risk factors.

The Digestive System: The Gastrointestinal Tract

The digestive system is not as dramatic as the cardiovascular system, and it may not be the most exciting system to discuss. Certainly it is not the most fun to see your doctor about. The whole system is important, however, because it is highly responsive to stress and abuse. Gastrointestinal complaints account for about 40 percent of all medical appointments.

From beginning to end, the gastrointestinal tract serves two primary functions—the absorption of nutrients and the elimination of wastes. The task of absorption of nutrients includes the breakdown of large carbohydrate, protein, and fat molecules into particles small enough to pass from the gastrointestinal (GI) tract into lymph and blood, and from blood into all the cells of the body. The GI tract continuously mixes and moves material along the entire route.

Protein in food is broken down into small packages by gastric enzymes, particularly **pepsin**, aided by **hydrochloric acid**. Because pepsin can initiate the digestion of all types of protein, including the protein of the stomach itself, the stomach and intestines produce thick mucus that protects them from digestion by pepsin and from erosion by hydrochloric acid.

To accomplish the task of mixing and movement, the entire tract has muscles that move material forward. The slow, rhythmic contractions are called **peristaltic waves**, and the process is called **peristalsis**. Other muscle activity controls mixing, forward and backward movement of material, the squeezing of material into segments, and the rate of movement in different sections of the tract during the various stages of digestion.

Like the heart, the stomach and intestines have mechanisms that enable them to do their work without input from the central nervous system. However, like the heart, the stomach and intestines are innervated by the sympathetic and parasympathetic nervous systems.

The process of digestion does not begin with eating. The GI tract responds to the **anticipation** of eating. When you think about food, signals travel from the cortex to the hypothalamus, initiating parasympathetic activity. The hungrier you are, the greater the response. This is another good example of mind $\longrightarrow$ body. Unlike other systems, the GI tract is activated by the parasympathetic nervous system and is inhibited by the sympathetic system. When food is anticipated, the parasympathetic system stimulates cells in the stomach lining that secrete gastric juices.

When food enters the stomach, increased secretion of gastric juices occurs because of increased parasympathetic stimulation of cells in the lining of the stomach. These cells release more pepsin, hydrochloric acid, and **gastrin**, a hormone that causes the gastric glands to increase secretion of pepsin and acid even more. Gastrin flow is also increased by distension of the stomach wall and by the presence of certain foods, particularly meat and partially digested proteins, by caffeine and alcohol, and by spices such as pepper or chili.

The GI tract has mechanisms for controlling the rate of digestion and the rate at which material moves from the stomach into the small intestine. Fats may stay in the stomach for several hours and slow the emptying of the stomach. As material enters the small intestine, the pancreas, liver, and gallbladder are stimulated to secrete a variety of enzymes and bile salts to promote the digestion of proteins, fats, and carbohydrates.

The large intestine, or colon, has the primary functions of removing water and sodium from waste material and storing the waste until the "go now" signal hits in a socially appropriate situation. To protect the colon from abrasion by undigested substances and from digestive enzymes, mucus is abundantly produced by cells in its lining. The production of mucus is stimulated by the presence of

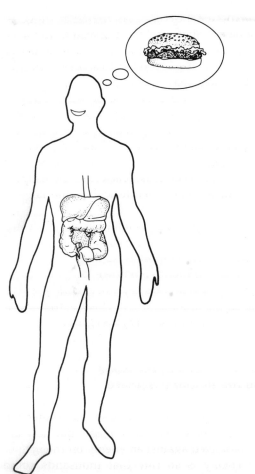

Figure 4.7 The Digestive System Responds to the Anticipation of Food, an Excellent Example of Mind-Body Interaction.

The Stress Response of the Gastrointestinal Tract

Although the GI tract does not play a role in the fight-or-flight response, it responds to stress in unusual and paradoxical ways.

The GI tract has at least five primary responses to stress: (1) reduction of protective mucus secretion; (2) vasoconstriction of the blood vessels in the lining of the stomach and intestines; (3) inhibition of peristalsis and other movement; (4) increased sympathetic activity in the colon, which increases constriction and decreases normal movement; and (5) a paradoxical rebound effect in which parasympathetic activity increases, increasing motility and acid secretion. This is paradoxical because the digestive system is designed to function during relaxation and to shut down during stress. The paradoxical increase in parasympathetic activity with stress, which often occurs when there is not enough food in the system to neutralize acid, plagues only some people and only with certain kinds of stress. Other people have the opposite GI stress response in which movement stops.

During short-term stress, the inhibition of the digestive system is not harmful. Humans, of course, have the ability to eat and be stressed at the same time and to prolong stress. The GI tract responds with a variety of symptoms.

Stress-Related Disorders of the Digestive System and Gastrointestinal Tract

Ulcers. Stomach (gastric) and duodenal peptic ulcers are the most common stress-related disorder of the GI tract. The duodenum, the first section of the small intestine to receive material directly from the stomach, is an area of high concentration of acid or pepsin. An ulcer is a sore in the mucus lining of the stomach or intestine that develops when the tissues are weakened and destroyed. The precise mechanisms of ulcer formation are not fully understood, but the process may be related to several factors—hypersecretion of acid and pepsin

material in the colon and by the parasympathetic system.

Amazingly, the continuous activity of the digestive system is unnoticed except at the very end point, when pressure in the rectum definitely makes its way into consciousness. This lack of consciousness is a blessing, but when things go wrong, the entire GI tract seems capable of distress. From swallowing to elimination, the sensations of pain, nausea and general discomfort can be nearly overwhelming.

when the stomach is empty, vasoconstriction of the blood vessels that nourish the lining of the GI tract, and decreased mucus production.

Irritable Bowel Syndrome. The irritable bowel syndrome is a pain in the gut. Besides pain, common symptoms are diarrhea alternating with constipation, "bloating," and gas. About 50 percent of all GI illness in the United States is diagnosed as irritable bowel syndrome. The cause of irritable bowel syndrome is unknown. "Spastic colon" and "irritable colon" are other names for the same symptoms.

In all patients, the basic problem is disregulation of muscle activity, affecting the small intestine or the colon or both. When the contents of the small intestine are moved into the colon too quickly, carrying unneutralized acid and undigested food, the colon reacts with diarrhea. When the circular muscles of the colon—which normally act like a gentle food compactor—become inactive, constipation results.

Stress, with components of anxiety or depression, is a well-known factor in irritable bowel syndrome. In a recent medical text on GI disorders and stress, the author, a gastroenterologist, states that after diagnosing irritable bowel syndrome, the physician "must inform the patient about the body-mind connection of the disorder" (Dotevall, 1985, p. 120).

The pain of irritable bowel syndrome is caused by increased pain sensitivity and distension in segments of the tract.

Colitis. "Itis" refers to inflammation or swelling, so colitis means inflammation of the colon. Ulcerative colitis is inflammation and ulceration of the colon, characterized by attacks of bloody diarrhea. Pathologic changes include blockage of the capillaries in the lining of the colon; ulcer-like destruction of the mucus membrane that protects the colon; and in advanced disease, destruction of the muscular layer. Complete recovery from ulcerative colitis is possible, but often the disease is chronic.

Esophageal Spasm. As the term suggests, esophageal spasm refers to spasm in the muscles of the esophagus that enables swallowing and movement of food to the stomach. Esophageal spasm makes swallowing difficult and painful. The spasm may occur with eating or as a stress response. Esophageal spasm can also occur as a conditioned response following the frightening experience of choking on food. Esophageal spasm often occurs when acid from the stomach leaks back into the esophagus, which cannot tolerate acidic material.

Globus Hystericus. Globus hystericus is the technical term for the feeling of having "a lump in the throat." The physical cause of this unpleasant sensation is unknown, and there is no organic disease. The symptom is clearly stress-related, and it is easy to hypothesize that it may be related to a need to express grief.

The Defenses of the Body and the Immune System

The fight-or-flight response is protection against threats from the outside, but how are you protected against an enemy on the inside? The enemy is so tiny that thousands could crowd onto the head of a pin and still not be seen, and can take up residence anywhere in the body. The answer: Create a defense that is equally tiny and can meet the enemy head-on, a defense system that can move anywhere in the body and that can overpower the enemy by sheer numbers. In fact, the body has 1 trillion cells that destroy **pathogens** (disease-causing agents) either directly or by creating substances that destroy them. Many of these cells migrate throughout the other trillions of cells in the body, and all have remarkable abilities.

If you were designing a defense system for your body, what would you want it to do? An obvious answer: Kill bacteria and viruses and cancer cells, and get rid of debris in blood and in tissue, and not just on Mondays. The defenses would need to know the difference between normal and abnormal cells—that is, between "self" and "not self" so that it would not destroy its own body. The ability to know the difference between self and not-self is perhaps the most important aspect of immunity, although the mechanism for this is not known.

The defense systems would also have to know where the battle is, how big an army is needed, and when the battle is won, and would need a way of remembering enemies. You would also design a defense system that is fast, vicious, and vigilant.

The body has many defenses, including the skin; the acid in the gastrointestinal tract that destroys bacteria; the tears of the eyes; the mucus of the GI tract; the nose and lungs that trap particles; and the millions of tiny hair-like cilia that move particles out of the lungs. By far the most dramatic and effective defense, however, results from the constant and coordinated activity of cells that arise from common ancestors in bone marrow. These cells develop into several types of specialized cells that work together. The main cell types that defend the body are **macrophages, neutrophils, T lymphocytes** and **B lymphocytes**. These cells and their interactions are diagrammed in Figure 4.8. Familiarize yourself with the diagram at this time.

Another word for defense is immunity, and all of these cells provide immunity. Lymphocytes destroy specific pathogens that they have "learned" to recognize. This type of immunity is referred to as **acquired immunity**, or as **specific immunity**, because the ability to recognize specific pathogens is acquired during the development of the lymphocyte. **Immune system** refers to the lymphocytes and their activities. Macrophages and neutrophils are capable of destroying pathogens without prior preparation; the immunity of these cells is referred to as **innate immunity**. Innate immunity also includes the various defenses such as the skin and acids in the stomach. Neutrophils and macrophages are the scavengers of the body. They destroy unwanted material by digesting it,

a process called phagocytosis (*phago* = to eat, *cyt* = cell, *osis* = intensive).

Neutrophils and macrophages can also move to the site of infection and play a role in inflammation and the destruction of foreign material. The swelling or inflammation around the infected area prevents the infection from spreading. Neutrophils can squeeze through pores in capillary membranes and move from blood circulation into tissue. Before maturing, macrophages are called **monocytes** and are small; once a monocyte slips through the vascular wall, it swells into a large cell called a macrophage, which can destroy bacteria and particles—even bits of wood or parasites—that are too large for a neutrophil to handle. Some macrophages, called tissue macrophages, dwell permanently in the lymph nodes and air sacs of the lungs, where the likelihood of encountering foreign material is high. Tissue macrophages can live in tissue for years and are the first line of defense against infection. Neutrophils that are not in circulation reside in bone marrow. They begin to multiply and to move toward the site of infection when infection occurs. Please read Box 4.2 now.

Neutrophils and macrophages defend the body against disease by destroying bacteria, viruses, virus-infected cells, and cancer cells through phagocytosis, but the body has other methods of defense that are the function of T lymphocytes and B lymphocytes, called "lymphocytes" because they reside primarily in the lymphatic system. Like neutrophils and monocytes, (the precursor of macrophages), lymphocytes are called white blood cells because they evolve from the same type of "master cell" in bone marrow as red blood cells and appear "whitish" under the microscope.

The defenses of the body can be described as a team. We can think of the four main players as the neutrophils, the macrophages, the T lymphocytes, and the B lymphocytes. Now we focus on these major classes of lymphocytes and their immune system activities. The immune system has two divisions: a **cellular division**

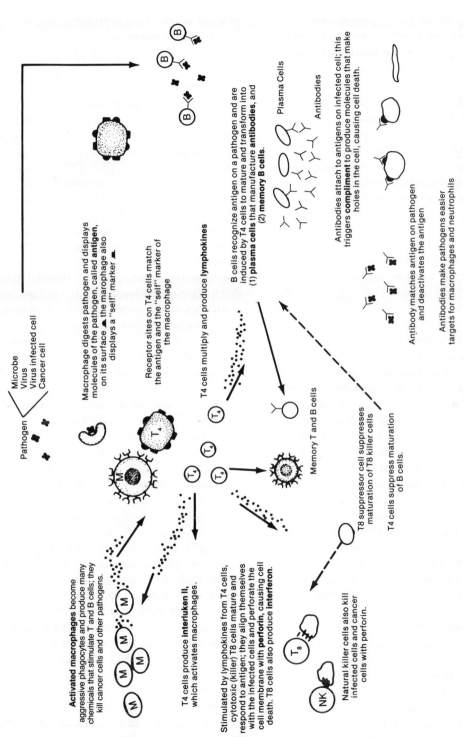

Figure 4.8 **The Principal Cells of the Immune System and Their Functions. These Cells Communicate Through Chemicals and Are a Defensive Team.**

Pathogen

Microbe
Virus
Virus infected cell
Cancer cell

Activated macrophages become aggressive phagocytes and produce many chemicals that stimulate T and B cells; they kill cancer cells and other pathogens.

Macrophage digests pathogen and displays molecules of the pathogen, called **antigen**, on its surface ▲ the macrophage also displays a "self" marker ■.

Receptor sites on T4 cells match the antigen and the "self" marker of the macrophage

T4 cells produce **interluken II**, which activates macrophages.

T4 cells multiply and produce **lymphokines**

Stimulated by lymphokines from T4 cells, cytotoxic (killer) T8 cells mature and respond to antigen; they align themselves with the infected cells and perforate the cell membrane with **perforin**, causing cell death. T8 cells also produce **interferon**.

Memory T and B cells

T8 suppressor cell suppresses maturation of T8 killer cells

T4 cells suppress maturation of B cells.

Natural killer cells also kill infected cells and cancer cells with perforin.

B cells recognize antigen on a pathogen and are induced by T4 cells to mature and transform into (1) **plasma cells** that manufacture **antibodies**, and (2) **memory B cells.**

Plasma Cells

Antibodies

Antibodies attach to antigens on infected cell; this triggers **compliment** to produce molecules that make holes in the cell, causing cell death.

Antibody matches antigen on pathogen and deactivates the antigen

Antibodies make pathogens easier targets for macrophages and neutrophils

115

THE LYMPHATIC SYSTEM

The body is really a giant balloon filled with fluid. When the fluid is in blood vessels it is called blood, and when it is in the kidneys and bladder it is called urine; when it is bathing the cells of the body it is called cellular fluid, and when it is in the lymphatic system it is called lymph.

Like the vascular system, the lymphatic system extends throughout the body and is a system of vessels and organs. Unlike the vascular system, it has no pump and does not circulate through a continuous circuit as blood does. Extracellular fluid seeps into the lymphatic vessels and is moved along through the system when the lymphatic vessels are squeezed during body movement and muscle contraction. The lymphatic system empties into blood circulation.

The lymphatic system has two main functions—it carries molecules from digestion that are too large to be absorbed directly from the gastrointestinal tract and empties them into blood circulation, and it

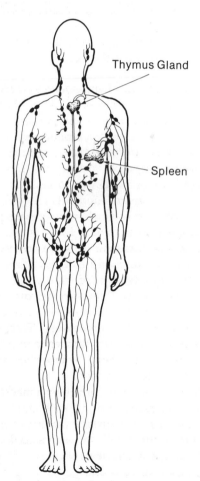

Thymus Gland

Spleen

Figure 4.9   The Lympathetic System and Organs Involved in Immunity.

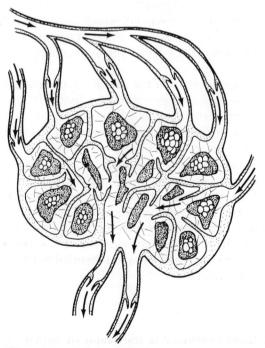

Figure 4.10   A Lymph Node.

is a primary site of the defense of the body against pathogens.

The parts of the lymphatic system that are particularly involved in defense are the lymph nodes, the spleen, the thymus gland, and areas in the gastrointestinal tract called Peyer's patches. Before birth and for several months after birth, the thymus processes undifferentiated cells into the basic types of lymphocytes that will provide protection for life. The lymph nodes, spleen, and Peyer's patches house masses of macrophages and lymphocytes. Debris, toxins, and abnormal cells are transported in lymph, and they are destroyed as the lymph moves through these special tissues.

Note the intricate channels in which lymph flows through a lymph node. The branching channels carry debris, toxic substances, bacteria, cancer cells, and other pathogens past the tissue macrophages and T and B lymphocytes that dwell in the node, a clever device for catching pathogens. When a battle is raging in a lymph node, it may become tender and swollen.

composed of a variety of T lymphocytes that recognize a pathogen by its specific molecular trademark, called an **antigen**, which destroy unwanted cells through cell-to-cell interaction; and a **humoral division**, composed of B lymphocytes that recognize specific antigens and produce specific mole-cules called **antibodies** (also called **immunoglobulins**—*immuno* = immune function, *globuline* = glob), which cause the destruction or deactivation of the pathogen. Like good team members, the players support each other.

The processes of the immune system begin when a macrophage destroys a "not-self" cell or a cell that is harboring a virus, or destroys other foreign matter. After digesting a cell or other material, the macrophage puts a partly digested protein, the antigen, from the material onto its own surface for recognition by T lymphocytes and B lymphocytes. Macrophages also release a substance called lymphokine, which activates lymphocytes and stimulates the brain to raise body temperature. A fever speeds cellular activity, and it may inhibit viral and bacterial growth.

Cellular Immunity

Cellular immunity is the result of teamwork among T cells and the special communication between a particular T cell, the T4 helper/inducer cell, and macrophages.

T Lymphocytes.   Lymphocytes emerge from bone marrow "unprocessed." About half these cells go to finishing school in the thymus, where they become T lymphocytes. They are named T cells because they are processed in the thymus gland. In the thymus, T cells are prepared to recognize the thousands of antigens that a human encounters in a lifetime. This is achieved through an ingenious process in cell division in which DNA is rearranged and a million different cells are created. Each cell is capable of recognizing a different antigen. The mechanism of recognition is the receptor site on the T cell surface, and the rearrangement of DNA creates cells with different receptor sites. After processing, T cells leave the thymus and take up residence in lymphoid tissue all over the body, where they wait for the signal to go into action.

When an antigen, carried by a macrophage, matches the receptor of a T cell, and when the macrophage's own surface molecules match a receptor on the T cell, the activated T cell begins to divide. T cells mature into two types, T4 helper/inducer cells and T8 killer cells. Much of the cellular immune response is orchestrated by the T4 helper/inducer lymphocytes, so named because they help other cells do their job and because they induce other cells into action, as indicated in Figure 4.8. They also enhance or suppress B cells and the production of antibodies. T4 helper/inducer cells are the primary target of the human immunodeficiency virus, the cause of acquired immune deficiency syndrome (AIDS), described in Box 4.3.

The types of T lymphocyte cells are: killer T8, helper/inducer T4, suppressor T, and memory T. These cells communicate through several types of powerful proteins called **lymphokines**, which they manufacture and release as needed.

Helper/Inducer T4 Cells. As noted above, these cells are the quarterbacks of cellular immunity; they help macrophages, killer T8 cells, and B cells in their jobs, although they do not kill cells or produce antibodies themselves. After recognizing an antigen that is displayed on a macrophage, helper/inducer T4 cells release lymphokines that stimulate the multiplication of other helper/inducer T4 cells, killer T8 cells,

---

BOX 4.3

ACQUIRED IMMUNE DEFICIENCY SYNDROME

AIDS was detected in the United States in 1981 when an unusual number of uncommon diseases were reported to the Centers for Disease Control—a rare form of pneumonia, a rare cancer, and certain central nervous system disorders. These diseases have an underlying feature—they are the result of impaired immunity, and in 1981 they were found only among homosexual men. Based on these observations, it was determined that the impaired immunity resulted from a process that could be transferred from person to person. It was named acquired immune deficiency syndrome, and although the cause was unknown, a virus was suspected.

Clues to the nature of the transmission and cause of AIDS accumulated as it was discovered that AIDS is most prevalent among people who engage in homosexual behavior with many partners; among people who receive blood transfusions, notably hemophiliacs; among children whose mother has AIDS; and among intravenous drug users sharing needles. The consistent finding was a depletion of T4 helper/inducer cells.

It took nearly three years of intensive research to discover that AIDS is caused by a virus called human immunodeficiency virus (HIV). HIV has a particular affinity for T4 helper/inducer cells. The virus invades these cells, and as a response, the immune system creates antibodies in an attempt to eliminate the infected T4 cells. The presence of antibodies is the first indication that a person is infected with HIV, and it provides a means for detecting infection and for screening blood donated for transfusion. Typically, T4 cell production increases as a response to infection, but within one year, T4 cell count begins a slow decline. Apparently, the immune system destroys the infected cells, and when the virus—triggered by unknown factors—rapidly propagates within T4 cells, the host cell is destroyed. Clinical signs of AIDS may not appear for several years, but the majority of people who have HIV will eventually develop AIDS. They will be vulnerable to diseases that the severely impaired immune system cannot prevent, as T4 cells are destroyed and HIV begins to replicate uncontrollably (Redfield & Burke, 1988).

As of December 31, 1988, a total of 82,764 AIDS cases had been reported to the Centers for Disease Control, and it is estimated that 1.5 million people in the United States are infected with the virus. Since reporting began in 1981, more than half the people with AIDS have died; of these, 63 percent were homosexual men who were not IV drug users, and 19 percent were heterosexual men and women who were IV drug users. Three percent of the victims were infected by blood transfusion. More grimly, 86 percent of people diagnosed with AIDS before 1986 have died (Centers for Disease Control, 1989). As of July 1988, 1,054 children under 13 years of age with AIDS had been reported (Heyward & Curran, 1988). As of July 1, 1988, 100,410 cases of AIDS from 138 countries had been reported to the World Health Organization. Based on this figure and on the latency period between infection and the development of symptoms, it is estimated that 5 million to 10 million people are infected worldwide, and that at a minimum, 1 million additional cases will be reported in the next five years (Mann & Chin, 1988).

The latency period between infection and appearance of symptoms makes AIDS particularly difficult to control because an infected person may not be aware of the danger and may transmit the virus unknowingly. To date, there is no medical cure for AIDS and no vaccine against HIV. For this reason, behavioral prevention of the spread of HIV—based on voluntary screening for the virus in people at risk for AIDS, the use of condoms, the use of uncontaminated needles, and other precautions—is the only solution to the spread of the virus.

and B cells. When B cells have increased sufficiently, helper/inducer T4 cells then release a lymphokine that instructs some of the B cells to become plasma cells and produce antibodies. Helper/inducer T4 cells also produce **interferon**, which has similar effects, and also keeps macrophages at the site of infection.

Killer T8 Cells. Killer T8 cells (also called T8 cytotoxic cells; *cyto* means cell and *toxic* means poisonous) have a more refined method of killing virus-infected cells and cancer cells than the macrophages and neutrophils that employ phagocytosis. Killer T8 cells align themselves with the cell and secrete a cylinder-shaped molecule called **perforin**, which punches a hole in the membrane of the virus-infected cell. The perforation allows the contents to spill out and water and salts to flow in, and the cell bursts (Young & Cohn, 1988). Killer T8 cells also secrete several other substances that recruit uncommitted T cells, attract macrophages to the site, stimulate macrophages to greater activity, and prevent them from leaving the area. Killer T cells also secrete a type of interferon that inhibits viral replication and enhances killer T cell activity.

Suppressor T8 Cells. Suppressor T8 cells turn off some of the activities of T cells and B cells when the immune response is no longer needed to fight against a particular antigen. Without suppression, the immune response could escalate out of control.

Memory T Cells. Some T4 cells stop multiplying and become memory cells that survive with the receptor-site "memory" of the antigen; when the antigen is encountered again, the response will be faster. Often the second response is so fast that the pathogen is destroyed before signs of the disease occur. Memory T cells enter circulation and can patrol the body for many months. Memory T cells are the basis of vaccination and immunity that arises from having an infection once.

Natural Killer Cells. Another type of cell was discovered in 1974, the natural killer cell. The natural killer cell is a lymphocyte of unknown origin. It is like the killer T cell but does not arise from the antigen response of T cells. It can kill certain cells spontaneously, without needing an antigen as a guide. Natural killer cells are the first defense of the immune system against virus-infected cells and cancer cells.

Humoral Immunity

B Lymphocytes. Lymphocytes that become B cells reside in lymphoid tissue. These cells are called "B cells" because when discovered they seemed to be the human equivalent of cells that are produced in the bursa of birds, which is specialized tissue near the tail. Like T4 cells, the DNA of multiplying B cells can be rearranged so that millions of B cells are produced, each capable of recognizing a different antigen. Through the random arrangement of DNA in T and B cells, these cells develop millions of receptors, making the immune system able to recognize all the antigens that nature and humans create.

When a B cell recognizes an antigen on a macrophage and is stimulated by a T4 helper/inducer cell, it begins to multiply; some of the new cells become memory B cells, and some become **plasma cells**. Plasma cells, the factories of antibody molecules, produce a specific antibody for the antigen that the original B cell recognized. Antibodies are proteins and are called immunoglobulins; there are five major classes of immunoglobulins, and two of these comprise about 93 percent of all antibodies. Those two are immunoglobulin G (IgG), which is found in blood and tissue fluids and is particularly effective against bacteria, viruses, and toxins; and immunoglobulin A (IgA), which is found in the respiratory tract and mouth, tears, stomach, and intestines for control of bacterial and viral infections.

A plasma cell can produce about 2,000 antibody molecules each second for several days until the cell dies. Antibody molecules travel to the site of the invasion through lymph and blood. When antibody molecules link up with the matching antigen on an unwanted cell, a complex is formed that activates an antimicrobial protein in blood, called **complement**. Complement is actually several types of protein that have different functions. Complement causes cell death by punching holes in the cell's membrane when it combines with the antigen-antibody complex. Complement proteins also increase phagocytosis and cause the release of histamine in damaged tissue, which increases the permeability of capillaries so that neutrophils, monocytes, and lymphocytes can get into tissue and fight infection or deactivate molecules that cause allergies. Antibody molecules also make cells easier targets for phagocytes and apparently make them "tastier" so that phagocytosis is increased. B cells, like macrophages, display antigens and can induce T cells to respond to the antigen.

The immune system is a complex, highly interactive system that allows us to rest easy, knowing that 1 trillion cells are ready to work as a team to protect us. So powerful is the system that even during the twelfth-century plague, when one third of the population of Europe died, two thirds lived.

The Nervous System and the Immune System

The brain and the immune system interact. If we were writing about any other system in the body, this would be obvious. The connection between the nervous system and the immune system has not been obvious. Research on the connections between the two has blossomed only in the last twenty years.

"But," you might say, "the connection is obvious, because when I'm really stressed I am more likely to catch the next bug that comes along, and stress gets into the body through the nervous system, so the nervous system must influence the immune system." This makes sense, but for years neurologists and immunologists believed that the nervous system and the immune system could not interact, because there was no known mechanism for it and because the immune system seems to do very well on its own. This short section is included because nervous system-immune system interaction is a mechanism for the relationship between stress and disease and for the affect of mind on immunity. Without this interaction there could be no "case of Mr. Wright."

For research evidence about nervous system-immune system interaction, we turn immediately to the work of Robert Ader, a psychologist who made an accidental discovery while studying conditioning in rats. Ader discovered that T lymphocytes of rats can be conditioned in the same way that Pavlov's dogs were conditioned to salivate at the sound of a bell when the bell was repeatedly paired with meat powder in the dog's mouth.

In 1974 Ader was conducting a standard aversive conditioning experiment with rats. The rats were first deprived of water and then allowed to drink water flavored with saccharin. Immediately after drinking, the animals received an injection of a drug that causes nausea and diarrhea. After this single pairing of the flavored water and the drug, the rats would not drink the saccharin water again when repeatedly exposed to it. This response is no surprise, because animals quickly learn to avoid noxious stimuli—the rats probably felt nauseated when they smelled the water. This happens to humans, too, as we know from the effects of chemotherapy described in Chapter 2. The surprise was that some rats died during the period of repeated exposures to the water. Searching for a reason for the unusual deaths, Ader found that the drug used to create the aversion suppresses the immune system. But it wasn't the single dose that suppressed the immune system and killed the animals—it was the re-exposure to the water after the pairing. Instead of the autonomic nervous system being conditioned, as in the case of

chemotherapy or Pavlov's dogs, this was *conditioning of the immune system,* an unheard of response. (Ader found similar research by two Russian scientists published in the 1920s.) This explained the death of the rats (Ader & Cohen, 1984).

Experiments such as this have been repeated many times and the results are consistent—the immune system responds to conditioning; immunosuppression occurs when the rat is re-exposed to the aversive conditioned stimulus, because immunosuppression occurred when the drug and water were first paired. *Conditioning is a feature of the nervous system,* so Ader argued that conditioning of the immune system must be mediated by the nervous system. Ader suggested that the term psychoimmunology be changed to **psychoneuroimmunology** to indicate the role of the nervous system in immune system functioning.

The fact that immune system conditioning is repeatable and consistent is evidence for the connection between the nervous system and the immune system, evidence that opens the door for the effect of mind on immunity. If conditioning occurs, it can occur only through the nervous system, and the nervous system is connected to the mind.

Discovering exactly how the nervous system affects the immune system is another matter. The difficulty in studying the link between the two systems is that the mobile armies of cells of the immune system cannot have nerves connected to them as the rest of the body does. The nervous system communicates with the cells of the immune system through mobile molecules, but assessing the interaction at the cellular/molecule level involves sophisticated technology and generous research funding.

The clearest link between the central nervous system and the immune system is the effect of the adrenal corticosteroids on many components of the immune system, a connection that has been observed since the 1930s but is not fully understood. The adrenal steroids are under the control of the pituitary and hypothalamus, which are regulated by "higher brain centers." Today it is known that glucocorticoids from the adrenal cortices affect cell-mediated immunity by (1) moving T cells out of peripheral circulation; (2) reducing the ability of T cells to produce certain lymphokines, thus inhibiting cell proliferation; (3) inhibiting suppressor cells; and (4) blocking the process of sensitization of uncommitted T cells. The ability of B cells to produce antibody (immunoglobulin) is also reduced by glucocorticoids. However, glucocorticoids have been shown to enhance natural killer cell activity (Tsokos & Balow, 1983).

The hypothalamus is also involved in immunity through mechanisms not related to the adrenal glands. In rats, at least, destruction of portions of the hypothalamus impairs immune function, and when the immune system is challenged with disease, electrical activity in the hypothalamus changes. In addition, it is known that the organs of the immune system—the thymus, spleen, bone marrow, lymph nodes, Peyer's patches in the intestines, and the tonsils—receive nerve fibers from the autonomic nervous system (Bulloch, 1985).

The most intriguing and least understood link between the immune system and the nervous system is the presence of receptor sites for neurotransmitters, hormones, endorphins, and enkephalines on lymphocytes. These substances are all synthesized in the brain and nervous system. The presence of these receptors for "recognizing" these nervous system substances suggests that the nervous system can "talk" to lymphocytes through these substances. In fact, it has been demonstrated that morphine and morphine-like substances can enhance natural killer cell activity against certain cells and that substance P (a substance involved in pain sensation) can stimulate T cells to multiply (Hall & Goldstein, 1985; Solomon, Kay, & Morley, 1983; Wybran, 1985).

The interaction of the nervous system and the immune system is also suggested by the fact that virus-infected lymphocytes and macrophages can produce ACTH and

COMMENT

Study of the immune system is complicated by the fact that most of the work is done with rats because the research methods cannot be used with humans. For example, to study the effect of various tissues and organs on immunity, the tissues or organs are removed; the effect of the adrenal glands on immunity is studied by removing the adrenals. To study the effect of various substances on immunity, such as glucocorticoids, usually the substance is injected into the animal at doses that are larger than the body normally produces. To study the ability of the immune system to reject tumors, tumor material is implanted into the animal. The laboratory animal is killed and examined to determine tumor growth.

endorphin-like substances that are similar to brain substances; perhaps in this way the immune system "talks" to the nervous system.

The Stress Response of the Immune System

That stress affects the immune system has long been assumed. The correlation of stress and disease has been observed by laypersons and physicians for ages, and it is logical to assume that stress affects immunity. Yet the mechanisms by which stress affects immunity, and thus disease, were not studied intensively until the birth in the 1970s of neuroimmunology, followed by psychoneuroimmunology.

The gap between the observation and investigation of the link between stress and disease resulted from the belief that the immune system was independent of the nervous system; since the stress response is mediated through the nervous system, there was no known way in which stress could affect immunity. As noted above, the links between the nervous system and the immune system are being revealed.

In addition, the stress response of the immune system is difficult to study because it occurs at the level of cells and molecules. Isolating and examining the activity of cells and antibody molecules, and cell products such as interferon, is vastly more complicated than measuring a physiology phenomenon such as blood pressure or blood cholesterol.

At this time, there is no clear road map for understanding the stress response of the immune system. The field of psychoneuroimmunology is too young, and the complexity of each system—psyche, nervous, and immune—is so great that we anticipate years of research before the basics of the effects of stress on immunity are known. A few landmark studies, however, have been done.

In humans, research on the immune system's response to stress is limited to stressors that occur naturally and that humans can be subjected to ethically. Because the death of one's spouse is a major stressor, several researchers have studied immune responses to bereavement. The data show that although many elements of the immune system are not changed, the T lymphocytes of bereaved persons have a suppressed response to mitogen challenge (see Box 4.4) (Bartrop, Lockhurst, Lazarus, Kiloh, & Penny, 1977; Schleifer, Keller, McKegney, & Stein, 1979). Irwin, Daniels, Smith, Bloom, and Weiner (1987) found that women who were recently bereaved had lower natural killer cell activity than women in a control group of similar age.

Divorce also takes a toll on the immune system. Kiecolt-Glaser, Fisher, Ogrocki, Stout, Speicher, and Glaser (1987) found that recently separated women have increased antibodies to Epstein-Barr virus (the agent for infectious mononucleosis, which 80 percent to 90 percent of adults carry without symptoms), indicating that the cellular immune system is

---

BOX 4.4

COMMENT

Immune system functioning is studied **in vitro** or **in vivo.** Literally, *in vitro* means "in glass"; studies *in vitro* measure the activity of immune system components "in the test tube" after they have been removed from the body. For example, the ability of T lymphocytes to destroy bacteria can be studied *in vitro*. The fact that lymphocytes and macrophages will destroy foreign cells outside of the body, *in vitro*, contributed to the belief that the immune system is independent of the nervous system. Another commonly used *in vitro* technique challenges lymphocytes against a mitogen, a substance that stimulates cell multiplication. The multiplication rate of lymphocytes when challenged by a mitogen is a measure of immune competence.

In vivo means "in the living organism." *In vivo* studies of immunity include implanting tumor cells within the animal and using tumor suppression or growth as an indicator of immune competence.

Immune system functioning can also be studied by measuring the amount of antibody present in blood and body fluids such as saliva. For example, IgA is the primary immunoglobulin for defense against respiratory disease and is present in lungs and saliva. IgA level can be obtained from saliva samples and is an indication of antibody activity.

---

less competent and has allowed the virus to multiply. Men have a similar response to separation and divorce (Kiecolt-Glaser, Kennedy, Malkolf, Fisher, Speicher, & Glaser, 1988).

Final examinations in school are another stressor familiar to many. Janice Kiecolt-Glaser, a psychologist, and her husband, Ronald Glaser, an immunologist at Ohio State University Medical School, have conducted several studies on the immune system responses of medical students just before, during, and several months after final exams. Their data show that the stress of exams weakens the immune system's suppression of the herpes virus, which was dormant in their subjects. This change in immunity was demonstrated by significant increases in levels of the antibody against the virus when the students were preparing for and taking their examinations. The increase in antibody activity indicates that the virus was beginning to proliferate and that the components of the immune system that suppress the virus were weakening. In addition, students who rated themselves as high on a loneliness questionnaire had the greatest antibody response during exams (Kiecolt-Glaser, Speicher, Holliday, & Glaser, 1984).

In another study, Kiecolt-Glaser and Glaser found that natural killer cell activity decreased during the stress of final exams in medical students (Kiecolt-Glaser, Glaser, Strain, Stout, Tarr, Holliday, & Speicher, 1986). In a similar study, Steven Locke and his colleagues at Harvard University found that college students who reported feeling very anxious and depressed about school had decreased natural killer cell activity (Locke, 1986).

Another approach to the puzzle of stress and immunity is to study patients who are already sick with a disease such as mononucleosis or a respiratory infection. Several studies have found that students with mono or upper respiratory disease report more life stressors and stress than do matched control subjects. A possible mechanism is suggested in research on IgA production during stress (Jemmott, Borysenko, Borysenko, McClelland, Chapman, Meyer, & Benson, 1983). IgA is found in secretions of the mouth, nose, and lungs and is a primary defense against infections, particularly upper respiratory infections. Studies with students show that IgA, measured in saliva, decreases with increased stress.

An early study on stress and immunity subjected volunteers to a combination of unusual stressors. Female subjects were kept awake for 77 hours with the task of repeatedly firing an electronic rifle at a small target while being bombarded with battle sounds. During the vigil, phagocytosis of bacteria was diminished and interferon production increased (Palmbald, Cantell, Strander, Froberg, Karlsson, Levi, Gronstrom & Unger, 1976).

The study of a rare stressor helped launch the interest in the effects of stress on the immune system. In 1972, NASA published the first report of immune system reactivity during splashdown. Immediately after splashdown, astronauts had decreased white blood counts compared with preflight and inflight levels. Astronauts report that splashdown is the most stressful event in space flight (Fisher, Gill, Daniels, Cobb, Berry, & Ritzman, 1972).

We have clear evidence that some components of the human immune system are susceptible to stress, as this brief survey shows. Many more studies have been done and continue to be completed. In volume, however, human research is minor compared with research using nonhuman animals, particularly rats.

Since the work of Hans Selye, laboratory rats and mice have borne the brunt of humans' interest in stress. In immune system research, animals are subjected to a stressor or series of stressors, and then components of the immune system are studied *in vitro* just as in human research. To hasten and amplify the immune response, stressors are often intense and not related to anything that the animal would experience in the natural environment. In one study, rats were forced to swim until exhausted, exposed to a loud noise for six hours, and immobilized for six hours over a seven-day period (Ader & Cohen, 1984). Other studies subjected animals to overcrowding or isolation, or to housing with "strangers"; this is said to create "psychosocial" stress in the animals. In another research design, the effects of helplessness on immunity were studied by putting the animal in a "no control" situation in which it could not control or escape electric shock.

Whether or not the stress induced in laboratory animals through these techniques is analogous to human stress is not known, and the parallels between rat and human immunity are not clear. Nonetheless, laboratory animal studies show that stress has many effects on the immune system, including altered response to pathogens such as viruses and tumor cells. The results of these studies, however, are not always consistent. In some situations, stress impairs the immune component being studied, while in other conditions the same component is enhanced. Sometimes the component is enhanced only to decrease over time, and sometimes the reverse happens. In other situations, one component of the immune system may be enhanced while another component is suppressed by the same stressor. We expect that inconsistent findings will be a puzzle and a part of immune system research for many years.

Now you might raise a reasonable question: *Are these various changes in immune system functioning related to disease?* Did the medical students with increased antibodies to herpes virus develop herpes? Did the widowers with suppressed T lymphocyte response to a mitogen challenge become ill? In short, are the immune system changes clinically significant? To date, long-term studies have not been conducted to answer this question. We can hypothesize that the effects of stress or loneliness seen in these short-term studies impair immunity and increase the likelihood of disease over time. The evidence comes from the retrospective and prospective studies described in Chapter 18. If personality affects immunity, the effect occurs over time—there is a delay between a crisis or a series of major life events and the onset or discovery of disease (Kiecolt-Glaser & Glaser, 1988).

Stress-Related Diseases of the Immune System

There are no known disorders mediated by the immune system that are clearly caused by stress in the way that tension headache, for example, is caused by stress. By definition, infectious diseases are caused by infectious agents. Yet, theoretically, every disease involving the immune system could be influenced by stress, and some are clearly triggered or made worse by stress.

The infectious diseases that have been linked to stress in research are mononucleosis, strep throat, and tuberculosis. Of the noninfectious disorders that involve the immune system, asthma has been most clearly linked with stress.

Asthma.   Asthma, referred to as bronchial asthma, is the result of an immune system mistake. To understand asthma, a quick review of the lungs is in order.

The lungs are like an upside-down tree, in which the trachea is the trunk. The right and left bronchi are the first major branches going into the right and left lungs; the branching continues, and the tubes become increasingly narrow. They end in a grape-like cluster of air sacs, the alveoli. A latticework of capillaries surround the alveoli through which oxygen and carbon dioxide are diffused. During inspiration, the elastic tubes of the bronchial tree expand, and during expiration, they relax. Smooth muscles, like those of the vascular system, surround the smaller bronchi and bronchioles.

The smooth muscles are a primary culprit in asthma. When the antibodies of the immune system mistakenly react to the allergen, such as harmless pollens, molds, or dust, the smooth muscles react with constriction, called bronchial spasm, as if to protect the lungs from further invasion. The constriction makes expiration particularly difficult. Breathing becomes labored, and wheezing occurs.

The second culprit is the mucus-forming cells that line the bronchial tree. Mucus is

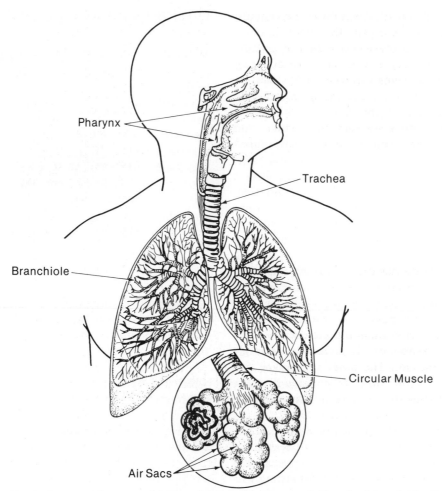

Pharynx

Trachea

Branchiole

Circular Muscle

Air Sacs

Figure 4.11   The Pulmonary System with Bronchioles, Air Sacs, and Circular Muscles in the Inset.

necessary to trap particles that enter the lungs, but during an asthma attack, these cells become hyperactive. They produce an excessive amount of mucus, which clogs the tubes and increases the severity of the attack.

Although there is no clear pattern of psychological variables in asthma, it is clear that stress can trigger attacks in some people, and the stress of an attack can make the attack worse. In addition, a few cases have been reported in which a person, consciously or unconsciously, initiates attacks to get a need met, such as avoiding a dreaded situation.

Autoimmune Diseases.   The immune system makes another error when T cells turn against the tissues of the body. This may happen because, given the millions of T and B cells that can recognize antigens, occasionally a receptor site matches "self" molecules. The match of the receptor with normal molecules causes the cell to respond as if the molecule were an antigen, and an immune attack is launched against healthy tissue (Cohen, 1988). Rheumatoid arthritis (destruction of cartilage and bone in joints), systemic lupus erythematosus (destruction of DNA, blood vessels, skin, and kidneys), myasthenia gravis (destruction of the muscle cell receptor for the transmitter acetylcholine), multiple sclerosis (destruction of the myelon sheath of nerves in the central nervous system), and juvenile diabetes (destruction of insulin-producing cells in the pancreas) are autoimmune disorders. Of these, the symptoms of rheumatoid arthritis, systemic lupus, and multiple sclerosis are known to be exacerbated by stress.

The Muscle System

Skeletal Muscles

The human body has more than 600 muscles. Three hundred muscles are called **skeletal** because they are attached to the skeleton; they are used for movement and posture. **Striate** is another name for skeletal muscle because, under the microscope, bands (striations) are seen in skeletal muscles. The other 300 muscles of the body are called **smooth** muscles because they appear smooth, not striated. Smooth muscles are involved in body functions such as digestion and elimination and control of blood flow and blood pressure through vasoconstriction and dilation. The heart muscle, called cardiac muscle, has properties of both striate and smooth muscle.

Skeletal muscles are innervated by nerve pathways that begin in the primary motor area of the cortex and travel uninterrupted to the medulla, where many fibers cross over to the opposite side and continue into the spinal cord. En route to the medulla, nerve fibers branch off the main motor nerves and travel to brain areas involved in muscle tone, fine motor movement, balance, and posture; some of the branching fibers go back to the cortex and enhance coordination of movement. In the cord, motor nerves travel to the appropriate level, where they synapse with a short interneuron in the cord; the interneuron synapses with the neuron that travels to the

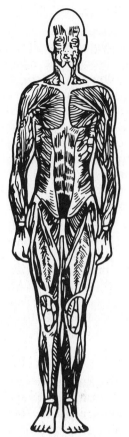

Figure 4.12   The Muscle System. There Are More than 300 Striate Muscles in the Body.

muscle innervated by the motor nerve. At the final synapse (the neuromuscular junction), the neurotransmitter acetylcholine is released, which initiates the changes in the muscle cell membrane that ultimately lead to contraction.

Skeletal muscles are considered part of the voluntary nervous system and are capable of being consciously controlled. However, we are not aware of most of the striate muscles and most are controlled indirectly only through movement.

Anatomy of a Muscle.   Skeletal muscles take the prize for having structures within structures within structures. From the outside, a large skeletal muscle looks like an elongated bag made of tough material called **fascia**. A cross-section through the muscle reveals all its structures, down to the chains of molecules called filaments that are the final step in contraction. With contraction, the filaments, **actin** and **myosin**, connect and move past each other like cog wheels, and the muscle shortens; with relaxation they release and slide back, lengthening the muscle.

The Muscle Fiber.   When you think of a cell, you probably think of a cute round thing with a nucleus and various organelles. A muscle cell, called a fiber, is different. The muscle cell is long and thin, and it houses the thousands of myofibrils and filaments. Individual muscle cells connect at both ends to a lattice of connective tissue that surrounds the bundles of fibers that make up the muscle.

Innervation of Muscle.   Muscle contraction occurs when hundreds of muscle fibers in a muscle are activated at the same time. The individual fibers are activated by a motor nerve, and each motor nerve stimulates several fibers. The motor nerve and the muscle cells that it innervates are called a **single motor unit**.

How Muscles Generate "Electricity." When receptor sites on a muscle fiber are stimulated by acetylcholine released from the motor nerve, reactions within the cell cause movement of **ions** across the cell membrane. The movement of ions is the "electricity" of physiological systems, just as the movement of electrons is the electricity in electrical systems. When muscle fibers contract, the electrical impulse generated by the fibers is added together and can be picked up by electrodes placed on the skin over the muscle. The total amount of "electricity" that a muscle generates is proportional to the number of fibers that are contracting; the greater the contraction, the greater the total electrical potential. This is the basis of biofeedback training for muscle control described in Chapter 8.

The Stress Response of Skeletal Muscles

Muscles get involved in stress because they are the bottom line of the fight-or-flight response. All the autonomic changes of the stress response would be of no use if we could not activate muscles to save us. This is probably why muscles are so quick to react to stress, even when fight or flight are not options. Muscles also have a third option—they can tighten without movement. Barbara Brown, a pioneer in biofeedback training, calls the muscle response to stress the "fight-or-flight-or-freeze" response (Brown, 1977).

Some animals, such as rabbits, freeze before they run. Freezing is one way of not being noticed. Humans also freeze with fear, but the mild version of this response is tension without movement. Often the tension is so mild that it is not noticed. Short-term mild tension in striate muscle is not a problem, but chronic mild tension in striate muscle is. Chronically tense muscles are deprived of proper blood flow and become painful from the build-up of lactic acid. In addition, chronically tense muscles can pull bones out of line, such as the vertebra of the neck, pinching nerves and causing additional pain. Nerves that pass through tight muscles are also injured and can become inflamed (neuritis).

Stress-Related Disorders of Skeletal Muscles

Because muscles are the bottom line of the stress response, they are highly susceptible to all kinds of stress.

Muscle Contraction (Tension) Headache. Headaches that result from muscle tension are experienced as dull, localized or general, and constant. Usually a tension headache does not

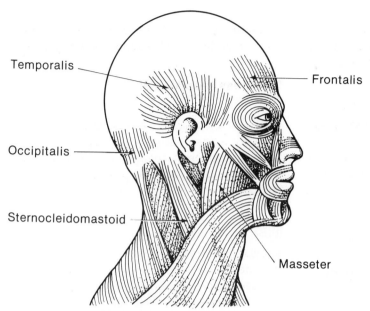

Temporalis

Frontalis

Occipitalis

Sternocleidomastoid

Masseter

Figure 4.13   Major Muscles Involved in Tension Headache.

have the intensity of migraine and is not preceded by an aura. Often the affected muscles feel sore and the points at which the muscles join bone may be especially tender. In some cases, the muscles are in spasm and feel like knots. Sometimes the muscles feel loose, but the pain persists.

A muscle contraction headache can result from muscles that are abused by poor posture or work habits that put the head off balance and force the neck and shoulder muscles to constantly contract. Usually, a muscle contraction headache results from muscles tightening with stress. The muscles of the neck and jaw are highly susceptible to stress, and they can lead to generalized headache by chronic contraction of the scalp muscles.

Clenching and Bruxism.   Tightening the muscles of the jaw and clenching the teeth are common reactions to stress. In a large crowd of Christmas shoppers, you may spot one or two people who continually tense and relax the jaw muscles; you can see the masseter muscle bulging and relaxing as the person presses the

teeth together and relaxes. Stress responses such as this can become a habit and continue unconsciously, even when the person is not stressed.

Bruxism refers to grinding the teeth together, and occurs primarily during sleep. If you have slept in the same room with a

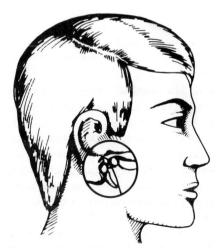

Figure 4.14   The Temporomandibular Joint (TMJ).

"grinder," you know how loud the sound can be. The force of this grinding can be enough to damage the temporomandibular joint (TMJ) and the teeth, and dental patients are often fitted with a plastic guard that fits over the teeth and is worn at night. Bruxers often waken with a sore jaw and may have trouble opening the mouth wide enough to eat a glazed donut because the jaw muscles are so tight.

Clenching during the day is also a common habit that creates pain in the jaw muscles, and can produce a temporal headache. While malformation of the temporomandibular joint or poor alignment of the teeth (malocclusion) can cause muscle tension and pain, it is clear that these problems are exacerbated by stress-related facial muscle tension.

Low Back Pain. Low back pain is a common problem that temporarily disables 5.4 million Americans each year, at a cost of at least $16 billion annually (Frymoyer, 1988). Low back pain may result from injury or from minor muscle strain. A back that is vulnerable because of poor posture, lack of muscle strength and flexibility, and obesity or psychological stress is more likely to sustain injury and muscle strain. Once injury and strain have occurred, these variables may contribute to poor recovery and chronic pain. Stress hits a body's weakest link, and if the back has been injured or is susceptible to strain, stress can contribute to the pain.

The Pain-Tension Cycle. The cycle of muscle tension and spasm–pain–increased tension–more pain is a common problem in muscle spasm/pain disorders. Muscle tension is a typical response to pain of any type. We all remember the brave soldier in the old western movie who bites on a block of wood as his leg is amputated. Bracing is another part of the tension/pain pattern. Often people respond to pain, especially chronic pain, by bracing—holding the body rigidly, as if to protect injured muscles. In fact, bracing creates more tension and pain.

Torticollis. Torticollis is a rare but dramatic disorder in which the head is chronically rotated to one side by the contraction of neck muscles on the side to which the head turns and the weakening of the muscles on the opposite side. Often a tremor accompanies the rotation, especially when the person tries to bring the head back to center. The causes of torticollis are unknown, although it is clear that stress is an aggravating ingredient and may at times be the cause.

CONCLUSION

The effect of stress on physiology can be fleeting and unnoticed, or it can be chronic and lethal. Acute stress triggers the fight-or-flight response, and the response subsides when the stress subsides. The stress response to an acute stressor is not damaging unless the stress is extreme and the body is already compromised by disease, destructive lifestyle habits, or genetic predisposition. Chronic stress, however, is a risk to health. With chronic stress, the body must continually react. Over time, chronic activity of the sympathetic nervous system and muscle tension impede the ability of the body to return to healthy homeostasis, and symptoms develop.

The estimate that most visits to a physician are for stress-related complaints illustrates the pervasiveness of stress and the stress response, as does the amount of medication used in this country to treat these complaints. In 1986, the three most commonly prescribed nonantibiotic drugs were for hypertension, anxiety, depression, and gastrointestinal disorders (*Drug Utilization in the U.S.–1986*, Office of Epidemiology and Biostatistics, FDA). The toll of stress on mental and physical health, and on our communal pocketbook, places stress in a unique category. It is epidemic, and yet there is no pathogen to eradicate and no inoculation against it. That is the bad news. The good news is that stress and the complications of the stress response are preventable. Combating illness and disease by understanding and combating stress is the focus of Part Five.

|||||▶

APPENDIX: TERMS FOR THE NERVOUS SYSTEM

We have a unified nervous system that functions as an integrated whole. The labels that describe the various branches of the nervous system are based on anatomical differences and on the specialized functions of the branches. Each branch is sometimes referred to as a nervous system, such as "the autonomic nervous system." With the exception of the reflexes, however, the nervous system functions as a whole and is not really composed of separate nervous systems. As you turn the pages of this book, the somatic branch of the peripheral nervous system and the central nervous system interact. If you feel stressed as you read, the sympathetic branch of the autonomic branch of the peripheral nervous system and the central nervous system interact, and you might detect an increase in heart rate. The interaction of the brain and the rest of the body enables us to control somatic and autonomic processes.

Central Nervous System: The Brain and the Spinal Cord

The spinal cord has been compared to a cable system that carries messages back and forth between the body and the brain, and the brain has been compared to a computer. It is an enormously complex system of interacting "circuits" that can monitor and integrate "inputs" from the mind, from itself, and from the body, and can initiate "outputs" to the rest of the nervous system, the body, and the mind. As knowledge of the intricate workings of the brain grows, the "connectedness" of the whole brain is more apparent.

Peripheral Nervous System

This nervous system comprises all nerve pathways lying outside (peripheral to) the brain and spinal cord. The peripheral nerves carry signals between the brain and cord and the rest of the body. The peripheral nervous system is divided into two major systems according to function, the **somatic** and the **autonomic**.

Somatic Nervous System

The somatic nervous system has two functions: (1) It mediates the movements and tone of the skeletal muscles, and (2) it mediates the sensory systems of the skin such as touch and pain. The motor aspect of the somatic nervous system is called the "voluntary nervous system" because it can be voluntarily controlled. If your motor nerves are intact and communicate with the brain and spinal cord, you can get up and move around because you can voluntarily control the motor nerves. Except for the spinal reflexes, which make you hop off a nail, the motor system is under your control. Your body will not go to the refrigerator and eat chocolate cake unless you direct it to. Fortunately, we can be conscious of the somatic nervous system and can control it. If you wish to, at this moment you can become conscious of the pressure of your rear against the chair; if you wish to, you can consciously move. Our ability to become conscious of and voluntarily control the somatic nervous system has, undoubtedly, saved us many times. The term "voluntary nervous system" is incorrect, however, because humans can develop varieties of muscle habits that become involuntary and unconscious. You have seen people with bad posture, their heads thrust forward or chests caved in, or who bite their nails, or who continually clench the jaw. You might say "relax your jaw," and for a moment the clenching comes into consciousness, and the person voluntarily relaxes; but as soon as the attention shifts away from the jaw, the

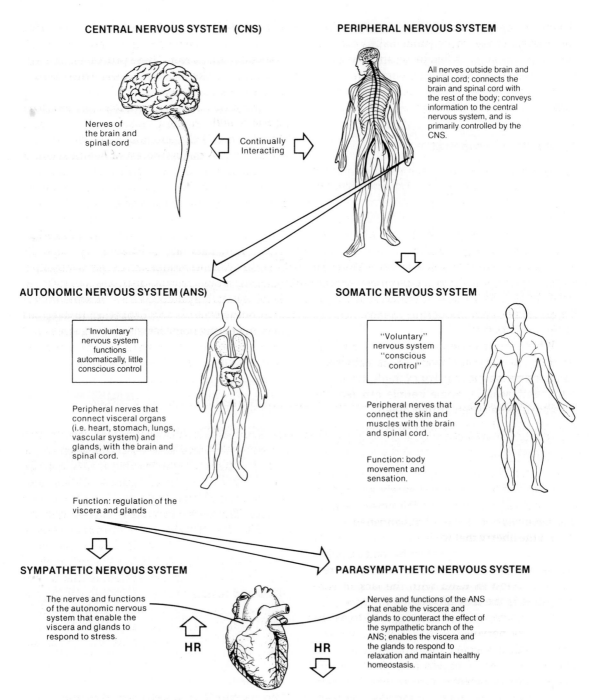

CENTRAL NERVOUS SYSTEM (CNS)

Nerves of
the brain and
spinal cord

Continually
Interacting

PERIPHERAL NERVOUS SYSTEM

All nerves outside brain and
spinal cord; connects the
brain and spinal cord with
the rest of the body; conveys
information to the central
nervous system, and is
primarily controlled by the
CNS.

AUTONOMIC NERVOUS SYSTEM (ANS)

"Involuntary"
nervous system
functions
automatically, little
conscious control

Peripheral nerves that
connect visceral organs
(i.e. heart, stomach, lungs,
vascular system) and
glands, with the brain and
spinal cord.

Function: regulation of the
viscera and glands

SOMATIC NERVOUS SYSTEM

"Voluntary"
nervous system
"conscious
control"

Peripheral nerves that
connect the skin and
muscles with the brain
and spinal cord.

Function: body
movement and
sensation.

SYMPATHETIC NERVOUS SYSTEM

The nerves and functions
of the autonomic nervous
system that enable the
viscera and glands to
respond to stress.

HR

PARASYMPATHETIC NERVOUS SYSTEM

Nerves and functions of the ANS
that enable the viscera and
glands to counteract the effect of
the sympathetic branch of the
ANS; enables the viscera and
the glands to respond to
relaxation and maintain healthy
homeostasis.

HR

Figure 4.15 Terms for the Nervous System.

clenching begins again, unconsciously and involuntarily. These unconscious habits can create symptoms such as headache and myofacial pain. Fortunately, because the somatic nervous system can be consciously controlled, we can consciously unlearn bad habits.

2. Autonomic Nervous System

The autonomic nervous system was so named because it can function autonomously without direction from the mind. It could also have been called "the automatic nervous system" because it runs automatically. The autonomic nervous system innervates the organs, called the viscera, and the glands that run themselves. All the internal organs, from the pupillary sphincter of the eyes to the anal sphincters, as well as the exocrine and endocrine glands, are on "automatic" control.

When the autonomic system is running smoothly, we are not aware of its activity; it functions unconsciously. For example, try to feel your heart beating. Some people can feel the heartbeat, even when sitting quietly. Now put your attention into your liver to feel what your liver is doing. This is not possible. You have a liver, but it is "in the unconscious," fortunately. If we were constantly bombarded by signals from the viscera, we would surely go mad, or we would learn to tune out the noise; perhaps through evolution this is what happened.

Yet the liberty that we have from demands of the autonomic nervous system becomes a liability, as we see in the section on the stress response. Hand in hand with the lack of consciousness is the lack of voluntary control. The autonomic nervous system is referred to as the "involuntary nervous system," because when it was named, it seemed that humans could not control the internal organs and glands. If you wished at this moment to change your liver output, decrease blood sugar, or increase the reabsorption of sodium from the kidneys, you would find the task difficult, if not impossible. And in any case, how would you know whether you had

succeeded? You would not know, because being unconscious of these processes really means getting no feedback from these processes. The significance of lack of feedback will be discussed in the chapters on biofeedback training.

The good news is that *the autonomic nervous system is only relatively "involuntary."* It was a mistake to call the autonomic nervous system involuntary. A major interest of health sciences is to use our ability to regulate the autonomic nervous system. Two ways that we can regulate the autonomic nervous system will be clear when we examine two of its primary functions, response to stress and response to relaxation. These functions are mediated by separate neuronal pathways that are called the sympathetic nervous system and the parasympathetic nervous system. During normal conditions, these systems work together to keep the body in healthy homeostasis. During stress and deep relaxation, these systems function more dramatically, for survival and revival.

2A Sympathetic Nervous System

The sympathetic nervous system is the system of nerves that mediates the preparation of the body for flight or fight; in other words, it mediates the stress response. Figure 4.16 illustrates the major functions of the sympathetic nervous system. The term *sympathetic* can be remembered by this thought—when you are stressed, this branch of the autonomic nervous system is in sympathy with you. The general principle of the sympathetic nervous system is that it prepares and sustains the body in threatening situations. Some of its actions are discussed in detail in this chapter. We can control the autonomic nervous system because we can control stress and relaxation. *Counteracts:*

2B Parasympathetic Nervous System

If nature had evolved only the sympathetic nervous system, we might have "burned out"

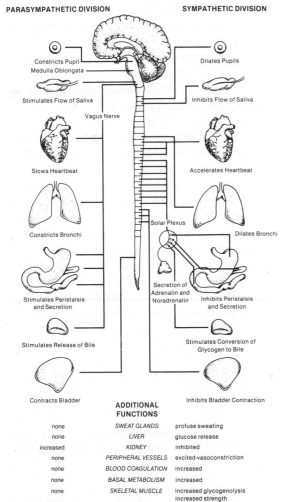

PARASYMPATHETIC DIVISION   SYMPATHETIC DIVISION

Constricts Pupil
Medulla Oblongata

Stimulates Flow of Saliva   Inhibits Flow of Saliva

Vagus Nerve

Slows Heartbeat   Accelerates Heartbeat

Constricts Bronchi   Dilates Bronchi

Solar Plexus

Stimulates Peristalsis   Secretion of   Inhibits Peristalsis
and Secretion   Adrenalin and   and Secretion
                                   Noradrenalin

Stimulates Release of Bile   Stimulates Conversion of
                                   Glycogen to Bile

Contracts Bladder   Inhibits Bladder Contraction

Dilates Pupils

ADDITIONAL FUNCTIONS

none	SWEAT GLANDS	profuse sweating
none	LIVER	glucose release
increased	KIDNEY	inhibited
none	PERIPHERAL VESSELS	excited-vasoconstriction
none	BLOOD COAGULATION	increased
none	BASAL METABOLISM	increased
none	SKELETAL MUSCLE	increased glycogenolysis increased strength

Figure 4.16   The Functions of the Sympathetic and Parasympathetic Nervous Systems.

long ago. Survival also depends upon recovery from stress and return to homeostasis. The parasympathetic nervous system mediates recovery and the relaxation response. Figure 4.16 illustrates the main functions of the parasympathetic system. The fact that body processes such as digestion, heart rate, and respiration are regulated by the parasympathetic system during normal conditions suggests that this system evolved as the primary homeostatic mechanism (see "Homeostasis" below)

and perhaps preceded the development of the sympathetic pathways. The rapid and extreme reactivity of the sympathetic nervous system may be the result of evolution—the folks with a sluggish fight-or-flight response never made it up the trees. In any case, we can control the autonomic nervous system because we can control our state of relaxation and our recovery from stress.

Basic Mechanisms and Principles

Mechanisms

Familiarity with the basic mechanisms and principles of the nervous system will help you understand the dynamics of the nervous system in illness and in health.

Neurons and Neuronal Transmission.   The basic element of the nervous system is the nerve cell, called a **neuron**. The central nervous system comprises billions of neurons in the brain and spinal cord. In ways that are not fully understood, neurons make possible all the activities of the body and the activities of the mind that are manifested through the body. The body (peripheral nervous system) "talks" with the brain (central nervous system) through neuronal activity. "Neuronal activity" refers to the communication between neurons.

Neurons do not touch; they communicate with each other by a chemical messenger called a **neurotransmitter**, which is released from a neuron when it is activated. The transmitter molecules travel across a minute gap between the neurons called a **synapse** and activate **receptor sites** on the adjacent neuron.

There are perhaps as many as 50 neurotransmitters in the central and peripheral nervous systems. The nervous system has many transmitters, which allow systems of neurons to have different functions. For example, the terminal neurons of the sympathetic and the parasympathetic systems—the neurons that connect to organs and glands—have different transmitters; if they had the same transmitter, then the two systems might be turned on at the same time, creating chaos in the body.

Adrenaline (epinephrine) is a neurotransmitter released from nerves of the sympathetic nervous system and a hormone released from the medullae of the adrenal glands. Adrenaline has effects that are similar to those of noradrenaline, although adrenaline has a stronger effect on heart rate and force of contraction and less vasoconstriction effect on blood vessels than noradrenaline. In fact, adrenaline causes vasodilation of large skeletal muscles and cardiac muscle. Adrenaline increases the metabolic rate of cells, and it can affect every cell in the body, increasing the cell metabolic rate by 100 percent. Adrenaline also increases glycogenolysis (conversion of glycogen into a simple sugar) in the liver and muscle and enhances the release of glucose into blood. In addition, adrenaline increases the rate of fat metabolism in fat cells, and it can increase free fatty acids in blood by as much as 15 times the normal amount (Guyton, 1977).

Noradrenaline (norepinephrine) is a neurotransmitter of the sympathetic nervous system and a hormone released from the medullae of the adrenal glands. Most of the final nerve endings of the sympathetic nervous system release noradrenaline. Norepinephrine disregulation in the brain may be associated with major depression (Gold, Goodwin, & Chrousos, 1988).

Another term that is used for adrenaline (epinephrine) and noradrenaline (norepinephrine) is **catecholamine**; epinephrine and norepinephrine are catecholamines.

Acetylcholine is the transmitter of the parasympathetic nervous system and for the nerve innervation of skeletal muscle.

Serotonin is a neurotransmitter that is found in the brain, in tissues of the GI tract, and in blood platelets. Serotonin may be either a vasoconstrictor or vasodilator. Axons that release serontonin are found in the hypothalamus and spinal cord. This transmitter seems to be involved in sleep cycles, temperature regulation, and emotional state, particularly depression.

Other transmitters that are important to our discussions throughout this text will be described when appropriate. In addition to the well-known neurotransmitters, there are also **neuropeptides**, a class of neurotransmitter that includes enkephalines, endorphins, and substance P, which are involved in pain transmission and sensation.

When a neuron has received transmitter substance from a sufficient number of neurons simultaneously, an **action potential** is created. The action potential is an electrical gradient change that flows along the cell membrane as sodium ions (Na+) rush into the cell and are pumped out again. As the term suggests, an action potential is an electrical change (potential) that stimulates the neuron into action. The shift of positively charged ions across the membrane is like a tiny current of electricity. When the current reaches the axon terminal, the transmitter substance is released. After the neurotransmitter has been released and has been received by the adjacent neuron, enzymes in the synapse return the unused transmitter substance to the axon terminal. Some transmitters are **excitatory** and increase the likelihood that an action potential will be generated in a neuron. Others are **inhibitory** and, by increasing the amount of electrical potential needed to activate an action potential, they reduce the likelihood that an action potential will occur.

From this brief description of neuronal activity, several principles are clear:

1. A neurotransmitter substance must be available in the axon terminal. Anything that changes the amount of neurotransmitter substance, or its release, will affect neuronal transmission, that is, the ability of the neuron to stimulate the adjacent neuron.
2. Anything that changes the enzyme that returns the transmitter to the original

neuron, called **reuptake**, will change the amount of free transmitter in the synapse, the amount that is taken up, and the amount that is present to stimulate the adjacent cell.

3. Anything that affects the breakdown of the neurotransmitter will change the effect of the transmitter. For example, norepinephrine is broken down (deactivated) by catechol-O-methyl transferase and is deactivated by monoamine oxidase after reuptake. Drugs that block these enzymes prolong the effects of norepinephrine. Antidepressants block the reuptake and breakdown of transmitters.

4. Receptor sites must be available to receive the transmitter substance; if the sites are blocked, the transmitter cannot affect the cell.

Principles

Homeostasis.   Homeostasis is the term created by the American physiologist Walter B. Cannon (1871–1945) to describe the ability of the body to maintain a steady internal balance. The body has hundreds of homeostatic mechanisms that keep the internal environment fairly constant. All the vital body processes, organ systems, and hormone levels are maintained in a normal range through homeostatic mechanisms. The ability of the body to maintain healthy homeostasis is a recurring theme in physiology, and it was described in Chapter 2 as a dynamic in health and wellness. Unfortunately, humans have an amazing ability to throw the body off balance. When the body is unable to return to healthy homeostasis, illness develops.

Feedback.   Homeostasis works through feedback, also discussed in Chapter 2. When appropriate cells sense that a process is off-balance, the deviation is corrected by reversing the processes or counteracting it through feedback of signals to the appropriate organs or systems or glands. When the temperature sensors detect overheating, sweat glands are stimulated and cooling begins; this is called negative feedback because it reverses the process. Without feedback, the body could not maintain homeostasis.

Purpose.   The body is not a haphazard enterprise; everything has a function. Sometimes the purpose of a particular physiological process is difficult to determine, but in studying physiology, it is helpful to continually ask, "What would be the usefulness of this. . . ."

The Bottom Line.   Molecules are the bottom line of all physiological processes. No matter how complex an activity might be—running, digestion, breathing, or heart-rate acceleration—the bottom line is activity at a molecular level. Therefore, when mind ⟶ body, the ultimate effect is at a molecular level. For example, fear does not affect the heart by magic; fear affects the heart through known mechanisms, including communication between neurons through neurotransmitter molecules, communication between neurons and heart muscle cells, and molecular activity within the heart muscle cells.

CHAPTER 5

Evaluating Research and Physiological Data

IIII➡

Jim was an athletic young man who went to see his physician for a routine physical. The exam included a resting electrocardiogram (ECG). After examining the ECG, the physician asked Jim about his heart attack. Jim was stunned. "I have never had a heart attack," he said.

The physician pointed to the patterns on the cardiograph and said, "It never lies. Since you never experienced any chest pains you must have had a silent coronary."

That night Jim had chest pains. Jim returned to the doctor and took a treadmill stress test. The test showed clear abnormalities. The next day an angiogram was done. A radioactive dye was injected into Jim's bloodstream through an artery in his leg; when the dye reached the coronary vessels of his heart, they appeared on the imaging screen. Jim's angiogram revealed blockage in the coronary arteries. Coronary bypass surgery was recommended.

To Jim, the shock of the diagnosis, of "going in well and coming out sick," and the anticipation of surgery were extremely stressful. Jim was so anxious that his doctor suggested that he talk to Norman Cousins before having surgery. Norman Cousins, who teaches at UCLA School of Medicine, is keenly interested in mind and disease, having overcome a life-threatening disease and heart attack. Jim's doctor thought that Cousins could help Jim overcome the anxiety.

After talking with Jim for a while, Cousins pointed out that the interpretation of the cardiograph could be wrong, that athletes sometimes have tracings that look like heart damage. Cousins also talked to Jim about the treadmill test. When the person on the treadmill is fearful, the results may be invalid because fear affects the heart; in this case, the stress test measures the physiological effects of fear rather than the ability of the heart to tolerate exercise. Indeed, Jim had been frightened when he took the treadmill test. Cousins arranged for Jim to take the treadmill test again, but this time he would be in charge of his own test and would determine the speed and length of time that he would run. With an attitude of hope, and feeling "in control," Jim took the test again.

You can imagine the result. The second treadmill test showed no abnormality; it revealed a healthy, normal heart. The surgery was canceled. Six months later Jim had another angiogram, which was normal. (Jim's story is told in Cousins' book, *The Healing Heart*, 1983).

Jim's original ECG and angiogram produced a "false positive" report. He was diagnosed as "positive" for heart disease, and the diagnosis was false. False positive results occur when tests are not accurate or are misinterpreted.

The physician incorrectly diagnosed Jim as having heart disease because that is what the treadmill test and angiogram measures indicated. The measures were not valid, however, because the physician failed to take into account the emotional state of the patient. To avoid false positives, measurements must be highly reliable and valid, and they must be correctly interpreted. Jim's case illustrates the importance of reliable and valid measures. In the study of health, instruments and tests are used to measure physiological and psychological variables. Physiological data are derived from instruments that measure physiological variables, such as blood cholesterol and blood pressure. Psychological data are often derived from "instruments," such as pencil-paper tests, that measure sociological and psychological variables. Two examples are the Holmes-Rahe Schedule of Recent Experience and the Jenkins Survey, which measures Type A Behavior Pattern, a personality pattern characterized by anger, aggressiveness, and competitiveness.

How do we know that data from these instruments actually reflect whatever the instrument was designed to measure? How do we know that the data are accurate and meaningful, and that they predict what they are supposed to predict? In evaluating your own physiological measures, such as blood cholesterol, blood pressure, heart rate, or white cell blood cell count, the same questions apply. For example, when your blood pressure is taken in the doctor's office, three questions can be asked about the measure:

1. Is the blood pressure reading accurate, or was there an error in the reading, perhaps because of a faulty blood pressure cuff?
2. Does the reading in the doctor's office correctly reflect daily blood pressure?
3. Does the reading indicate good or bad health or predict it?

These questions concern **reliability** and **validity**. If Jim's experience were common, then the ECG and angiogram would be neither reliable nor valid because there was error in the measurement of the heart (not reliable) and would not predict health status (not valid). In Jim's case, the ECG and angiogram indicated that he was sicker than he really was. In evaluating research data and personal measures of health, we must know how reliable and valid the measures are; without high reliability and validity, measurements are meaningless or cannot be interpreted. In Sections One and Two we discuss the reliability and validity of measurements; these are important topics because measurements of one kind or another are used extensively in the health sciences. In Section Three we present several criteria for evaluating research and research results, and we guide you through a series of questions that can be asked of all research. After reading this chapter you will not be a statistician; in fact, you may be relieved to know that we do not present statistical formulas. Our intention is to introduce several important concepts for understanding research and physiological data.

Research is the primary tool of science, and it is the basis for testing theory and developing an empirical foundation in any field. We include this chapter on research evaluation because asking the right questions about research is invaluable in any field that relies extensively on research.

How are validity and reliability determined? To answer these questions, we take you on our own pursuit of reliability and validity. For the past 12 years we have studied the reliability and validity of physiological measures such as heart rate, blood pressure, muscle tension, perspiration, and skin temperature. Our studies have taken us on a puzzling and fascinating quest in which many mysteries still remain.

||||➡

SECTION ONE: THE PURSUIT OF RELIABILITY

Reliability refers to "the degree to which test scores are free from errors of measurement" (*Standards for Educational and Psychological Testing*, 1985, p. 19). For example, we can ask whether or not the measurements from a blood pressure cuff are reliable. If an error occurred in taking blood pressure, then the readings would not be reliable.

High reliability is important for all measures whether medical (such as the measurement of blood pressure), laboratory (such as the measurement of blood cholesterol level), psychological (such as the measure of Type A behavior), or psychosocial (such as the measurement of life change).

Now we begin our story.

In 1982, we received research funds from the Colorado Commission on Higher Education to assess the effectiveness of our biofeedback and stress-management classes (Shellenberger, Turner, Green, & Cooney, 1986). We had four ways of measuring effectiveness: health records, student reports, pencil-paper tests, and results on a stress profile given before and after the class. A stress profile is a 50-minute procedure for measuring a person's physiological responses during relaxed and stressed conditions. The physiological measures are muscle tension, measured from forehead muscles with an electromyograph (EMG) in millionths of a volt (microvolt); finger temperature, a measure of peripheral blood flow using a thermometer; and galvanic skin response (GSR), a measure of moisture on the fingers. These physiological processes are measured in the stress profile because they are particularly responsive to stress and because the instrumentation for measuring these processes is often equipment used in biofeedback training.

Physiological measurements are recorded continuously during 10 phases of the stress profile, and the measurements are averaged for each phase: (1) a baseline period in which the subject sits quietly; (2) a relaxation period; (3) the presentation of a math stressor; (4) giving the answer to the math problem; (5) a second relaxation period; (6) end of relaxation period; (7) imagining a severe stressor; (8) a relaxation period; (9) a startle stressor; and (10) a final relaxation period. The stress profile is used in many biofeedback therapy clinics and in research because it is thought to indicate a person's reactivity to stressors and ability to recover when stressed (Arena, Blanchard, Andrasik, Cotch, & Myers, 1983; Waters, Williamson, Bernard, Blouin, & Faulstich, 1987).

In 1979 we began giving students a stress profile before and after taking a class in biofeedback and stress management. Goals of the class were to teach people to be less reactive when stressed, to recover faster from stressors, and to be able to deeply relax. We hoped that by comparing stress profile measures before and after the class, we could demonstrate that students had learned to be less reactive and to recover faster when stressed. If many students showed significant improvement, then we could conclude that students learned to cope with stress as a result of taking the class.

This conclusion would be true, however, only if the stress profile were reliable and valid. Our first task then, was to determine the reliability of the stress profile.

The standard method for determining the reliability of measures that are generated by a test or instrument is to give the test or use the instrument repeatedly with the same subjects in the same conditions. This procedure is called "test-retest." If the scores on the test and retest are similar, then the test is reliable. If the scores are not similar, then some error is present and the test is not reliable. It is assumed, for example, that children's intelligence, as measured on an IQ test, does not change. This means that if an IQ test is reliable, the scores on the test and retest should be similar when given to the same children twice.

The importance of reliability is in the fact that tests are given only once. Tests are not repeated many times with each person to determine reliability. Once a test is created and its reliability is determined, other researchers use it with subjects, but they do not determine reliability again. Usually, blood cholesterol is determined only once and may not be taken again for many months or years; some physicians take a single blood pressure reading and may prescribe medication on a basis of that one reading.

When only one measurement is made, it is essential to know how much variation normally occurs in the measure. If great variation is common, then there is not much confidence that a single reading is accurate; if there is little variation when the measure is repeated, then one can be confident that the single reading was quite accurate.

The same test-retest procedure is used to determine the reliability of measurements made from an instrument such as a thermometer. To determine the reliability of temperature measurements, the thermometer is repeatedly placed in water of known and constant temperature. If the readings are always the same, the readings are reliable; if the readings are always different, they are unreliable, and we would discard the thermometer knowing that there was a source of error in the instrument. Once the thermometer is determined to be reliable, then we can take a single reading and be confident that it is correct.

How similar do test and retest measures have to be, to be reliable? Do the measures have to be identical, or can there be some difference? Measurements do not have to be perfectly matched. There is a way of determining how similar the scores are and a criterion for determining reliability. The statistic used for determining similarity of measures is called a **correlation coefficient**. The correlation coefficient indicates how similar the scores are. Scores that are perfectly correlated have a correlation coefficient of 1.0. The closer a correlation coefficient is to 1.0, the more reliable the measures are; the closer to zero, the less reliable. Test-retest scores with a correlation of zero are not correlated at all.

How high must the correlation be to conclude that a measure is reliable? A correlation coefficient of .80 is a rigorous criterion for reliability that has been used, particularly when a measurement is used to make inferences about an individual (American Psychological Association, American Educational Research Association, & National Council on Measurements Used in Education, 1954). For example, a test used to place a child in a remedial learning program should have a correlation coefficient of at least .80. A minimal criterion states that the correlation coefficient must be high enough to be statistically significant (described in Section Three). A third method for determining reliability is called the "standard error of measurement," described below.

To determine the reliability of the measures on the stress profile, we gave 85 students the stress profile twice at an interval of nine weeks; this matched the interval of time between profiles in the stress management class. We compared data on each physiological parameter to determine how consistent they were. Table 5.1 shows the correlation coefficients for each of the three physiological measures, during the phases of the stress profile.

We were discouraged by the results. All the measures were statistically significant (the minimum criterion), but only the EMG measures taken during relaxed conditions met the maximum criterion of .80 or more.

Table 5.1   Test-Retest Correlation Coefficients (N = 85)

Phase	EMG	GSR	Temperature
Baseline	.72	.48	.39
Relax	.80	.53	.41
Math Stressor	.40	.52	.43
Math Answer	.37	.56	.43
Relax	.72	.53	.46
End Relax	.87	.43	.51
Visualize Stressor	.67	.38	.51
Relax	.76	.45	.54
Startle Stressor	.56	.36	.54
Relax	.71	.46	.60

To improve the reliability of our measures, we conducted another study in which we gave stress profiles to the same subjects on four days over one month—days 1, 2, 14, and 28 (Shellenberger & Lewis, 1986). We also changed the math problem each time so that subjects could not adapt to the stressor. In addition, we attempted to hold constant many factors that might influence the subject's physiological measures. Subjects were asked not to drink, eat, exercise, or smoke for 60 minutes before the profile. Subjects were informed of the importance of maintaining constant conditions for 24 hours before each profile. Constant humidity and temperature were maintained in the testing room, and subjects had the same reclined posture during each profile. Subjects had a 20-minute adaptation period in which they sat quietly in the testing room before beginning the profile, so that we would not be measuring physiological adaptations. Subjects were scheduled to take the profile at the same time of day and day of the week. In addition, the recording instruments were tested and found to be accurate. Subjects filled out a questionnaire before each profile that asked about use of street drugs, medications and cigarette use, last aerobic exercise, mood, and stress level at the time of taking the profile. In other words, we attempted to hold constant as many variables as we could to reduce variations in the measurements.

The results were again disappointing. The correlation coefficients were no higher. In examining the individual subject data, however, we found a clue—*individual differences.*

Some people are "physiologically stable," with little variation in their measures, and some people fluctuate greatly from day to day. Figure 5.1A shows the electromyograph (EMG) measures of a person with a fluctuating physiology; because of this variation, the correlation coefficients average .26, and the measure is unreliable. Figure 5.1B shows the EMG readings of a person with stable readings and coefficients that average .97, and the measure is reliable.

Like many researchers, we assumed that measures of human physiology are fairly stable. Obviously, measurements of variables that are constantly changing cannot be reliable. Much to our surprise, human physiology can be very unstable in some people. Our measures were unreliable not because there was error in the measurement or experiment, but because physiological processes fluctuate naturally and are affected by situational and cognitive variables. Other researchers have also noted the variability of many physiological measures (Arena, Blanchard, Andrasik, Cotch, & Myers, 1983).

After obtaining the correlation coefficient, we analyzed the data using the standard error of measurement. In the term *standard error of measurement,* error simply refers to the difference in scores between a test and retest. Error does not mean making mistakes, although if a researcher made a mistake in giving a test or in a procedure, that would be an error and could influence the difference between test and retest measures. "Error of measurement" simply refers to the fact that we are talking about variation in measures, or scores. "Standard" means average, so the standard error of measurement is a statistic or number that represents the average amount of variation in repeated measures. If the standard error of measurement is large, then the variation among measures is large; if the standard error is small, then the variation is small. If we refer to correlation coefficients, then in the first case, the correlation would be lower, and in the second, it would be higher.

The standard error of measurement gives a *range* in which an individual's true score on a test might fall. Consider blood cholesterol again. When I (RS) have my blood cholesterol taken, I always wonder whether the measurement for that day, at that time, is typical of every day and truly represents my blood cholesterol. I know that there are many sources of "error"— personal and laboratory variables—that make it unlikely that the single reading is accurate. I would like to know the range of scores in which

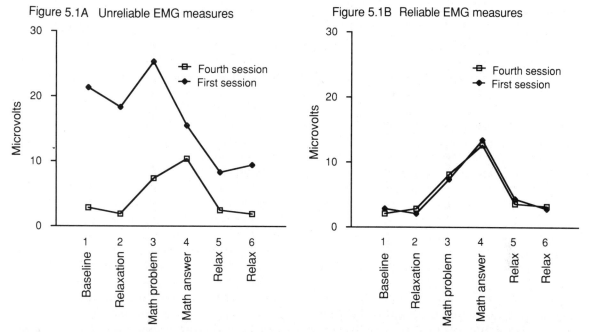

Figure 5.1A Unreliable EMG measures

Figure 5.1B Reliable EMG measures

Figure 5.1   Stress Profiles of Two Students, One with Unreliable Measures (5.1A) and One with Reliable Measures (5.1B). Four Stress Profiles Were Given during One Month. The Graphs Show Measurements on the First and Fourth Profiles. EMG Averages Are Shown for Six Conditions: 1-Baseline, 2-Relaxation, 3-Math Problem, 4-Math Answer, 5-Relax, 6-End of Relaxation.

my true cholesterol level is likely to be. If the range is small, then my cholesterol will be close to the level measured for that day; if the range is large, I know that the reading could actually be much higher or much lower than the measurement for that day.

When I get my blood cholesterol results, I ask for the standard error of measurement. Unfortunately, it is not available and the laboratory personnel do not know what I am talking about. With the standard error of measurement, I could determine the range of scores in which my true blood cholesterol level is likely to be. The range is based on the standard variation in blood cholesterol that occurs when cholesterol is measured repeatedly over many days with many subjects, which is how the standard error is determined. With the standard of error of measurement, I would calculate a range above and below my actual reading, and I would be confident that my cholesterol

level was within that range. The range is called a **confidence band**.

Figure 5.2 shows a confidence band for my last blood cholesterol reading. The reading was 170 milligrams per milliliter. Assuming that the standard error of measurement was 5 mg, I create a range—the confidence band—by adding 5 to 170 and subtracting 5 from 170. An accurate interpretation of my cholesterol would be to say that it falls between 165 and 175. Although it is customary to say "My blood cholesterol is 170," this is not accurate; in fact, there is only a 68 percent chance that it is in the 165–175 range.

The band for ±5 is called a 68 percent confidence band. There is a 32 percent chance that it is outside the 165–175 range. To be 95 percent confident that my cholesterol level is within a given range, I double the standard error of measurement, to ±10, getting a range of 160–180. With a 95 percent confidence band there is only

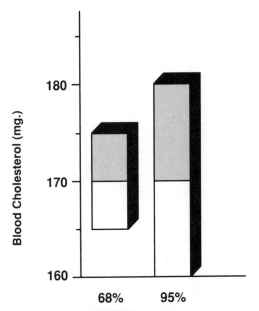

Figure 5.2 Hypothetical Confidence Bands for Blood Cholesterol.

a 5 percent chance that my scores are outside this range, but the range in which my cholesterol level is likely to fall is larger. (For the purposes of this chapter, you may ignore this bit of statistical magic. If you have taken statistics, you may remember the description of the normal distribution of a set of scores. You can account for 68 percent of the scores by adding or subtracting the standard deviation of the scores from the mean of the scores and can account for 95 percent of the scores by doubling the standard deviation. To derive the 68 percent and 95 percent confidence bands, the standard error of measurement, like the standard deviation, is simply added to or subtracted from the mean, or twice the error term is used.)

If, in fact, the standard error of measurement for blood cholesterol were actually only 5 mg, I would be 95 percent confident that my cholesterol was in the range 160–180. I would be satisfied because 180 is a satisfactory level, and it could be as low as 160. If cholesterol measurements were unreliable, with a large

standard error of measurement, say 20 mg, then I would be 95 percent confident that my actual level was between 210 and 130, that is, 170 ± 40. In this case I would not know whether my cholesterol was too high or quite low.

Now what if my cholesterol is measured at 210, and I decide to lower cholesterol by maintaining a strict diet? For many weeks I stick with the diet, and then I have blood cholesterol measured again. This time the reading is 180. I am delighted and immediately believe that the diet lowered my cholesterol until the laboratory tells me that the standard error of measurement is 20 mg/ml, and, therefore, the 95 percent confidence range for the prediet reading is 250–170 and is 220–140 for the second reading, as seen in Figure 5.3A. Looking at Figure 5.3A you can see that both readings could have been between 220 and 170 and, therefore, it is possible that my level has not changed at all. The area in which the bands overlap is the range in which the scores could have been the same. So in fact, I do not know for sure that the diet lowered cholesterol. The diet may have lowered cholesterol, but I do not know because the bands of the first and second reading overlap. I decide to stick with the diet. If the measurement had been reliable, with a small standard error of measurement, then the story would be very different, as seen in Figure 5.3B. In this case the range of possible cholesterol levels do not overlap; this means that whatever my level was on the first reading, it was definitely higher than on the second. I am confident that the diet has lowered blood cholesterol.

In summary, because there are so many causes of variation—or "error"—in blood cholesterol, it is impossible to know whether a single reading is correct. Since this can never be known, we can estimate a range and be confident that the true level is in that range. This is the best that can be done with psychological and physiological variables. The standard error of measurement should be included

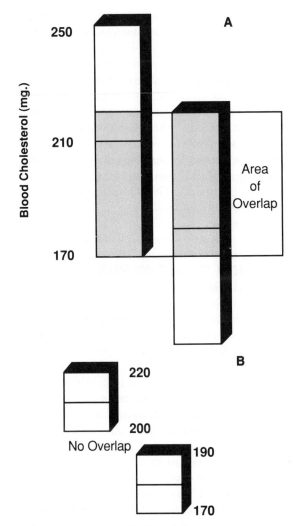

Figure 5.3   **Data with Confidence Bands That Overlap (5.3A) Are More Difficult to Interpret than Data with Confidence Bands That Do Not Overlap (5.3B).**

However, we realized that a reduction was not necessarily an indication of relaxation. We needed to know what "normal" relaxation measures were so that we could compare the "norms" with our data, just as we need to know what "normal" blood pressure is for comparison with an individual's reading. We examined the data from 200 profiles. We knew that we could not simply take an average of the reading and call that normal. We knew that since readings always involve some "error," the standard error of measurement was necessary to tell us the range of measures that are normal. Using the standard error for the normal data, we placed confidence bands around the individual measures of each subject. The range of normal variation in physiological measures was great, so the confidence bands were very large.

Figure 5.4 is an example of 68 percent confidence bands for EMG readings in microvolts for one student. Examine the confidence band

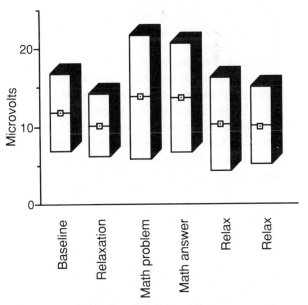

Figure 5.4   **68 Percent Confidence Bands for EMG Readings. The Wide Bands for the Stressors Indicate That People Differ Greatly in Response to These Stressors.**

when reporting psychological and physiological data so that the data can be interpreted correctly.

Now we return to research on stress profiles. As we said, one goal was to show that students had learned to relax, and we used physiological indicators of relaxation: a reduction in muscle tension, an increase in finger temperature, and a reduction in skin perspiration.

for phase six, the final relaxation. The person's response may have been anywhere from 5 microvolts up to 15 microvolts. Here is the problem: If we had given her a stress profile after she took the class, we would be unable to show that she had learned to relax. The range is so great that, even if she went from 15 microvolts on the preclass profile to 5 microvolts on the postclass profile, we could not claim with certainty that the change was due to her learning relaxation. The subject could have had this amount of change because of normal variation alone.

If we claimed that the student had learned to relax, based on changes in EMG measures, we might be wrong. Claiming that the student had learned to relax when in fact she had not, is analogous to a false positive in medical testing. Clearly, when measures are highly variable, the data cannot be interpreted.

We use our research on stress-profiling to illustrate the basics of reliability and the importance of determining the reliability of measurements. Had we used stress-profile measures to determine success of the stress-management and biofeedback class, we would have misinterpreted the data.

We also use the stress-profile research to illustrate reliability because physiological measures are common data in the health fields. They must be evaluated with care and some skepticism, especially when physiological measures are used to demonstrate learning. In our field, biofeedback therapy, in which physiological measures are used, we are developing ways of demonstrating learning that are not based on simple before-and-after physiological measurements that might be unreliable.

Now we return to Jim and the case of the false positive. The angiogram and treadmill led to a false positive, not because there was error in the instrumentation or procedure, but because there is variability in physiological processes. Jim is a good example of the variability of human physiological functions, particularly the cardiovascular system, which is very sensitive to stress. Jim's physician misinterpreted the test results because he failed to consider the effect of stress.

Measurements that are highly reliable, however, may not necessarily measure what they are supposed to measure. For example, a reliable IQ test may tell us nothing about intelligence. Although subjects who take the test repeatedly may have a similar score, the test itself may be flawed—instead of measuring basic intelligence, it might be measuring reading ability or cultural influences. The IQ measures would be reliable but not valid.

||||➡

SECTION TWO: THE PURSUIT OF VALIDITY

"Validity refers to the appropriateness, meaningfulness, and usefulness of the specific inferences made from test scores" (*Standards for Educational and Psychological Testing*, 1985, p. 9). A test or instrument is said to be valid when the measurements from it are useful and meaningful and measure what they are supposed to measure. If measurements did not predict anything or relate to health in any way, then the measurements would have no validity. One could have reliable blood pressure readings, but if the readings had no relationship to health, they would be meaningless and not valid.

There are different kinds of usefulness and meaningfulness, and, therefore, different kinds of validity. In this chapter, we discuss concurrent and predictive validity.

The stress profile measures only physiological reaction to stressors and recovery during relaxation. The underlying assumption is that health and responsivity to stressors and recovery, as measured by the profile, are related. If this is correct, then the stress profile would have concurrent validity and/or predictive validity. We examined both the concurrent and predictive validity of the stress profile.

Concurrent Validity

Concurrent means "at the same time." A test has **concurrent validity** if it indicates the presence of the variable being studied, such as health. If measures on the stress profile indicated whether or not a person was healthy at the time of taking the profile, the profile would have concurrent validity because the profile indicated the person's state of health at the time that it was given.

To determine the concurrent validity of the stress profile, we examined the data of 200 subjects who took one stress profile but did not participate in a stress-management class. All 200 subjects completed a comprehensive medical history (the Cornell Medical Index). In addition, all 151 of the students in the stress-management class and the 85 control group subjects had taken the Cornell Medical Index. This gave us a large population of 436 subjects who had stress profiles and completed the medical history.

We identified six groups of subjects who reported having heart disease, essential hypertension, ulcers, diarrhea, cancer, or headaches. We also identified a group of subjects who reported no health problems. We compared the stress profiles of each symptom group with the stress profiles of the symptom-free group. No significant difference emerged. The results of this study showed that the stress profile lacks concurrent validity. The stress profile could not distinguish symptom-free subjects from subjects with symptoms at the time that they took the profile.

Predictive Validity

Predictive validity refers to the relationship between the test measures and a future condition. We examined the ability of measures on the stress profile to predict the health of a subject two years after taking the stress-management class. We conducted a two-year follow-up study on 149 students who took the stress-management class and on the 200 control subjects who had one stress profile (Shellenberger, Turner, Green, & Cooney, 1986). The subjects received an extensive health questionnaire of current psychological and physiological health, the Holmes-Rahe Schedule of Recent Experiences, and the State-Trait Anxiety Inventory. Fifty questionnaires were returned from the stress-management group and 78 from the control group. In comparison to the control group, the members of the stress-management group showed a statistically significant reduction in physical symptoms and symptom severity, reported fewer physician visits, and perceived themselves as mentally and physically healthier.

Next we compared results on the stress profile with symptoms, physician visits, and self-perceptions of physical and mental health. The stress-profile measures did not predict any of the health changes. Even the most reliable measure, EMG during relaxation, had no predictive value.

The stress profile, as we used it, lacked predictive and concurrent validity and had only moderate reliability. Another attempt to demonstrate concurrent validity of the stress profile in our laboratory used "purer" subject groups than students from our classes. Subjects in the symptom groups were not using medications and had long-term symptoms. The stress-profile measures could not discriminate between symptom-free subjects and subjects with tension and migraine headaches (Clarke, Morris, & Cooney, 1987). We had to conclude that the stress profile is not valid; it cannot be used to predict or indicate health status. This was not a great surprise, because measures on the profile are not highly reliable.

Summary

We have taken you through our stress-profiling research to highlight the importance of establishing the reliability and validity of measures, to describe the meaning of these terms, and to indicate the difficulty of establishing reliability and validity of measures. When you study research results based on a measurement, whether psychological or physiological, you will want to know how the researcher established the reliability and validity of the measure. It is an important question to keep in mind when you evaluate research or your own physiological measures. When measurements are not reliable or valid, conclusions based on the measurements may be faulty.

IIII➡

SECTION THREE: QUESTIONS AND ISSUES—A CHECKLIST FOR RESEARCH EVALUATION

The primary concern of research is always the same: to generate data that accurately reflect the variables under investigation. This is crucial because conclusions based on erroneous data will be erroneous also. Research must be evaluated to determine whether or not the design or execution introduced errors or bias that could invalidate the results and conclusions. This section presents a checklist for evaluating the design and execution of research. The checklist includes determination of reliability and validity discussed in the previous section.

Credibility of the Source

Do the authors of the funding agency have a vested interest in the results? Does the experimenter have a particular "ax to grind" or a personal investment in the results? It is important to know who the experimenter is and how the research was funded. We received funds from a neutral organization, the Colorado Commission on Higher Education, to hire an independent researcher not familiar with the stress-management program and with no investment in the

outcome. The researcher and one assistant analyzed all the data. Laboratory assistants unfamiliar with the research projects administered the stress profiles. In contrast, a study of cigarette smoking as a risk factor for cancer and heart disease funded by the American Tobacco Institute could be biased. While funding and affiliation of the researcher are considerations in evaluating research, an appropriate research design, the use of reliable and valid measures, and conclusions that do not "go beyond the data" ensure the integrity of the research.

Subjects

Several questions and issues are relevant to the selection of subjects in research.

(1) What is the age, sex, ethnic background, occupation, and health status of the subjects, and will these variables affect the results? If the subjects are from a select subject population, is it possible to generalize from the results? Studies in psychology are often conducted on a convenient subject population: freshmen and sophomores in college who are taking general psychology classes; often these students earn extra credit for participating in research. Do the results of research on this select population apply to the general population? In some cases the answer is clearly "no," as we discover in the next chapter on studies of hardiness and health.

(2) How many subjects were tested? The number of subjects is referred to as "sample size" or "N" (N = 15 means that there were 15 subjects in the group). In general, the larger the N, the greater the likelihood that the results of the study will represent true findings, although larger samples do not guarantee significant results. The appropriate sample size depends on the goals of the research; the primary issue is that the conclusions be in keeping with the sample size. For example, if a study of 20 psychology students resulted in the conclusion that life changes do not affect health, the sample size would be meager for such a conclusion. In

contrast, studies of the Holmes-Rahe survey used thousands of subjects.

(3) How were the subjects selected? Subjects can be randomly chosen or can be volunteers who are randomly assigned to the experimental and control groups. The size of the sample is often less critical than how well it represents the population that the researcher wishes to describe. If a study generalizes about college freshmen in the United States, the sample must be representative of college freshmen across the country.

(4) How does the research account for individual difference? In most cases, the purpose of research is to discover trends and estimate probabilities based on group data. For example, research on smoking and lung cancer must examine hundreds of smokers to determine the incidence of lung cancer among smokers. From these data, a probability of getting lung cancer

from smoking is generated. But some smokers develop lung cancer early in life, while others smoke a lifetime without disease. Why? Individual difference.

Individual difference refers to the fact that no two people are alike, a continuous problem for research and for interpretation of results. Individual differences create three major problems: First, results may be "watered down," because research based on population samples "smooth out" individual responses by averaging the individual responses together. Second, studies with great variation in individual responses may be less meaningful, because the averaged data do not represent the subjects in the study. And third, results based on group data cannot predict the response of an individual.

To obtain a purer sample, in which individual differences are reduced, researchers try to create homogeneous samples by selecting

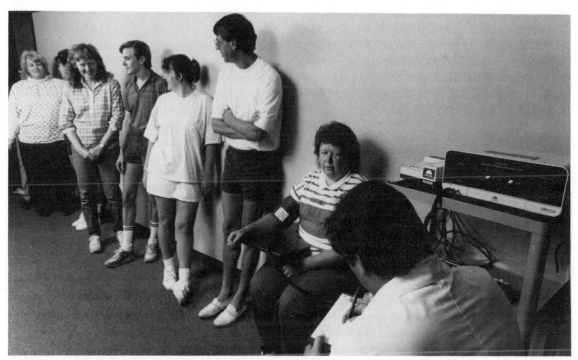

Individual Differences Are Clearly Seen in This Line of Students Waiting to Have Blood Pressure Taken. The Variation in Individuals Makes Group Data Difficult to Interpret.
Source: Robert Waltman, Aims Community College, Greeley, CO.

subjects who have similar sex, age, social background, and socioeconomic status. Another method for reducing individual differences is selection of subjects who are "pure" responders. For example, studies of the Holmes-Rahe survey and sickness could follow the health histories of only those with 300 or more points and compare the results to those with 50 or fewer points.

A good study will address the issue of individual difference and will try to reduce subject variation. Please read Box 5.1 now.

Independent and Dependent Variables

The language of experimental and laboratory research is of "independent" and "dependent" variables. In experimental and laboratory research, the independent variable is the variable that the experimenter manipulates to determine the effect on some other variable, called the dependent variable. For example, a researcher might study the effects of relaxation training on the stress level of college students. The relaxation training is the independent variable and stress level the dependent variable, because stress level hypothetically depends upon relaxation training.

Some types of research, such as epidemiology, do not involve experimentation. In **epidemiological** research, data are gathered on large groups of people and variables are correlated, but no experimentation is done—no variable is changed to determine the effects on another variable. As an example, the Jenkins Survey of Type A behavior, created by psychologist David Jenkins, was designed to measure Type A behavior. Type A behavior is associated with coronary heart disease. When the relationship of Type A behavior and coronary heart disease is studied, large groups of people are assessed for Type A characteristics, and these characteristics are correlated with the disease. In this case, Type A behavior is referred to as a "measured" independent variable, meaning

BOX 5.1

INDIVIDUAL DIFFERENCE

Individual differences make each human unique and make human research very difficult. To overcome these difficulties, some researchers work with laboratory animals, particularly rats. Genetically similar, identically reared laboratory rats may have few individual differences, but the relevance of the data for humans is always uncertain.

Human variation enabled Norman Cousins to speak of recovery from serious disease in this way: "No one knows enough to be pessimistic." But this wonderful variation makes it difficult to gather group data and then predict for a particular individual.

Of course, individual difference enables people to ignore research results: Smokers look at the data, note that only some people who smoke get lung cancer, and think "It will never happen to me."

Sometimes it is the unusual single case that alerts the researcher or clinician to a previously unnoticed variable. Carl Simonton, a pioneer in cancer treatment, became curious about the influence of the mind on cancer when a patient had an unusual recovery. This led to the development of a new approach in cancer treatment, discussed in Chapters 9 and 18.

that it is measured but not manipulated, as in a laboratory experiment. Type A can also be referred to as a quasi-experimental variable, again meaning that the behavior is not actually changed or manipulated. Coronary heart disease is the dependent variable, because the hypothesis is that the disease depends upon the presence of Type A behavior. Any other variable may be either independent or dependent, depending on the purpose of the study. One way to distinguish the two is by the phrase "If _____ (independent, or measured variable), then _____ (dependent variable)." If Type A personality is present, then coronary heart disease will be present. If Type A personality pattern is decreased, then the likelihood of coronary heart disease will decrease.

When the independent variable is a personality characteristic or trait, how is the trait defined and determined? How many Type A characteristics does a person have to have to be classified as Type A? How many positive items on an anger scale does a person need to be classified as an angry person? In evaluating research, it is important to know the criteria that are used to define the trait being studied. The criteria must be stringent enough to eliminate subjects who do not actually have the characteristic being studied.

Correlation and Causality

In health research, we are interested in the strength of the relationship between variables such as personality and health. For example, we can ask, "Is there a strong relationship between Type A personality and coronary heart disease?" **Correlation** is often used as a synonym for "strength of a relationship." This is the same concept that we used in discussing test-retest scores and correlation coefficients. A **positive correlation** means that rising scores on one variable are associated with rising scores on another variable. Scores on the Holmes-Rahe survey are positively correlated with scores on a sickness inventory if the Holmes-Rahe hypothesis about life changes and sickness is correct. A **negative correlation** means that rising scores on one variable are associated with falling scores on another variable. For example, age over 65 years and

income are negatively correlated, because for the population in general, as age over 65 increases, income decreases.

The previous section discussed the use of correlation coefficients for determining the reliability of a test. Correlation coefficients are also used for determining the validity of a test. A perfect positive correlation is written +1.00, and a perfect negative correlation is −1.00. If all the Type A men in a study have coronary heart disease and if all the Type B men have no heart disease, there is a +1.00 correlation between Type A and coronary heart disease and a −1.00 correlation between Type B and coronary heart disease. The test for measuring Type A and Type B behavior would have concurrent validity.

Following this hypothetical example, in which there is a perfect positive correlation between Type A behavior and coronary heart disease, can we conclude that Type A behavior causes coronary heart disease? No. Correlation cannot be used to infer causality. There are other possible explanations: Coronary heart disease (H) may cause Type A behavior (A). The physiological changes that occur in heart disease may cause anxiety, irritability, and time pressures, and thus change the personality of individuals, H → A; or, a third factor may cause both Type A behavior and coronary heart disease. For example, a competitive social environment (S) may cause both Type A behavior and coronary heart disease. The frustrations and competitiveness of twentieth-century America may cause changes in physiology that in turn cause coronary heart

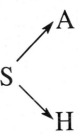

Figure 5.5

disease. Because correlation does not prove causality, how is causality determined?

Some researchers argue that in research with human subjects, establishing causality is impossible because of the differences among individuals, the multiplicity of causes for human behavior, and the uncontrolled variables that humans bring to a study. Nevertheless, there are guidelines and methods that provide a degree of certainty regarding causality. We examine these methods in the next section on research design.

Research Design

One method for improving determination of causality is the **prospective** research design. In the prospective design, subjects are measured on whatever variable is thought to be the cause of the behavior of interest, before the behavior or disease occurs. For example, the Western Collaborative Group Study conducted by Friedman and Rosenman, the originators of the Type A concept, was prospective. Healthy subjects were classified as Type A or Type B; the health records were examined 8 1/2 years later to determine which subjects had coronary heart disease. In studying personality and disease, the prospective study eliminates the possibility that the sickness itself caused the personality pattern, because the subject's personality pattern is determined to be present before the disorder develops. The results of the Western Collaborative Group Study disproved the alternative hypothesis that Type A behavior is caused by coronary heart disease.

Alternative explanations of results can be eliminated through experimental and control groups. For example, even if Type A behavior predicts coronary heart disease, there may be alternative explanations. One alternative is that a bad marriage is the real cause of coronary heart disease and the real cause of Type A behavior. To find out whether a bad marriage

is a likely cause, we could set up an elaborate prospective study with four groups: Type A individuals with a poor marriage (experimental group); Type A individuals with a good marriage (control group); Type B individuals with a good marriage (control group); and Type B individuals with a poor marriage (control group). If Type A individuals have coronary heart disease regardless of the quality of their marriage, and Type B individuals have less coronary heart disease regardless of the quality of their marriage, then we could confidently exclude the hypothesis that a poor marriage is the cause of both Type A behavior and coronary heart disease.

Control groups can rule out possible explanations for results that are not related to the independent variable. Even so, it is often impossible to claim that a causal relationship between two variables has been established with certainty. It is always possible to think of another possible cause. If you are a Type A person and do not want to change, you may be able to imagine many other causes of coronary heart disease that do not relate to you.

Elimination is another method for establishing causality: Eliminate the presumed cause of the variable being studied and observe the results. A standard procedure in brain research is to eliminate the part of the brain that is presumed to cause a particular behavior; if the behavior stops, this is evidence for the causal relationship of the brain area and the behavior.

Using the elimination approach, how would you design a study to determine the effects of Type A behavior? You would reduce or eliminate Type A behavior in Type A people and study disease patterns. Several studies have taught Type A people to have Type B behaviors—they feel less hostility and less time pressure. In one study, Type A individuals significantly lowered their blood cholesterol levels by developing Type B behaviors (Suinn, 1980). (Chapter 17 describes a program for changing Type A behavior.)

Statistical and Practical Significance

How significant are the results? *Significance* has two meanings. One is defined statistically, and the other is our common use, "important."

Statistical significance is a measure of the probability that the differences between two groups are due to the independent variable and not to chance. For example, studies show that Type A individuals have more coronary heart disease than Type B individuals. But we need to know whether this difference is due to chance or to important Type A characteristics that cause heart disease that Type B individuals do not have. Statistical significance is a way of talking about the probability that the results of research—more Type A people have coronary heart disease than Type B people—are really due to characteristics of Type A's and not to chance.

A research result is statistically significant when it is extremely unlikely that it occurred by chance. The accepted criterion for saying that a result is significant is when chance could account for the result only 5 times out of 100, expressed as $p < .05$ (p = probability and $<$ means less than). Results are of even greater statistical significance if chance could account for the data only 1 out of 100 times, expressed as $p < .01$. If chance could have created the result more than five times, say 20 times out of 100, then the results are not significant because the probability that the results occurred by chance is high. In general, research findings are not reported unless the statistical significance is at least $p < .05$. Because sample size is included in the formula for determining significance, the larger the sample, the greater the likelihood that the results will be statistically significant.

An important point is that data can be statistically significant but have no significant meaning or practical importance. For example, a study of heart-rate reduction with biofeedback training reported statistically significant results at the $p < .05$ level of significance. In fact, subjects lowered heart rate an average of eight-tenths of a beat per minute. This is not physiologically significant—heart rates can vary more than five beats per minute during a normal resting period (Banderia, Bouchard, & Granger, 1982). The issue of statistical versus physiological significance applies to other health research, such as research on personality variables and components of the immune system. An immunologist states: "Many research studies show a statistically significant difference between control and experimental groups but the differences are too small to be of biological significance. . . . 'Statistically, but not biologically significant' is a phrase immunologists love to use" (Cohen, 1985, p. 168).

A research report needs to provide an explanation of the practical as well as the statistical significance of the results. The criterion of statistical significance, however, must be met before determining practical significance.

Replication

Has the study been replicated by other researchers and were the results similar? Before I change my lifestyle after taking a personality test for Type A behavior, I want evidence from many studies that Type A behavior is a risk factor for coronary heart disease. Am I unreasonable in this requirement? No. Support of hypotheses builds slowly in the health sciences. Conclusions based on research results are definite only after similar results occur repeatedly.

Demonstration of Learning

When the independent variable involves a skill, does the research indicate that the skill was learned, and how was learning measured? We include this item because several health professions, such as psychotherapy and biofeedback training, involve skills. Throughout this text we report research that involves skill acquisition. When research attempts to evaluate the effectiveness of a skill, it must first be demonstrated that the skill was learned. For example, results of a biofeedback training study designed to assess the effectiveness of hand temperature training for reducing migraine headache might lead to the conclusion that hand-warming is not effective in the treatment of migraine. In evaluating the research, two questions are asked: First, did the subjects learn to raise hand temperature high enough and consistently enough to be clinically significant, to reduce their headaches? Second, how is learning measured? If subjects did not master the skill, then no conclusion can be made about the efficacy of hand-warming for reducing headaches.

The demonstration of learning is not always easy. The earlier section on reliability and validity shows that physiological measures may be so variable that a change from test to retest may be the result of natural variation and not the result of learning. When physiological measures are used to demonstrate learning, the interpretation of results is uncertain.

The Law of Initial Values (Benjamin, 1963; Lacey & Lacey, 1962) is another complication in demonstrating that a skill is learned, based on physiological data. The law states that the magnitude of the change of any physiological response is a function of the beginning level. For example, the upper limit of finger temperature achieved through biofeedback training is approximately 97°F. A trainee with a starting temperature of 94°F may raise the temperature only two or three degrees, because of the high initial value. A second trainee beginning at 70° could increase the temperature as much as 25°. Has the second trainee significantly learned to relax and increase blood flow in the hands, while the first trainee has not? Not necessarily. Without accounting for initial values, the data could be misinterpreted.

In evaluating studies that involve acquisition of a skill, it is important to determine whether the researcher considered the initial values of the subject in measuring learning.

Interpretation

Correct interpretation of results is the goal of research and is a difficult and complicated task. Research results depend on many variables, and interpretation must take these variables into account. Failure to evaluate research design and measurement procedure when evaluating results is a common error. A second error is unwarranted generalization and conclusions that "go beyond the data." You will not know that conclusions are in error unless you know how to critically evaluate a study. A good researcher will include these issues in the discussion of results.

The purpose of the research must also be considered in the interpretation. Was the research designed to prove a particular point, or was it purely exploratory? Research that is designed to prove a point or settle a controversy must be critiqued with particular care because the research design may inadvertently bias the results in favor of the hypotheses.

IIII➡ CONCLUSION AND CHECK LIST

Research is an integral part of the health sciences, and research is complex. The results of a study depend on many variables that must be carefully evaluated before the results are accepted or rejected. These variables include research design, the reliability and validity of the measurements, and statistical and clinical significance. We have suggested several questions that you should raise when evaluating research. Box 5.2 is a checklist of the variables that we described.

When you read a research study, use the checklist to evaluate it. If a study is low on any item, then the results of the study may be in

BOX 5.2

RESEARCH CHECK LIST

	Low	Moderate	High
1. Credibility of the source			
2. Subject selection			
3. Independent and dependent variable			
4. Strength of correlation or causality			
5. Research design			
6. Statistical and practical significance			
7. Replication			
8. If the independent variable is a skill, was the skill learned?			
9. Reliability			
10. Validity			
11. Interpretation			

doubt. For example, imagine that you are evaluating a study on the use of subliminal tapes to help people lose weight. Who funded and conducted the research? Did a company that sells subliminal tapes pay for and conduct the research, or is the project funded by an independent institution? Who are the researchers? Are they invested in the results? Could researcher bias affect the results or the interpretation? If you are not certain, suspend judgment about the effectiveness of the tapes for helping people lose weight until other studies conducted by independent researchers have found similar results.

Suppose that you are reading a study showing that children who learn to relax improve academically. Item eight on the checklist would be an important consideration. Did the research demonstrate that the children significantly learned to relax, or did the researchers merely report that children listened to relaxation tapes for 15 minutes every day for five weeks, for example, and assume that the children learned a relaxation skill? Exposure to relaxation tapes does not mean acquisition of relaxation skills. If the researchers did not measure relaxation skills, suspend judgment about the affect of relaxation on academic performance.

On subject selection, you would rank a study "high" if the subjects were randomly selected and were appropriate for the conclusions. For item three, independent and dependent variables, you would determine whether the variables were well defined and appropriately isolated. As you evaluate research, go through the checklist and determine whether the criteria discussed in this chapter are met.

We have included a chapter on research because research is important in the health sciences. Research is a tool for demonstrating relationships between variables—such as Type A behavior and coronary heart disease—and as an experimental process in which the effects of the independent variable are demonstrated—such as the effects of changing Type A behavior and reduction in risk for coronary heart disease. Although common sense, personal experience, and intuition are all ways of knowing, and often contribute to knowledge, the ultimate test of the validity of an idea or procedure is research validation. We might have a clear and correct hunch that certain behaviors are a risk for disease, for example, but the hunch is not likely to be accepted as correct until it is demonstrated through research.

The concepts introduced in this chapter are rather general: test-retest, reliability, correlation coefficient, standard error of measurement, and validity of various types. We do not intend to turn you into a statistician; our intention is merely to introduce several important concepts and issues in research. You do not need to be completely skeptical or accepting about every research finding; you can ask intelligent questions about health sciences research, and you can seek some of the answers yourself.

Now we must tell the whole truth. We have taught you the ideal method. You now know that it is important to know how high the correlation coefficient is on test-retest scores when the reliability of a test is determined; you now know that it is important to know how much variation there is in a measure. The truth is that few researchers report these statistics. The confidence band approach to describing variation and uncertainty in a particular measure is a recent innovation, and it is not usually reported. This means that we are unable to present confidence bands for the data in this text, although we describe many studies in which physiological measures are the dependent variable, and it would be useful to have this information in evaluating the data.

If you are designing instead of evaluating research, the same questions and issues apply. Research is fun, and it is hard work. It involves mysteries and puzzles that may take many years to solve. In the chapters on personality and health, for example, we discuss studies in which researchers spent 30 years conducting one longitudinal study on a population from birth to adulthood in order to determine the stability of personality traits.

As you can imagine, a career in health research is challenging.

The Dynamics of Stress Resistance

Part One examined two innate and fundamental dynamics of health and wellness, mind → body and homeostasis. Part Two described a force in life, stress, that is so pervasive and potentially destructive that coping effectively with it is a dynamic of health and wellness. The content of Part Three presents a solid foundation for effective coping, a foundation for personal health and for effective therapy.

In the Preface we suggested that health is not a matter of "just good luck." The content of Part Three takes you beyond good luck to the development of skills and resources for health and wellness.

In Chapter 6, Psychosocial Dynamics of Stress Resistance, we describe psychological and social factors that promote stress resistance, which helps people stay well in spite of stressful life events. In Part Three you will discover that like illness and disease, health and wellness have patterns, conditions, and variables, and that people who are psychologically and physically healthy have characteristics and resources that distinguish them from unhealthy people. Knowledge of a stress-resistant personality type, the hardy personality, is emerging through extensive research on healthy people. The characteristics of hardiness are described in detail. After examining the psychological characteristics and social supports of stress-resistant people, we focus on the next question "What skills do stress-resistant people have that enable them to remain healthy?" The concept "learned resourcefulness" nicely states the idea that stress resistance results from using resources that can be learned.

The remaining chapters in Part Three describe a variety of skills and resources, beginning with another fundamental dynamic in health and wellness, relaxation, in Chapter 7, Relaxation. Relaxation has the status of a dynamic because it promotes healthy psychological and physiological homeostasis. Chapter 8, Biofeedback Training, describes the principles and rationale for this unique tool for psychophysiological self regulation. We discuss the conceptual model and provide a brief history, including controversies that make the study of biofeedback training particularly interesting. Chapter 9, Imagery for Health and Wellness, describes a resource that people are born with but rarely taught to use. We present many uses of imagery and visualization, including stress management, enhancing performance, self-exploration, and healing. Like many other "natural resources" imagery is a dynamic that can be a powerful tool in health and wellness.

Chapter 10, Cognitive and Multicomponent Approaches to Stress Resistance, describes cognitive skills that facilitate stress resistance and tells how these skills are taught. These include skills for cognitive restructuring, to overcome negative thinking, and stress inoculation, a complex set of skills for coping with all stressors. We also discuss applications of stress-inoculation training for reducing anger and for enhancing performance in sports and education.

We begin Chapter 10 with a diagram of the techniques for gaining stress resistance discussed in Part Three. We recommend examining Figure 10.1 now.

CHAPTER 6

Psychosocial Dynamics of Stress Resistance

IIII➡

"I can't believe this report!" exclaimed Lawrence Hinkle to his colleague and medical partner, Norman Plummer. "Listen to this."

> M. L. was the daughter of a teenage girl and an alcoholic longshoreman. She grew up in an atmosphere of poverty and constant squabbling, punctuated by the deaths of four of her nine brothers and sisters. When she was three years old her father deserted the family; when she was five her mother was judged unfit to raise her, and she spent the next eight years in a series of orphanages. At the age of 13 M. L. was put to work as a domestic servant, but three years later she embarked upon a series of other jobs and casual love affairs carried on, as she put it, "all over town." Then, at 23, she went to work for the telephone company, and at 27 she married a plumber's helper who was neurotic, chronically sick, and usually out of work. They had no children, and when she was 44 he died in her arms; at the time she was interviewed she had been a widow for 10 years.
>
> (Tanner, 1976)

"That life history would make a psychiatrist blanch," said Dr. Plummer.

"Yet M. L. was the most stable, highly respected, and well-liked of all the 2,000 company employees," said Dr. Hinkle. "The only illnesses she suffered during 31 years as a telephone operator were a few common colds—though she did admit to a spell of 'nervousness' after her husband's death."

Lawrence Hinkle and Norman Plummer, physicians for the New York Telephone Company, were trying to identify the causes of absenteeism in the employees. They examined the life histories, quality-of-work evaluations, and health histories of 2,000 employees. To their surprise, some employees had an unusual number of stressful life events but remained healthy, like the longshoreman's daughter (Hinkle, 1974). This contradicted the research of Holmes and Rahe on the relationship between stress and illness.

To determine the effect of stress on health, Holmes and Rahe created the Social Readjustment Rating Scale, which gives a stress "score" to various life changes. Holmes and Rahe found that if a person's total score is more than 300 points in a single year, there is nearly an 80 percent chance of illness in the following two years. Yet the telephone company study and other research shows that people can accumulate life-change units of 300 or more and remain healthy (Kobasa, 1979). The correlation coefficient between the number of life-change units and number of illnesses in the two years after taking the questionnaire, in the Holmes and Rahe study, was 0.78. In another study, however, the correlation coefficient was 0.10, and in Rahe's study of naval officers, the correlation was 0.12. The low correlations in these studies reflect the fact that some people had high life-change scores and few illnesses (Kobasa, 1979; Neugebauer, 1984).

Obviously many people experience stressful life changes and hardships and do not get sick. Many people work night and day at stressful jobs and do not become ill. Prisoners have survived concentration camps and stayed well. The longshoreman's daughter survived a very stressful childhood and marriage and remained healthy; in fact, of 2,000 telephone operators she was the healthiest. What are the characteristics of these people? What enables them to remain healthy in spite of stressful events?

In the search for the dynamics of health and wellness, answers to these questions are important. We learn about health by studying healthy people. Research on healthy people and the dynamics of health reflect the growing awareness that to promote health and develop successful treatments, we must know what health is. Knowledge of health and wellness is the foundation of treatment.

The application of the dynamics of health and wellness in therapy and teaching concerns two major issues regarding stress: how to eliminate stress, and how to cope with stressors and be stress-resistant when stress cannot be eliminated. This chapter concentrates on the psychological and social factors that contribute to stress resistance—staying well in spite of stress.

Stress resistance is precisely what the term suggests, being resistant to the negative effects of stress. The basic research approaches to understanding the dynamics of stress resistance are to study the characteristics of people who are stress-resistant and to teach people to be stress-resistant, and then follow their health history.

Stress resistance is a global concept that does not specify exact mechanisms. In fact, there are probably as many ways of being stress-resistant as there are ways of being stressed. In this chapter we introduce the major elements of stress resistance.

Section One examines the research of Suzanne Kobasa, a pioneer in the study of healthy people. Kobasa created the concept "hardy personality" to describe the characteristics of people who stay well in spite of stressful life changes.

In Section Two, we discuss "meaning in life." Meaning, or purpose in life, is a force that enables people to overcome great stress and gives the "staying power" needed to cope with the hassles of everyday life. The importance of meaning in life has been studied most thoroughly in circumstances in which life is threatened. We examine the research on people who survived concentration camps, torture, rape, abuse, and deprivation, and remained healthy.

In Section Three, research on the importance of social factors for physical health is

examined. Social resources such as positive marital relationships, friends, and participation in religious groups are invaluable buffers against stress and illness.

In Section Four, we examine ways that ordinary people deal with the stress of ordinary situations, including the "ultimate" coping style, called transformational. Finally, we ask: "What specific skills do people have who are behaviorally well?" Because we describe self regulation as the essence of wellness, we are asking "What skills are needed for self regulation?" In answering this question we describe the concept "learned resourcefulness," which means that to be stress-resistant, people must have resources, and that these resources can be learned. The topic of self regulation is so extensive that a chapter is devoted to it in Part Five.

IIII➡

SECTION ONE: HARDINESS

While flipping through a popular woman's magazine in her doctor's waiting room, psychologist Suzanne Kobasa noticed an article on stress. The article included the Holmes and Rahe Social Readjustment Rating questionnaire. The author said that if a person scored 300 or more points on the test there was an 80 percent chance of becoming seriously ill, and a 60 percent chance if the score was 200 or more points. The author advised readers who scored high to avoid stressful events by avoiding touchy issues with one's spouse, friends, or colleagues.

Kobasa was bothered by the fact that the scientific basis for a link between stressful life changes and illness is weak. From her own studies, she knew that the correlation between scores on the Social Readjustment Rating questionnaire and sickness is low. Kobasa was also disturbed by the advice. Avoiding stressful events by ignoring problems seemed limiting; opportunities for personal and professional growth could be lost. Kobasa also thought that the author's view of the person as a passive victim of stressful events was misleading and overlooked the fact that people have considerable potential for creatively handling stressful life change.

Kobasa's dissatisfaction with these popular ideas about stress motivated her to change her career and enhanced our understanding of the dynamics of health. It was obvious to Kobasa that people can experience many life changes and stay healthy. She reasoned that physically healthy stressed people are psychologically different from physically unhealthy stressed people, so she set out to discover the personality characteristics of people who are healthy in spite of stressful life events.

For many years, Kobasa has tackled this topic through extensive studies with a variety of subjects: executives, lawyers, bus drivers, cancer patients, military personnel, and students. This work has created an entirely new area of research, the study of hardiness.

Take a minute: Let come into your mind the image of a hardy person.

Do It Now.

What did you think of? A pioneer woman striding across the prairie, a child on one hip and a rifle on the other? A Sylvester Stallone with bulging muscles? Yourself, studying all night for an exam? A 1-year-old getting up again after falling down for the hundredth time? Was your person the "image of health"?

To study people who stay healthy in spite of stressful events, Kobasa needed a large number of subjects who were stressed. The executives at Illinois Bell Telephone Company were a perfect group. Middle- and upper-level executives were confronted with many stressors. A major stressor was the reorganization of the company, with the possibility of promotion, demotion, or loss of job.

Kobasa's first task was to identify high stress/high sickness and high stress/low sickness subjects. In other words, instead of using a random sample of executives in which all combinations of stress and sickness would be found, she selected subjects so that in one group the correlation between stress and sickness would be low (high stress/low sickness) and in the other group the correlation would be high (high stress/high sickness). With this sampling technique, Kobasa created groups that would characterize the extremes, thus highlighting the differences between the healthy subjects and the unhealthy subjects.

Kobasa mailed a stress and sickness questionnaire to 837 executives. Of those who responded, 116 executives had high stress/low sickness scores and 150 executives had high stress/high sickness scores. Kobasa randomly selected 100 subjects from each group for her study. Subjects took three standardized psychological tests (see Box 6.1). Analysis of the tests revealed significant differences between the sick and the healthy people.

Kobasa found that people who are physically well in spite of stress have a particular constellation of personality characteristics that she labeled "hardy." Hardy people (1) have a strong **commitment** to work, family, friends, religion, political or altruistic endeavors; (2) view **change as a challenge**; and (3) experience a sense of **personal control** over their lives. The three C's—commitment, sense of control, and challenge—are the essential ingredients of psychological hardiness (Kobasa, 1979).

Did your image of "the hardy person" include these characteristics?

Each of the personality tests that Kobasa used had questions related to commitment, sense of control, and perception of change as a challenge. The set of questions on a test that relate to a particular characteristic is called a "scale," so Kobasa refers to the sets as "hardiness scales." To determine the ability of the hardiness scales to predict sickness, Kobasa gave the three tests to an additional 80 executives. Using only the data from the hardiness scales, she correctly determined the health status of 62 of those executives. Please read Box 6.1 now.

To determine the stability of the hardiness traits over time, Kobasa retested the executives twice in two years. The traits were stable, and over the two-year period hardy executives

BOX 6.3

REPLICATING RESEARCH

The work of Kobasa and colleagues was careful and lengthy. Investigators attempting to verify research results must maintain these high standards. In fact, this does not always happen. Investigators who attempt to repeat original work may shorten the techniques or simplify measures, using a pencil-paper test to replace a lengthy interview, for example. The shortcuts may lead to results that erroneously cast doubt on the original concepts and research findings.

When results seem to conflict, it is important to examine the studies in detail. For example, Feist and Brannon (1988) state, "Kobasa's hardiness hypothesis has received only mixed support from other investigators" (p. 131). We examined the two studies that were used to support the "mixed support" comment. Both studies were retrospective (Ganellen & Blaney, 1984; Schmied & Lawler, 1986), and Ganellen and Blaney did not include all five hardiness scales. In another study of undergraduate students (research for a master's thesis), Wiebe and McCallum (1986) conclude, "In our study, hardiness

does not appear to affect sickness by changing the effects of stress. Thus, it may be misleading to view hardiness as a stress-resistant resource" (p. 436). The results of this two-month prospective study cannot negate the results of a five-year prospective study. However, as Hull, Treuren, and Virnelli (1987) point out, further research is needed to refine the hardiness scales. In addition, replication of Kobasa's prospective studies with working people is needed. Current research, even that supporting hardiness as a buffer against illness, has been primarily retrospective and has used college students as subjects (Rhodewalt & Zone, 1989).

Often, conflicting or nonsupportive results follow methodological errors and failure to exactly replicate original studies. This has been a recurring problem in research on Type A behavior, hardiness, hypnosis, transcendental meditation, autogenic training, progressive relaxation, and all types of biofeedback training. This issue is discussed further in the chapters on biofeedback training and behavioral medicine.

---

the behaviors, beliefs, and skills that enabled inmates to adapt to imprisonment. Frankl noted that those who could not adapt and perished from sickness and despair had lost all meaning in life and were unable to make sense of the present or to see any future. Prisoners who hung on to "meaning" seemed to have a thread that kept them from despair and fatal disease. From these observations, Frankl formulated the concept "will to meaning" described in his first book, *Man's Search for Meaning* (1963).

Will to meaning refers to the universal human need for a meaningful purpose in life and the will to create meaning. Frankl believes that the will to meaning is a primary drive similar to thirst and hunger. It was their will to meaning, Frankl says, that kept prisoners from committing suicide—"throwing oneself on the high voltage wire" (Frankl, 1963). "He who has a why to live for can bear with almost any how" was the guiding motto behind Frankl's efforts to help his fellow prisoners. The specific focus of each person's "why" varied among the survivors of the Nazi Holocaust. For some, meaning in life came from the desire for revenge; for others, it was to be reunited with family members; some prisoners endured in order to inform the world of the atrocities; and others endured to establish a national homeland.

In the concentration camp, the will to create meaning helped Frankl gain a sense of control by providing a focus for his inner life that he could control. Frankl writes that when he was disgusted and overwhelmed:

> I forced my thoughts to turn to another subject. Suddenly I saw myself standing on the platform of a well-lit warm and pleasant lecture room. . . . I was giving a lecture on the psychology of the concentration camp. . . . All that oppressed me at that moment became objective, seen and described from the remote viewpoint of science. By this method I succeeded somehow in rising above the situation, above the sufferings of the moment, and I observed them as if they already had become a part of the past. . . .
>
> (Frankl, 1963, p. 117)

On the basis of his experiences in the Nazi death camp, Viktor Frankl concluded that a fundamental motive is at the basis for human existence—the will to create meaning, fueled by the fundamental need for meaning.

Is "will to meaning" a basic motive? Let us look at some evidence. Most teenagers who commit suicide have the basic necessities: food, clothing, and security. Is the real problem a "crisis in meaning"? Is meaning, or the will to create meaning, so lacking in these teenagers that when an apparently minor crisis arises—like a poor grade or a disloyal friend—the event cannot be put in perspective. Personal experience and research suggest what most people intuitively know— meaning in life promotes life. A cancer patient may live beyond life expectancy to attend a daughter's wedding; patients may live beyond medical expectations when living becomes the purpose in life (Achterberg, Matthews-

Simonton, & Simonton, 1977; Phillips & Feldman, 1973).

If this is beginning to sound familiar, it should. Kobasa acknowledged the influence of Frankl and other existential thinkers who emphasize the importance of meaning (Wood, 1987). In this respect, hardiness research is a verification of Frankl's insight on the importance of a meaningful purpose in life, except that Kobasa used the term commitment.

Professor Radil-Weiss, at the Institute of Physiology in the Czechoslovakia Academy of Sciences and a survivor of Auschwitz, describes the importance of meaning in life in the following way:

> Under these exceptional conditions, where the stress was maximum and the reserves were subject to maximum depletion, it was more apparent than under normal circumstances to what an extent the neural and neurohumeral regulation of internal processes in the organisms depends on the psychic processes. . . . Men of strong will, convinced of the importance of the principles they consistently followed, and imbued with a unified world conception, endured better than persons who vacillated in their points of view.
>
> (Radil-Weiss, 1983, p. 259)

The observations of Frankl and Radil-Weiss on the importance of the will to meaning for surviving extreme conditions is confirmed by several researchers. Aaron Antonovsky has spent many years studying the importance of a meaningful purpose in life, which is based on a "sense of coherence" (Antonovsky, 1987).

The Sense of Coherence

Aaron Antonovsky, professor of medical sociology at Ben Gurion University of the Negev in Israel, studied 77 European women who had been in a concentration camp during World War II. Most of the survivors were poorly adapted to life compared with other women, but some were well adapted. Antonovsky observed that although these women had lived through inhuman experiences, they were fairly healthy, had raised families, and had a social network. Many held jobs and were involved in their communities. How did these women stay mentally and physically healthy? Like Frankl, Antonovsky found that the well-adapted survivors maintained a sense of coherence based on the belief that life is meaningful. They had mobilized their inner resources to resist the extremely stressful environment. The sense of coherence results from the belief that something in life is worthy of commitment. Antonovsky says that people with a sense of coherence can turn unhappy experiences into a challenge and will be determined to overcome the situation with dignity.

To understand how the sense of coherence enables people to survive extreme conditions, Antonovsky studied 51 people who had experienced major trauma and were coping well. He included people who had been interned in concentration camps and people who had undergone trauma such as severe disability, loss of a child or spouse, or poverty. Antonovsky's lengthy interview began with the request: "Please tell about your life." In answering this, a 90-year-old man with a strong sense of coherence said:

> How we overcame all the difficulties in our lives? You need patience. You have to believe in the Promise, a word I learned in Bulgaria. . . . It doesn't have to be God. It can be another force, but you have to have faith. Otherwise you can't suffer so much and go on. . . .
>
> (Antonovsky, 1987, p. 68)

To measure a person's sense of coherence, Antonovsky developed the Orientation to Life questionnaire. A number of studies have shown the instrument to be highly reliable. There is increasing evidence that people who score high on sense of coherence are healthier than people who score low.

Sense of coherence, meaning in life, and commitment refer to the same phenomena— the importance of a meaningful purpose in life for maintaining health and surviving stressful experiences. Kobasa compared Antonovsky's

---

BOX 6.4

ORIENTATION TO LIFE QUESTIONNAIRE

The following questions are examples from Antonovsky's Orientation to Life questionnaire. Each question has seven possible answers.

1. When you talk to people, do you have the feeling that they don't understand you?
   1 never have this feeling–2–3–4–5–6–7 always have this feeling
2. Do you have the feeling that you don't really care about what goes on around you?
   1 never have this feeling–2–3–4–5–6–7 always have this feeling
3. Life is:
   1 full of interest–2–3–4–5–6–7 complete routine
4. Until now your life has had:
   1 no clear goals–2–3–4–5–6–7 very clear goals
5. Do you have very mixed-up feelings and ideas?
   1 very often–2–3–4–5–6–7 very seldom or never
6. Do you think that there will always be people whom you'll be able to count on in the future?
   1 you're certain there will be–2–3–4–5–6–7 you doubt there will be
7. Many people—even those with a strong character—sometimes feel like sad sacks (losers) in certain situations. How often have you felt this way in the past?
   1 never–2–3–4–5–6–7 very often

Orientation to Life questionnaire with the hardiness scales and found a high correlation between commitment and sense of coherence (Wood, 1987).

We do not need research evidence, however, to know that the importance of meaning applies also to the small stressors and hassles of life. If going to school is meaningful to you, you will tolerate the daily stress of school; if raising a family is meaningful to you, you will tolerate the stress of raising children; if having money is meaningful to you, you will tolerate the stress of making money. When you give even the most mundane things in life some meaning, you will tackle them with more cheer and energy than when you convince yourself that mundane chores are meaningless.

You probably realize that having meaning in life and having goals in life are related; meaning comes from having goals. After years of demonstrating the destructive physiological effects of stress, Hans Selye created the idea of eustress to express the fact that some stress is good, as described in Chapter 3. An important element in eustress, Selye said, is having personal goals (Selye, 1978). The stress that comes from achieving personal goals can be eustress. Trying to live according to someone else's goals is stressful.

Everyone has heard a story of a dying person who had one more goal to live for and, in the process of achieving that goal, became healthier and did not die. The powerful effect of goals on health is well known to therapists who work with cancer patients. (See Chapter 18, Personality and Cancer.) The cancer treatment includes a lengthy questionnaire on goals, and the patient establishes clear goals for the next week, the next month, the next year, and the next three years (Simonton, Matthews-Simonton, & Creighton, 1978). The meaningfulness of goals pulls people along with less stress and with greater tolerance of stress than when life has lost meaning or one's goals are not one's own.

The importance of meaning in life to physical and psychological health cannot be

---

HOW MEANINGFUL IS THE GARBAGE?

Baba Ram Dass (formerly Richard Alpert, Harvard psychologist and student of Eastern philosophy) says: "When you carry the garbage, just carry the garbage." Then he added: "And bring honor to the garbage."

Bring honor to the garbage? Was the man crazy? Not really. Ram Dass meant that our attitude makes a difference in the way that we feel about a task. And he meant: Do not judge the garbage, do not moan and groan about how awful the garbage is and how unfair it is to have to carry it— just carry out the garbage. This is a good metaphor for many tasks in life.

---

underestimated. How purpose in life develops is a topic in need of research.

Stoical Fortitude and Emotional Insulation

Poverty is a major stressor in life. The poor suffer from cancer, heart disease, ulcers, hypertension, mental illness, and brain damage more frequently than any other group (Antonovsky, 1987).

To understand the effects of poverty on people's health, a Columbia University researcher, Leo Srole, and his coworkers studied the residents of downtown Manhattan in New York City from 1954 to 1974. During this longitudinal study, Srole and Fisher (1980, 1984) found people who "came through the entanglement of deep poverty with few or no apparent symptoms." They discovered that people who transcend extreme poverty have three resources: (1) strong family ties, (2) a special group identity, and (3) a stoic fortitude ethos. A strong family and the sense of belonging to a unique group helped people in poverty overcome the deprivations of a poor environment. The attitude of "stoic fortitude" provided the psychological foundation needed to overcome difficult circumstances. By stoic fortitude ethos, Srole refers to a societal belief that the courage to persevere in spite of adversity is good and that people will prevail when they try. At the beginning of this chapter, you imagined a hardy person. We suggested a pioneer woman striding across the prairie with a child on one hip and a rifle on the other. This image represents a universal sense of courage, of stoic fortitude—the strength to persevere and survive. Stoic fortitude also suggests the strength to handle emotions, being neither overwhelmed by negative feelings nor repressing them. If you visualize the pioneer woman on the prairie, you will note that she is neither crying nor smiling; nor is she stonefaced or sullen. How can we describe the face that sometimes an artist captures— is it courageous determination tempered with an inner belief in success? Surviving extreme poverty demands stoic fortitude.

The characteristic of stoic fortitude is similar to the emotional insulation described by Hinkle. Hinkle studied poor refugees from China and Hungary as they adjusted to a new life in the United States. Hinkle was impressed by a stress-resistant characteristic of these people that he called emotional insulation (Hinkle, 1974). Emotional insulation is the ability to emotionally detach from past relationships, groups, and goals, and to adapt to new relationships, groups, and goals. This ability protected refugees from overwhelming feelings of grief and loss.

Resilient Children

Some of my (RS) patients had parents who were abusive, crazy, or uncaring. I assumed, like many other psychologists, that children of bad parents would be seriously ill adults. I was amazed when I read the studies of resilient children, the children of crazy parents or destructive social environments who are psychologically and physically healthy.

Like many other psychiatrists, James Anthony (1987) believed that the best way to understand the development of mental illness is to study the children of mentally ill parents. In 1966, Anthony identified 300 children of schizophrenics in St. Louis, Missouri. He followed the development of these children for 12 years, hoping to unravel the etiology of schizophrenia. Anthony expected to find emotionally disturbed children, and indeed he did. To his surprise, however, 10 percent of the children were unusually well adapted. As an example, Anthony describes a 7-year-old boy who ate at home every day although his schizophrenic mother believed that someone was poisoning the food at home. His 12-year-old sister believed the mother and refused to eat at home. When Anthony asked the boy why he ate the food at home, the boy shrugged and said, "Well, I'm not dead yet" (Pines, 1984). Anthony believes that the boy's success in staying healthy is his emotional detachment from his mother. Anthony found that the less emotionally involved a child is with a sick parent, the less likely the child is to have emotional problems (Anthony, 1987).

Another stress-resistant boy was 11 years old and in the fifth grade. He had an alcoholic father, a disorganized dyslexic mother, two brothers involved in crime (one of whom was in prison), a hyperactive brother, and a mentally retarded brother. They lived in a messy shack that smelled of urine. Both parents were despondent and depressed. The school principal described the child in this way:

> He is a boy who gets along well with others. He is a good athlete and has won several trophies in different sports. Everyone in school likes him because he is well-mannered and a bright student. He never misbehaves and so he has never

come to the attention of the police or the juvenile court. He comes to school in worn but presentable clothing. He tells us that he prepares his own breakfast in the morning. He is a good kid.
(Garmezy & Tellegren, 1984, p. 240)

Garmezy describes these children as resilient. "They know how to make something out of very little. And they bounce back! It's the recovery phenomenon after stress that's so characteristic of them. They just have a tough bite on life" (Garmezy, cited in Pines, 1984, p. 61).

The unusual capacity of resilient children to detach from "sick" people and from a "sick environment" is coupled with the ability to develop a good relationship with a healthy adult. Both Garmezy and Anthony found that resilient children have "warm, satisfying, one-to-one relationships to set them off in life" (Garmezy, 1986).

Emmy Werner and her colleagues (Werner & Smith, 1982; Werner, 1989) studied several hundred children on the Hawaiian islands over a period of 30 years. One of their subjects was Mary. Mary's mother was chronically anxious and periodically hospitalized for mental problems. Her father was an unskilled farm laborer with a fourth-grade education who could not provide adequate clothing and food for his family. Between the ages of 5 and 10, Mary was physically and emotionally abused. Yet at age 18, she had survived these hardships and was successful in school with a happy and optimistic attitude about life. Mary had a positive self-image and many friends and was sensitive and caring to others (Werner & Smith, 1982).

These researchers found many stress-resistant children who survived chronic poverty, family conflict, abuse, and parental mental illness. Werner (1984) describes four characteristics typical of these children:

1. Resilient children are able to "recruit" a nurturing surrogate parent who could be a teacher, baby-sitter, nanny, member of the clergy, parent of a friend, relative, coach, or housemother in an orphanage.

2. Resilient children have good social skills and a strong desire to help others. They are friendly and well-liked by their classmates and usually have one or several close friends (Garmezy, 1983; Werner & Smith, 1982). In the extreme conditions of poverty, war, or concentration camp, resilient children help other children (Garmezy & Tellegren, 1984; Moskovitz, 1983; Segal, 1985) and resilient children take care of their siblings when a parent is absent or abusive.

One survivor of Auschwitz, Menashe Lorenczy, described how he helped his twin sister, Leah, obtain extra food. Menashe had the job of taking soup from the kitchen to the children in the barracks. At the risk of punishment or death, he often hid Leah in the empty soup container on the return trip to the kitchen, where she ate extra bits of food from the floor and sinks. Another time Menashe helped Leah escape from the hospital, where she was sick with an infection. Because she was sick, there was imminent danger that Leah would be sent to the crematorium. Menashe complained of a painful toothache. He was sent to the hospital. Menashe's healthy tooth was removed, but he helped Leah escape by joining a group of children who were returning to the barracks. Many children had this kind of courage and resilience in the camps.

3. Resilient children have hobbies and creative interests. A 9-year-old son of a schizophrenic father and emotionally disturbed mother retreated to a small basement room for refuge. His basement room was stocked with books, records, and food. David, age 8, had a depressed father and a schizophrenic mother. He and his friends escaped to the attic to play with model airplanes and railroads. On the island of Kauai, resilient children fished, swam, and danced. "Their hobbies, and their lively sense of humor, became a solace when things fell apart in their lives. . ." (Werner, 1984).

4. Like stress-resistant adults, resilient children seem to have faith that things will

work out as well as can be reasonably expected, and that the odds can be surmounted (Werner, 1984).

Resilient children demonstrate the tremendous capacity of human beings to survive difficult conditions. Resilient children have resources for maintaining psychological homeostasis. The hallmarks of resilient children are a healthy detachment from the disturbed environment or parent; a supportive relationship with an adult; and activities that provide meaning, such as hobbies, sports, and friendship. These qualities, and the courage of resilient children, are examples for everyone.

Social Support and Extreme Conditions

You may have noted that positive interaction with other people is a hallmark of successful coping in extreme circumstances. Social support is a significant factor in helping victims recover from the guilt, self-doubt, and depression that result from severe psychological and physical abuse.

Social Support and Torture

How can anyone survive the extreme psychological and physical effects of torture? The struggle to maintain sanity in the face of isolation, interrogation, and torture was an everyday experience for many Vietnam prisoners of war. David Jones (1986) studied Vietnam veterans who had been POWs for at least six years, as he had been. Guilt and loss of self-esteem were major problems for these men when they were pushed beyond their limit of endurance. "With rare exceptions, the POWs placed a great deal of value on resisting interrogation. Much of the content of their books deals with this matter. They all agreed that any of them could be 'broken' by torture, and so they had to deal with two issues: how to

best resist and how to regain their positive self-esteem once they had broken under torture" (Jones, 1986, p. 401). Jones found that the healthiest survivors were in camps in which prisoners developed intense loyalty and support for one another and who understood and forgave those who leaked information when tortured.

In spite of the goal to resist torture indefinitely and to give nothing of value to their captors, many men were pushed beyond their limits. Once they broke, they had to overcome feelings of shame and guilt and re-establish a stance of resistance. Many POWs found that telling the other prisoners what was said under duress was cathartic (an emotional release). By telling everything to their fellow prisoners, POWs experienced forgiveness and continuing acceptance by the group (Jones, 1986, p. 400). The most important factor that sustained the prisoners was the knowledge that they could "roll with the situation," could recover from the torture just as other POWs had, and would not be condemned for breaking under torture.

The studies of Vietnam POWs show that social support was a significant factor in helping tortured prisoners recover self-esteem and maintain mental health. But we do not need to look so far from home for parallel conditions in our own environment. Positive social support is also crucial for many women who have suffered the horrors of sexual abuse and battering.

Social Support and Abuse

Traditionally, domestic violence has been ignored or silenced. Yet it is estimated that at least one out of three women in this country will be battered by a man she loves (Russell, 1982; Straus, Gelles, & Steinmetz, 1980; Walker, 1980). Many battered women have low self-esteem and blame themselves for being battered (Frieze, 1979; Walker, 1980). They worry that if they try to escape the situation or end the relationship, they may be killed or their children abused.

People who work with abused women are struck by the fact that some women stay in the abusive relationship for many years. A study of 287 battered women found that the women stayed in the relationship for an average of four years before seeking divorce (Fields, 1978). However, some women muster the courage to leave the relationship and create a new life. In a study of women who left an abusive relationship, it was found that the key motivator was the support of another person who helped them escape (Giles-Sims, 1983). One woman "made the break" after many talks with a friend who had also been abused. "I talked to her a lot because we could communicate about the things that had happened to her. She is the one that really helped me a lot—being able to talk to somebody that it had happened to, too. And she would always say, 'I don't know why you stay'" (Giles-Sims, 1983, p. 135).

Crisis hot lines, support groups, and shelters for women in abusive relationships are based on the importance of social support for coping with the stress of an abusive relationship.

Summary

We have looked at five factors that help people survive extremely stressful conditions, the essential factors in stress resistance.

1. Purpose in life (will to meaning and sense of coherency). Concentration camp prisoners survived dire circumstances and maintained their psychological and physical health by having a meaningful purpose in life that was a faint light at the end of a dark tunnel.
2. Stoical courage. People who do well in spite of poverty have a stoical courage to persist in the face of difficult conditions. This aptly describes resilient children and concentration camp survivors.
3. Emotional insulation. Hinkle found that the most important characteristic of stress-resistant people is their emotional detachment from extremely stressful situations that would devastate most people. Resilient children detach themselves from crazy parents, and immigrants detach themselves from past relationships and communities.
4. Concern for others. Resilient children helped their siblings, parents, or friends; Vietnam prisoners helped one another.
5. Social support. Resilient children found support from a surrogate parent or friends, abused women found support from friends or counselors, and Vietnam prisoners received support from one another.

These elements of stress resistance are intertwined and are probably present in all survivors, although researchers may focus on only one element.

Research on the characteristics of stress-resistant people who survive extremely stressful conditions provide insight into our own potential for coping with stress and becoming stress-resistant. Of equal importance, when the ingredients of stress resistance are known, the task of enhancing stress resistance by facilitating the development of these ingredients can begin.

|||▶

SECTION THREE: SOCIAL SUPPORT AND HEALTH

If you have encountered a stressful life event such as the death of a family member, loss of your job, or divorce, you probably found that good friends or a strong family were important in getting through the most difficult periods. You may not have realized, however, that social support also acts as a buffer against disease and illness. In tough times good friends and family are invaluable for psychological and physiological well-being.

Studying the effects of supportive interaction on health and wellness exemplifies the biopsychosocial approach and the interdisciplinary nature of the study. Anthropologists, sociologists, epidemiologists, and psychologists contribute to our understanding of global variables such as social structures and particular variables such as love, and how they affect health.

A layperson's definition of social support would probably focus on positive interaction. However, researchers define social support in many different ways and describe many different aspects of social support (Cohen, 1988). In this chapter, we link several areas of research in a way that highlights the many facets of the jewel of positive human interaction.

The language and terms used to describe these facets are many: social ties, social interest, social support, friendliness, affiliation motive, love. Some studies focus on the health benefits of receiving positive support; others focus on the benefits of giving support to others; and in some research the relative effects of being the recipient or the provider of support, or both, cannot be evaluated. We can safely speculate that both giving and receiving support strengthens one's inner resources and that the foundation of the positive effects of something as global as social ties is the positive give-and-take of mutual interaction.

We begin with two major studies that attempt to identify the most important global social variables that affect health.

Social Support and Social Ties

Alameda County, California

In 1965, 6,928 residents of Alameda County (Alameda County includes the University of California at Berkeley) responded to an extensive questionnaire on personal health practices, psychosocial variables (focusing on social support), and demographic characteristics. Mortality data for this sample population were collected in 1974.

Berkman and Syme (1979) examined the 1965 data, which included health variables (smoking, exercise, obesity, and use of alcohol), socioeconomic status (education, type of job, and income level), and social support (marital status, friendships, family ties, and participation in social and religious groups—a constellation of variables that the researchers called social ties). These data were correlated with deaths from all causes in the sample population.

Of all the variables, social ties had the highest correlation with health and longevity. Based on number of social ties and their relative significance (marriage and close friends and relatives were judged as more significant than church and social organization membership), an inverse relationship was found between social ties and risk of death from all causes. People with many close social ties had a risk of death that was low, relative to people with few social ties. Social isolation was a clear risk factor. It was also found that people with close social ties and unhealthy lifestyle behaviors such as smoking, excessive drinking, and no exercise lived longer than people who had healthy lifestyle behaviors but lacked close social ties (Berkman & Syme, 1979; Berkman & Breslow, 1983; Reynolds & Kaplan, 1986). The positive effects of close social ties appeared to compensate for bad habits.

The study also found that men and women who had close social ties were less likely to get cancer and were at much lower risk of dying when diagnosed with cancer. After examining these data, Charles Arnold, physician for the Metropolitan Life Insurance Company, commented: "As shown here, these social relationships may even be more therapeutic than those dosages to which patients' adherence is faithfully urged" (Arnold, 1985, p. 2897).

TECUMSEH, MICHIGAN: A REPLICATION STUDY

A replication of the Alameda study was conducted in Tecumseh, Michigan. In 1967, 2,754 people were given medical exams, questionnaires, and an extensive interview. Ten years later the researchers found that, of the variables studied, social ties had the highest correlation with health and longevity. People with close social ties lived longer than those who lacked close social ties.

(House, Robbins, & Metzner, 1982)

Roseto, Pennsylvania

Another major study on social support and health involved Roseto, a small Italian-American community in eastern Pennsylvania. In 1964 Stout and coworkers (Stout, Morrow, Brandt, & Wolf, 1964) reported their finding of an unusually low death rate from myocardial infarction in Roseto. Rosetans had no heart-related deaths for people under the age of 47 for six years (1955–1961), and the death rate from heart attacks was half that of neighboring communities and of the United States as a whole.

Intrigued by this finding, Bruhn and coworkers (1966), attempted to discover the cause. They found that in general, Rosetans were overweight, consumed more total fat than the average American, had a high rate of cigarette smoking, lived a sedentary life style, and had serum cholesterol levels comparable to the average American. Clearly these variables were not contributing to death from myocardial infarction. Bruhn hypothesized that the low number of heart attacks was not due to dietary, ethnic, or genetic factors but to the mutual social support that Rosetans gave one another (Bruhn, 1965; Bruhn & Wolf, 1978). To test this hypothesis, Bruhn and coworkers studied the citizens of a neighboring town, Bangor, that had a death rate equal to the national average. They found that Bangor and Roseto differed in many ways. To a greater extent than the residents of Bangor, Rosetans were ethnically uniform, maintained their cultural traditions including diet and religion, participated in social affairs, conformed to the cultural norms, and were mutually supportive during crises. Bruhn concluded that these social variables protected the Rosetans from early heart attack.

Bruhn and coworkers predicted that as the Rosetans became Americanized (more mobile, materialistic, and individualistic), the social support system would break down and myocardial infarction would approach the national rate.

The prediction was validated in the 1970s when Old World values lost their importance and the social structure of the Rosetans began to dissolve (Bruhn & Wolf, 1979). Pursuing individual advancement and status, younger Rosetans had little time for religious activities, community clubs, or social interaction, and they gradually became more dependent on outsiders. This is precisely the period in which premature deaths from heart attack increased and finally matched the death rate of Americans under age 47. This longitudinal study of the Rosetans provides evidence for the importance of social support as a buffer against a major cause of death, myocardial infarction. Please read Box 6.5 now.

A major criticism of large population studies using broad categories such as "social ties" is the failure to precisely identify the kind of social support that is beneficial for resisting stress. There are many types of social support—emotional, financial, motivational, educational, moral. All of these may be

BOX 6.5

OLIVE OIL? A RESEARCH ISSUE

Looking at the Roseto data in the late 1980s, we can ask, "What about olive oil?" Recently, the consumption of olive oil has been shown to be a protector against coronary heart disease. Did the Rosetans consume large quantities of olive oil and did this change in the 1970s? Was it olive oil rather than social support that protected the Rosetans?

The point is that there are many variables that must be accounted for before factors can be causally related. Epidemiological studies are difficult because so many variables are involved in health and illness. After determining that the Rosetans did not have fewer health risks or health advantages than most Americans (the investigators probably did not measure olive oil consumption because at the time olive oil was not known to be a variable in reduced risk of coronary heart disease), the comparison of the social structures of Roseto and Bangor was the next step in systematically attempting to account for the unusually low number of myocardial infarctions in Roseto.

It is always possible to postulate alternative explanations and to ask "olive oil" type questions in analyzing any study, and this is good. It is important to postulate other variables that the researchers failed to account for. Before a study is questioned or repudiated because a theoretical variable was not accounted for, however, it must be determined that there is good reason to believe that the variable did occur and could explain the data. For example, another possible explanation of the Rosetans' health is that they had a guardian angel who looked after them and protected them from myocardial infarction as long as they remained true to their religious traditions. When the Rosetans became more secular and Americanized, the guardian angel departed.

The guardian angel hypothesis is an unreasonable explanation and cannot be used to cast doubt on the social support hypothesis. One reason is that there is no way to determine whether it is true or false. In contrast, the olive oil hypothesis is reasonable, and it is testable—a survey of olive oil consumption in the 1960s and 1970s could have been conducted.

Another criterion for assessing the reasonableness of an alternative hypothesis is whether or not there is supportive evidence for the hypothesis from other studies. There is no evidence from other studies that guardian angels will protect a city from cardiovascular illness. We do know, however, that olive oil reduces triglycerides and blood pressure and is consumed by southern Italians in Italy, but this does not necessarily mean that the Rosetans used olive oil in greater quality than the people of Bangor. In fact, many southern Italians live in Bangor. Regarding our olive oil hypothesis, there is not enough evidence to suggest that social support is not the correct explanation for the low rate of myocardial infarction in Roseto.

Periodically, we raise an "olive oil" question, meaning that we consider an alternative explanation for research findings.

involved in the beneficial effects of social ties. Studies have been conducted to identify the type of social support that is most beneficial for resisting the effects of stress.

Type of Social Support

Social support can be comforting or helpful or both. Parry (1986) refers to the type of support that brings emotional comfort as **emotional support**, meaning empathy and caring. Support that provides help is referred to as **instrumental support**, meaning financial support, advice, and information. The kind of social support that is most useful depends upon the situation and the needs of the receiver. Kobasa found that friends, spouses, and coworkers of the Illinois Bell executives were not always supportive in a way that was helpful. For example, in response to their husband's complaints about the difficulties of divestiture, some spouses gave emotional support, saying, "Don't worry. No matter what happens at work, we will always love you." Or the executive's friends might say, "Come have a beer and forget about it." The nonhardy executives reported that this type of emotional support did not make them feel better because it did not help solve the problem. More than emotional support, these executives needed instrumental support from the boss. The bosses who helped the executives solve problems at work provided the best support. Kobasa found that the executives who had a helpful boss tended to be healthier than executives with an unhelpful boss. In fact, executives with helpful bosses were healthy regardless of whether or not they were hardy (Kobasa & Puccetti, 1983).

That the executives judged instrumental support from the boss to be of greater importance than emotional support from the family is understandable because the boss is the key to the resolution of the stressful situation. The greater importance of instrumental support would be true of many stressful situations, as when a car breaks down on a highway.

Sympathy from passing motorists is nice but not needed. Instrumental support—the expertise and resources for repairing the car—is needed. In other situations, emotional support may be more important. In a study of 193 working-class employed mothers, Parry (1986) found that employed mothers who had instrumental support but lacked emotional support had more psychiatric symptoms and greater severity of symptoms than employed mothers who had emotional support but lacked instrumental support.

After receiving the diagnosis of cancer, many patients do not want to be told that they will be all right or hear about another patient's remarkable progress. Their first need is for emotional support—comfort as they grieve and adjust to the bad news. When the grieving is over, they are ready for instrumental support—advice and treatment alternatives. Cancer patients feel better after talking to other cancer patients who understand their needs and know how to give emotional support (Dunkel-Schetter, 1984).

Pregnancy and Emotional Support

The value of emotional support was dramatically demonstrated by physicians Sosa, Kennell, Robertson, Klaus, and Urrutia (1980) who were concerned about the lack of social support for mothers during delivery that characterizes the birthing practices in modern hospitals. To study the significance of support, Sosa and colleagues selected 136 pregnant women at the Social Security Hospital in Guatemala City, Guatemala. During admission for delivery, the women were randomly assigned to an experimental group or a control group. In addition to routine hospital care, the women in the experimental group were attended by a *doula*, a laywoman who provided constant support from admission through delivery. The *doula* rubbed the mother's back, held her hands, provided conversation, and functioned as a friendly companion. After delivery, doctors who were unaware of the nature of the

Table 6.1 Social Support and Effects of Stress

| Critical Life Stress | High Social Support | | Low Social Support | |
	n	Number and Percentage of Women with Complications	n	Number and Percentage of Women with Complications
High	15	5 (33.3)	11	10 (90.9)
Medium	44	17 (38.6)	44	20 (45.4)
Low	28	15 (53.6)	28	13 (48.2)

study assessed the health of the mothers and the newborns.

The mean delivery time was 8.7 hours for the experimental group mothers versus 19.3 hours for the control group mothers. The women in the experimental group had fewer complications during delivery and snuggled with their infants more than did women in the control group. The women with support smiled, stroked, and talked to their babies much more than the control mothers did. Our great grandmothers were probably not aware that the support and comfort they received during the delivery at home reduced some risks of childbirth and apparently enhanced emotional bonding with the newborn.

In another study, Nuckolls, Cassel, and Kaplan (1972) classified 170 pregnant women as under high, medium, or low levels of stress and as having high or low levels of social support during pregnancy and delivery. As seen in Table 6.1, a greater percentage of women in the high stress/low support group (N = 11) had complications (stillbirth, prolonged labor, neonatal death within three days) than all other groups. Apparently, the buffering effect of social support is greatest when stress is high, as seen by the numbers highlighted in Table 6.1 Please read Box 6.6 now.

Several current childbirth methods emphasize the participation of family members in the delivery. In the Lamaze method, social support is provided by a "coach" who attends classes with the mother and provides support

BOX 6.6

OLIVE OIL QUESTION: A RESEARCH ISSUE

Ten of the 11 women in the high stress/low social support group of the Nuckolls, Cassel, and Kaplan study had childbirth complications. This suggests that a lack of social support is actually detrimental when stress jeopardizes health, as seen by the fact that relatively fewer high-stress women with high social support had complications. However, do other variables account for the high number of women with birthing complications who had low social support? It might be the case that women with low social support were also poor and malnourished. Perhaps they had little prenatal care, or perhaps they used drugs or were abused. Any of these variables could account for birth complications, suggesting that lack of social support may not be the primary variable. Until we know more about these women, we cannot conclude definitively that lack of social support in high-stress women causes complications during pregnancy and delivery.

during delivery. Today many hospitals include husbands in prenatal classes and encourage their participation during delivery. The trend to midwifery and home delivery are clear indications that women want social support during pregnancy and delivery. In this case, returning to an older tradition seems to be beneficial for the health of the mother and the child, and, it is hoped, for the father as well.

How does a supportive person during delivery reduce complications for mother and child? How did close social ties protect the Rosetans from early heart attack and the Alameda County residents from cancer and death? Why does social isolation increase the risk of mortality? There are no clear answers to these questions, except the obvious. Social support reduces stress by providing comfort and help. In the next section on love and health, we find additional clues.

Love and Health

> If I told patients to raise their blood levels of immune globulins or killer T-cells, no one would know how. But if I can teach them to love themselves and others fully, the same change happens automatically. The truth is: Love heals.
>
> Love, Medicine and Miracles,
> Bernie S. Siegel, M.D.

For centuries, poets, philosophers, and theologians have written about the virtues of love, but only recently has love become a topic of scientific study. The study of love is valuable because it verifies what humans have always known—love heals both psyche and soma. To set out to prove what humans have always known may seem somewhat misguided. In fact, proving the obvious scientifically is often necessary before the obvious becomes part of medical treatment and procedures.

Love and Cardiovascular Health

In Israel, 10,000 married men 40 years or older participated in a five-year prospective study.

For each subject, blood cholesterol, blood pressure, anxiety, and family and psychosocial problems were measured. Each subject received an electrocardiogram. It was found that anxiety, family problems, age, total serum cholesterol, blood pressure, ECG abnormalities, and diabetes mellitus were independent risk factors for angina pectoris (angina is chest pain resulting from inadequate blood supply to the heart muscle).

The family problems questionnaire included this question: "Does your wife show you her love?" Response to this question was the best predictor of the development of angina pectoris in the following five years. Most interestingly, men who already had risk factors such as hypertension, high serum cholesterol, ECG abnormalities, or high anxiety levels were insulated from the development of angina pectoris when they felt their wife's love and support. "The wife's love and support is an important balancing factor, which apparently reduces the risk of angina pectoris even in the presence of high risk factors" (Medalie & Goldbourt, 1976, p. 910). For example, the average incidence of angina pectoris is 5.7 per 1,000 men. High anxiety, without a loving and supportive wife, increases the incidence of angina to 93 per 1,000.

BOX 6.7

OLIVE OIL QUESTION: A RESEARCH ISSUE

The Israeli researchers did not ask, "Do you show your wife your love?" Did the reduced incidence of angina result from receiving love, giving love, or both? We do not know. A fact of life in research is the impossibility of anticipating all the variables that might influence the outcome.

However, the incidence rate for angina was reduced from 93 to 52 per 1,000 when the highly anxious subject felt the love and support of his wife. Please read Box 6.7 now.

This research complicates the simple explanations of illness and health that focus primarily on physical causes of illness and physical factors in prevention, like lowering blood pressure and blood cholesterol. Bernie Siegel, M.D., assistant clinical professor of surgery at Yale Medical School, states, "Someday we will understand the physiological and psychological workings of love well enough to turn on its full force more reliably. Once it is scientific, it will be accepted" (Siegel, 1986).

The buffering effect of love is also seen in a study of Type A people. The Type A behavior pattern includes aggression, competitiveness, and chronic time pressure, and is a risk for coronary heart disease. Attempting to understand why some Type A individuals do not develop coronary heart disease, a team of researchers examined the relationship between Type A behavior, arterial blockage, and emotional support of friends and family. They found that Type A individuals with emotional support from friends and family have less arterial blockage than Type A individuals who lack emotional support (Burg, Blumenthal, Barefoot, Williams, & Haney, 1986).

FISH CHOWDER

The elderly patient was not recovering from a routine appendectomy. She felt weak and could not eat. The nurses noticed that she had few visitors and spent most of her time staring out the window. Her young physician was worried and baffled, finding no cause for her increasing lethargy and deteriorating health.

After several days of witnessing this downward trend and beginning to feel quite desperate, the physician approached his elderly patient and took her hand. He asked, "Is there anything at all that I can do for you?"

Immediately the woman lifted her head, eyes brightening. "Yes, there is something," she said. "If you could just get some fish chowder, the chowder that they make on the sea coast in Cornwall."

"Fish chowder from Cornwall?"

"Yes," she replied, "I would love some fish chowder. When I was young I lived in Cornwall. I haven't had fish chowder from Cornwall in many years."

On his next day off the physician drove to a seacoast town many miles away, purchased a liter of the fish chowder, and returned immediately to the hospital. He heated the chowder and took it to his patient.

The following day the woman's condition was considerably improved. Color was in her face and she was chatting with the nurses when her doctor entered the room.

"I am so much better," she said holding out a thin hand. "See, I am not trembling anymore." Within three days the woman was released from the hospital in good health.

The young doctor was puzzled. He began to wonder what was in the fish chowder that had hastened his patient's recovery. He told the head nurse of his decision to investigate the ingredients of the fish chowder. The nurse, who had seen many deaths and births in her long career, put her arm around the young physician's shoulders and said:

"It wasn't fish chowder, Doctor, it was love."

Told by the physician, years later, and wiser

How does positive human interaction function as a buffer against cardiovascular illness, in this case arterial blockage? James Lynch, a psychophysiologist at the University of Maryland Medical School, provides another clue: the "person effect."

Lynch began his career as a psychophysiologist in the laboratory of Gantt who had studied with the Russian physiologist, Ivan Pavlov. To study classical conditioning, Gantt worked with dogs in isolation chambers. The chamber is designed to eliminate all external stimuli during conditioning. During the experiments, Gantt monitored several physiological responses, including the animal's heart rate. One day Gantt told Lynch that he wanted to show him a discovery. He asked Lynch to watch the electrocardiograph of a dog that was hanging in its sling in the isolation chamber as he entered the room and began stroking the dog's head. The polygraph record was dramatic; the dog's heart rate increased rapidly to 170 beats per minute when Gantt entered the room and then dropped to 30 beats per minute when Gantt petted the dog's head. Gantt, an ardent Pavlovian, said, "I call this the person effect. The effect of person is one of the most ignored phenomena in all of modern medicine. . . . Perhaps it is ignored because its influence is so pervasive. It is much like the air we breathe, taken for granted unless it is poisoned or polluted" (Lynch, 1985, p. 62). Gantt hoped that in Lynch's lifetime medical science would understand the importance of "the effect of person" on health and illness.

After this fascinating demonstration, Lynch began to study the person effect in different settings. In one study, Lynch recorded the physiological effects of interactions between nurses and coronary care patients. Lynch also studied the interaction between pets and humans. Lynch measured the blood pressures of 36 children when a friendly dog sat next to each child and when it was absent. When the dog was present, the child's blood pressure was significantly lower than when the dog was absent.

Next Lynch studied pet owners and their dogs. When pet owners talked to the experimenter, blood pressure rose significantly, but when they talked to their dogs the pressures remained at baseline or dropped. In a similar study with 60 undergraduate students, Vormbrock and Grossberg (1988) found that blood pressures were significantly lower for students while they petted a dog than when the dog was absent. Please read Box 6.8 now.

Lynch found that threatening interactions elevate cardiovascular responding (heart rate, blood pressure, and peripheral resistance), while nonthreatening interactions can lower cardiovascular responding below baseline. The most crucial factor, said Lynch, is "Who is speaking?" From his research, Lynch found that if the person speaking elicits defensive listening, then heart rate, blood pressure, and peripheral resistance will be elevated. If the person speaking elicits a calm response, the cardiovascular responses will be lowered. When Lynch read peaceful poetry to hypertensive patients, blood pressures fell to low levels. For some patients blood pressure reached the lowest level in the patient's medical history.

Positive interaction, human and nonhuman, has positive effects on the cardiovascular system as seen in "gross" measures such as blood pressure, reduced incidence of angina, reduced death rate, and increased longevity. The microscopic benefits that account for these measurable effects are not known. One area of research, however, does measure benefits at the cellular level.

Love and Immunity

A study of the relationship of intimacy and immune functions was conducted by Janice Kiecolt-Glaser and Ronald Glaser at Ohio University Medical School. The Glasers studied 38 married women and 38 women who had been divorced in the year before the study. In the sample of 38 divorced women, those who had

BOX 6.8

PETS AND CARING

Imagine that you live alone. You are coming home from a very frustrating day, discouraged and depressed. As you open the door, your loyal pet rushes to meet you, bouncing with excitement, your pet who never talks back and is always loving. You tell your dog about your crummy day. You play with it and give it love. You feel a lot better.

Pets can be the most loving creatures on earth. They love to love, and just as importantly for their two-legged companions, they love to be loved.

After returning home from hospitalization for a heart attack, patients who have pets live longer than those who do not. This finding was replicated in several studies. Patients who had pets had half the mortality rate of those who did not have pets (Friedman, 1980, 1983).

Caring also works for pets: Caring helps the pet's cardiovascular system. Two groups of rabbits were fed a high-fat diet. One group was ignored while the other group was talked to and petted. The comforted group had significantly lower levels of blood cholesterol and atherosclerosis than the ignored rabbits (Beck & Katcher, 1983).

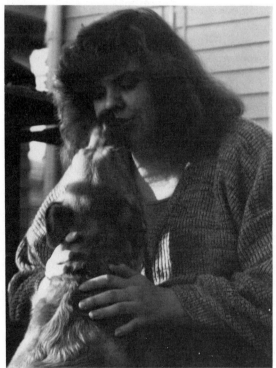

Pets Are Good Friends.
Source: Gordon Steward, Denver, CO.

unhappily married (Kiecolt-Glaser, Fisher, Ogrocki, Stout, Speicher, & Glaser, 1987).

Kiecolt-Glaser and Glaser and their coworkers also compared quality of marital relationship and immune functioning in 473 women. The more supportive the relationship, the more competent the immune system; the poorer the relationship, the less competent the immune system as measured by natural killer cell activity. Based on these data, Kiecolt-Glaser and Glaser and coworkers concluded that supportive interpersonal relationships act as a buffer against stress by promoting immunocompetence (Kiecolt-Glaser, *et al.*, 1987).

Affiliative Motive, Love, and Immunity

For many years, David McClelland of Harvard University has studied human motivation, being one of the first research psychologists to

been most attached to their husband had the lowest levels of natural killer cell activity. Of the 38 married women, those who were happily married had significantly higher levels of natural killer cell activity, lower levels of antibody titers to Epstein-Barr virus, and a higher percentage of helper T cells than the break away from the traditional discussions of motives as the impetus for fulfilling basic physiological instincts. McClelland's first contribution to understanding motivation was his work on "need achievement," the universal human need to achieve. McClelland has also studied another important dimension of human motivation that he calls "affiliative motive."

The affiliative motive refers to the desire to be with other people. He wrote, "The word love is commonly used to describe various types of affiliative ties" (McClelland, 1985, p. 334). McClelland found that people who score high on affiliative motive are unselfish, cooperative, sociable, and thoughtful; they develop relationships, or "affiliative ties," characterized by openness, caring, concern, reciprocal dialogue, joy, and conviviality (McClelland, 1985).

McClelland has found a relationship between affiliative motive and two physiological measures, blood pressure and S-IgA concentration. S-IgA is an immunoglobulin found primarily in saliva. People who score high on the affiliative motive have higher levels of S-IgA and lower blood pressure than people who score low. A longitudinal study initiated when male graduates were in their 30s and completed 20 years later showed that subjects with high affiliation scores had significantly lower diastolic blood pressure than the average American (McClelland, 1979).

In a study of first-year dental students, Jemmott, McClelland, and coworkers compared illness reports, S-IgA levels and affiliation scores. Illness reports and S-IgA levels were correlated with periods of high and low academic stress, as other studies have shown. The healthiest students, however, scored the highest on affiliative motive. These students had fewer colds and significantly higher concentrations of S-IgA throughout the year than all other students (Jemmott, et al., 1983).

Knowing that people with a high affiliative motive have higher levels of S-IgA than people low on the affiliative motive, McClelland wondered whether by arousing a person's affiliative motive, S-IgA would increase. To test this interesting idea, McClelland created a method for arousing the affiliative motive—using movies.

McClelland and Kirshnit (1982) examined the relationship between motive scores, S-IgA, and response to two situations, one uplifting and one degrading. The films used to expose subjects to these situations were *Triumph of the Axis*, a grim documentary about Hitler's early triumphs in World War II and his treatment of the Jews, and *Mother Teresa*, on the life and work of the Benedictine nun who won the Nobel Prize for her care of the sick and dying outcasts in the slums of Calcutta.

McClelland and Kirshnit (1982) measured motives and S-IgA several days (assessment day) before and just after subjects viewed the films. Emotional response to *Triumph of the Axis* had no effect on S-IgA concentrations of subjects high on the affiliation motive (but it lowered S-IgA concentrations in subjects high on the power motive), with minimal effect for the entire sample. *Mother Teresa* produced an immediate and significant increase in S-IgA concentrations on the average for all subjects (Figure 6.1).

Exposure to Mother Teresa's compassionate love evoked a beneficial response in the subjects' immune system defenses against disease.

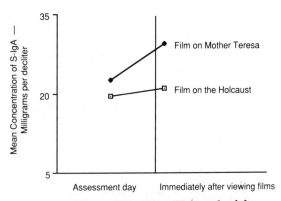

Figure 6.1 Effects of Watching "Triumph of the Axis" and "Mother Teresa" on Immunoglobulin A. From McClelland, 1984, *Human Motivation*, p. 368. Reprinted with Permission.

lacking close social ties, and the Roseto study found that people with close social ties are less susceptible to coronary heart disease than people lacking close social ties.

2. The studies by Hinkle and Plummer show that people who are empathic, friendly, cooperative, and feel connected to other people have fewer illnesses than people who do not have these attributes.

3. Positive social interactions with people and pets can reduce cardiovascular risk factors such as high blood pressure and are a buffer against arterial blockage in Type A individuals.

4. Positive interpersonal relationships can enhance immune functioning, as seen in the studies by Kiecolt-Glaser and Glaser on marital relationships and in McClelland's research on the affiliative motive and S-IgA.

5. The core of social support is empathy, which is the ability to understand and respond affectively to another person.

These studies demonstrate that positive interaction has a significant impact on a person's ability to resist stress and stay well.

||||➡

SECTION FOUR: COPING SKILLS AND LEARNED RESOURCEFULNESS

You may not have suffered abuse, rape, torture, schizophrenic parents, or poverty. Your concern may be with more everyday hassles such as exams, deadlines, jobs, or conflicts with people. In Chapter 3, Stress, we described the work of psychologist Richard Lazarus, a pioneer in the study of ordinary stressors of life and who developed the Hassle Check-List. Lazarus is also a pioneer in the study of how ordinary people cope with the ordinary stressors of life (Lazarus & Folkman, 1984).

Coping, as in the sentence, "We are coping with the stress of exams by forming a study group," means using cognitions and behaviors to manage stressful situations. This section describes skills that lead to successful coping.

Take a minute: Let come into your mind the last time you had to cope with a stressful situation. Be in the situation and experience yourself coping. Try to experience your coping style.

Do It Now.

How do you normally cope? What coping skills do you use? Many people do well; we might use the term "behavioral wellness." Students do well on exams in spite of anxiety; people recover from the loss of a loved one without chronic depression; people overcome severe addictions; and people resist temptations such as high-fat, high-cholesterol foods, cigarettes, drugs, and alcohol. These people are undoubtedly hardy and resilient and have a transformational coping style. The question now is: "What skills do these people have?"

To answer this question, Michael Rosenbaum (1980a, 1980b, 1983) of Haifa University in Israel synthesized the work of several clinical researchers (see Box 6.10) and created an umbrella term to capture the essence of these skills, **learned resourcefulness**. Just as Martin Seligman found that a major cause of depression is learned helplessness, Rosenbaum suggests that a major cause of health and wellness is learned resourcefulness. By "learned resourcefulness," Rosenbaum means a learned repertoire of basic skills that people use to successfully regulate their lives and confront daily hassles. Rosenbaum believes that learned resourcefulness is the foundation of self regulation, the basic skill.

In Chapter 1, we said that self regulation is the key to health, meaning self regulation in all domains: physical, mental, emotional and behavioral. Self regulation enables stress-resistant people to stick to their goals, to *not* eat a piece of chocolate cake just because it is being served, to *not* become handicapped by depression after being fired, to *not* smoke a cigarette after a stressful day, to *not* become overwhelmed by

---

BOX 6.10

SELF REGULATION

In the 1960s and early 1970s, clinical researchers began to study and develop self-management techniques that people could use for making pro-health lifestyle changes, including diet control, increased exercise, and overcoming cigarette and alcohol addiction. Some of these researchers use the term "self-control," and others use "self regulation." Often the words are used interchangeably.

Clinical researchers and colleagues who have developed self regulation techniques, and the focus of their work, are:

Bandura (1977, 1986)   Self-efficacy, phobias
D'Zurilla & Goldfried (1971)   Problem-solving
Janis & Mann (1977)   Decision-making, weight control, smoking
Goldfried (1971, 1977)   Problem-solving, relaxation, decision-making
Kanfer (1970)   Depression, weight control, smoking
Leventhal (1970)   Smoking, fear, anger
Mahoney (1974)   Anxiety
Meichenbaum (1977, 1985)   Pain, anger, anxiety
Stuart (1977)   Weight control
Suinn & Richardson (1971)   Anxiety
Thoresen & Mahoney (1974)   Smoking, weight control

---

deadlines; to *not* feel and act helpless in stressful situations; and to *not* give up when social support is absent. We emphasize *not* to accentuate the struggle and the choices that self regulation involves. For example, many people have difficulty losing weight, and for them eating fruit for dessert means not eating cake. Many people become overly stressed when events do not happen as expected. For them, staying flexible and cheerful means not becoming rigid and depressed.

So we are actually asking, "What are the basic self regulation skills of behaviorally well people?" Pulling together the ideas of therapists, theorists, and researchers, Rosenbaum (1983) describes skills in four areas.

Cognitive Skills

Cognitive skills are the use of perceptions, thoughts, and self-talk to regulate emotional and physiological responses. Rosenbaum includes in his learned resourcefulness model a set of cognitive coping skills based on the work of cognitive therapists Mahoney (1974) and Meichenbaum (1977, 1985). These psychologists emphasize the importance of cognitive coping skills: positive imagery, positive thoughts, positive expectations, and positive self-talk. Positive cognitions help people achieve goals. Negative cognitions hinder achievement. For example, "I will study for my exam every day this week" is a positive cognition. "I never score higher than a C on an exam, so why bother to study" is a negative cognition. People who reduce anxiety, cope with exams, and overcome phobias decrease negative thinking and increase positive thinking (Schwartz, 1986).

Problem Solving

Problem-solving includes planning, evaluating alternatives, anticipation of consequences, and defining problems. We are constantly confronted with problems that require solutions, such as car trouble, lack of money, deadlines, and interpersonal conflict. Problem-solving skills are part of the behavioral repertoire of learned resourcefulness. For example, one technique called "brainstorming" is the suspension of judgment while generating many alternatives for solving the problem at hand. Several studies have demonstrated that brainstorming increases the probability of finding good solutions (D'Zurilla & Goldfried, 1971).

Delayed Gratification

Delayed gratification is the ability to postpone immediate rewards for long-term benefits. To cope with school and work stressors, people must be able to pursue long-term goals at the expense of immediate pleasures; for example, they study instead of party. To reap the long-term benefits of health and wellness, people must reject immediate pleasures such as high-cholesterol food and cigarettes. The idea that the ability to delay gratification is a skill may seem unusual, if not perverse since sometimes it feels like suffering. However, if you have ever witnessed the destructive results of the inability to reject momentary gratification, in yourself or in others, then you can understand why this skill is an essential element in self regulation. Delay of gratification skills, for example, visualizing the rewards of behaviors such as studying and work, are essential for long-term

well-being (Mischel, Shoda, & Peake, 1988; Rosenbaum & Smira, 1986).

Self-Efficacy

Self-efficacy is having confidence that you can accomplish what you set out to do. Rosenbaum says a sense of self-efficacy is the foundation for learning and applying skills for coping with stress. People who have a strong sense of self-efficacy will work longer and harder at learning and applying coping skills (Bandura, 1986).

A sense of self-efficacy is the type of characteristic that supports itself—it enables people to tackle difficult situations and learn new skills, leading to a greater sense of self-efficacy. The sense of self-efficacy is not a skill per se, but it is based on skills. The relationship of sense of self-efficacy to self regulation is clear: People will try to regulate themselves when they sense that their efforts will be effective or when they sense that they can generate the effort in the first place. The first step to the positive upward spiral of self-efficacy is mastery of basic skills, such as replacing negative thoughts with positive thoughts.

Stanford psychologist Albert Bandura has contributed to knowledge of the dynamics of self-efficacy by studying people who have overcome phobias—intense fears of such things as snakes, spiders, dogs, heights, water, and public places. Bandura found that a sense of self-efficacy distinguishes phobics who courageously overcome their fears and those who do not (Bandura, 1986). When people see themselves as efficacious, they believe that they can control the things that they fear and they take the necessary steps to overcome the fear.

To assess these four components of learned resourcefulness, Rosenbaum created the Self-Control Schedule (1985). Please read Box 6.11 now.

Rosenbaum's first task was to assess the reliability of the Self-Control Schedule. In studies involving more than 600 subjects, he gave the

---

BOX 6.11

SELF-CONTROL SCHEDULE

The following items are on the scale. Responses are +3 very characteristic, +2 rather characteristic, +1 somewhat characteristic, −1 somewhat uncharacteristic, −2 rather uncharacteristic, −3 very uncharacteristic.

1. When I do something anxiety-arousing, I try to visualize how I will overcome my anxiety.
2. When I am feeling depressed, I try to think about pleasant events.
3. When I am faced with a difficult problem, I try to approach its solution in a systematic way.
4. I prefer to finish a job that I have to do and then start doing the things I really like.
5. My self-esteem increases once I am able to overcome a bad habit.
6. In order to overcome bad feelings that accompany failure, I often tell myself that it is not so catastrophic and that I can do something about it.
7. Even when I am terribly angry at somebody, I consider my actions very carefully.
8. When I realize that I cannot help but be late for an important meeting, I tell myself to keep calm.
9. When I am short of money, I decide to record all my expenses in order to plan more carefully for the future.
10. Once I am hungry and unable to eat, I try to divert my thoughts away from my stomach or try to imagine that I am satisfied.

Rosenbaum, M. (1980). "A schedule for assessing self-control behaviors: Preliminary findings," *Behavior Therapy, 11,* 109–121. Copyright by the Association for the Advancement of Behavior Therapy. Reprinted by permission of the publisher and the author.

---

schedule at two different times and compared the results. On the first test the mean score was 25.1, and on the second test the mean was 24.4. The correlation coefficient was .86, reflecting high reliability. The validity of the Self-Control Schedule has been examined with a variety of subject populations and conditions. In a laboratory setting, Rosenbaum (1980a, 1980b) conducted a number of studies using pain, aversive noise, and nausea stressors as challenges. He hypothesized that people who score high on the Self-Control Schedule are less likely to be affected by stressful stimuli. The pain stressor was placing one hand in a bucket of ice water. Subjects who scored high or low on the scale reported the same degree of pain, but the subjects who scored high on learned resourcefulness tolerated the pain longer than subjects low on resourcefulness. In a field study (Rosenbaum, 1983), Israeli sailors were assessed on their tendency to become seasick and on their ability to function on the ship. During a storm at sea, the sailors who were high on learned resourcefulness performed better than low resourceful sailors. The same results were found with subjects exposed to an aversive noise while attempting to complete a complicated task. High learned-resourcefulness subjects coped more effectively than low learned-resourcefulness subjects. In another study, the Self-Control

Schedule predicted those hemodialysis patients who were able to control liquid intake despite intense thirst, a behavior essential for the treatment of patients with kidney failure (Rosenbaum & Smira, 1986).

"Learned resourcefulness" is an excellent term because it embodies two important concepts: Coping with stressors demands resources, primarily skills; and these skills can be learned. Research on the development and use of these skills by healthy people is still sparse, but the concept is worthy and will lead to extensive research. In Chapter 10 we describe ways of teaching learned resourcefulness.

||||➡

CONCLUSION

For centuries, science and medicine have concentrated on the prevention and treatment of disease. Today, however, we are in the midst of a dramatic transformation. We are beginning to study the antecedents and dimensions of health and wellness, with this question in mind: "Who stays well, and how—what are the dynamics of health?"

In this chapter we have described many psychological and social factors that predispose a person to health and wellness. We examined research on people who survived stressful situations and remained healthy, people who are stress-resistant—executives, lawyers, bus drivers, army officers, concentration camp survivors, telephone operators, poor people, immigrants, rape victims, abused women, and children who survived poverty and abuse. In addition we reviewed large population studies that link psychosocial variables and health, and we gathered evidence showing that positive human interaction promotes health and well-being.

The dimensions and dynamics of health and wellness are complex because humans are complex. Human health and well-being are affected positively by the biological, psychological, and social variables that influence human behavior. No single variable stands out as the key to health and wellness, and no single study has examined all the variables. The complexity

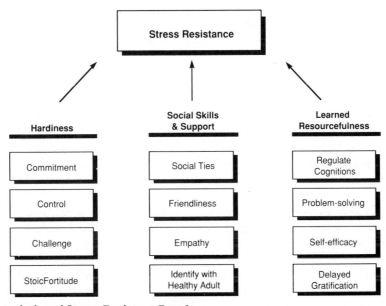

Figure 6.2 Characteristics of Stress-Resistant People.

is increased because these variables interact and for each person may have greater or lesser importance.

In the study of the dynamics of health and wellness we use many sources to answer the question "Who stays well?" When we look at the data as a whole, four patterns emerge: (1) Healthy people have a constellation of attributes such as fortitude, a sense of control, commitment to personal values, and goals, and they can transform stressful situations into opportunities and challenges for personal development. (2) Healthy people have the qualities of friendliness and empathy, which foster friendship and social support. (3) Social support provides meaning in life and is a buffer against stress. (4) In extreme situations, hardy people detach from the destructive environment in a healthy way. We also see a pattern of specific skills that are resources for coping with major events and everyday hassles. These skills, like problem-solving and controlling thoughts and feelings, engender a sense of self-efficacy and self-control.

When we put the pieces of the puzzle together, we create a picture of the healthy person that is "bigger than life." Healthy people do not necessarily have all the characteristics presented here, but we have identified the factors that help people stay healthy. Figure 6.2 summarizes the characteristics of stress-resistant people.

By studying the struggles and courage of many people we are learning that

> There is a more hopeful way of looking at stress—you don't have to accept a victim's fate. There are ways to change from helpless to hardy.
>
> (Suzanne Kobasa, 1984, p. 64)

CHAPTER 7

Relaxation

IIII➡

Recall the story about the snake and the garden hose. When you became aware that the snake was the garden hose, what happened? You laughed at yourself and relaxed. What happens physiologically when you relax? With relaxation, heart rate and blood pressure drop, the pupils of the eyes constrict, the adrenal glands "turn off," muscles relax, breathing returns to normal, the stomach begins to digest again, vasodilation begins, and sweat glands turn off. Relaxation reverses the stress response and helps the body return to healthy homeostasis.

Just as nature created the stress response, so nature created the **relaxation response**. If there were no way to physiologically turn off the sympathetic nervous system following fight or flight, the human race would have fared no better than Hans Selye's rats, which died from exhaustion. Relaxation is a powerful dynamic in health and wellness.

But relaxation does not make the headlines. As a tool for maintaining homeostasis, relaxation has been given little consideration until recently, with two notable exceptions discussed in this chapter. Perhaps relaxation has been neglected because people do not get sick from it and because the power of relaxation has been easy to overlook in a medical science that has focused primarily on the study of disease and disease mechanisms. In addition, the use of medical remedies for stress and stress-related illness has a powerful ally in the pharmaceutical companies that promote the use of medications rather than self regulation techniques. And too, when told "you need to relax" by a physician, the patient is rarely given specific instruction in relaxation.

We devote an entire chapter to relaxation and relaxation training, because relaxation can be learned and used to enhance health and overcome disease and illness. Relaxation training plays a prominent role in treatment of stress-related illnesses, in stress management, in performance enhancement, in biofeedback training, in imagery and visualization techniques, and in hypnosis. In addition, relaxation training is an important element in taking self-responsibility for health, and sometimes it is the first step.

What is "relaxation"?

Take a minute: Let come into your mind the last time that you were relaxed. Get into the situation; be in it; relive it. Feel what your body is doing; feel what your mind is doing.

Do It Now.

In this culture, relaxation usually means doing something fun—going to a movie, exercising, reading a book, having a cigarette, getting high on drugs, hanging out in front of the TV, hitting the nightclubs, cruising the streets.

Another meaning of relaxation is getting your mind off your work or not worrying by doing something diverting. When therapists and stress-management specialists teach relaxation, this is not what they teach, because relaxation as fun-play-diversion is not enough to turn on the relaxation response. Something more is needed: profound psychophysiological relaxation.

Profound psychophysiological relaxation is powerful; it is this type of relaxation that brings the body back to homeostasis. Yet, profound relaxation is a new idea. Profound relaxation has been a source of guilt or a sign of laziness. If you thought of yourself as experiencing profound relaxation during the exercise above, you are off to a good start.

■ **Reminder:** Relaxation is always psychophysiological. To achieve profound relaxation, mind and body are relaxed simultaneously. ■

Popular books on relaxation, meditation, and stress management in general outnumber books on stress. As awareness of the importance of relaxation training for stress management and health grows, old techniques are being revived and new techniques are being created.

This chapter begins with a discussion of a fundamental physiological procedure—breathing. Correct breathing is the cornerstone of health and relaxation, and breathing exercises are an integral part of most stress-management techniques. In Section Two, we describe two relaxation methods that were created early in this century and that have been rediscovered, progressive relaxation and autogenic training. Progressive relaxation and autogenic training lead the trainee to a state of deep relaxation. In Section Three, simple and short techniques are described, focusing on the relaxation response technique, the quieting reflex, and other techniques that are used many times a day. Section Four briefly describes the physiology of relaxation with a look at a new area of study—the effects of relaxation and stress management on components of the immune system.

Therapists are familiar with a variety of techniques and usually teach several to every client, allowing the client to decide which is best. The four relaxation methods described here have some common features, but they were created for different purposes. Mastery of the four techniques and proper breathing make a solid foundation for stress management and healthy homeostasis.

‖‖‖➡

SECTION ONE: CORRECT BREATHING

Breathing? Correct breathing is the foundation of relaxation, and some say that it is the foundation of good health. All relaxation exercises begin with a focus on breathing.

The first time that breathing was brought to my (JG) attention was when my voice teacher told me to stretch out on the floor, to put one hand on my chest and one hand on my abdomen, and to relax my elbows. She stared at me awhile, noting that the hand on my abdomen was moving up and down as I breathed, while my chest hand remained absolutely still. She said that my breathing was "in the right place."

I was in India the next time that I heard about the importance of correct breathing. The intimate relationship between breathing and health came to my attention in India during three months of psychophysiological research with yoga teachers and practitioners. I knew that many forms of yoga and meditation use breathing techniques to still the body and mind. I did not know that one type of yoga—called Pranayama Yoga, or the Science of Breath—is devoted to the study of the effects of breathing exercises on physical and mental health. Our Indian friends explained that breathing is connected to the body and that the body is connected to the mind, so if one learns to control the breath, one can control both body and mind. They also said that when we breathe we do not just breathe oxygen, we breathe prana, the universal energy that is in all things; by gaining control of the breath, we gain control of prana.

I did not study Pranayama Yoga in India, but returned to the United States with an idea: The first task of every client would be to learn to breathe correctly, and the first exercise would be a breathing technique for relaxation.

In correct breathing, air flows easily to the bottom of the lungs with inhalation, which expand as the diaphragm moves down. The stomach lies just below the diaphragm and moves gently out. During all normal daily activities, this is the correct way to breathe. The stomach should always gently move out with inhalation and in with exhalation, while the shoulders and chest are still and relaxed.

When sitting or standing, there is greater blood flow to the lobes of the lungs. Thus more oxygen is absorbed when breathing is

A STORY FROM INDIA

There was once a minister to a great king. He fell into disgrace. As a punishment, the king ordered him to be shut up in the top of a very high tower. This was done, and the minister was left there to perish. He had a faithful wife, however, who came to the tower at night and called to her husband at the top to know what she could do to help him. He told her to return to the tower the following night and bring with her a long rope, some stout twine, packthread, silk thread, a beetle, and a little honey. Wondering much, the good wife obeyed her husband and brought him the desired articles. The husband directed her to attach the silk thread firmly to the beetle, then to smear its horns with a drop of honey and set it free on the wall of the tower with its head pointing upward. She obeyed all these instructions, and the beetle started on its long journey.

Smelling the honey ahead it slowly crept onward, in the hope of reaching the honey, until at last it reached the top of the tower, when the minister grasped the beetle and got possession of the silk thread. He told his wife to tie the other end to the packthread, and after he had drawn up the packthread, he repeated the process with the stout twine, and lastly with the rope. Then the rest was easy. The minister descended from the tower by means of the rope and made his escape. In this body of ours the motion of the breath is the silk thread; by laying hold of and learning to control it we grasp the packthread of the nerve currents, and from these the stout twine of our thoughts, and lastly the rope of the prana, controlling which we reach freedom.

From *Raja-Yoga* by Swami Vivekananda, pp. 29–30

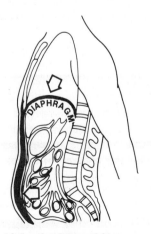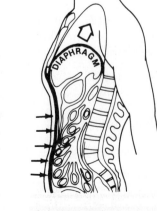

INHALATION

The bottom of the lungs fill and the diaphragm moves down, compressing the abdominal organs; the abdominal muscles relax, and the stomach moves gently out.

EXHALATION

As the lungs empty and contract, the diaphragm moves upward; the abdominal muscles continue to relax and the stomach moves in.

Figure 7.1. Correct Abdominal Breathing.

done correctly. The high chest breath is shallow and does not provide sufficient oxygen, so the breathing rate is automatically increased and tension is created in the body. People who have breathed incorrectly for years are often unaware of these changes until they experience correct breathing. Read Box 7.1 now.

Strained, shallow breathing and stress go together. Deep, relaxed breathing is an effective destressor. Deep breathing says to the body, "No tiger here." When one consciously controls the breath, the mind is automatically controlled. A useful breathing exercise is described in Box 7.2.

Two-stage breathing is a rapid destressor, a promoter of homeostasis, an easy-to-use relaxation technique that you carry with you at all times. No special training is needed, and no one knows when you are doing it.

Breathing is the body's first effort in this world; it is the basis of life and energy, and it has the unique characteristic of being an automatic function that can be voluntarily controlled. Control of breathing is one handle that we have on physiological functioning. In addition, in the process of controlling breathing and thus the body, the mind is also brought under control. For this reason, a variety of

---

BOX 7.1

CHECK YOUR BREATHING

You can check your breathing by placing one hand on your chest and one hand on your abdomen at the level of your beltline. If you are breathing correctly, the chest hand does not move and the abdomen hand moves out when you inhale and moves in when you exhale.

BOX 7.2

BREATHING EXERCISE: THE TWO-STAGE BREATH

This exercise builds upon correct breathing, so correct breathing must be mastered first.

Stage 1: Fill the bottom of the lungs, slowly.
Stage 2: Fill the top of the lungs, slowly.
Exhale slowly, through the nose, feeling the tension flowing out.

In teaching this exercise I guide the trainee as I watch the breathing by saying: "Starting low . . . adding the top . . . now easily out through the nose, feeling the tension flowing out; and starting low . . . adding the top . . . now easily out through the nose, feeling all the tensions of the day flowing out, not so fast that you miss the feeling and not so slowly that you run out of air; and starting low. . . ."

Many students and clients tell us that of all the stress-management techniques that they have learned, this simple breathing exercise is the most effective for quickly turning off the stress response and turning on the relaxation response.

---

concentration and meditation techniques use breathing as the object for focusing attention during mind quieting.

One advantage of knowing how to use breathing as a destressor is that it is brief. Next, we describe two relaxation procedures that were meant to take time.

IIII➡

SECTION TWO: RELAXATION TECHNIQUES—COMPLEX

Progressive Relaxation

It started with an interest in the startle response. Everyone remembers the involuntary jump that instantly follows a surprising stimulus, such as a door slamming. Edmund Jacobson, a student of Walter Cannon at Harvard University in 1910 (Cannon was the physiologist who named the fight-or-flight response and homeostasis), was intrigued by the startle response and by his observation that the intensity of the startle depends upon how tense a person already is when startled (Cannon, 1932). A relaxed person will be less startled than a tense person. Because the startle response is difficult to measure accurately, Jacobson investigated a response that is easier to quantify, the knee-jerk reflex. Jacobson created an elaborate mechanical device for delivering the hammer blow to the patellar tendon and measuring the degree of deflection of the knee. He found that the intensity of the knee-jerk reflex is also affected by relaxation; total relaxation eliminates the reflex. The implication of this finding did not escape Jacobson. Years later he wrote: "These observations suggested the possibility that all subjective irritation or distress might be reduced if the individual were to become sufficiently relaxed; and this hypothesis remains today a beacon-light for further experiments and observations" (Jacobson, 1929, p. 109).

After graduating from Harvard University, Jacobson went to medical school. As a physician, he was aware that the stress of modern life contributes to a variety of disorders, including gastric ulcers, ulcerative colitis, hypertension, heart attack, and anxiety. Actually, Jacobson used the word "effort," because "stress" and "stressor" were not yet commonly used. Jacobson's knowledge of muscle tension convinced

him that muscle tension is a primary manifestation of effort. He wrote:

> All day long you will carry on in a series of efforts within efforts. Whether you are a housewife, a school-girl or a child; whether a businessman, a mechanic or a farmer, this will be true. Whatever your occupation, to be sure, the direction of your efforts will vary. In any event the maze of them will be indescribably complicated. Often you will not know of them at all, as they occur largely mechanized by habit. Often they will shade one into another inseparably, and often you will not even become aware of your efforts and their aims, although very vaguely you will recognize some of yours, marking the significance of your day and your life.
> (Jacobson, 1934, p. 21)

Knowing that efforts create tension and tension creates illness, and having studied the extraordinary effect of relaxation on processes as seemingly automatic as the knee-jerk reflex, it made sense to Jacobson that profound muscle relaxation might counteract the effects of efforts. Over several years Jacobson developed a systematic relaxation technique that he called **progressive relaxation**. Progressive relaxation was designed to help people eliminate and prevent the muscle tension created by their efforts.

From the beginning of his long career, Jacobson sought to study and apply progressive relaxation scientifically. To achieve scientific legitimacy it was essential to develop a way of measuring muscle tension and relaxation so that the effectiveness of the techniques could be verified. With the help of Bell Telephone Laboratories, an oscilloscope was developed that could detect the minute electrical voltages that muscles generate. The changing voltages were displayed on a fluorescent screen. Jacobson could observe muscle tension and relaxation as fluctuations of the signal on the screen. (Had Jacobson thought to turn the oscilloscope toward the patient and instructed the patient to use the information to achieve greater relaxation, biofeedback training would have been developed decades earlier than it was.)

Jacobson worked with subjects in his clinic and in a laboratory that he established for the scientific study of relaxation. Over several years of experimentation and observation, he clarified the principles of relaxation and tension that are the foundation of progressive relaxation. In *Progressive Relaxation,* published in 1929 for physicians, Jacobson describes his research and gives elaborate instructions for teaching progressive relaxation to patients (Jacobson, 1929). In 1934 the book was published for the public with the intriguing title *You Must Relax.* It has been reprinted four times. The principles of relaxation described in these books are as true today as when they were written, indeed, as true as they were centuries ago:

1. Relaxation is the opposite of "nervous excitement," the "direct negative" of muscle tension. "To be relaxed is the direct physiological opposite of being excited or disturbed" (*Progressive Relaxation,* p. ix).
2. "Nervous disturbance is at the same time mental disturbance" (*Progressive Relaxation,* p. ix).
3. Excess tension is a waste of energy.
4. Relaxation turns on the "built-in tranquilizer" that is in everyone.
5. Striate muscle relaxation generalizes to the internal muscles, affecting the cardiovascular system and gastrointestinal tract.
6. Muscle relaxation induces mental relaxation.
7. Overactivity is a habit that can be unlearned.
8. Relaxation is the opposite of doing; relaxation is not doing.
9. Relaxation in the presence of difficulties is the goal.
10. Any disturbance, from without or from within, can be used as a signal to relax.

COMMENT

A person who receives therapy from a professional for a physical or psychological disorder is usually referred to as a patient, particularly when the person is being treated in a traditional medical setting.

Traditionally "patient" connotes a passive recipient of treatment. Because this connotation is not appropriate for therapies in which the person is an active participant, therapists who use a teaching model of therapy and who focus on the essential power of the person to promote self-healing, might not refer to the person as a patient. Many therapists have adopted psychologist Carl Rogers' term "client," which he used for the therapy that he developed and called "client-centered therapy." Some therapists prefer the term "trainee," because it emphasizes the role of the person as a learner and active participant in therapy.

In this textbook, we use these terms according to the context, although the best term for someone receiving professional help for a psychophysiological problem might be learner or student.

The Technique

Jacobson was convinced that every "effort," including thinking, is accompanied by muscle tension, and that to be truly relaxed even the slightest tension must be released. He developed a method for achieving total muscle relaxation by experiencing and then releasing very subtle tension in muscles. To facilitate awareness of muscle tension, the first step in progressive relaxation is to create tension consciously and try to feel it for several minutes. The exercise is done while lying down, arms at the sides. The first exercise is deceptively simple:

> Bend the left hand back at the wrist. Focus on the subtle feeling of tenseness in the upper portion of the forearm, below the elbow (the feeling of the bent wrist is not the sensation to be observed). After several minutes relax completely and observe the sensation of "not doing."

This is the basic exercise of progressive relaxation. The person creates gentle tension in a muscle group, and feels the tension for several minutes, then relaxes completely for the remainder of the session. The goal is to learn to relax each new muscle group while simultaneously relaxing previously trained muscles. Progressively the entire body will be consciously relaxed. Please read Box 7.3 now.

Regarding the experience of subtle tension in muscles, Jacobson wrote:

> This sensation is the signal mark of tension everywhere in the body. It deserves your interest, for it can prove of daily help to you. Vague as it is, you can learn to recognize and to distinguish it from other sensations. This will enable you to know at any moment when and where you are tense.

> (Jacobson, 1934, p. 100)

It must have been clear to Jacobson that extreme muscle tension is easily felt and that people can become "relatively" relaxed, but that it is the subtle tension over time that creates problems. This is certainly our experience with clients who say, "I don't know why my muscles are so sore and I have a headache. I wasn't doing anything." In fact, a lot was going on in the striate muscles, but the tension was subtle and the person was not consciously aware of it.

The program that Jacobson guided his patients through was lengthy: six days on each arm; nine on each leg; three on the trunk; two on the neck; forehead, brow, and eyelids one day each; seven days on the eyes; cheeks and lips one day each; jaws and tongue two days; muscles of speech three days; seven days learning to relax while imagining speech; and seven days

---

BOX 7.3

FEELING SUBTLE TENSION

You are reading this box.

Your neck muscles are tense unless your head is balanced perfectly on the vertebra in your neck and you have this book at eye level.

Your neck muscles are tense because your head is off balance. The tension is subtle; you can read for hours without noticing it. You notice the effects of tension only when muscles begin to hurt or you get a headache.

With your head in the reading position, put your attention into your neck muscles. Do you feel anything?

Gently move your head back to a balanced position over the vertebra of the neck. You will find a spot that feels very different, as the muscles in the back of your neck begin to relax. Now gradually rock your head back to your reading position. Repeatedly move your head back and forth from the place where it is perfectly balanced on the spine and no muscles are needed to hold it up, to your reading position. You will begin to feel subtle muscle tension.

It was awareness of this degree of tension that Jacobson was trying to enhance through the methods of progressive relaxation.

---

practicing various mental images while noting and reducing muscle tension in the eyes and face, and ceasing mental activity. Total: sixty-eight days. Jacobson recommended one or two sessions per week with the physician and one to two hours of daily practice at home. The patient then practiced relaxation while sitting, and finally while working. Learning to relax while working was an important part of the total program. Jacobson referred to the skill as **differential relaxation**, meaning that while some muscles were being used, all the other "different" muscles would remain relaxed.

Jacobson came to the conclusion that muscle tension is the cause of our ills—and therefore the cause is within us—even though we may attribute tension to an external agent, as in, "That final exam sure made me tense." In everyday living, tight muscles do not "just happen." Muscles are used in ways that create tension. Jacobson reasoned that people can learn to counteract the tension with deep relaxation; in other words, people can do something about tension and thereby improve health. This was an important insight, and today the self regulation concept is a recurring theme in stress literature. Progressive relaxation has been reborn because it fits well into the new orientation of skills for health and wellness. Although Jacobson's program of progressive relaxation was lengthy, he emphasized that the skill of relaxation would benefit people for life.

In *Progressive Relaxation* and *You Must Relax* Jacobson describes many cases in which the use of progressive relaxation resulted in the amelioration of physiological symptoms including insomnia, a particular interest of Jacobson's. Jacobson believed that insomnia could be overcome by total muscle quieting. His personal experience convinced him that it is impossible to think and be totally relaxed at the same time. Insomniacs often attributed sleeplessness to uncontrollable mental activity, so Jacobson taught total muscle relaxation as a way of quieting the mind. If you are curious about this, try it.

Jacobson also found that deep muscle relaxation, practiced daily, ameliorated psychological problems such as anxiety and phobias, even though the cause of the problem was not addressed in therapy.

Progressive relaxation is the development of the skill of deep relaxation of muscles, based on awareness and release of subtle muscle tension.

ANTIANXIETY

Three psychiatrists, Haugen, Dixon, and Dickel, trained patients in muscle relaxation, using feedback from an oscilloscope, before beginning psychotherapy. After relaxation training, patients were invited to begin therapy for the original problem. About 90 percent of the patients claimed that the problem had disappeared or no longer seemed so overpowering.

A Therapy for Anxiety Tension Reduction, Haugen, Dixon, and Dickel, 1963

Jacobson observed that learning to remain relaxed even during difficulties could take weeks, months, or even years.

Today progressive relaxation has been shortened into a 30-minute exercise that is only remotely related to the original. The current types of progressive relaxation involve extreme tensing and relaxing, and progress through the major muscles of the body in a single session; focus on sensitivity to subtle sensations of tension is lacking. For many people, today's progressive relaxation is a favorite technique and does promote awareness of muscle tension and its opposite, muscle relaxation.

Autogenic Training

Take a minute: Follow these instructions:

1. Put the book down and sit up in a comfortable position.
2. Place your hands in your lap.
3. Say silently to yourself, "My hands are heavy and warm."
4. Repeat this phrase three times, about a minute apart. Try to feel the sensations

of heaviness and warmth flowing into your hands.

Do It Now.

You have just begun **autogenic training**. You did it yourself and that is why it is called "autogenic" (*auto* = self, *genic* = generated).

At the same time that Edmund Jacobson was developing the techniques of progressive relaxation in the United States, Johannes Schultz, a psychiatrist and neurologist in Germany, began the development of the relaxation procedure that he called autogenic training.

Schultz conceived of the idea of self-generated training out of his interest in hypnosis and self-hypnosis and from his knowledge of the techniques of Europe's leading hypnotherapist and brain researcher, Oskar Vogt. Vogt thought of the hypnotic state as a type of artificial sleep that the patient could learn to induce in himself, and he had developed a technique for teaching the patient to do so. Like Vogt, Schultz understood the value of freeing the patient from dependency on the therapist.

Schultz knew that hypnotized subjects commonly report sensations of heaviness and warmth and that these sensations seem to correspond to a state of deep relaxation. Schultz discovered that these sensations can be created voluntarily, without hypnosis, when a person passively repeats verbal statements focusing on these sensations. More importantly, Schultz discovered that by focusing on feelings of heaviness and warmth, people could guide themselves into a state of deep relaxation. Like Jacobson, Schultz understood the value of relaxation, and he understood the value of self-training. He called the training autogenic because the patient repeats the verbal "formulas" to herself; a hypnotist is not needed after the technique is learned.

To help patients completely relax, Schultz developed two types of exercises, one for quieting physiological processes and the other for mental processes. The physiological verbal exercises focus on feelings of heaviness in the skeletal muscles, warmth in the hands and feet (vasodilation), a calm and regular heartbeat, calm breathing, warmth in the abdomen, and coolness in the forehead.

Unlike progressive relaxation, in which the experience of tension is used to promote the skill of deep relaxation, autogenic training phrases—called verbal formulas—are used. The trainee directs the mind and body by repeating the phrases mentally, while trying to feel the sensations suggested by each phrase. For example, in the first exercise for heaviness, the person repeats, "My right arm is heavy." Attention is directed to the right arm, and the person attempts to create the sensation of heaviness.

As with the original form of progressive relaxation, the patient using autogenic training as taught by Schultz progressed very slowly. A patient would spend several weeks gaining the skill of heaviness in the arms and legs, and only then progress to the sensation of warmth in arms and legs, which took another few weeks. The program for physiological relaxation lasted several months.

Schultz and his student, Wolfgang Luthe, M.D., who became a world authority on autogenic training, elaborated on the original procedure by adding an "organ specific" formula with which the patient directs attention to a particular organ. For example, the phrases used for bronchial asthma are: "My throat is cool," "My chest is warm," and "It breathes me." Schultz and Luthe also created phrases that focus on the patient's cognitions or behavior; they called the phrases "intentional formula." These phrases were designed to reinforce a behavior—"Now I am tired and I fall asleep"—or to neutralize a worry or overconcern with the training—"It does not matter." Today we refer to this technique for directing the self as "positive self-talk" or "positive coping statements," and therapists are well aware of the usefulness of internal verbalization for self-directed change.

Autogenic training evolved into a formal therapy, and a therapist certification process was established by the International Committee for the Coordination of Clinical Application and Teaching in Autogenic Therapy. Work with hundreds of patients convinced Schultz and Luthe that the therapist must be highly skilled in guiding the patient to self-directed change. They were concerned about the skills of the therapist because they discovered that this type of deep relaxation can release buried trauma that may erupt as physiological disturbance and anxiety, a process that they called autogenic discharge. They believed that therapists should be competent to handle such events. In 1932, after many years of experimentation with autogenic training, Schultz published a thorough description of the procedures and clinical results, *Das Autogene Training.* Nearly 30 years passed before the therapy and results were known in America. By 1959, when *Autogenic Training* was published in English by Schultz and Luthe, more than 600 articles on the therapy had been published in European journals.

The introduction to *Autogenic Training* begins: "Psychophysiologic psychotherapy is based on the assumption that psychologic functions cannot occur independently of physiologic processes or without the involvement of some organic structure. . . . In accordance with this orientation, and in contrast to so-called 'mental methods' (for example, psychoanalysis), autogenic training approaches mental and bodily functions simultaneously" (Schultz and Luthe, 1959, p. 1). Now another 30 years have passed, and we can say that psychophysiologic psychotherapy is a good description of many new therapies that work with mind and body simultaneously.

Schultz and Luthe were certain that homeostasis is the underlying physiological process that enables autogenic training to be so effective. It was clear to them that the body tends to return to healthy homeostasis, regardless of the disorder, when the skills of physiological and mental relaxation are learned and practiced regularly. The methodical approach to somatic and autonomic nervous system relaxation proved to be effective in the treatment of many disorders.

Today, therapists who teach autogenic training use a brief 20-minute autogenic training exercise of 24 phrases, combining suggestions for heaviness, warmth, and mind quieting. This brief exercise, practiced daily, is an excellent technique for general relaxation training and for increased blood flow in the periphery. Control of blood flow is used in the treatment of several vascular problems, described in the next chapter on biofeedback training, and in the chapters on behavioral medicine. Please read box 7.4 now.

BOX 7.4

AUTOGENIC PHRASES

I am beginning to feel quite quiet.

My feet feel heavy and relaxed.

My ankles, knees and hips feel heavy, relaxed and comfortable.

My stomach and the whole middle portion of my body feel relaxed and comfortable.

My arms and hands are becoming heavy and warm.

I can feel the heaviness and warmth flowing down my arms into my hands and fingertips.

My shoulders, arms and hands are becoming heavy and warm.

Deep within my mind I can experience myself as relaxed, comfortable and still. My mind is becoming calm and quiet.

I withdraw myself from the surroundings and I feel serene and still.

Adopted from the original phrases by Alyce Green, The Menninger Foundation

Meditation

The practice of meditation begins with body quieting and induces body quieting as a prelude to stilling and focusing the mind. Meditators who practice regularly report an experience of inner calm and "centeredness" that promotes physiological and psychological relaxation.

Teachers of meditation are quick to say that meditation has nothing to do with religious dogma or persuasion, which is true. Yet meditation is often associated with Hinduism or Buddhism because these religions consider meditation a path for spiritual growth and the ultimate experience of oneness with God.

In fact, seeking union with God through self-discipline and focusing within is common to all religions. In Raja Yoga, a system of self-discipline that developed in India centuries ago, the student must master six steps before beginning the practice of meditation. The first four involve moral training, purity of the body, and breath control; the fifth is called "withdrawing the senses from their objects"; the sixth is concentration, or learning to focus the mind on a single object; and the seventh is meditation. Moving through these steps to meditation may take many years.

In the West, meditation often refers to concentration, the quieting of the mind by focusing on a religious or quieting object or a thought, mental image, or on breathing. The basic technique is easy to describe but difficult to practice. The body is quieted through stretching, muscle relaxation, and slow diaphragmatic breathing. A comfortable sitting position is taken in which the spine is straight (limber-legged people sit in the lotus posture, with the legs folded "Indian style" but with the feet on top of the thighs—this posture automatically straightens the spine and creates a solid triangular base that makes it impossible to fall over during meditation, should the meditator lose body consciousness). The mind is focused on the object, eventually so completely that awareness of all else fades away, and consciousness merges with the essence of the object.

In beginning meditation the person experiences a striking inability to focus the mind for more than a moment. The "drunken monkey been stung by a bee" mind flits about from one sensation to another—the knees hurt, the back is uncomfortable, there are sounds outside—and from one thought to another, and from one memory to another. Meditation teachers all have the same advice: When the mind wanders off, gently bring it back to the object. Be patient and persevere. It is said that when the mind is perfectly controlled, it becomes a powerful tool for knowledge and insight and is a channel to the gems of wisdom in the unconscious mind.

There are varieties of meditation techniques and experiences. When the mind is quieted by causing it to rest upon a single object, it is freed from its bondage to the physical senses and from ordinary consciousness of worries and attachments. Meditators report that the experience is of freedom, "going beyond the self to a greater Self," or a blissful sense of being one with God or the universe.

The practice of meditation and its effects are of interest because meditation is a type of self regulation training that promotes psychophysiological health. In addition, as in prayer or contemplation, meditation can be practiced as part of one's spiritual development. The spiritual domain, like the physical, emotional and mental domain, is important in human experience and well-being, and for some people it is the driving force for growth.

Summary

In this section we describe two relaxation techniques and meditation that were designed to take time. Progressive relaxation focuses on relaxation of striate muscles, and autogenic training focuses on relaxation of

BOX 7.7

THE CONTROLLED STUDY

Research designs often include a control group or groups for comparison to the experimental group. A "controlled" study controls for variables that might affect the control and experimental groups differently and lead to false results. In the study of immune system functions, it is important to "control for" the variables that are known to affect the immune system, such as medications, sickness, sunburn, alcohol, aspirin, strenuous physical exercise, weight, and time of day that blood samples are taken.

To *control for* these variables means to make sure that they cannot contribute to the differences in measures, for example from one blood sample to another or from one group to another. These variables are controlled for by eliminating them or by making sure that they are always the same. For example, a subject's blood samples can always be taken at the same time of day. This controls for "time of day" as a variable in differences in blood samples for each subject. Subjects who use alcohol could be eliminated from the study, and so forth. The object is to create subject groups that are as identical as possible, to keep the testing procedures as constant as possible, to eliminate any variable that could affect the results of the research, and to cancel the effect of any variable that cannot be eliminated by making sure that the variable applies equally to both experimental and control groups.

Designing a well-controlled study is a difficult task, but it is the only way to be certain that the difference in experimental and control group results is due to the independent variable (stress management and relaxation training in Peavey's study) and not to some other variable.

The study by Peavey et al. was "well controlled" because variables that might affect neutrophil activation capacity were eliminated, monitored, or the same for the experimental and the control group subjects. The term *held constant*, like "controlled for," is used to describe the fact that a variable is the same for both groups. We could say, "Age was held constant for both groups," meaning that the average age was the same for both groups. If average age is held constant, then differences in neutrophil capacity between the experimental and control groups cannot be because of age. In immune system studies, if a variable such as age— which affects the functioning of the immune system—is not controlled for, and if by chance the average age of subjects in the experimental group is very different from that of the control group, then age and not the experimental variable could account for the differences between the groups.

Research with humans, on complex physiological systems, is difficult because controlling for all the variables is difficult.

Actually, this difficulty applies equally to research with laboratory animals but was overlooked for many years. Today it is known that many laboratory variables affect immune functioning, including living conditions such as temperature and noise level, and the manner in which the animals are handled and transported. Unless these variables are controlled for in animal research, data on immune functions are questionable.

(Cohen, 1985)

patients and nonpatients how to reduce the physiological and psychological impact of daily stress. The dedication of these people to the development of their ideas, to research, and to teaching is a testimonial to the importance of relaxation skills for health and wellness.

The four systems have more similarities than differences:

1. People can overcome and prevent stress-related disorders by learning the skill of deep relaxation and directing the body mentally.
2. Relaxation skill involves a sequence of steps that progress slowly.
3. As skills are gained, relaxation techniques are used in more difficult situations, defusing stress and thereby the stress response.
4. An essential ingredient in learning and using relaxation skills is a passive approach. It is not possible to force mind and body to relax; striving to relax becomes a stressor in itself, and both the autonomic and the somatic nervous systems react with increased tension. Conscious, willful relaxation is a process of "letting go" or doing without trying, a unique experience for people who are continually trying to make things happen. The concept of a passive approach has been referred to as passive concentration, passive attention, passive volition, and effortless effort.
5. The power to counter stress is in the person.
6. Relaxation facilitates the return to healthy homeostasis.
7. Relaxation is a skill that must be learned and practiced; a therapist or teacher can be a guide, but the work lies with the trainee.

Finally, meditation and the relaxation programs described here are unique, but they have three elements in common: muscle relaxation, quieting the mind, and conscious deep breathing.

We cannot underestimate the role of stress in illness, and we cannot underestimate the role of relaxation in health.

We are impressed by the fact that relaxation techniques for physiological and psychological well-being have been available for many decades, and yet relaxation training for treatment and prevention is only now gaining recognition. In 1929, in the preface to *Progressive Relaxation,* Jacobson wrote:

> Oddly enough, in spite of the apparently vast importance of rest, and although several books have been written on the subject, the field has remained practically unexplored from a scientific standpoint. While devoting huge efforts to the development of other investigative and therapeutic measures, Medicine has used this, perhaps her oldest remedy, naively and with little attempt at systematic study. However, if straws show which way the wind blows, there are signs of awakening curiosity.
>
> (Jacobson, 1929, p. x)

The new disciplines—health psychology, behavioral medicine, and behavioral health—are challenged to study the power of relaxation as a tool in stress management, healing, and prevention. We immediately add that gaining the skill of relaxation may be as important as relaxation itself. The skill brings a sense of personal power, of control, and is a tool for achieving self-responsibility.

In this chapter we described several relaxation techniques and gave many tips for personal training. If you are reading this book for a college course, your instructor has given you relaxation training exercises in class and relaxation practice homework. Do not fail to practice.

As public awareness of the impact of stress on health increases, and as health costs increase, therapeutic techniques and programs for teaching people how to manage stress through relaxation skills also increase. Therapists and stress-management consultants teach a variety of relaxation techniques.

Some of these techniques, such as progressive relaxation and autogenic training, have been used for many years, and some are created by the therapist on the spot. Some techniques, such as the quieting reflex, become systematic therapy programs that are taught to other therapists and to teachers. We anticipate an increasing use of relaxation training as an integral part of daily life in schools for teachers and students, in business for executives and the rank and file, and in medicine for professionals and patients.

Do not take a ho-hum attitude about relaxation. Relaxation is powerful. Profound relaxation is the process that brings the body back to healthy homeostasis and helps to keep it there. Brief relaxation, a hundred times a day, helps the body maintain homeostasis. The relaxation response is there to use. People need only learn how.

CHAPTER *8*

Biofeedback Training

IIII➡

Pin the tail on the donkey was a disastrous party game if one wanted to maintain one's dignity. Of course, the idea was to look silly and make everyone laugh. No one ever got the tail on the right part of the donkey, because you had to be blindfolded and spun around a few times. You staggered off toward the donkey, paper tail in hand, trying to guess where you were. Now isn't that just like life: blindfolded and spun around a few times.

It isn't really. The emphasis of this text is clear: Human beings have inborn mechanisms such as homeostasis, the relaxation response, and mind → body that are powerful dynamics for health, and skills for resisting stress can be learned. People can develop resources for coping with crises and everyday hassles. Biofeedback training is a tool for developing skills and resources.

In a nutshell, **biofeedback** means exactly what the term suggests, the feedback of biological information. Biofeedback is the process of monitoring a physiological response such as heart beat, blood pressure, or muscle tension, turning the physiological signal into meaningful information, and feeding back the information. To whom? To the person being monitored. For example, when a doctor listens to your heart, that is not biofeedback; when the doctor puts the stethoscope to **your** ears, that is biofeedback. When you use the information to learn to change your heart rate, you are using biofeedback training. As the word *training* suggests, you make the change over time with practice, using the feedback as a guide. Because the body responds to stress and relaxation, and both are under your control, and because mind → body, you have power to change your physiology. This seemingly simple

process has stirred the foundations of medical science, rekindled an interest in mind → body, and added a powerful tool to the armamentarium of therapists of all types.

In Section One we introduce two principles of biofeedback training: **consciousness leads to control,** and **feedback.** Consciousness is the basis for self regulation. Without being aware of the need to change and knowing how to change, a person cannot make change occur. This principle is true for all types of self regulation—cognitive, emotional, or physiological. We introduce "consciousness leads to control" in this chapter because biofeedback training is primarily a tool for becoming aware of how mental and physiological processes interact and how they can be controlled. The importance of feedback of information for learning is clear when we ask "How does a person become more conscious?" The answer is: with feedback. "Consciousness leads to control" and feedback are dynamics in health and wellness because they enable the self regulation of physiological and psychological states.

In Section Two the varieties of biofeedback training and the rationale for biofeedback training are described, concluding with an essential dynamic of health and wellness that we have mentioned several times—self-responsibility. We give self-responsibility the status of a dynamic because without a healthy sense of self-responsibility, people do not make the effort needed for health.

In Section Three we go back in time to the beginnings of biofeedback and biofeedback training in research laboratories around the country. You will learn of the controversy among the pioneers. Researchers who had worked primarily with laboratory animals and those who espoused behaviorism thought of biofeedback as operant conditioning, but other researchers thought of biofeedback training as a tool for teaching psychophysiological self regulation based on consciousness and volition. Yet, in spite of conflicting models and research results, biofeedback training emerged from the laboratory and evolved into a powerful therapeutic technique for self regulation training that is used in the clinic, classroom, and workplace.

IIII⬤

SECTION ONE: UNDERLYING PRINCIPLES OF BIOFEEDBACK TRAINING

Consciousness Leads to Control

Ms. Jones comes to the clinic for treatment of chronic headache. She thinks that the headaches might be related to muscle tension, although she feels relaxed most of the time.

"Ms. Jones, why are your shoulders up around your ears?"

"They aren't."

But Ms. Jones' shoulders are high. Through coaching, she becomes aware that her shoulders are up around her ears. Can she immediately drop her shoulders into a relaxed position? No. High shoulders have become an unconscious body habit. Although the skeletal muscles are part of the voluntary nervous system, body habits are habits because we lose consciousness of them. We are aware only of the symptom, such as headache.

Through a variety of training techniques, Ms. Jones becomes conscious of the fact that her shoulders are high, and she learns to relax them enough to feel the difference.

"I see what you mean. They really were high. Now I can feel the difference."

After the session, will Ms. Jones continue to keep her shoulders relaxed? As soon as she gets into her car and shifts her attention to driving,

her shoulders are back up around her ears. The process of becoming conscious is gradual. Gradually Ms. Jones will learn to focus attention on her shoulders, become conscious of the tension, and relax. Sometimes, when her attention shifts or she is stressed, the behavior will return. As Ms. Jones becomes increasingly aware, however, she will learn to relax her shoulders, *even before they begin to tense*. Ms. Jones cannot control the tension and, more importantly, she cannot *prevent* the tension until she becomes conscious of the behavior. Please read Box 8.1 now.

"Consciousness leads to control" is a dynamic in health and wellness because consciousness is an essential ingredient in gaining self regulation of physiological and psychological processes. In fact, "consciousness leads to control" is a truism worth attending to in all aspects of life—political, ecological, social, and particularly in health. People who are not conscious of the need for change, or who do not know how to change, cannot gain control of life. This is true for such simple things as controlling hypertension with salt reduction after becoming conscious of the role of sodium in hypertension, and for such complex processes as changing irrational belief systems after becoming aware of the role of irrational thoughts in stress.

Biofeedback training is sometimes called consciousness training because consciousness of psychophysiological processes is the core of psychophysiological control. The question is "What leads to consciousness?" The answer is feedback of information.

The Power of Feedback

"Give me feedback, or give me death." That is about the truth of it. Your body constantly uses feedback to maintain homeostasis. People without feedback systems have difficulty surviving physiologically, and people without the ability to use feedback of information have great difficulty learning.

BOX 8.1

THE POTTY STORY

Step 1: Tif discovers a puddle on the floor and says, "Janie did it." He has no consciousness.

Step 2: Tif notices a strange feeling in his diapers. The dawning of consciousness tells him that the feeling might be connected to him; consciousness comes after the fact.

Step 3: Tif is definitely aware that his body is about to do something. He wets his diapers, saying, "I did it." Tif is conscious of body signals before and during the act, but he has no alternative behavior.

Alert parent decides that it is time for potty training.

Step 4: Alert parent rushes Tif to the potty at the first sign of imminent peeing and shows him what to do, saying, "Good boy." The parent reinforces Tif's growing awareness.

Step 5: Tif is conscious of body signs. He has control and rushes himself to the potty, but he pees over it. He is conscious, he has control, and he is working on the appropriate behavior.

Alert parent praises Tif for his first attempt and continues praising him as he learns the behavior.

Step 6: Tif is playing in the yard, fully conscious of body signs. Tif "holds it" for just one more chance to catch the ball. Then he says, "Go potty," and rushes off. He scores a direct hit. "Yea, Tif. See what you did. You did it." Now Tif has consciousness, sphincter control, and appropriate behavior. No more wet diapers.

Step 7: The family is getting ready for a trip. Parent says, "Everybody go before you get in the car." Tif says he doesn't have to go. Parent says, "Try anyway." **Prevention.**

Potty story created by Carol Schneider, Ph.D., Director, Colorado Center for Biobehavioral Health, Boulder, Colorado (Schneider, 1983).

Consciousness leads to control. Is this not obvious? Would you try to control something of which you were not aware? This is not to say that consciousness causes control. As the potty story illustrates, control is gained through practice and through all the other ingredients that are involved in learning, such as feedback.

The power of feedback of information was described to Mr. Wright in the first chapter with the example of learning to play darts. It was clear to Mr. Wright that learning to hit the bull's-eye depends on getting information from the dartboard and using the information to make a better throw. Obviously, if the player were blindfolded, learning to hit the bull's-eye would be very difficult.

Skills are learned with feedback of information. Some skills, such as playing darts, have information built into them; the dart board has score rings that give numerical and spacial information. Other skills, such as running or swimming competitively, are learned with the aid of feedback from instruments such as a stop watch. Some skills, such as ballet, are learned with feedback from a mirror or video. Some skills, such as riding a bike or walking a tightrope, rely primarily on continuous feedback from the body itself. In sports or dancing, another important source of feedback is the coach. Good coaches know how to give clear feedback. Poor coaches do not know how to analyze or feed back the bits of information that can guide the athlete to a better performance. Some athletes are excellent despite their coaches because they can create feedback for themselves.

Sports, academic learning, social learning, theatrics—all depend upon feedback of information. You can tell a joke that you think is funny, but if no one laughs, you won't tell that joke again. Social feedback determines more of our activity than we probably know.

The necessity of feedback is well known to parents, teachers, coaches, animal trainers, and even rat psychologists, although in operant conditioning with rats, the information is usually called the reinforcer. From the animal's point of view, the bit of food that reinforces the behavior being learned says "That is correct," which is vital information for learning. When the reinforcement ends, the behavior ceases (called extinction in operant conditioning jargon) because the new information (no reinforcement) says "Not correct."

Skills cannot be "given" the way that facts can be given. Unless you are a Mozart or Michelangelo with an innate talent, you learned your skills through information feedback. In learning a skill, feedforward is useful—"Do it this way, try this. . . ." The foundation of learning a skill, however, is feedback—information that tells you immediately how you did. This is the information that increases consciousness.

Note that feedback of information actually has two functions: it verifies, and it increases consciousness.

Suppose that you are trying a new pole-vaulting technique, and you want to know whether the technique increases the height of your jump. Feedback of information from the crossbar verifies whether or not the new technique helped. Suppose that you are trying a new weight-loss program. Information from the scale verifies the effectiveness of your program.

Now imagine that you have a new dart board. You are going to learn to play darts, in private. What is your procedure? You simply throw the first dart, see where it lands, and use the information to adjust your behavior. You throw again, again getting information from the dart board (or wall), and again adjust your behavior. With every throw-feedback sequence you become more conscious—conscious of your body, your technique, the distance to the board, the weight of the dart, and even conscious of your mental stance. As you become more conscious of what you are doing, of what to do, and of how to do it, your skill improves.

Feedback leads to consciousness, and consciousness leads to learning and control. This process has been occurring in you since birth, unnoticed. This type of learning—action, feedback, new action, feedback—is called **trial and error**. Please read Box 8.2 now.

Summary

"Consciousness leads to control" and feedback of information are the underlying principles of almost all learning, certainly all learning of skills. Learning occurs when information feedback is available to guide behavior change and simultaneously increase consciousness. Without consciousness and feedback, learning cannot occur; it would be impossible to learn to hit the bull's-eye of the dartboard without feedback. "Consciousness leads to control" and feedback are principles that underlie biofeedback training because biofeedback training is skills training.

BOX 8.2

TRIAL-AND-ERROR LEARNING

So you want to teach a pigeon to bowl? No problem. Put the pigeon in the pigeon bowling alley with a ball, set up a reward system so that whenever the pigeon approaches the ball it will get a food reward, and wait.

Why wait? Because you cannot tell the bird, "Your task is to learn to roll the ball down the alley and knock over the pins. The best technique is to. . . ." You cannot give the pigeon this kind of feedforward instruction because it does not speak the language.* Being naturally active, however, the bird eventually approaches the ball and is rewarded. The bird, being fairly smart, approaches the ball again. Step by step the pigeon's behavior is shaped by reinforcing its approximations to hitting the ball and finally knocking over the pins.

The bird does not know what the task is or why it is being rewarded, and we can assume that it does not create a strategy— "Well, this turkey wants me to roll the ball down the alley, so the best approach is. . . ." But learning does occur. Eventually the bird will roll the ball down the alley, knock the pins over, and get its reward.

This type of learning is called trial and error because behavior change occurs through a series of attempts (trials) that are not quite right (error). With feedback of information (reward), the behavior becomes progressively more accurate if the person giving the reward knows what the goal is and when to inform (reward) the animal.

In learning to play darts, you use trial-and-error learning. You throw the dart (trial), see where it lands and judge the error; then, you adjust your behavior and throw again. As you become more conscious of what you are doing, the trials become more accurate. Unlike the pigeon, you know what the task is, and you develop strategies to reach the goal. Even so, learning solely by trial and error can be slow, frustrating, inefficient and perhaps dangerous. People who learn to ski by trial and error take a lot of falls.

Most skills are learned with a combination of good coaching and trial and error. A good coach can save a lot of learning time by helping the trainee overcome errors quickly through feedforward and feedback.

*We hasten to say that some animals do speak a kind of emotional, voice-tone language and do seem able to use feedforward information. When you teach a dog to shake hands, you first shake the dog's paw for it— feedforward.

IIII➡

SECTION TWO:
BIOFEEDBACK TRAINING

There is a problem with the body: Generally we are not conscious of most functions unless something is wrong. A healthy body gives little feedback. A sick body gives feedback as symptoms. Between nothing and symptoms, the body provides little information. Mr. Wright was asked to feel his heart beating, and he could. Then he was asked to feel his blood sugar, and he, of course, could not. People are unaware of most internal body processes. Even the skeletal muscles, which are controlled by the voluntary nervous system, are primarily unconscious and are controlled only by controlling movement. Fortunately, the skeletal muscles can be tensed voluntarily, and we can feel the tension. Feeling muscle tension helps bring muscles into consciousness and enhances the opposite of tension, relaxation.

As an experiment, lean back and relax your arms and shoulders, and try to feel the trapezius muscles across the top of your shoulders. Unless these muscles are very sore or someone just gave them a good squeeze, you feel nothing. Even when the trapezius muscles are tight, unless you consciously tighten them further, you may feel nothing.

Without feedback, and without consciousness of body processes, the body is difficult to control. Enter biofeedback.

Dr. Biofeedback explained to Mr. Wright that "bio" refers to body, and "feedback" refers to the feedback of information, so "biofeedback" refers to feedback of information about one's body. The feedback is provided by an electronic instrument that monitors the body process, converts it into meaningful information, and presents the information to the trainee. **Biofeedback training** refers to the use of the information to gain self regulation of the body process being monitored. **Biofeedback therapy** refers to the use of biofeedback training in conjunction with several other techniques to help treat a disorder or for stress management. Biofeedback therapy is a type of behavioral medicine, which is described in Part Five.

Turn to the photographs on pages 428 and 430 in Chapter 14. In the first photo the trainee is receiving feedback for tension in the masseter muscle of the jaw. She is learning to relax her jaw muscles. The electrical activity in the muscle is picked up by the electrodes over the muscle and the biofeedback instrument beneath the video display unit amplifies the electrical activity and converts it into the

feedback signal. The instrument feeds back an auditory and a visual signal. As tension in the masseter muscle changes, the auditory tone and the visual feedback change. The trainee also has a coach who uses teaching aids and suggests techniques for relaxing the muscle, as seen in the second photograph.

You will immediately understand why the biofeedback instrument is often referred to as a psychophysiological mirror. Like a mirror, the instrument provides information; like a mirror, the instrument reflects without judgment; like a mirror, the instrument has no power to change behavior. In biofeedback training, *the power to create change lies solely with the person.* We emphasize this seemingly obvious point because in the past, research on biofeedback training often attempted to study the power of the feedback signal rather than the ability of the person using the information. This research quirk is discussed in Section Three.

Removing the Blindfolds

Learning to play darts blindfolded would be impossible. If the player removes the blindfold and gets feedback from the dart board, trial-and-error learning can begin; add a good coach, and learning progresses faster. Biofeedback instrumentation removes body blindfolds. With information from the body, trial-and-error self regulation can begin; add a good teacher or therapist, and learning progresses faster. The methods of learning any skill apply to the skill of self regulation of psychophysiological processes: feedback → increased consciousness → change behavior → feedback → control. Biofeedback instruments provide the feedback of information that facilitates learning.

Varieties of Biofeedback

Any physiological process that can be detected, amplified, and converted into information can

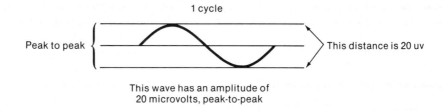

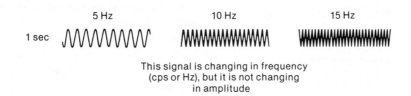

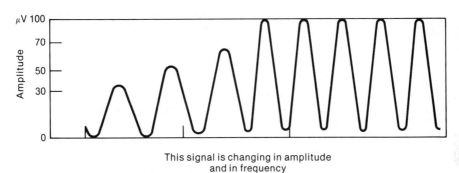

Figure 8.1   Brainwave Signals (EEG) and Muscle Potentials (EMG) Are Measured on Two Dimensions, Frequency and Amplitude.

be the focus of biofeedback training. The only limits seem to be technology and funding to develop the technology. Please read Box 8.3 now.

When biofeedback training is used for stress management and to treat psychosomatic illnesses, three basic modalities are used: muscle tension feedback, skin temperature feedback, and sweat gland activity feedback (also referred to as electrodermal feedback).

Muscle Tension Feedback

You remember from Chapter 4, The Stress Response, that muscles generate electrical potentials as ions move in and out of muscle cells when the cells contract and relax; with contraction the potentials increase in amplitude; with relaxation they decrease. The electrical potentials are detected by electrodes placed over a muscle. A biofeedback instrument amplifies the signal, averages the amplitude of the signal, and feeds back the signal to the person connected to the instrument. In the early days of physiological recording, signals from the body were recorded on moving paper. As recording techniques became more sophisticated, lines printed on the paper made it easier to measure the amplitude of the signal being recorded, creating a graph. Although feedback equipment now does not create a graph or

BOX 8.3

BIOFEEDBACK VOCABULARY

Modality: the physiological response being monitored by the biofeedback equipment, such as muscle tension, blood flow, heart rate, brainwaves. "What biofeedback **modality** is used in the treatment of hypertension? Skin temperature (blood flow)."

Signal: the electrical activity of the body monitored by equipment. "The brainwave **signal** indicates that the subject is sleeping."

Feedback signal: the type of feedback used. "The auditory **signal** is too loud."

Refer to Figure 8.1 for the following terms.

Amplitude: the size of the physiological signal. "Alpha brainwaves have greater **amplitude** than beta brainwaves." "The **amplitude** of the muscle signal is much larger than the amplitude of the brainwave signal."

Microvolt (μv): one-millionth of a volt; the basic unit for measuring the amplitude of electrical potentials in the body. "The brainwave signal averaged 20 **microvolts**."

Cycle: a single oscillation of an electrical signal from baseline.

Peak-to-peak (p-p): a method of measuring the amplitude of a signal, from the highest point to the lowest point of a cycle. "The **peak-to-peak** amplitude is 50 μv." "The amplitude is 50 μv (**p-p**)." There are several methods of measuring the amplitude of EMG signals, and it is customary to indicate the method used when reporting data. "Subjects in the experimental group had a decrease of 15 MV (p-p)."

Frequency (cps or Hz): the number of times that an electrical signal oscillates every second. It is shown in cycles per second (cps), or in hertz (Hz), which is cycles per second but named after the inventor, Heinrich Hertz, who was a pioneer in radio. "The brainwave record showed 25 **cps** and the subject was alert." "What is the predominant brainwave **frequency** when a person is sleeping?"

feed back information on paper, the word is still used. Feedback of muscle tension is referred to as *EMG feedback*. EMG stands for "electromyograph." *Electromyograph* means recording the electrical activity of muscles (*myo*) on a graph.

In biofeedback training, "EMG feedback" refers to the feedback of information about muscle tension, through visual or auditory signals; a graph is not made. EMG training is used in general relaxation training and in the treatment of disorders involving either excessive muscle tension, such as tension headache, low back pain, and spasticity, or reduced muscle activity, as in paralysis.

Temperature (Blood Flow) Feedback

Skin temperature is directly related to the amount of blood flowing through arterioles and capillaries. Blood flow is controlled by vasoconstriction and vasodilation of smooth muscles that encircle the arterioles. The instrument for temperature feedback can be a simple 45-cent weather thermometer or an expensive device with many types of feedback. To measure skin temperature, the bulb of the thermometer or the thermister (the temperature sensor on electronic feedback instruments), is taped to the skin. Temperature is a direct measure and is usually fed back in Fahrenheit degrees.

In my (JG) private practice, finger temperature feedback is usually the first biofeedback modality that I introduce to the client. I introduce temperature training first because it is easy to learn to increase temperature, it is correlated with relaxation, and it is a good demonstration of mind → body. In addition, hand temperature training can be practiced anywhere with an inexpensive weather thermometer. Temperature feedback is used for general relaxation training and in the treatment of vascular problems such as Raynaud's disease, migraine headache, vasoconstriction secondary to diabetes and connective tissue disease, and hypertension.

Electrodermal Response (EDR)

The sweat glands of the hands, feet, and armpits are responsive to stress. People who respond to stress with sweaty hands know how embarrassing this is, and "breaking out in a cold sweat" is a classic stress response. Sweat gland activity is commonly measured on the fingers, but it is not measured directly as amount of sweat. From a battery inside the instrument, a tiny current flows through two metal discs connected to the fingers. Conductance of electricity increases as skin moisture increases, because current flows more easily through the salty moisture on the skin, and conductivity decreases as moisture decreases. Very dry hands are quite resistant to the flow of electricity. The instrument feeds back information about the flow of current. Electrical conductivity of the skin is called the **electrodermal response**, and the feedback instrument is called an EDR. Sweat gland activity was the first physiological response measured in lie detection; today lie detection usually includes a measurement of heart rate, blood pressure, respiration, and EDR.

The EDR is used for general relaxation training and in the treatment of hyperhydrosis, which is excessive sweat on the hands. EDR feedback is also used with patients who have irritable bowel syndrome, because they commonly have an elevated EDR (Schneider, 1983). A few therapists use EDR during therapy sessions because it is an indicator of the emotional responses of the client.

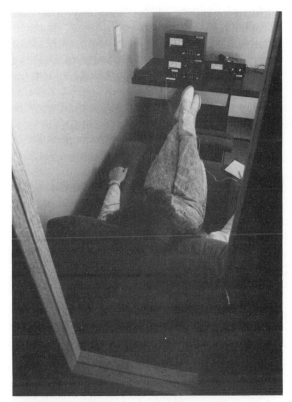

The Student Taking a Biofeedback Class at Aims Community College Uses EMG and Temperature Feedback for Relaxation Training.
Source: Robert Waltman, Aims Community College, Greeley, CO.

DETECTING LIES?

Can an EDR instrument detect a lie? Not always, but the idea is correct. A person can fool other people, but cannot fool himself. The mind knows the truth; the lie causes an emotional reaction and the body responds. Of physiological responses, sweat gland activity is one of the most responsive to emotions.

Results of the lie detector test do not stand up in court, however, because human physiology and emotional responses are too varied to unerringly reflect a lie, or to separate the response of lying from the fear of being falsely accused. The Council on Scientific Affairs of the American Medical Association recommends that the lie detector test be abandoned for employment testing and security clearance because it is not reliable or valid.

(*Journal of the American Medical Association,* Council on Scientific Affairs: Polygraph, 256; 1172–1175.)

Thermal, EMG, and EDR feedback are standard equipment in most clinics and for most uses of biofeedback training, in which relaxation and self regulation are primary goals. The use of these feedback modalities in treatment will be discussed in detail in Part Five.

Brainwaves

Brainwave feedback was developed early in the history of biofeedback training, but it is not standard in most settings. The electrical activity of the brain is called *brainwaves* because when the activity of the brain is monitored by electrodes on the scalp, amplified, and recorded on

paper, it looks like waves (see Figure 8.2 and Table 8.1).

Brainwaves are divided into four main categories, based on frequency. Each category is associated with a general state of consciousness and has a characteristic amplitude range.

A brainwave feedback instrument is called an EEG, for electroencephalograph (*encephalo* = brain). As with the EMG, no graph is made unless a paper record is needed for research or the EEG is being used to diagnose a brain disorder. An auditory signal indicating the presence of a particular brainwave category, particular amplitude, or both, is usually used in brainwave training. Brainwave feedback training can be used for general relaxation training or for states-of-consciousness training, because different brainwaves are associated with different states of consciousness. It is also used in the treatment of epilepsy, hyperactivity, narcolepsy, learning disorders, attention deficit disorders, and insomnia. The use of brainwave feedback training for treatment of epilepsy is described in Part Five.

Brainwave feedback training is not part of the usual biofeedback armamentarium because accurate equipment is expensive and brainwave training may be lengthy. Several specific applications of brainwave feedback training, such as the treatment of epilepsy, require specialized equipment and training and are not in the realm of the average clinician or stress-management consultant.

Other Feedback Modalities

Other biofeedback modalities include blood volume in the fingers, monitored with a plethysmograph; blood volume (also called pulse volume) in the temporal arteries of the head, for treatment of migraine headache; heart rate; heartbeat (ECG); blood pressure; gut sounds; tension in the anal sphincter muscles; stomach acidity; breathing sounds; respiratory functions such as lung capacity; tongue position on the

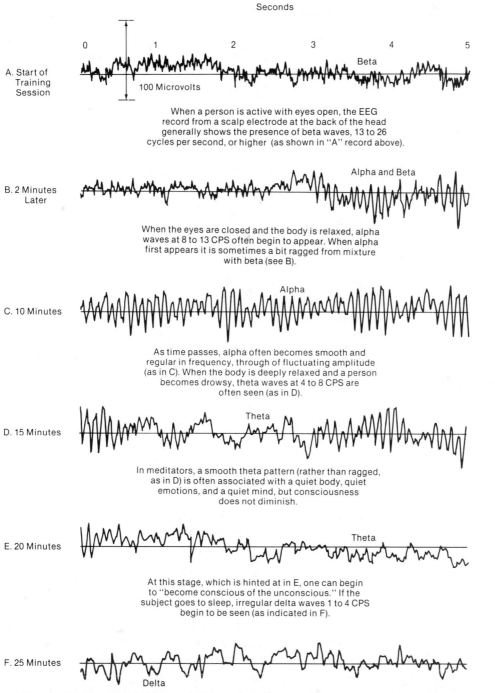

Seconds

A. Start of Training Session

100 Microvolts

When a person is active with eyes open, the EEG record from a scalp electrode at the back of the head generally shows the presence of beta waves, 13 to 26 cycles per second, or higher (as shown in "A" record above).

B. 2 Minutes Later

Alpha and Beta

When the eyes are closed and the body is relaxed, alpha waves at 8 to 13 CPS often begin to appear. When alpha first appears it is sometimes a bit ragged from mixture with beta (see B).

C. 10 Minutes

Alpha

As time passes, alpha often becomes smooth and regular in frequency, through of fluctuating amplitude (as in C). When the body is deeply relaxed and a person becomes drowsy, theta waves at 4 to 8 CPS are often seen (as in D).

D. 15 Minutes

Theta

In meditators, a smooth theta pattern (rather than ragged, as in D) is often associated with a quiet body, quiet emotions, and a quiet mind, but consciousness does not diminish.

E. 20 Minutes

Theta

At this stage, which is hinted at in E, one can begin to "become conscious of the unconscious." If the subject goes to sleep, irregular delta waves 1 to 4 CPS begin to be seen (as indicated in F).

F. 25 Minutes

Delta

Figure 8.2   Brainwave Record of a Trainee Progressing from Wakefulness to Sleep.
Source: Elmer and Alyce Green, *Beyond Biofeedback*, Delacort Press, 1977. Reprinted with Permission of the Authors.

Table 8.1   Brainwave Categories and Characteristics

Category	Frequency Range	Amplitude Range	State of Consciousness
Beta	13–26 cps	5–25 µv	alert, active mind
Alpha	8–13 cps	20–200 µv	relaxed, eyes closed
Theta	4–8 cps	15–100 µv	reverie
Delta	.5–4 cps	100–300 µv	deep sleep

palate for speech disorders; angle of the knee in walking; head position; and heel-toe sequence in walking.

If it can be monitored, it can be fed back. Unfortunately, biofeedback instruments are not available for several important physiological processes, more from the difficulty of monitoring and from lack of funding than from lack of creativity or need. Instruments are still to be developed for easily monitoring and feeding back many physiological processes—kidney functioning, the activity of the components of the immune system, pressure in the eyes, liver functions, blood sugar, muscle activity of the gastrointestinal tract, coronary artery diameter, and blood flow to the lining of the stomach.

QUESTION

There is no instrument to feed back information about blood flow in the lining of the stomach, and the instrument that feeds back stomach acidity information is beyond the budget of most practitioners. Nonetheless, biofeedback training is used successfully with ulcer patients. Why?

If you were treating a client with ulcers, what modality or modalities would you choose for feedback?

The Rationale for Biofeedback Training

You know that:

1. Mind→body.
2. The body knows how to maintain healthy homeostasis.
3. The cortex talks to the limbic system, the limbic system talks to the hypothalamus, the hypothalamus talks to the pituitary and to the medullae of the adrenal glands, the pituitary talks to all other glands and to the kidneys. This is a primary pathway for the stress and relaxation responses.
4. Stress throws the body off balance, and relaxation brings the body back to healthy homeostasis.
5. Relaxation is a mind/body skill.
6. Feedback→consciousness and consciousness→control, meaning self regulation of psychophysiological processes.

Knowing all this, you can now piece together the rationale, the explanation of how biofeedback "works." We use quotes because biofeedback training does not "work"; the trainee "works." Figure 8.3 illustrates the process, and the text describes it.

The goal: Increase hand temperature.

After an introduction to biofeedback training in which the principles and the mind → body dynamic are explained, and after an introduction to autogenic training, the coach says: "I am going to say a phrase, and you repeat it silently to yourself. As you do, try to feel the

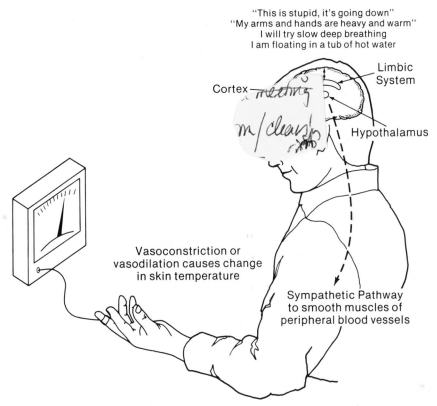

Figure 8.3   The Rationale for Biofeedback Training, Using Skin Temperature (Blood Flow) Feedback as an Example.

sensations suggested by the phrase—'My hands are heavy and warm.'" The trainee might immediately think, "This is stupid, and it's impossible anyway." If this self-talk creates stress, the cortex sends signals to the limbic system that initiate or facilitate a feeling of frustration; the message continues to the hypothalamus, where the centers for vasomotor control are located; the signal proceeds to the smooth muscles of the peripheral vascular system, initiating vasoconstriction; the vasoconstriction causes reduced blood flow in the fingers, and finger temperature goes down; the decrease in finger temperature is fed back to the trainee through the instrumentation. Seeing this feedback, the coach says, "You are probably trying too hard. Don't try; just repeat the phrase easily without trying to do anything." When the trainee stops

trying and begins to feel the sensations suggested in the phrase, vasodilation begins. The hands begin to warm, and the trainee sees the increase on the temperature feedback meter.

Learning in biofeedback training is like learning to play darts. The trainee receives information from the feedback instrument, uses the information to adjust mental and physical behavior, becomes more conscious of what is needed to increase hand temperature, and eventually gains control. When mind and body are directed toward relaxation, the body automatically creates the various physiological changes of the relaxation response.

The key step in the process of learning psychophysiological self regulation with feedback is adjusting mental and physical behavior. This is where a coach can help with suggestions and where trial-and-error learning occurs, using the feedback as a guide. When the goal is increasing hand temperature, the trainee might begin with deep breathing, then use autogenic phrases, then switch to imagery of a warm beach, and then experiment with the word *warm*, receiving feedback to verify the effectiveness of each strategy. Learning how to increase hand temperature progresses in the same way that all skill-learning progresses: through trying what the coach suggests, through experimentation, through feedback, through becoming increasingly conscious of how to accomplish the task, and through practice. Please read Box 8.4 now.

Physiological control is possible because mental/emotional control is possible. Turning on the relaxation response at will, changing perceptions, turning off negative self-statements, and visualizing a positive outcome are examples of this special talent.

Biofeedback training rests on key dynamics of health and wellness. Without mind ⟶ body there would be no rationale, without homeostatic processes the body would be unable to balance itself through relaxation, and without consciousness there would be no change in behavior and no control of psychophysiological processes.

Take a minute: Imagine that you meet a friend that you have not seen in some time. Your friend asks, "What classes are you taking now?" You immediately say that you are taking a terrific class called The Dynamics of Health and Wellness, and just now you are studying biofeedback training. Your friend responds, "Biofeedback. I thought that biofeedback was a fad, and anyway, no one knows how it works."

How would you explain biofeedback training to your friend? Without referring to the rationale, imagine that you are explaining what biofeedback training is and how it "works."

Do It Now.

We hope that you took this suggestion seriously. Probably a question such as that will be on your next exam.

BOX 8.4

CONSCIOUS OF WHAT?

If you try to explain how you achieve movement, such as raising your right arm, you will get up to the point at which you raise the arm, and then you will be unable to describe exactly how you do it. You will finally say, "I just do it."

We are not conscious of the neuronal activity that mediates between the mental initiation of an action and the outcome. Between these points is a vast realm of unconscious processes. And yet we move.

This is also true in controlling the autonomic nervous system. We are not conscious of neuronal activity, and yet we can control processes such as blood flow in the periphery. This is because we can control mental and physiological processes that change blood flow: deep breathing, imagery, creating feelings of heaviness and warmth, and relaxation.

Brainwave feedback training is particularly interesting because the brain has no sensory systems whatsoever. We cannot feel activity in the brain. Yet brainwave control is possible because brainwaves are correlated with states of consciousness (alert, relaxed, reverie) and we can become *conscious of consciousness*. We can learn to control consciousness and, therefore, we can control our brainwaves.

When you understand the rationale for biofeedback training and self regulation and can explain it to someone, you will be amazed at what you know. When you think a moment further, you will realize that phenomena such as the placebo effect are also explained by the rationale. You will be impressed by the implications of the rationale.

What does the rationale mean? It means that people have power to promote health through internal resources. As you ran through your explanation of biofeedback training, however, perhaps you noticed an ingredient without which all fails: self-responsibility.

Self-Responsibility

A hardy sense of self-responsibility is another key dynamic in health and wellness. Without it no change takes place, and self regulation will not occur. Self regulation is a skill, and like any skill, self regulation takes both knowledge and practice. Knowledge and practice take work, and work takes self-responsibility. Thus, without a strong sense of self-responsibility, nothing will happen. Conscious homeostasis is meaningless without self-responsibility. All the information in this book has no power in itself to create change and has no value unless it is put to use, and that takes self-responsibility. As therapists, we are continually challenged by clients who cannot or will not take self-responsibility. Donald Ardell, a pioneer and leader in the business of promoting wellness, describes self-responsibility in this way. "It is the mariner's compass, the ring of power to a life of high level wellness" (Ardell, 1977, p. 102).

Due to circumstances beyond my control,
I am the captain of my ship
And the master of my soul.

||||➡

SECTION THREE: BIOFEEDBACK TRAINING: A SHORT HISTORY

We doubt that any other discipline has ever evolved with such speed from "founding parents" who had so little in common. The people who got together in 1969 to form a new professional organization that they named the Biofeedback Research Society did have two things in common. They were all involved in research in which a physiological function was monitored and was in some way fed back to the subject, whether rat, cat, or human. And they were all enthusiastic about the horizons that this procedure would open up. Interestingly, everyone had a different horizon in mind. For this reason, the history of biofeedback training has a different slant, depending upon who is telling it. The researchers who thought of biofeedback as operant conditioning describe the operant conditioning work with laboratory animals as the foundation of biofeedback. The researchers who thought of biofeedback as a tool for helping humans gain self regulation of psychophysiological processes describe the foundations of biofeedback very differently. Please read Box 8.5 now.

With the complexity of applications and implications seen in Box 8.5, it is no wonder that the people who came together to form the Biofeedback Research Society spoke different languages.

Pathways to Biofeedback Therapy

A detailed account of the history of biofeedback training is not necessary for understanding the principles and applications of biofeedback training. However, as we noted in Chapter Two in discussing the demise and rebirth of the mind in science, history brings meaning to the present. *Biofeedback* has had different meanings to different people, and therefore the field has not been without internal controversy. The different viewpoints are useful to understand, particularly when evaluating research on the efficacy of biofeedback training. In addition, we use the history of this unique field to discuss several issues that pertain to the development of therapeutic techniques and to the study of the efficacy of these techniques.

BOX 8.5

THE DIMENSIONS OF BIOFEEDBACK TRAINING

Consider all the fields that contribute to biofeedback training (BFT) and to which biofeedback training contributes:

Learning theory	BFT involves learning.
Operant conditioning	BFT was thought to be a type of operant conditioning.
Physiology	Biofeedback instruments reflect physiological processes.
Psychophysiology	Biofeedback instruments reflect psychophysiological processes.
Experimental psychology	Biofeedback instruments provide instant data, useful in research.
Cognitive psychology	Cognitions affect physiology and thus play a role in BFT; BFT affects cognitions.
Humanistic psychology	BFT is a demonstration of human potential.
Transpersonal psychology	BFT demonstrates the power of the will and is therefore a tool in human evolution.
Personal growth	BFT is a tool for self-exploration.
Stress management	BFT is a tool for relaxation and becoming stress resistant.
Therapy (psychotherapy, neuromuscular rehabilitation)	BFT is an adjunctive technique in many therapies.
Education	BFT is a valuable tool in the classroom and as a subject of study.
Medicine; behavioral medicine	BFT is a tool in the treatment of disease and illness.
Prevention	BFT is a tool for gaining stress resistance and maintaining homeostasis.
Biomedical engineering	BFT uses instrumentation.
Computer science	BF systems can be computerized.
Business	Instruments, computer programs, tapes, instruction materials, and books on BFT can be sold for professionals and laypersons.

That feedback enhances learning was not a new idea in the mid-1960s, nor was physiological feedback, which had been used, although rarely, in the 1950s. However, when several researchers around the country independently developed instrumentation for monitoring and feeding back physiological information through tones, lights, and other signals, it was an idea whose time had come. The first meeting highlighted the controversy over just what the idea was. It became clear that although the common element was physiological feedback, researchers disagreed on whether or not the physiological changes were the result of voluntary control or conditioning, and whether or not the mind was involved. Many behaviorists investigating the process were not interested in the self regulation aspect of biofeedback training, coming as they did from traditional experimental psychology and animal conditioning laboratories in which self regulation has no meaning. Other pioneers felt that self regulation is the heart of biofeedback training (Green & Green, 1977). In other words, these researchers had different **models** of biofeedback. Please read Box 8.6 now.

Researchers who accepted the operant conditioning model for biofeedback, akin to operant conditioning with laboratory animals, naturally attempted to study biofeedback training and its effects through the research methods of operant conditioning. They adopted for biofeedback the language and the goals of operant conditioning. Researchers who accepted the self regulation model for biofeedback training, in which biofeedback instrumentation is a tool for teaching self regulation skills, naturally used research methods that facilitate self regulation and adopted the language and the goals of self regulation training. The differing research methodologies and goals of these models often led to conflicting results.

Because biofeedback attracted such a variety of researchers, often quite opposed in models and interests, there is no direct route that leads to the use of biofeedback training today in behavioral medicine. Following is a brief tour of several pathways to clinical biofeedback training.

Operant Conditioning with Laboratory Animals

To understand the contribution that operant conditioning with rats made to biofeedback, a quick review of conditioning is in order.

Pavlov demonstrated that the autonomic nervous system can "learn" in the sense that processes such as salivation can be elicited by a stimulus that does not normally elicit salivation, such as the ringing of a bell. The process of

---

BOX 8.6

THE IMPORTANCE OF THE MODEL

A model is a conceptual framework for understanding a process being investigated. For example, Freud had a particular model of the human psyche; in his model the id, the ego, and the superego are components of the psyche. In the textbook *Introduction to Experimental Psychology,* the authors state: "The model or set of models a psychologist believes in determines to a great extent the kind of research he does, and the type of explanations he develops" (Matheson, Bruce, & Beauchamp, 1974). We emphasize *the kind of research he does.* The romantic image of the open-minded scientist is a myth primarily because scientists design research according to their models of the phenomena they are studying. The research design determines the data, and the data determine the conclusions about the phenomena being studied.

Because the model sets in motion this sequence—research methods ⟶ data ⟶ conclusions—it is important to have the correct model for the phenomena being studied. As you continue in your studies, continually ask: "What is the model being used, and is the model correct?" Inappropriate models lead to false conclusions and confusion. Sometimes a researcher does not state the model that is the basis for the research, but often the model can be deduced by examining the research methodology.

---

linking salivation to the ringing of a bell is called classical conditioning and happens when the bell is rung simultaneously with presentation of meat powder into the dog's mouth, which does elicit salivation automatically and is called the unconditioned stimulus. This process was described in Chapter 2. The language used to describe this phenomenon is "The autonomic nervous system can be classically conditioned." Note that the idea that the dog learns to associate the bell with food is not considered, because anticipation is a "mentalistic" concept. When the dog's emotional or mental response to the bell is ignored, it does appear that the bell causes salivation. In other words, it looks as though an external stimulus, the bell, causes a change in the autonomic nervous system, salivation, and the dog's mind is bypassed altogether.

Operant conditioning (also called instrumental conditioning) is the process of teaching an animal to perform a task or operation by rewarding the animal when it approximates and finally performs the task, such as pressing a bar that triggers the release of food. The reward is also called the reinforcer because it strengthens the likelihood that the behavior will be performed again. Learning through operant conditioning is based on trial and error. Trial and error is the only method of learning in laboratory animals, because they cannot be verbally coached or instructed. The model for this type of operant conditioning states that behavior is controlled by rewards or by the stimulus that signals the animal to perform the rewarded behavior. A researcher using operant conditioning would say, "The response came under the control of the stimulus." It is thought that the behavior of the animal or human is controlled by external variables, the stimulus or the reward. In operant conditioning this appears to be true, at least with laboratory animals, because the experimenter controls all the variables. The animal has no choice of stimuli and rewards, and it appears to have no conscious control; the behavior seems to be the result of the variables chosen by the experimenter.

■ **Note:** Operant conditioning has always involved overt behavior that is performed with skeletal muscles (the somatic nervous system).   ■

Now we can return to our history of biofeedback training. In the mid-1960s the question that had always been answered "no" came up again: "Can the autonomic nervous system be operantly conditioned?" It was clear that the autonomic nervous system could be classically conditioned, but it was thought that functions of the autonomic nervous system could not be operantly conditioned, that is, changed by rewarding changes in the desired direction. For example, it was thought that rewarding an increase in heart rate would not affect heart rate unless the person or laboratory animal tensed the skeletal muscles to increase heart rate, in which case the reward went to the somatic nervous system and not the autonomic nervous system. But in the mid-1960s, a new method was discovered. Through a series of experiments with curarized rats (curare is a drug that paralyzes all skeletal muscles, thus eliminating the somatic nervous system from the experiment), Neal Miller of Rockefeller University in New York and several of his students demonstrated that by rewarding rats for a particular physiological change, the animals could do an amazing variety of autonomic nervous system feats such as increasing blood flow in one ear only, and changing urine output and blood pressure (Miller, 1971; DiCara, 1972). This procedure was called operant conditioning because the physiological change, such as blushing in one ear, was gradually acquired when the response was rewarded (the reward was electrical stimulation of the pleasure center in the rat's brain) and when the animal could produce the response when signaled to do so, usually by a tone.

These studies demolished the rigid conceptualization of the autonomic nervous system as involuntary and outside the the domain of learning (for those who had never questioned that concept), and it also diminished the idea that if autonomic functions could be manipulated, it was only through control of striate muscles, such as holding the breath and tightening the chest muscles to raise blood pressure.

Although Miller and DiCara and other researchers were unable to replicate these striking results, for some experimental psychologists, the operant conditioning experiments with rats opened the door to research with humans. This research also gave support to the operant conditioning model of biofeedback in human research. Lacking from the operant conditioning approach with rats, however, were several elements that are the heart of biofeedback training with humans: the use of volition, the goal of voluntary psychophysiological regulation for health, skills training, generalization of training to many situations, and cognitive restructuring. Even so, many reviewers of the field cite the Miller and DiCara research as a foundation of biofeedback training with humans.

Biofeedback with Humans: Operant Conditioning and Drug Models

Researchers who came into biofeedback research from operant conditioning research, quite naturally adopted the model of operant conditioning and the research methodology of operant conditioning for biofeedback.

Perhaps this model was accepted for biofeedback training because when biofeedback is viewed with operant conditioning glasses, some aspects of the procedure appear to be operant conditioning. The signal from the biofeedback instrument, usually a tone or light, looks like the typical stimulus of operant conditioning. In some experiments, rewards were given for correct responses, because it was thought that the reward would increase the likelihood that the *target response* would be repeated. Following the operant conditioning model, the feedback signal was thought of as a stimulus that controlled the trainee's physiology, rather than as information *created by the trainee* and used for learning self regulation. We highlight "created by the trainee" because this is a key element in biofeedback training that sets it apart from operant conditioning. The biofeedback signal is generated by the

BIOFEEDBACK OR BIOFEEDBACK TRAINING?

The word *biofeedback* refers to many different processes—operant conditioning with rats; operant conditioning with humans using biofeedback instrumentation; and self regulation training using biofeedback instrumentation as a tool, a therapy in which biofeedback training is one element. Clients sometimes use the word to mean anything learned in biofeedback therapy, as in "I used my biofeedback" when in fact the person used deep breathing learned in therapy.

You may have noticed that we use biofeedback, biofeedback training, and biofeedback therapy. We use biofeedback training to mean the use of information from a biofeedback instrument for the purpose of learning a self regulation skill, and biofeedback therapy to refer to a multimodal therapy in which biofeedback training is a part. We use biofeedback to refer to a procedure in which signals from a biofeedback instrument are presented to the trainee, or laboratory animal, and trial and error is the only learning strategy available because instructions, coaching, and other important variables in self regulation training are omitted.

trainee, not by the instrument or the experimenter, and reflects what is going on inside the person. As the physiological process being reflected comes under the control of the trainee, the trainee gains control of the signal.

You saw in Box 8.6 that the model that a researcher has of the phenomenon being studied determines the research methodology. The operant conditioning model of biofeedback training involves a particular methodology for studying biofeedback training. In the typical operant conditioning study, subjects were connected to the instrumentation and told in which way the feedback signal (called the stimulus) should be changed. Minimal or no instructions were given on how to make the desired physiological change. Trial and error was the strategy that subjects had to use. Often the training sessions were only 3 to 16 minutes long, and often only 1 to 4 sessions were given (Shellenberger & Green, 1986).

As you can imagine, learning to control an autonomic nervous system process such as heart rate, blood pressure, or blood flow (skin temperature) would be very difficult in these conditions, and many operant conditioning studies failed. Subjects were unable to gain control and learning did not occur, and when the subjects were patients, symptoms were not reduced. But because human physiology naturally fluctuates, sooner or later the physiological process fluctuated in the correct direction, and the feedback and the reward would indicate the correct change, just as sooner or later the rat presses on the food bar and is rewarded. Occasionally, subjects did learn how to change the physiological process when given feedback. The successful heart rate, blood pressure, and skin temperature (blood flow) studies impressed many people because they demonstrated that humans can gain a degree of control over sections of the autonomic nervous system, which previously was thought to be involuntary.

The operant conditioning model of biofeedback has a partner that we call the **drug model**. The drug model suggests that if biofeedback is effective, it must have specific effects on physiological functions and reduce symptoms, and that these specific effects must be demonstrated independently of placebo effects. We refer to this as the drug model because the concern for demonstrating specific effects and eliminating placebo effects comes directly from drug research in which the specific effects of

the active ingredient in the drug are studied. This seems like a strange model for something that has no more power to affect physiology than a mirror, and in fact it is not an appropriate model for biofeedback training. Nonetheless, it has been quite popular (Furedy, 1985).

The research methodology of the drug model attempts to eliminate everything from the experiment that might affect the outcome except exposure to signals from a biofeedback instrument. Thus, to study only biofeedback and to eliminate the placebo effect, variables such as relaxation training, homework exercises, imagery, positive expectations, and positive interaction with the experimenter are eliminated. These variables are eliminated because they are thought to create placebo effects, making it impossible to determine the specific effect of biofeedback. Some researchers have also used double-blind methodology to study biofeedback. As explained in Chapter 2 on the placebo effect, the double-blind design is used in drug research. Neither the person giving the drug nor the subject knows whether the subject is getting the medication or the placebo. When this design is used in biofeedback training, neither the person "giving" biofeedback nor the person "receiving" biofeedback knows what is being fed back. Nonetheless, a few researchers thought that this was the appropriate design for biofeedback research. They thought that being exposed to biofeedback should change physiology, just as being exposed to a drug changes physiology, and that the effects of biofeedback must be separated from placebo effects (Furedy, 1985). Please read Box 8.7 now.

The attempt to study the specific effects of biofeedback was like trying to study the specific effects of a mirror. The information from a mirror has no power to affect behavior, and neither does the signal from a biofeedback instrument, or even the information itself. The person using the mirror controls the reflection, just as the person using the biofeedback instrument controls the information from the machine. Fortunately, humans can learn in

BOX 8.7

ISOLATING THE INDEPENDENT VARIABLE

When a researcher wants to determine the effect of a single variable, called the independent variable, the effect of that variable must be isolated from the effect of other variables. One way to isolate the independent variable is to eliminate any other variable that could affect the outcome of a study. Any other variable is said to confound or contaminate the data and is called a **confounding variable**.

Believing that biofeedback has a specific effect that must be demonstrated in order to claim that biofeedback is effective, researchers using the drug model tried to eliminate all variables from biofeedback research except the "active ingredient," meaning exposure to signals from the biofeedback instrument. Therefore, in this research all of the important ingredients in biofeedback training—breathing exercises, relaxation training, homework, motivation, and interaction with the experimenter— where thought to be confounding variables and were eliminated. In operant conditioning research these variables were simply not included because they were not considered important, but in drug model research they were eliminated because they were thought to be confounding variables.

A recurrent theme in health fields is that to enhance health and well-being, people need to learn skills—relaxation, stress-management, stress-resistance, cognitive, child-rearing, assertiveness, and lifestyle skills. These skills are learned through a variety of tools that interact to promote learning. It is not possible to separate a single active ingredient, the independent variable, and attempt to show the effect of that one variable on learning. When this is attempted in biofeedback research, and the independent variable is thought to be exposure to signals from a biofeedback machine (excluding all the "confounding" variables), the study usually fails.

Research that studies multicomponent processes may be criticized, and the results may be discounted because the effect of a single independent variable was not isolated. We suspect that in the study of health, in which biological, psychological, and social variables interact, very few single variables can be isolated.

As health sciences evolve, new research methods for studying complex processes will be developed and will be recognized as scientifically legitimate.

spite of the research methodology, and sometimes positive change occurred even in drug model research. Most commonly, however, no learning occurred, and the conclusion was that biofeedback training is not useful for symptom reduction and that people cannot learn to control physiological functioning (Lang, 1977; Nielsen & Holmes, 1980; Guglielmi, Roberts, & Patterson, 1982; Kewman & Roberts, 1980).

In summary, the operant conditioning and drug models of biofeedback training led to research methodology in which the signals from the biofeedback instrument were thought to be a stimulus that could control behavior or to have a druglike power that could affect physiology and reduce symptoms. Researchers who used these models did not think of biofeedback as merely a tool to help the trainee learn a skill, and often no learning occurred. When no physiological change occurred or symptoms were not reduced, it was generally concluded that biofeedback training was not effective. Rarely did these researchers conclude that the model of biofeedback and the research methodology were faulty.

The moral of this story is that in designing research and evaluating research results, it is important to critically examine the model and the methodology being used. The operant conditioning and drug model methodologies are appropriate in some situations, but not in biofeedback training in which the methodology hinders learning.

Humans can learn in spite of the research methodology, as we noted. Sometimes positive change did occur in the conditioning-drug model research, and these results were valuable in offsetting the results of the negative studies.

Biofeedback Training: Research

Biofeedback training research spread like wildfire because the idea behind it is so sensible and easy to grasp—information feedback makes learning easier. Feedback of physiological information for psychophysiological self regulation was novel, but the implications were immediately recognized. The implications were as simple and homey as learning to have warm feet in bed and as complex as awakening humans to their potential for volition and self-healing.

The organizer of the 1969 meeting and the first president of the Biofeedback Research Society, Barbara Brown, wrote: "Bio-feedback is simple in concept only. It is probably the most complex of all of the discoveries about man's being, for it points straight to the greatest mystery of all: the ability of the mind to control its own and the body's sickness and health (Brown, 1974, p. 11).

We now introduce you to a few of the pioneers because they highlight the variety of interests and personal histories of the people who found themselves under one roof in 1969, trying to decide what to call the new process.

Joe Kamiya and Brainwave Feedback. Imagine a sleep researcher staying up nights to watch the EEG record of a sleeping subject. Tiring as that sounds, one of the first and dramatic feedback studies came from the all-night vigils. In 1958 Joe Kamiya was working in the sleep research laboratory at the University of Chicago. During the tedious task of monitoring the brainwave records, he saw the smooth high-amplitude slow waves of alpha come and go as the subject drifted from wakefulness toward sleep and back to wakefulness. Kamiya wondered whether the subject had any awareness of the shifts in alpha.

Because the brain has no sensory system, Kamiya knew that he was really wondering whether the subject could feel a shift in consciousness as alpha waxed and waned. Kamiya devised a simple way to find out. Periodically he rang a bell, with the instruction to the subject to guess whether brainwave A or brainwave B was present just before the bell. Subjects were told immediately that they were right or wrong. Kamiya found that after several hours of training, many subjects could guess correctly at least 80 percent of the time, and some always knew which brainwave they were producing. By 1961, at the Langley Porter Neuropsychiatric Institute in San Francisco, Kamiya had automated the procedure. An instrument filtered the alpha frequencies from other brainwave frequencies, measured the amplitude of the waves, and produced a tone when the amplitude was of a predetermined level. Again it was found that subjects could increase the amplitude and the amount of alpha.

When Kamiya reported this work at the Psychophysiological Research Society in 1965, the impact was immediate. To the scientists, controlling brainwaves seemed improbable, and to the public, it bordered on the mysterious.

The idea that humans could control this silent organ was revolutionary. Today the fact that brainwaves can be consciously controlled seems obvious. Humans can control the activity of the mind and the activity of the mind is correlated with brainwaves, so humans can control brainwaves (Kamiya, 1971; Kamiya, 1979).

Elmer and Alyce Green, Pioneers in Thermal, EMG, and EEG Feedback. Elmer and Alyce Green were already studying voluntary control through feedback of blood flow in the hands (temperature feedback) and muscle tension (EMG feedback) when they heard Joe Kamiya's presentation on EEG feedback in 1965. Elmer Green tells us that while listening to Kamiya he immediately realized that brainwave training would complete the feedback package, because EMG and thermal feedback are reflected in the periphery and represent autonomic and somatic nervous system functions, while EEG is a central nervous system process only. Through these three types of feedback, subjects would gain control over sections of the entire nervous system. This sparked the idea for what was later called the "triple training program," in which subjects tried to increase alpha and hand temperature and to lower forehead EMG simultaneously.

One of us (JG) had the opportunity to interview the Greens, and we include their personal story here, as told in the interview.

A Conversation with Founding Parents

Judy: You might say that I grew up along with biofeedback training, professionally, I mean, but how did you two get into it? Tell me about the early history, before biofeedback got its name.

Alyce: Looking back, it seems that many of our interests came together in the development of biofeedback training—our interest in the role of the mind in healing, our interest in volition and the ability of humans to gain self regulation,

Elmer's background in physics, engineering and biopsychology, and my background in counseling and creativity research, even our interest in yoga and Eastern philosophy. These things influenced the way in which we developed biofeedback training in our laboratory and later in the clinic, but in 1964 when we left the University of Chicago and began setting up the psychophysiology lab at The Menninger Foundation we had a particular idea in mind. We planned to study the physiological correlates of autogenic training.

Judy: Why autogenic training?

Elmer: Well, a physiological study of autogenic training seemed like a good way to begin research on the broader area of mind-body and psychophysiological control that we were interested in. Perhaps I should say "a scientifically legitimate way." Getting support to study techniques like yoga or meditation would have been difficult in 1964, but autogenic training is different: It is a well documented Western self regulation technique developed by a German physician.

Judy: That's true. Autogenic training is certainly legitimate, as you say, and it is a technique for psychophysiologic regulation. But how did the idea of feedback come in? Autogenic training doesn't include feedback.

Alyce: It just made sense. When we read *Autogenic Training* by Schultz and Luthe in 1962 we realized that they were teaching a skill, and that it took so long to learn because the trainee had no feedback, no way of knowing what was happening. We were pretty certain that the training would go much faster if people could watch their own finger temperature change as they used the phrases for heaviness in the body and warmth in the hands.

Elmer: Feeding back physiological information did not seem revolutionary at the time. While I was studying biopsychology in Chicago in 1960, I had a polygraph that recorded heart beat, brainwaves, respiration, and skin voltage. Out of curiosity I occasionally used the polygraph to monitor my heart beat. I watched the paper record as it was made, and I experimented with changing my heart rate, using the record to tell me how I was doing. As I say, feedback wasn't revolutionary. The revolutionary ideas were more complicated.

Judy: What ideas?

Elmer: Two primarily—the idea that the body is a reflection of the unconscious mind and that feeding back unconscious body processes to a person would enable the person to confront the psychological unconscious and thus gain conscious self regulation. When I first met Gardner Murphy in 1964, he had the idea that physiological feedback might be useful for becoming conscious of unconscious muscle tension.

Judy: That was a novel idea. Several other pioneers in biofeedback training have talked about Murphy, and I know that he gave the keynote address at the first meeting in 1969. Tell me about him and how he got involved in biofeedback.

Elmer: Gardner Murphy was the director of research at The Menninger Foundation who hired me. He was a scholar. He wrote some of the early textbooks on psychology and he was interested in psychophysiological research. He was also open minded about things like ESP. His main interest though was in what he called "self-confrontation." Gardner firmly believed that the best way to solve personality problems was through self-confrontation. It happened that Gardner had neck pain and he was certain that it was caused by unconscious muscle tension. He also believed that unconscious tension in striate muscles reflects unconscious psychological tension. He felt that if he could confront the muscle tension in his neck, he might be able to reduce the tension and pain, and equally importantly, that the unconscious cause of the tension might dissolve as he worked on the physical manifestation of it. Gardner also thought that through striate muscle feedback, a person might possibly gain insight into the cause of the muscle tension. That really was a new idea, a revolutionary idea—that by confronting muscle tension, which meant getting feedback, and becoming conscious of the

tension and figuring out how to reduce it by using feedback, both the tension and its cause might be overcome.

Judy: So that explains why you, more than other pioneers in biofeedback training, have emphasized the fact that biofeedback training is consciousness training. And by that you mean becoming conscious of unconscious body processes and thus becoming conscious of unconscious psychological processes.

Elmer: Exactly. But we went beyond Gardner's idea about striate muscles. We realized that the functions of the autonomic nervous system reflect unconscious psychological processes even more than striate muscles and are more responsive to stress. Feedback of autonomic processes as a way of correcting unconscious psychological processes usually reflected in the autonomic nervous system as a symptom made sense. And this idea fit well with our plan to feed back finger temperature during autogenic training, because temperature is correlated with blood flow, and blood flow is controlled by the sympathetic branch of the autonomic nervous system.

Judy: Did many people believe that the autonomic nervous system could be voluntarily controlled?

Elmer: Very few. People believed that it was not possible to control the autonomic nervous system directly. They believed that the only way to change autonomic functioning was through the striate muscles. For example, it was thought that heart rate could be controlled only by tightening the chest muscles or changing breathing, or something like that. That is why Miller and DiCara paralyzed their rats, and why it seemed so amazing that the rats could change autonomic functions even when the striate muscles were out of the picture.

Judy: But anyone who thought about the implications of hypnosis or the placebo effect, or the reports from India, or the physiological effects of stress and relaxation for that matter, would have suspected that the autonomic nervous system is controllable, independently of striate muscles.

Alyce: That is right, but no one thought about it. Phenomena like these weren't of interest to many of the researchers who began investigating biofeedback, especially those who had been working only with laboratory animals. And the medical texts still referred to the autonomic system as the "involuntary nervous system."

Elmer: In any case, Gardner's idea about "confronting" unconscious muscle tension through feedback, and the fact that the first exercise in autogenic training focuses entirely on the sensation of heaviness for reducing muscle tension were intriguing, so we built equipment for monitoring and feeding back muscle tension. We first experimented with forearm muscle tension. We were surprised to find that subjects could reduce muscle tension to nearly zero. Actually, we thought that there was something wrong with our equipment until we searched the literature and found that John Basmajian had already done this kind of work and discovered that with feedback subjects could learn to control the firing of single motor units, exactly what we found. Our first paper was written about this research, and we titled it "Feedback Technique for Deep Relaxation." That was 1969.

Alyce: Just before doing this research, we had begun the autogenic training study, first without temperature feedback and then with feedback of finger temperature as the indicator of blood flow in the hands.

Elmer: We recorded more than finger temperature, however. After reading *Autogenic Training* we were convinced that the great variety of medical applications of autogenic training implied that much more was going on physiologically than just striate muscle relaxation and increased blood flow in the hands. So in addition to measuring blood volume in both hands and finger temperature, we also recorded brain waves, galvanic skin potential, heart rate, and respiration to find out how the practice of autogenic training affected these processes. To avoid the "about to be electrocuted" feeling that so many electrodes and wires might create in research subjects, we sewed all the wires for

recording the physiological processes into the sleeves of a jacket that was worn during the training. We did not want stressful feelings about the recording procedures to interfere with the training and cause us to misinterpret the records.

Judy: That was a great idea. I wonder how often research results are inaccurate because the subject's emotional response to the situation affects the physiological recordings. But what you said about broad medical applications of autogenic training reminded me of the fact that Schultz and Luthe believed that autogenic training promotes homeostasis, so in that sense there was a lot more going on.

Alyce: In fact, the first clinical discovery in our lab is a good example of how relaxation enhances homeostasis.

Judy: You must mean the migraine headache discovery.

Alyce: Yes, but Elmer, you were in the control room at the time, so you tell what happened.

Elmer: Okay. After the autogenic training session the subjects sat quietly in a darkened room while the physiological parameters were still being recorded. One afternoon while I was monitoring the record of a subject as she sat in the darkened room I noticed that her hand temperature, which was quite low, suddenly increased 10 degrees in about two minutes, an unusually rapid change. This occurred about three minutes before the end of the session, so when it was over I went into the training room and asked her what had happened about three minutes ago. She said, "How did you know my migraine went away?" That bit of startling information could not be ignored, and as you know, that chance finding led to the use of biofeedback training, meaning autogenic feedback training, as part of the treatment for migraine headache.

Alyce: Within a month two people learned how to stop migraine headaches using a temperature feedback device that Elmer invented. The use of autogenic training and feedback of increasing finger temperature, which correlates with increasing blood volume in the hand, turned out to be a powerful combination for learning relaxation and vasodilation in the periphery.

Judy: In fact, autogenic training with temperature feedback is the first biofeedback exercise for most of my clients, and it is easy to practice at home with a little weather thermometer for feedback. I imagine that the discovery with the migraine patient really launched autogenic feedback training, as you call it, and hastened the use of biofeedback training as a treatment tool.

Alyce: Probably so, at least after Joe Sargent's first report on the research project with migraine patients at The Menninger Foundation in 1970. By that time we were involved in brainwave feedback training for enhancing creativity—you know about that research because you helped us with it. But that was two years after biofeedback got its name.

Judy: That's right, I wanted to know how biofeedback got its name. Tell me about the first meeting in 1969.

Elmer: It was certainly an interesting meeting. People from many different fields were attracted to feedback, and when it came time to decide on a name for the process so that the society could be named, people had very different ideas about what feedback was all about and what it should be called. It took a lot of discussion, sometimes heated discussion, before everyone agreed that the best thing to do was to create a single, simple word to describe the process. And so biofeedback was chosen, short for *biological feedback*. Some of us argued that the term chosen for the process and for the society should include "psychophysiological" and "self regulation" to reflect the fact that mind and body are always involved together in the process and that the goal of training is self regulation. Mind and body always interact, and so in one sense it is incorrect to think of the feedback as just physiological, as if the mind weren't involved. If it weren't for mind-body interaction, there could be no training, so "psychophysiological" makes sense. If you go

backward through the rationale, you might start out by thinking that you are feeding back finger temperature, for example. But then you realize that it isn't really temperature; the feedback really represents blood flow. But then you realize that it isn't really blood flow feedback; it really represents something that the hypothalamus is doing, modified by the limbic system. It really represents limbic system feedback. Then you realize that the feedback includes limbic system and cortex, because the use of phrases or images to change hand temperature is cortical activity. Of course, the conscious use of phrases and images, and the use of volition in general, are mental activities, activities of the mind, so the feedback is always psychophysiological.

Alyce: In 1969, however, many people at the meeting felt that there should be no reference to the mind or to the self. They felt that these concepts would be detrimental to the scientific tone of the society, and a few actually argued that the mind and consciousness are not involved in biofeedback. One physician maintained that the term "psychophysiological" was a distortion of the truth, since there is no psyche.

Judy: Good grief.

Elmer: These were the behaviorists and people involved in operant conditioning who apparently thought that Miller and DiCara's work with paralyzed rats was a good model for biofeedback with humans. You know that the work with rats was called "biofeedback." This created confusion about what biofeedback training with humans actually is.

Judy: Didn't they understand the rationale?

Elmer: No. Well, there was no written rationale at that time, and these people were not thinking beyond the laws of operant conditioning. But for many years my goal was to find out how the mind manipulates the body. Not "does it" but "how does it." That is why I left physics and went back to graduate school in biopsychology. As part of my graduate work I read the early research on the limbic system and emotions. I was also interested in ethology and the fact that sensory perception governs behavior in lower animals. To explain how human can gain voluntary control of physiological processes, especially through their own perceptions, I put several lines of research together and added feedback as part of the process. I remember discussing the rationale at the first meeting in '69, and we described it in detail by about 1973. Even so, for many years a number of researchers argued that the mind was not involved, and the sceptics claimed that there is no explanation for how biofeedback works. Of course, there is a misunderstanding right there, since biofeedback doesn't "work"; the person using the feedback "works." But I am sure that you are writing about that. Anyway, the basics of how mind influences body have been understood for many years now. We have known for many years that the "wiring" for psychophysiologic self regulation is nicely laid out in the brain and makes it possible for people to consciously change physiological—I should say psychophysiological—processes.

Alyce: It is pretty interesting that almost 20 years after the first meeting, in 1988, the society changed its name to **Association for Applied Psychophysiology and Biofeedback.** The name now reflects the facts more accurately, both in research and in clinical practice.

Judy: Actually, this was the second name change for the society. You originally named it the Biofeedback Research Society, but biofeedback training grew out of the laboratory and into the clinic so rapidly that by 1976 the clinicians and educators in the society felt that the name was too limiting, and it became the Biofeedback Society of America. I wonder what the next name change will be!

Alyce: Who knows. We changed the name of our work 15 years ago. We do no refer to it as biofeedback training. We use the term "psychophysiologic therapy" because we use many techniques, such as imagery and breathing exercises, that are not "biofeedback" per se. Biofeedback training, meaning the use of biofeedback equipment, is only one tool in psychophysiologic therapy.

Judy: In fact, in Part Five of the textbook we will introduce the basics of what we might call "psychophysiologic therapy for self regulation," the broad therapy that has evolved from biofeedback training and many other techniques. Now I have one more question for you. In all the years that you have been involved in the development of biofeedback training and clinical applications, what have been the most rewarding experiences for you?

Elmer: Probably the remarkable things that patients can do to recover from problems referred to as "chronic" or even "fatal." But in research it is probably theta brainwave training.

Alyce: I think we would agree that the brainwave training program for enhancing creativity was certainly the most interesting work for us, because it combined my interest in creativity and our belief that all people have a treasury of knowledge and creativity in the unconscious mind that can be used when the person learns how to open the treasure chest. I had read enough reports of creative people to know that inspiration or the solution to a problem, or an idea for a story, would often come when the person was in a state of reverie, that state between waking and sleep when the mind drifts and images seem to appear spontaneously in consciousness. Based on experience with preliminary EEG research and our own personal experiences with reverie, we hypothesized that theta is the brainwave correlate of reverie and that if people could learn to get into reverie through theta feedback, they would experience an increase in creativity. You probably remember all this because you trained the subjects to use the brainwave feedback equipment.

Judy: I also remember that creativity is very difficult to measure and that the most consistent finding was an increase in what you call "integrative" experiences. Over the 50 brainwave training sessions, the subjects got to know themselves better, so to speak, and some solved interpersonal problems.

Elmer: That is correct, and that is why we decided to explore the use of theta training with psychiatric patients. That research was intriguing and many patients benefited greatly, but there is much more to be learned, and we hope that we will be able to continue on with the research. You know how it is, research funds determine the direction of research in most labs.

Alyce: I think that in terms of clinical application, the work with hypertension is very exciting and certainly important, since hypertension is such a widespread problem.

Judy: That was another case of a surprise finding! I remember the woman who gave you the clue about temperature training and blood pressure reduction. Wasn't she a reporter for the *Kansas City Star?*

Alyce: Yes, and you remember that after several years of trying to describe biofeedback to reporters, we finally decided that the best way to understand biofeedback training is to do it. So we gave her an autogenic feedback session, and loaned her a temperature trainer for one week. When she returned the instrument she said, "You may be interested to know that I got rid of my hypertension last week." She had had borderline hypertension and was taking a tranquilizer for anxiety. She stopped her medication and had her blood pressure checked after one week of practicing hand warming, and it was normal.

Elmer: We would never have advised the medication change, but the results were interesting. A few months later a physician asked us if we could help a patient with uncontrolled hypertension. Of course we agreed to give it a try, using temperature feedback for increasing blood flow in hands and feet. We guessed that in order to increase blood flow in the periphery, peripheral resistance would have to drop, and therefore blood pressure would drop. The first trainee did extremely well, and so we were encouraged to continue. Over the next couple years we worked with about 10 patients, with good results. Then we began training patients in small groups of four or five and that worked well, and now Steve Fahrion is just finishing an extensive three-year research program, funded by the National Heart, Lung, and Blood Institute. The results look good, and we are making headway on understanding the dynamics of the cardiovascular system, and how self regulation is possible.

Alyce: Returning to Elmer's comment, I have to say that the greatest satisfaction in our work is seeing the change in clients as they gain self regulation skills—not just the changes in symptoms, but the changes in self-image, and beliefs, and hope. It is truly rewarding to help people awaken the power that they have for healing and health, and sometimes it is so amazingly simple—a few new ideas, a few new skills, and the person is in control again and on the road to being weller than well, to use Karl Menninger's term.

Judy: I guess that is why I love the work so much, too. This makes me think of one more question. Is there anything that you would like to say to the student reading this text?

Elmer: Something humorous or something serious?

Judy: Whatever.

Alyce: Let's just say, "You have picked a terrific topic, for you and all humanity, so stick with it. And good luck!"

Barbara Brown and EEG Feedback. In a laboratory at the Veterans Administration Hospital in Los Angeles, Barbara Brown came upon the idea of feeding back information in her own way. The year was 1967.

Biofeedback training evolved in Brown's laboratory out of her curiosity about imagery and whether or not the differences in how people image could be detected in brainwaves. Of particular interest to Brown was the fact that some people have intense and colorful visual imagery, while others do not have visual imagery.

Brown was an expert in analyzing the brainwaves of cats. Without much change in instrumentation, she and her colleagues began analyzing the brainwaves of humans, hoping to find differences between those who have visual imagery and those who do not. The experiment included flashing colored lights at the subjects while recording brainwaves. It was found that the same color elicits different responses from people who differ in their experience of visual imagery, perhaps a clue to the differences in the way that people image and recall in images, some vivid and some not.

Brown realized that the brainwave was somehow reflecting differences in subjective human experience, a domain rarely studied in "hard science." During the study of color, subjective experience of the color presented, and brainwave correlates, Brown conjured up "my most impossible, foolish thought, and stumbled upon bio-feedback" (Brown, 1974, p. 31). The impossible thought was to let the brainwave create the color of the light presented to the subject, so that the color would be a reflection of the subjective experience. The technological difficulties of converting brainwaves into a variety of colors was insurmountable at the time, so Brown simply turned alpha into a blue light and asked subjects to describe their subjective experiences as it increased and decreased in brightness as the amplitude of the brainwave fluctuated. This was biofeedback, without the name. The blue light indicated the presence of alpha in the brainwave. In subject after subject, alpha increased over time, and subjects reported feeling restful but never bored. In the first book written on biofeedback training by a pioneer in the field, *New Mind, New Body*, Brown says that the implication was immediately understood—if people could learn to control "an obscure brainwave" by identifying the presence of the brainwave subjectively, then people could probably learn to control any function. Brown wrote:

> What would medical science think? How would psychiatrists react? Could biology accept this new reality? Where were my scientific colleagues; did they know? Had they stumbled across the same bewilderingly unexpected ability of human beings? Where was everyone? The excitement cried to be shared.
>
> (Brown, 1974, p. 33)

And shared it was. Through a series of unexpected contacts, Brown learned that several researchers around the country had also discovered alpha feedback, and a newsletter was circulated among them. By 1969 many types of feedback were being explored and discussed, primarily at the meetings of the Psychophysiological Research Society. It was time to officially break away from traditional psychophysiological research and to think about creating a society devoted to the study of the new phenomena of physiological feedback. A letter of inquiry sent to people who had an interest in the process drew an enthusiastic "yes," and the first meeting was scheduled. One hundred and forty researchers came together to share their experiences and form the society. Brown was elected chairperson. The society and the term "biofeedback" were off and running.

John Basmajian and EMG Feedback.

Do you think that you could control a particular, individual cell in your body if you were given feedback about what the cell was doing? If you are like a lot of other people, you could. The cell that you can control is a long motor neuron that travels out of the spinal cord to the muscle fibers that it innervates.

If you did not mind having extremely fine needle electrodes inserted into a muscle (the electrode is small enough to pick up the electrical activity of a single motor unit) and you received feedback of the activity of the neuron, you could learn to voluntarily control the activity of the single motor unit being monitored by the electrode. According to Barbara Brown, when John Basmajian, a physician and at that time director of rehabilitation research at Emory University in Atlanta, presented his research on the control of single motor units, those in the audience at the 1969 meeting who were not familiar with this rather esoteric work were stunned.

Using feedback from the big muscle at the base of the thumb, Basmajian found that many subjects could learn to completely turn off

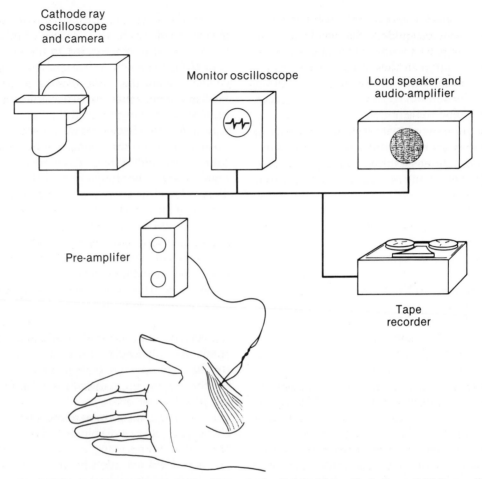

Figure 8.4 Feedback procedure for Gaining Control of a Single Motor Unit. From J. V. Basmajian (1974). *Muscles Alive: Their Functions Revealed by Electromyography.* © **1974 by Williams and Wilkins Co., Baltimore. Reprinted by Permission.**

the activity of the single motor unit, and then, on command, increase the activity so that the muscles cells would contract in a particular rhythm that could be reproduced. Some subjects could even control several motor units, individually, and gave them names. Basmajian called these subjects SMUGs, for single motor unit geniuses. The amount of muscle contraction produced by a single motor unit is infinitesimal and cannot be felt, and subjects could not describe how the units were controlled. This work was first described in 1963 (Basmajian, 1963).

The work with single motor unit control demonstrated the value of feedback and of the ability of humans to gain control of normally unconscious processes. This work also contributed to the development of feedback training in neuromuscular rehabilitation, an important application described in Part Five.

Tom Budzynski, Johann Stoyva, Behavior Therapy and Tension Headache. In 1963 the aerospace industry lost an engineer and psychology gained an untiring researcher. Aerospace engineer Tom Budzynski left the industry for

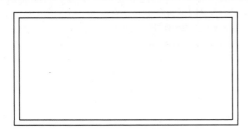

In this box put a red apple. Make the apple so vivid that you could reach into the box and get it. Now reach in, grab the apple and take a big bite of it—hear it crunch, taste the sweet juice. Now turn the apple into a green banana; now an orange with pink polka dots. Now stare at the box and see last night's dinner.

Most people can do this. If you are unable to create a visual image, just keep reading.

Now stare at the box and try to see nothing at all. How long can you see nothing before something appears?

Now read this instruction and then do the exercise. Using the blank box to focus your attention, or with your eyes closed, go back to a special day in childhood. When you find that special day, be there. Be a child again. Relive the moments that are special. Notice everything around you—what you are wearing, how you feel, how old you are, what you are doing. Enjoy being a child again. Be in the situation for a couple of minutes.

Now read this instruction and then do the exercise. Using the blank box or with your eyes closed, drift forward in time to one year from today. Experience yourself one year from today. Notice where you are, how you feel, what you are doing.

Now without moving, imagine tying your shoes, one and then the other.

Now feel the warmth of a wood-burning stove. Run your fingertips across sandpaper, and now silk. Hear the wind in the trees; smell fresh-baked bread.

Cereal box. Nude. Spaghetti. Paper airplane. Puppy. Love.

Now take one minute to create a cozy little apartment overlooking the sea. On one of the walls hangs a landscape painting. In the painting put some hills and trees, and a country road that winds over the hills and out of sight. Now create a car and drive along the road, over the hills and out of sight.

In these exercises you have used imagery and visualization. The terms *imagery* and *visualization* are used interchangeably by some authors. Others use *imagery* to mean pictures or sensations created spontaneously in the mind, as in "I was thinking about my asthma and suddenly the image of a black cloud came into my mind," and use *visualization* to mean the conscious construction or manipulation of images, as in "In my visualization I saw my bronchial tubes opening, and then I cleaned them out with a vacuum cleaner." Because these seem to be distinct experiences, we use these meanings of imagery and visualization.

Imagery and visualization are the forte of the mind. They are the primary tools for thinking, remembering, and fantasizing, and a medium for creativity. Many creative people have described an ability to use the image-making faculty of the mind for solving problems and developing ideas. The discovery of the benzine ring by the French chemist Frederic Kekule is a classic example. Kekule had cultivated the ability to watch as his mind played with images of atoms. On one occasion he watched in a state of reverie as his mind created atoms that joined into a chain that turned into a snake that took hold of its tail, forming a ring. From this spontaneous imagery Kekule worked out the mathematical formulas that proved the existence of the benzine ring (Koestler, 1964).

Imagery and visualization are essential for normal psychological and social development. Imagine trying to grow up without the ability to imagine being grown up. Imagine the boredom of childhood without fantasy (at least before television). Longtime imagery researcher Jerome Singer found that children with rich fantasy lives are better adjusted and less hyperactive than children who cannot fantasize and that adolescents who are unable to visualize the consequences of their behavior are more likely to commit crimes than their visualizing peers (Singer, 1976).

Imagery is also the language of the body and has powerful physiological effects. Bite into a juicy lemon, run from a vicious dog, fall off a high cliff, make love: do these things in fantasy and the body responds in proportion to the richness of the images and their emotional impact. Because the past lives in the present as images, traumatic experiences continue in the present, eliciting physiological responses that contribute to the experience of the trauma. In this chapter we describe techniques for defusing both the memory and the physiological response to the memory.

In spite of their omnipresence, imagery and visualization did not have a role in psychology or medicine, neither in theory nor in treatment, until recently. Like the mind itself, imagery was shunned by experimental psychology and was not considered a fit subject for scientific study, being subjective and unobservable.

This status has changed. As Robert Holt, psychologist at New York University, stated in a landmark article on imagery in 1964, "the ostracized has returned" (Holt, 1964). By the mid-1970s many academicians, researchers, and clinicians were interested in imagery, and two national associations and two publications devoted to imagery were established. Researchers such as University of Wisconsin psychologist Peter Lang (1979) studied the relationship between the emotional content and quality of images and physiological responses, working with phobic and nonphobic subjects. This research augmented the development and refinement of the use of visualization and imagery in psychotherapy.

Today, imagery and visualization are well-known ingredients in therapeutic techniques such as desensitization, flooding, hypnosis, stress-inoculation training, and healing. Experimental psychologists study the dream imagery of subjects in sleep laboratories, and others use imagery and fantasies to study human motivation. David McClelland of Harvard University, cited in Chapter 6, believes that imagery and fantasies provide the most reliable and objective indices of human motivation (1985). In fact, McClelland states that the most significant contributions of behavioral medicine research in the future will come from the study of imagery for healing and health (cited in Borysenko, 1985, p. 39). McClelland believes that imagery "affects things at a more fundamental level than action-based therapies" (Borysenko, 1985, p. 40). By action-based therapies McClelland means therapies that focus only on behaviors without examining the cognitions leading to the behaviors. What is needed, says McClelland, is "work at the deeper level" (Borysenko, 1985, p. 40).

The many uses of imagery and visualization range from the mundane, such as trying to remember all the items on a grocery list, to the potentially life-saving, such as trying to help the immune system destroy a cancer. In Section One we describe the use of imagery and visualization in relaxation training, biofeedback training, and stress management. In Section Two we describe the use of imagery and visualization for overcoming the stress of past events. In Section Three imagery and visualization techniques for self-exploration are described. In Section Four we discuss the use of imagery and visualization for healing, and in Section Five we review the limited but

BOX 9.1

CLINICAL DATA

Throughout this text we provide guidelines for analyzing health research. We have pointed out that research may fail to take into account important variables that affect research results and have referred to these as "olive oil" variables. We also have discussed the difficulties of attempting to conduct research on complex human behavior by isolating an independent variable with "divide and study" methodology. Now we focus on another issue that is particularly germane to this chapter on imagery and visualization: the work of clinicians in the development of concepts and tools for promoting health. This issue arises in a chapter on imagery and visualization because most of the work in this area is the result of creative clinicians who develop techniques and concepts while working with clients. These clinicians are not traditional researchers, and the clients are not research subjects.

To add to the difficulty of establishing a treatment modality such as hypnosis, imagery, or biofeedback training, research funding for these nontraditional treatments is sparse. It is particularly so for imagery and visualization in the treatment of medical problems such as cancer, and for psychoneuroimmunology, in which imagery and visualization are used.

As you read this chapter, bear in mind that clinical findings are valid, whether or not they are the results of research, and that the lack of extensive research is due to the difficulty of researching something as complex as imagery and health and to the lack of research funds and support. We emphasize these points to offset the tendency to discount clinical findings and techniques by referring to clinical results as anecdotal rather than as data. This is particularly important when you read the section on the use of imagery and visualization in healing.

---

intriguing research on the effects of imagery and visualization on the immune system. We conclude the chapter with an overview and a glance into the future. Please read Box 9.1 now.

||||➡

SECTION ONE: VISUALIZATION FOR STRESS MANAGEMENT

Our ability to visualize has tremendous survival value. If you were chased by a bear the last time that you rounded a particular bend in the trail, it would be useful to visualize

the bear (in other words, to remember) before rounding that bend the next time. You might make a decision not to go that way at all. Or, to use a more appropriate example, if you lose your class notebook, and you want to survive the next exam, you create an image of your notebook where you last had it and look for it there. Memory is an essential function of the mind, and images are the key to memory.

Memory through imagery is a talent that most of us have without practice. However, the use of imagery and visualization must be learned and practiced like any other skill. Relaxation, stress management, personal growth and self-exploration, problem-solving, improving performance, overcoming phobias and fears, creativity, and healing all involve the skill of using imagery and visualization.

Relaxation Training

Without·suggestions from us, students in our biofeedback training class use imagery when they are learning to relax with the feedback of finger temperature.

> I was on a long beach; the sun was pouring down on my shoulder; and I could feel the heat flowing down my arms.
> I put myself in a hot tub with my boyfriend.
> I imagined that I was in front of a warm fire, holding a cup of hot chocolate.

Visualization for relaxation often combines visual details and sensations such as the warmth of the sun, heaviness in arms and legs, floating, or being limp.

Clients and students who have never used visualization are often surprised by the richness and immediacy of their images. I (JG) will never forget a middle-aged client who was severely handicapped by asthma and the side-effects of several medications. This man was not particularly "psychologically minded" and had few words to describe his feelings. Midway through a visualization for creating a peaceful place, tears began rolling down his cheeks. When we concluded the visualization, his first words were, "I never knew I had a mind." He described a truly beautiful scene in which he sat, leaning against an old tree stump on a hillside overlooking a lake with tall reeds. Off in the distance were hills and woods, and as he watched, a flock of ducks glided in. The ducks amazed my client more than anything else because they just appeared, in perfect formation, making a graceful banking turn as they came down; there was no experience of creating them. Going to his beautiful place became a powerful tool for this client, and

the old stump became a symbol of his own strength and healing.

Visualization for relaxation is an excellent example of a psychophysiologic technique in which both mind and body are involved. Visualization for relaxation relaxes both mind and body.

Relaxation skills are a key to stress management, desensitization, cognitive restructuring, and healing. Imagery and visualization play an important role in these areas because they facilitate relaxation.

Biofeedback Training

Chapter 8 described biofeedback training as psychophysiological self regulation training in which information from biofeedback instruments enhances learning. Learning is enhanced through feedback, but the feedback itself has no effect on physiology. The trainee practices a variety of self regulation techniques, using the information from the biofeedback instrumentation as a guide. Imagery is a natural ingredient in biofeedback training, as noted above. In relaxation training, trainees spontaneously use relaxing visualizations. When the goal is handwarming, the trainees use kinesthetic imagery of heaviness and warmth. They may also visualize blood flowing into the hands or may create a setting, such as sitting by a hot fire. For muscle relaxation, trainees often visualize and kinesthetically experience themselves in situations involving no muscle tension, such as floating on a soft air mattress on a quiet pond or being a limp rag doll. To reduce moisture on the hands during EDR feedback, the trainee might imagine being in a desert or putting the hands under a sun lamp.

Stress Management

The mind has a penchant for rehearsal: It will rehearse anything—past, present, future, and the thoroughly impossible. Because visualizing the worst, and thus preparing for the worst, were once important for survival, the mind is especially good at rehearsing the negative. When anticipating a stressful event, most people visualize bad things happening: dropping the lecture notes, or forgetting the next line in a speech, slipping on the ice, driving off the road, looking foolish in front of important people, or getting bad news from the physician. However, because our physiology, feelings, and behavior reflect whatever we are rehearsing mentally, the new cognitive therapies and stress-management techniques naturally include **positive imagery rehearsal** (Meichenbaum, 1985).

Positive imagery rehearsal can be used for things as mundane as remembering everything on the grocery list to things as important as handling a crisis. The importance of positive imagery rehearsal was described years ago in Norman Vincent Peale's popular book *The Power of Positive Thinking,* and today it is taken seriously by such diverse professionals as psychotherapists, diving coaches, and sales managers. Regardless of the situation being rehearsed, the steps are the same: (1) Relax mentally and physically; (2) let the image of the stressful situation come to mind; (3) visualize handling the situation in precisely the manner desired; (4) visualize handling one or two unexpected aspects of the situation; and (5) visualize a positive outcome. For example, sooner or later you will have to speak in public. The process is simply to visualize oneself at the beginning, middle, and end of the presentation. You experience yourself speaking fluidly and slowly. You see the audience responding. You are standing confidently, glancing at the audience and your lecture notes with ease. You are relaxed. You give yourself a good round of applause.

The goal here is to take the edge off the stress of anticipation and to counter negative imagery. The goal is not to eliminate all stress, but rather to experience handling the stress well. In addition to excellent preparation, for which there is no substitute, imagery rehearsal gives us the leading edge. Imagery rehearsal increases the likelihood of success because success is rehearsed and because rehearsal reduces stress by enhancing a sense of confidence and competence.

||||➡

SECTION TWO: OVERCOMING THE PAST

When people begin stress-management training, they usually want to learn to cope with immediate stressors—interpersonal conflict, loss of job, time pressure. For many people, however, the stress of past events continues in the present. The past returns as memories and conditioned responses that trigger emotions and behavior, and yet there is no immediate situation to resolve. The extraordinary difficulty with the past is that it is past. People believe that they are doomed to feel bad forever because the past cannot be changed. Human experience supports this view, the neurosciences support it by suggesting that memory is encoded in the brain as a kind of "hardwiring" that cannot be changed, and to some extent traditional psychotherapy also supports it. We take the opposite approach, suggesting that because the past is gone and does not exist, it can be relived in a new way. It can be remade, detached from, and reconstructed, and memories can be reinterpreted. Concurrently, the behaviors and emotions that arise in the present can be dealt with in the present. In this section we present several techniques for overcoming the past by using imagery and visualization.

Systematic Desensitization

A good example of a past event that affects the present is the classic **phobia** in which a traumatic experience creates a conditioned fear response that is triggered long after the initial event is over. In classic phobias, the person has a vivid memory of the event that triggered the phobia. In other cases, the memory is vague or the fear seems to be related to no traumatic event and yet escalates over time. Systematic desensitization is an effective technique for helping people overcome a conditioned fear response that holds them captive to the past and a slave to the response itself.

Literally, desensitization means becoming insensitive to a stimulus to which one was sensitive. In allergy treatment, desensitization means becoming insensitive to the allergen. Allergy shots contain a minute amount of the allergen. The theory is that by being exposed to small amounts of the allergen, the body will become desensitized to it. Through systematic desensitization a person is gradually desensitized to a stressor by systematically receiving small doses of the stressor. (Stress-inoculation training, discussed in Chapter 10, is based on the same idea.)

Now, think of a phobia, for example, an elevator phobia. How would one get a "small dose" of an elevator? The answer is by imagining things associated with elevators. In systematic desensitization the trainee creates a hierarchy of situations related to elevators from least stressful to most stressful. For example, driving into a city in which there are tall buildings with elevators might be the least stressful situation on the hierarchy, and riding in an elevator to the top of a skyscraper might be the most stressful. Intermediate steps might include parking the car in front of a tall building, walking into the lobby, standing in front of the elevator, and pushing the up button. By imagining these little doses while relaxed, the person gradually becomes desensitized to the elevator. The panic response is replaced with coping responses: relaxation and positive self-talk.

Joseph Wolpe, a psychotherapist and creator of systematic desensitization, reasoned that by systematically pairing each step on the stressor hierarchy with relaxation, the stress elicited by each step would be extinguished. The first task in desensitization training is to learn to relax. Wolpe taught his clients a short form of Jacobson's progressive relaxation procedure in

about eight sessions. When the trainee had mastered relaxation, each stressful event on the hierarchy was paired with the relaxation response by simultaneously relaxing and imagining the stressful event. Wolpe claimed that desensitization was achieved when the trainee had relaxed while imagining all the stressful events on the hierarchy.

Joseph Wolpe reported a 90 percent success rate with 210 phobic patients using systematic desensitization and other behavior therapy methods such as assertiveness training (Wolpe, 1958). Wolpe's unusually high success rate stimulated extensive research on systematic desensitization over the next 30 years with a variety of phobias. Although later research has been unable to replicate this high success rate, controlled studies have shown that desensitization is an effective technique for treatment of phobias and other anxiety-related disorders (Masters, Burish, Hollon, & Rimm, 1987).

Biofeedback-Assisted Desensitization and Flooding

Biofeedback training pioneer Tom Budzynski, who you met in the last chapter, was fascinated by Wolpe's work on systematic desensitization. He realized that biofeedback instrumentation would help in systematic desensitization both as a teaching tool and as a way of verifying whether or not the patient had become desensitized. Desensitization is achieved when the client has mastered relaxation and replaced anxiety with relaxation while imagining the stressful events on the hierarchy. Using biofeedback instrumentation, the trainee monitors the stress response during the visualization of the stressful scene and knows when physiological relaxation is achieved. When desensitization training is guided by a therapist, biofeedback instrumentation enables the therapist to assess the client's state of relaxation; often clients are unaware of high levels of tension and report that they are relaxed. The addition of biofeedback training makes systematic desensitization more effective by ensuring relaxation and by verifying pairing of relaxation with the steps on the stressor hierarchy (Budzynski, 1973; Budzynski & Stoyva, 1972).

Budzynski found that occasionally a successful client would encounter the stressful situation again, panic, and become resensitized to the stressful stimulus. One of the first patients to whom this happened had overcome an elevator phobia. Two years after training, the client was in an elevator in a large hotel when a group of conventioneers crowded into the elevator. The man panicked and instantly relearned his fear of elevators; he returned to Budzynski for therapy. This time, in addition to the biofeedback-assisted desensitization procedures, Budzynski used another technique called **flooding**. As used by Budzynski, flooding is the process of repeatedly exposing the client to the worst conceivable situation through visualization, until the anxiety response is extinguished. After the client had again mastered relaxation and inhibited the anxiety responses, Budzynski had him imagine riding an elevator in the worst conceivable situation—in a crowded elevator with loud, drunken conventioneers who pushed him to the back of the elevator. The client repeatedly visualized this scene until he was able to stay relaxed (Budzynski, 1977). After that case, Budzynski adopted flooding as the last phase of desensitization training. The test of the training comes when the stressful stimulus is encountered, *in vivo*.

Some therapists who use flooding believe that relaxation is not necessary for overcoming a past stressor, suggesting that repeated exposure to the fearful stimulus in imagery automatically reduces fear (Marks, 1975). This may work for some people who are not extremely phobic, but repeated exposure to the fearful stimulus in imagination can also result in increased sensitization (Foa, Blau, Prout, & Lattimer, 1977). When fear of a particular stimulus

increases, it is usually because the stimulus is repeatedly imagined and fear is experienced but the person does not have cognitive or relaxation skills to counter the fear.

That people can desensitize themselves by pairing relaxation with visualization of the stressor makes good sense. Imagery and visualization experiences are real; visualization of an event, as in stress rehearsal, increases the likelihood that the event will occur as it was visualized. In desensitization training, relaxation is experienced simultaneously with visualization of a stressor and the trainee is not overwhelmed. Pairing relaxation with the stressor breaks the fear response and replaces it with the relaxation response. This is why desensitization training is a type of counterconditioning (Kazdin & Wilcoxon, 1976). When this response is learned well, the person can confront the actual stressor.

Imaginative Role-Playing

Systematic desensitization procedures are not always appropriate methods for overcoming a stressful event. For example, Joe came into therapy to me (RS) for treatment of insomnia two years after his daughter's death in a car accident. This was his story:

> I feel terrible. Two years ago my 17-year-old daughter asked to take the family car to a football game. She had been driving for only three months, and it was raining that day. I hesitated at first but she insisted. Finally, I relented. That night her car skidded out of control and she was killed. My minister and my friends tell me that I should forgive myself. But I can't. I should not have let her take the car.

In this example the problem is not a phobic response and yet a past event is controlling Joe's life; his thoughts, feelings, and behaviors in the present are shaped by the event. Joe knows that if he forgives himself, his feelings will change. But he feels stuck. How can Joe overcome this past event?

The death of Joe's daughter was a **referential experience** for Joe in that much of his life was "in reference to" the death. In fact, he had considered suicide. One way to undo a referential experience is to create a new referential experience that defuses the trauma. Joe needed a referential experience that would allow forgiveness. Trying to persuade Joe to forgive himself did not work, but the experience of forgiveness can be effective. **Imaginative role-playing** is a technique for creating new referential experiences.

In imaginative role-playing the person creates a new experience. Role-playing is a widely used and researched therapeutic technique (Decker & Nathan, 1985) that was originated by Joseph Moreno (1947) and was developed by the founder of Gestalt therapy, Fritz Perls (1969). With my guidance (RS), Joe used imaginative role-playing to create an experience for resolving his guilt.

Procedure

After establishing rapport and empathy so that Joe felt emotional support, an important catalyst in the process, I helped Joe unfold the following drama:

"Joe, tell me what your daughter was like."

"She was full of life. She loved school. She was excited about living. She loved music and she loved to read. The good Lord gave me a wonderful daughter. I felt so fortunate."

"You really had a special daughter, Joe, and you loved her deeply."

"Yes," Tears come to Joe's eyes.

After a few minutes of silence, I say to Joe, "I want to explore with you some of your deep feelings and thoughts about this event. The way I want to do this is have you act out some of your feelings and thoughts. To do this I want you to begin by imagining that your daughter is sitting in this chair and you are talking to her. What's her name?"

"Jennifer."

"Put Jennifer in the chair and tell her how much you have missed her these last two years."

"Jennifer, I have really missed you these last two years. You are really neat. I miss you so much sometimes that I just don't want to live."

"Joe, now sit in this chair and be Jennifer and respond to you."

Joe looks at me with puzzlement. "She's dead. I can't do that."

"Yes, I know that, Joe, but she still lives on in your thoughts and feelings. It is important that we explore your thoughts and feelings." Joe moves to the other chair.

"Dad, I miss you, too. You are a really neat father. I feel sad that you are so unhappy now."

Joe returns to his chair and responds, "Jennifer, I feel so guilty. I should never have let you take the car."

"But, Dad, I insisted. I'm not blaming you."

"But you should. If I had not let you take the car, you would still be here today."

I said, "Joe, this is crucial. Focus a minute. What do you think your daughter would want to say to you now if she could?"

After a few minutes of silence, Joe sits in the chair and responds as Jennifer would.

"Dad, I really want you to be happy. I don't want you to waste your life away. There are too many neat things to do in life. And Mom misses you. You're not the person you used to be. Everyone forgives you except yourself. I want you to forgive yourself and live life to its fullest."

Tears come to Joe's eyes. He says, "Thank you Jennifer. I will."

Joe turns to me and says, "You know, that is what she would really want. She was full of life. She would want me to be full of life."

"You really had a neat daughter, Joe, and she continues to be neat in spirit. She really helped you out today."

"Yes." Joe gives me a hug.

Through this procedure Joe had a new experience in which he accepted forgiveness from his daughter and began to forgive himself. Creating positive referential experiences through imaginative role-playing is an effective method for helping people overcome past trauma. Themes of love, forgiveness, hope, joy, and personal power are the ingredients in many referential experiences. A skilled, empathic facilitator helps the person create referential experiences that overcome past negative events.

In an emotional and healing visualization experience, I (JG) guided a chronic headache client through a childhood experience that had weighed upon him for 40 years. Hans was convinced that his father had not loved him. Hans told me that the last time he saw him, his father was cold and did not smile, and so he knew that his father did not love him. I asked for details and learned that Hans had seen his father for the last time in a Nazi concentration camp, and even though Hans had taken food and clothing to him, his father did not smile.

As adults we can understand that the father was distant because he was afraid for himself and for his family in town. By being distant, he was psychologically protecting himself and his son. The 12-year-old child had neither the psychological knowledge to understand nor the skill to help his father share his feelings. The child interpreted his father's behavior as lack of love. Because he never saw his father again and could never experience his father's love again, he carried that memory and interpretation as a deep sadness.

To overcome that event, Hans relived and changed the last visit with his father. Hans rode to the prison on his bicycle with the packages of food and clothing. He met his father and gave him the packages. His father thanked him but did not smile and turned away. The young boy asked his father what was wrong; was he afraid? The boy and father shared their fears, and they talked about the family and what might happen. Up to this point my client had not spoken but he was weeping. I held his hand and said, "What would you like to say to your father?" He then spoke, "I love you." After

a few moments I asked, "What would you like your father to say to you?" With great emotion he responded, "I love you, too." When the flood of tears subsided, I suggested that he say goodbye to his father and ride home on his bicycle. The visualization experience ended with my saying, "Slowly bring yourself back to the body in the chair, and when you are ready just open your eyes." For several minutes Hans relived the experience privately, and then he simply said, "He did love me."

The effect of the visualization experience was profound. An unfinished experience was finished, and Hans felt a deep sense of closure and certainty that he was loved by his father. The impact of visualization lies in the fact that the experience was real. As adults we had talked about the misinterpretation of the 12-year-old boy and the fact that young children are unable to understand the complex psychological problems of adults. But the intellectual knowledge of the adult could not undo the hurt of the childhood experience. By recreating the past and experiencing love as a child, Hans removed the hurt that had been with him for so long.

Summary

People carry great burdens from the past. Desensitization training and imaginative role-playing are effective techniques for overcoming and defusing the stress of past events. In desensitization training the trainee overcomes fear by experiencing in imagery the event or situation that triggered the phobic response. The imagery of the fear-evoking situation is coupled with relaxation in the present, and fear is not experienced. Biofeedback instrumentation helps in both teaching and verifying relaxation. When desensitization is successful, the stimulus that previously evoked fear now evokes relaxation. In addition, mastery of relaxation and desensitization skills enhances a sense of competency and resourcefulness.

With the emotional support and guidance of a skilled facilitator, people can overcome the past. People can learn to forgive themselves or accept the loss of a child or spouse by creating referential experiences of forgiveness and love in the present.

The ability to reconstruct the past by establishing new associations between images, thoughts, and feelings helps people gain power over their lives. Fear can be replaced with feelings of competency and support. Overcoming the traumas of the past is an important dynamic in health and wellness.

||||➡

SECTION THREE: VISUALIZATION FOR SELF-EXPLORATION

To thine own self be true,
and it shall follow as the night the day
that thou canst not then be false to any man
—Polonious, *Hamlet*

The wisdom of knowing oneself is a repeating theme in all cultures and in all times. In some contexts "know thyself" has a religious connotation of seeking God within oneself, as in the Christian concept "the kingdom of Heaven is within." All religions have honored the mystic who retreats from the mundane world to seek God through meditation and prayer. In other contexts, knowing oneself means knowing one's own values and goals. This is a characteristic of "commitment to self," the most important aspect of hardiness. Polonious advises his son, "To thine own self be true," meaning "follow your own principles; do not be influenced by what other people think and do." As a dynamic of health and wellness, knowing oneself incorporates these concepts and the knowledge of psychological and physiological processes.

People seem to have differing ability to focus within and to become aware of inner needs. And people have differing interest in doing so. Usually people get interested in knowing themselves better in the context of psychotherapy and illness, when it finally seems important to find out what's going on. In general, our culture does not encourage self-knowledge. Yet, self-knowledge is a part of health. To maximize psychological and physiological health and well-being, people need to know themselves.

Self-knowledge means to understand one's needs, goals, motivations, history, memories, hopes, fears, potentials, and spiritual values, and to understand the physiological domain—what the body needs, how it develops symptoms, and how it can be brought to perfect health.

A very large textbook could be written on the religious, philosophical, and cultural approaches to self-knowledge. In this section our task is much more humble; we discuss imagery and visualization techniques that can be used to gain self-knowledge, techniques that are western and modern.

Our human resource, the facility of the mind to yield information through images, has been known for as long as dreams have

---

BASIC PREMISE

Like knowledge of the outer world, knowledge of our psychological and physiological inner worlds can be actively sought. Just as knowledge of the outer world is gained through exploration of the outer terrain, so knowledge of the inner world can be gained through exploration of the inner terrain.

The basic premise of all self-exploration is that within each human is the potential to gain insight into aspects of the self that are not normally conscious. This can be as simple as remembering events in childhood or as mystical as meeting the God within.

taken the dreamer beyond ordinary thinking and knowing. Dream interpretation is similar to working with imagery and visualizations that arise spontaneously or are consciously created in the waking state. As fascinating and informative as dream interpretation can be, in this section we focus on the conscious elicitation of imagery and conscious work with visualization while awake.

The techniques that we describe were developed by therapists. However, imagery and visualization for self-exploration and self-knowledge are tools that anyone can use. Several therapists have written books on imagery and visualization for the public. One of the earliest was *Directing the Movies of Your Mind*, by Adelaide Bry (1978).

Freud

If you had to think of the name of a European psychotherapist, you would probably think of Sigmund Freud. Freud understood the power of images to reveal hidden fears and motives, and described dreams as "the royal road to the unconscious" (Freud, 1938). Early in his practice Freud used hypnosis to elicit images from memory. Freud and his mentor, physician Josef Breuer, found that when their hypnotized patients remembered traumatic events and relived and expressed emotions associated with the events, symptoms disappeared and a sense of emotional release occurred. Freud discovered that hypnosis itself was not crucial and began using a different technique. He placed his hand on the patient's forehead, with the suggestion that the essential memory would come to mind at that moment. Freud eventually replaced this technique with free association and analysis of dreams and ultimately decided that dreams and imagery represent primitive mental processes and came to rely more on verbal material, or secondary process material, as he called information and insight that comes to the patient through rational thinking.

Jung

While Freud was gradually relying less on imagery, his contemporary and expatriate of psychoanalysis, Carl Jung, was moving in the opposite direction. Jung is perhaps best known for his interest in universal symbols that appear in all cultures and religions and in myths, symbols that he called *archetypes*. For example, a wise old man symbolizes wisdom or the wise self. A dangerous beast symbolizes threat or the part of the self that sabotages growth, and a young maiden symbolizes purity. As Jung found, myths and fairy tales often use archetypal images that awaken in the reader the meaning of the symbol. From this fascination with symbolic imagery, Jung began to use visualization personally and over many years guided himself into the hinterland of his own unconscious. In his autobiography, *Memories, Dreams, and Reflections*, Jung (1963) describes a variety of imagery techniques that he used, including a descent into a deep abyss as a method for getting to the depths of the unconscious. In the abyss Jung conversed with beings that appeared there.

To help his patients use imagery and reap information from the unconscious, Jung developed a simple technique that he called **active imagination**. The patient was asked to relax, clear the mind, and then invite images to flow into consciousness. The images were to be watched as though the imager were watching a movie, but the person could interact with the images as Jung had learned to do. Jung expected that this technique would bring into consciousness issues that were unresolved, often hidden in archetypal images.

Other therapists in Europe, and eventually in the United States, were convinced that visualization and imagery are a more direct route to the unconscious than verbal discourse. The idea was that by the time a person had thought about an issue and talked about it, the mind had had an opportunity to censor and change the material. Imagery bypasses some of the

ARCHETYPAL IMAGES AND "STAR WARS"

The movie *Star Wars* uses archetypal images to portray the forces of good and evil. In fact, George Lucas studied Jung, and the characters Princess Lea, Obiwan Kenobi, and Darth Vader (Dark Father) are clear archetypal images. One of the beings that Jung met in the abyss was a little dwarf who talked with Jung from the entrance of a cave. This is Lucas' character Yoda in *The Empire Strikes Back.* The wonderful trilogy *The Lord of the Rings* by J. R. R. Tolkien—concerning the battle of good against evil and the adventures of the hobbits, elves, dwarves, humans, and wizards, and all manner of other creatures—is filled with archetypal images that inspire, and frighten, and thrill.

censors. To facilitate the process, several therapists developed visualizations that are more directed by the therapist than the active imagination technique of Jung. The techniques described here are examples of the variety of imagery and visualization exercises for self-exploration.

The Directed Daydream

A problem in trying to gain insight and knowledge through dream interpretation is that dreams are unpredictable. Daydreams are somewhat better because they are consciously created and usually focus on a topic, and perhaps the directed daydream is the best process for focusing the mind to gain insight on a particular topic. The technique was created by the French psychotherapist Robert Desoille and first described by him in 1938. The therapist begins by reminding the client that anything is possible in a dream and then gives a beginning image, which the imager describes in detail. For example, Desoille believed that a sword represents "maleness"; his first exercise for male patients was to create an image of a sword and describe it in detail. A tenet of this kind of work is that "the patient knows best" about the correct interpretation of the images, although Desoille and several others who developed imagery techniques had a Freudian orientation and created imagery experiences and interpretations that fit the orientation.

Over many years of experimentation Desoille formalized six imagery themes that he believed are related to basic issues in life. Two themes, ascending and descending, are used repeatedly because Desoille thought that these themes are related to "a basic law of the mind." He said, "It is expressed in everyday language when we speak of 'bright ideas,' 'warm feelings,' and 'lofty thoughts.' And on the other hand, we recognize 'shady deals,' a 'cool reception,' and 'low deeds'" (Desoille, 1965, p. 2). Ascending images seem to take the imager toward a "higher self" and feelings of peace or union with a wiser self or with nature, and descending images seem to direct the imager toward a "lower self" and feelings of conflict or awareness of a hidden self that Jung referred to as "the shadow." A common ascending image is climbing a mountain, and a common descending image is exploring a tunnel. Desoille's second imagery experience is descending to the depths of the ocean. This is how he describes it:

> I ask the patient to imagine a seashore, a rocky coast where the water is very deep. After the patient has described this scene, I suggest that he imagine putting on either a diving suit or a scuba outfit, and that he let himself slip into the water, descending as deeply as possible. As he does this, I urge him to tell me in detail what he sees in his mind's eye. In general, feelings of fear arise quite quickly, and if I suggest to the patient that something threatening is likely to appear, a monster may loom into view. I

encourage the patient to subdue the beast or tame it. . . . I then urge the patient to have the monster take him on a tour of his haunts, visiting a grotto, for example. If he finds anything special there, I have him take it with him. Then I ask the patient to imagine returning to the surface and bringing the monster with him onto the beach. At this point, I might suggest that the patient again tap the monster with his magic wand. He is told that the purpose of this act is to induce a metamorphosis in the (monster) so as to reveal its true identity.

(Desoille, 1965, p. 6)

Of this Desoille said, "This second directed daydream is a rather random probing of the patient's unconscious. It corresponds to the question, 'What is going on in the depths of your personality; what painful feelings are capable of upsetting you?'"

The imagery program includes creating a daydream on each theme, sometimes repeating them, in search of the problem behind the symptom and its **resolution**. Desoille found that when the imagery experiences became real for the imager, the accompanying emotions helped resolve the problem. A second tenet of this technique is that when the person reaches the crux of the problem in imagery and resolves it, such as slaying the dragon, then the psychic conflict is actually resolved and the person is stronger.

Guided Affective Imagery

Like the directed daydream technique, guided affective imagery uses structured imagery experiences to guide the person into self-exploration, self-confrontation, and problem-solving. The creator of this therapeutic technique, Hans Carl Leuner, a German psychiatrist, first described the technique in 1954. Leuner emphasizes the importance of deep relaxation as a prerequisite of imagery because, in his experience, relaxation facilitates imagery that is both vivid and affective.

Leuner created 10 imagery motifs. The beginning motif is a meadow in which the imager experiences safety and peace. The next motif is a brook that flows through the meadow; the imager follows along its course to the sea or to its source. Other motifs are: climbing a mountain; creating a house; entering the woods at the edge of a meadow; encountering relatives; plucking a rose; meeting the ideal person. Four additional motifs are used "only by the fully trained therapist" and not with patients with a "weak ego structure": standing near the opening to a cave and waiting to see what comes out; seeing a figure emerge from a swamp, coaxing it to solid ground, and feeding it; viewing a volcano that may erupt; and discovering an old picture book and looking at the pictures (Leuner, 1978). Leuner believes that imagery is valuable because the person moves slowly, uncovering conflict at a safe rate, and is protected from extreme anxiety by interacting with the therapist. He also recognized the value of testing actions, acting out in imagery, and getting in touch with unconscious needs.

Let's examine one motif briefly, to see how the visualization might flow, from the imager's perspective:

My meadow has a small brook that meanders along . . . it is moving slowly. The banks of the brook are sandy; animals come to the brook. I am following the brook into the woods. It flows over rocks and fallen logs. Sometimes it gets narrow and is rushing along, making a lot of noise as it tumbles down a hillside into a valley. In the valley it flows into a pond made by beavers. On the other side of the beaver dam, it flows again, out into the valley. Really it is now a river, flowing along between beautiful green hills. There are white houses on the river bank. Ahead I see a huge dam, this is a man-made dam for generating electricity, and a huge reservoir. I can't follow the river anymore; it is a part of the reservoir. There are many other rivers that flow into the reservoir. I guess it will make it to the sea, but not as the little brook.

If you had created this visualization, how would you interpret it? Imagine that you are suffering from a psychosomatic symptom. How would you interpret the fact that your river

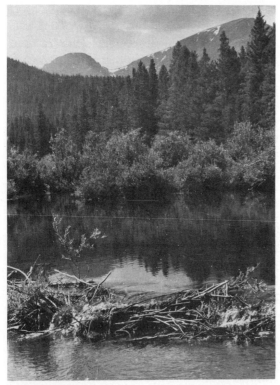

Sometimes Imagery Is So Vivid That the Experience Feels Real.
Source: Judith Green.

flowed into a reservoir, blocked by a dam? Would the meaning of the symbolic dam come into your mind? How would you have finished the visualization? Did you have a tendency to "be" the brook?

Gestalt Techniques

A dynamic addition to experiencing through visualization puts the imager into the object being imaged. In describing the above imagery, the person would say, "I am a brook. I am meandering through a meadow. I can feel my coolness and sandy banks. Now I am beginning to flow out of the meadow, I am moving faster and faster, over rocks. . . ." As you can imagine, being the object is much different from observing the object.

We refer to taking the perspective of the object imagined as a "gestalt" technique because it is akin to the role-playing technique developed by the founder of Gestalt therapy, Fritz Perls (1969). Perls emphasized the fact that the power of imagery for health and healing is enhanced when the imagery is acted out in a dramatic fashion. Perls would have a person using the meadow visualization act it as a monodrama, by acting the various parts and creating a dialogue between opposing parts. For example, the person might create the drama in this way:

Brook: "I am a small brook that moves slowly along. Sometimes I am narrow and move fast, but usually I am relaxed, peaceful, and quiet. I provide life to animals who drink me. I like flowing through this meadow, where it is beautiful and quiet. Oh, no! Up ahead I see a dam. What will happen to me?"
Dam: "I need your power, little brook, to help human beings."
Brook: "But if you take my power, I will no longer be a little brook. I will die. And you already have more water than you need."
Dam: "You will not die, little brook. You will become transformed and become part of a big reservoir."
Brook: "I don't want to be transformed. I don't want to die. I am not ready yet."
Dam: "You have no choice, little brook. I am a big dam."
Brook: "I don't want to die. I don't want to die."

At this point Perls would probably ask the person to repeat key phrases, such as "I don't want to die" or "You have no choice," and then to conclude the visualization.

Brook: "I don't want to die. I do have a choice. I will flow into the forest. I will take a different path."

After the drama is completed, there is often no need to analyze and interpret the drama, because acting out the various parts enables the person to experientially know the importance of the fantasy. Perls argues that certainty is not obtained through analytical thinking; real knowing, he argues, comes from *being* the elements of a visualization or dream, not from simply observing the elements and trying to interpret them intellectually. This is like the difference between being in a play and watching it. Please read Box 9.2 now.

Summary

This section has described imagery and visualization techniques that facilitate self-knowledge, a dynamic in health and wellness. These techniques are useful when you want to know yourself better, when you need more information about a problem, and when you want to have fun exploring the inner terrain.

BOX 9.2

SPONTANEOUS IMAGERY

Spontaneous images arise sometimes that are surprising, delightful, and informative. The image-making faculty of the mind occasionally pops images into consciousness when a person is thinking or engaged in routine activity, but you may have noticed that spontaneous images are more likely to occur when you are in the quiet state between waking and sleep. This "twilight zone" of consciousness is a reverie state in which the environment and sometimes your body disappear, and you are hanging out with your mind; you are conscious, but not thinking actively. In this state you become the passive observer of your own mind. Perhaps spontaneous images are likely in this reverie state because the mind and body are quiet enough for the soft voice of the unconscious to be heard.

Getting into the reverie state and calling upon the image-making faculty as an observer are skills that can be cultivated. The usefulness of this has been demonstrated repeatedly by creative people, such as the French chemist Kekulé, who was mentioned in the introduction. Many creative people have described their ability to produce a dreamlike state in which images arise from the unconscious.

Intrigued by these reports, biofeedback training pioneers Alyce and Elmer Green hypothesized that theta would be the brainwave correlate of reverie. They conducted research with college students on reverie and creativity through theta feedback (Green & Green, 1976).

If you are good at getting into this state between waking and sleeping, you may have noticed that sometimes your spontaneous imagery is related to something that has been on your mind, and it may provide creative insight. It seems likely that this capacity of the mind can also be used for gaining knowledge of the body, much like the inner advisor technique and talking to the symptom. In this case you would ask your mind to provide information about your body's needs, and then you would be attentive to your spontaneous imagery.

IIII➡

SECTION FOUR: IMAGERY AND VISUALIZATION FOR HEALING

Mr. Wright was asked to imagine drinking the juice of a lemon as a good example of mind → body, because the lemon is "only" in the mind and the body responds. The same example illustrates the power of images to affect the body.

You probably already know this. If you have ever daydreamed yourself through a hair-raising scenario, or an erotic experience, you are familiar with the fact that images and visualization produce physiological effects. In fact, if you have stepped on a garden hose and thought that it was a snake, you know the power that perceptions have to affect physiology. We hypothesized that the placebo effect may result from visualizing the desired effect of the placebo, and experts agree that the powerful effects of hypnosis are due to visualization. It is interesting that highly hypnotizable subjects report an extraordinary ability to create and be totally involved in their imagery, a talent that in many cases began in childhood (Wilson & Barber, 1983). In a study on immune system functioning described in Section Five, Howard Hall, professor of psychology at Case Western Reserve University, found that the most hypnotizable subjects had greater changes in immune system function as a result of visualization than less hypnotizable subjects (Hall, 1983). Perhaps the highly hypnotizable subjects were better visualizers.

Given the fundamental principle that images affect physiology, we need not be mystified by the fact that through visualization people can do seemingly incredible tasks such as change the body's immune reactions to challenges such as the tuberculin bacillus (Smith & McDaniel, 1983; Smith, McKenzie, Marner, & Steele, 1985) and other allergens. In a review article, Hall (1983) cites many studies on modification of immune system response to allergen challenge through hypnosis. In these studies, immune system functioning is changed not simply through relaxation, but by consciously directing the immune system to create the desired effect.

Many people know someone who had a tenacious wart that mysteriously fell off or disappeared after a bit of magic. We know a child whose father offered him a dollar for his wart; the wart, which had beaten all other remedies, fell off. Our colleague, Ed Wilson, M.D., tells of his fail-safe wart removal program. He painted a child's warts with fluorescent paint to make them glow under an ultraviolet light. Wilson told the child that after this special treatment the warts would disappear, and they always did. The track record for removal of warts with hypnosis is also good. But no one knows how the mind and emotions eliminate warts and the virus that causes them. If we understood the mechanisms by which the mind eliminates warts, knowledge of the immune system would be greatly advanced (Thomas, 1980).

The use of imagery and visualization for body healing is as natural as creating visual images of hot beaches and kinesthetic images of heaviness for increasing peripheral blood flow. In our therapy we include visualization for body change and healing, whether the physical disorder is clearly related to stress, is organic as in cancer, or is structural as in injury. We describe three visualization exercises that illustrate these uses.

Asthma

I (JG) have worked with several asthmatic children for whom medications did not eliminate sensitivity to allergens and chronic wheezing. Visualization is an important part of the treatment for these children. I call one visualization exercise "the cleanup and inspection tour." This tour begins by selecting various powerful cleanup tools and a bright light. The child imagines that she is standing at the place where the trachea divides into the bronchial tubes, one branch going to the right lung and one going to the left. The tour begins by shining the bright light into the right bronchial tube and seeing how open and healthy it looks, a healthy pink color, very open and relaxed. The child moves down the tube until she comes to the place where the tube divides. First she shines the light down the smaller branch, seeing how open that branch is and how relaxed the circular muscles are. Then she moves down the larger branch, shining the light all around and seeing the tube perfectly open, relaxed and a healthy pink color. Each time the tube divides, the child shines the light down the smaller branch, checking to make sure that it is open and clean and pink, and then she moves along the larger branch. Finally the tubes get very small, and the child can see the air sacs expanding and relaxing perfectly with each breath. The child is instructed to clean up anything that looks suspicious. Most children find some sort of gunk or slime that must be sprayed with Lysol and vacuumed up. The cleanup and inspection tour becomes part of the daily homework exercise.

The cleanup and inspection tour has clear psychophysiological benefits. Many asthmatic children are afraid of their lungs and feel powerless to control the asthmatic attack. Through this visualization they become familiar with their lungs and gain a sense of power. I am also convinced that the visualization is an instruction to the bronchioles to stay open.

Broken Bones

What would an orthopedic surgeon do in the winter in the heart of ski country in Colorado? Set broken bones, of course. Robert Swearingen set a lot of bones and sent a lot of people home with a cast, a relaxation technique, and a visualization to hasten bone mending. Swearingen began using this procedure after noticing that the injured skiers who needed less pain medication were more relaxed than others and that

they had been handled by a particular ski patrol team, a team that paid as much attention to the patient's psychological comfort as to physical comfort (Swearingen, 1978).

After taking X rays, Swearingen explained to the frustrated skier exactly how he would set the bone, how it would heal, and how relaxation and visualization would help the bone mend. Swearingen showed the patient drawings depicting four stages of bone-mending (Figure 9.1) and taught a simple relaxation technique suited to the patient. The patient was instructed to visualize Stage 1 for 10–14 days, Stage 2 for one week, Stage 3 for three weeks, and Stage 4 until complete healing occurred. The visualization is "anatomical" rather than symbolic.

> Stage 1: In this stage a beneficial blood clot (hematoma) surrounds the fracture. The tissue in the hematoma is not organized.
> Stage 2: The hematoma is organized into a lattice of fibrous scar tissue. This occurs about two weeks after the fracture.
> Stage 3: Calcium is being laid down within the fibrous latticework.
> Stage 4: New bone bridges the fracture.

Swearingen understood that mind and body interact and was convinced that the patient can enhance the body's natural healing processes. Carol Schneider, Ph.D., colleague and reviewer of this book, wrote the following note after reading this section:

> Tom Budzynski told me about Swearingen in 1975 when my broken leg was not healing. It was seven months after the fracture and the bones had not joined and no calcium had been deposited. The orthopedist was planning surgery with bone from my hip. Swearingen drew me the pictures and had me visualizing twice a day for 20 minutes that calcium ions were dropping on the network lattice so that I would go from images 2 to 3 to 4. One month later, I saw the orthopedist and he was surprised that I had so much calcium there where none had been before. It was unusual to occur spontaneously after so many months. I had also made the mistake of

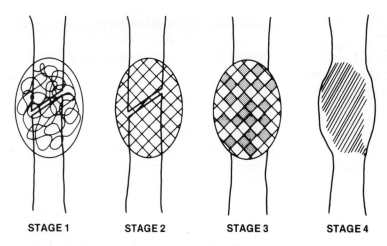

STAGE 1   STAGE 2   STAGE 3   STAGE 4

Figure 9.1   Visualization for Bone Mending in Four Stages. Adapted from *Bridges of the Bodymind* (Achterberg and Lawlis), Copyright © 1980 by the Institute for Personality and Ability Testing, Inc. Reproduced by Permission.

"tuning out" my leg so it was cold all the time. I needed to warm the broken limb so that the blood flow would go there, and I did this through visualization. I think that both visualizations helped. The orthopedist thought it just "happened."

Skin Grafts

Treatment of severe burns with removal of damaged tissue and grafting can be traumatic and painful. To help patients cope with the process and to enhance healing, Jeanne Achterberg and her colleagues (1980) created a relaxation and visualization procedure that guides the patient through the healing process. The procedure is used after the patient has learned about the healing process, and after the patient has had an opportunity to express all fears and beliefs about recovery and has gained relaxation skill through biofeedback training or other techniques. The drawings in Figures 9.2 a, b, and c, are used to aid the visualization.

Figure 9.2a shows the wound producing a "glue" that helps the graft stick and become part of the body. Figure 9.2b symbolizes the network of tiny blood vessels growing into the area of

the graft, bringing oxygen and nutrients. Figure 9.2c shows the blood vessels from the graft and blood vessels from the body connecting, permanently fixing the graft to the body.

This work breaks with a long tradition of putting the mind in the back seat in the treatment of physical disorders, where it could be ignored, tranquilized, or treated like a bad child that should not be negative or ornery.

The use of imagery and visualization in healing also taps a human resource that may

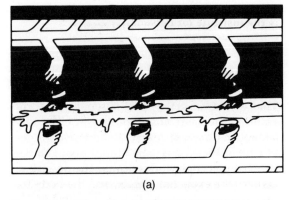

(a)

Figure 9.2a   Visualization for Skin Graft Healing. The Wound Produces a Glue That Helps the Graft Adhere to the Body.

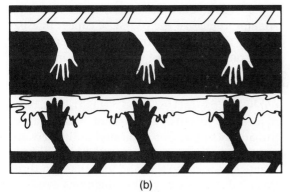

(b)

Figure 9.2b   In This Visualization for Skin Graft Healing, Blood Vessels Begin to Grow between the Graft and the Body.

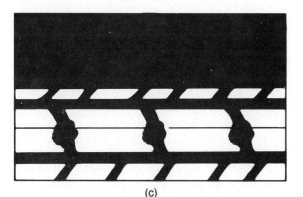

(c)

Figure 9.2c   In This Visualization for Skin Graft Healing, the Blood Vessels Connect and the Graft is Bonded to the Body. Adapted from *Bridges of the Bodymind* **(Achterberg and Lawlis), Copyright © 1980 by the Institute for Personality and Ability Testing, Inc. Reproduced by permission.**

have greater potential than yet known and may provide insight into a dimension of health and illness not yet explored. We write "than yet known," but is it not possible that the well known results of hypnosis and the placebo effect are in fact the results of positive imagery? Perhaps placebos work because the patient visualizes the expected effects, and the body follows the visualization. This might explain the fact that placebos often have only short-term effects. When taking the placebo becomes

RELAXATION AND IMAGERY

To explain the importance of relaxation with visualization, we use this analogy: Imagine that all the children in a classroom are out of their seats, running around and making a racket; when the teacher speaks, no one hears. But if all the children are in their seats, facing forward, paying attention, and not speaking, they hear the teacher. Your body is the classroom and your mind is the teacher, it is important to have your "classroom" quiet and paying attention before speaking to it with the mind. We believe that the reverse is also true—just as the teacher must be quiet and paying attention to hear the students, so must you have a quiet mind that will hear when the body speaks. Thus, relaxation of body and mind is important before using imagery to direct the body.

routine, the immediacy of the visualization and expectation may decrease, and the body responds accordingly. In the case of Mr. Wright in the first chapter, we can guess that the surprising swings in his progress were due in part to images that he created as he anticipated the positive effects of Krebiozen on cancer and as he reacted to the news of the failure of Krebiozen.

Cancer Treatment

The systematic use of imagery and visualization for cancer regression is a revolutionary area. To combat cancer, a disease that is synonymous with death in the minds of many people, nonmedical techniques that might beneficially alter the prognosis deserve investigation. These techniques become known to clinicians and the public long before they are accepted by the medical establishment. Visualization for cancer treatment is one such technique.

Most writers refer to the work of oncologist Carl Simonton and psychologist Stephanie Matthews-Simonton (now Stephanie Simonton-Atchley) as the first systematic attempt to use imagery and visualization in the treatment of cancer. They developed a treatment program for cancer patients with both traditional medical treatment and a self-help program that includes relaxation and visualization.

Usually patients in traditional medical settings are not asked about how they imagine themselves or the disease being treated; at least they weren't in the 1960s. Yet Carl Simonton paid attention to a common report of patients with spontaneous remission of cancer that "I always imagined myself as well." Simonton took this statement literally and appreciated its significance because it corresponded with his observations of his own cancer patients who outlived the statistics. To Simonton, a patient's statements about getting well and statements that implied a strong will to live suggested an intriguing new approach in the battle to fight cancer: Enhance the patient's will to live, and strengthen the patient's fight against cancer with visualization.

After studying a variety of visualization, motivational, and self regulation techniques, such as biofeedback training, the Simontons developed a generic visualization experience for combating cancer. The visualization uses the two known forces that combat cancer growth: the patient's immune system and traditional medical treatments such as chemotherapy and radiation. The visualization incorporates four elements: (1) seeing the treatment destroying cancer cells that are too weak and confused to repair the damage; (2) seeing the white cells of the immune system swarming over the cancer, killing cancer cells and cleaning up the debris; (3) seeing the cancer shrinking; and (4) seeing a return to perfect health.

In 1971 Carl Simonton made the first attempt to change the course of cancer in a patient by deliberately directing the patient's visualization. This patient is described in *Getting Well Again* (Simonton, Matthews-Simonton, & Creighton, 1978), the Simontons' book for the public on the imagery and visualization techniques and results. The patient was dying of throat cancer but was dedicated to the new approach, as shown by the fact that he faithfully practiced the relaxation and visualization three times a day, every day. The Simontons wrote:

> What happened was beyond any of Carl's previous experience in treating cancer patients with purely physical intervention. The radiation therapy worked exceptionally well, and the man showed almost no negative reaction to the radiation on his skin or in the mucous membranes of his mouth and throat. Halfway through treatment he was able to eat again. He gained strength and weight. The cancer progressively disappeared.
>
> (Simonton Matthews-Simonton, and Creighton, 1978, p. 8)

Within two months the cancer was gone!

With these results there was no turning back. Like all other therapies, the Simonton approach evolved with the ups and downs of the patients with whom the approach was used. Early in the development it was discovered that it is important to know exactly what the patient is visualizing, because, when given the general instruction to imagine the cancer and its destruction, some patients create images that suggest fear and a sense of powerlessness, imagery that does not promote healing. The Simontons began asking patients to describe their imagery, and even to draw it. They found that the imagery can be a diagnostic tool for analyzing the patients' beliefs about the power of the cancer and the power of the treatment and immune system to destroy the cancer. A systematic analysis of imagery based on research with cancer patients is described in *Image of Cancer* (Achterberg & Lawlis, 1978). Please read Box 9.3 now.

BOX 9.3

IMAGERY FOR PROGNOSIS

The Simontons began asking patients to draw a picture of their imagery and describe it in detail after discovering that a patient who was doing poorly had created a very negative visualization. The patient saw the cancer as a big rat and the chemotherapy as yellow pills that the rat ate; the rat felt sick but grew bigger.

The obvious implication was that the patient's imagery reflected his beliefs about the cancer and treatment. It was immediately clear to the Simontons and their colleagues that a person's imagery could be used to assess the patient's psychological status. Furthermore, it could be used as a springboard for helping the patient express fears and beliefs, which could be addressed in counseling.

Figure 9.3 is the drawing by a woman with bone cancer that reflects a sense of power and positive outcome. She imagines the cancer cells as small compared with the white blood cells, and she imagines the white cells as mobile, determined, and powerful. The drawing indicates that this patient believes that she can win.

Figure 9.4 is a much less hopeful drawing, showing little activity. The immune

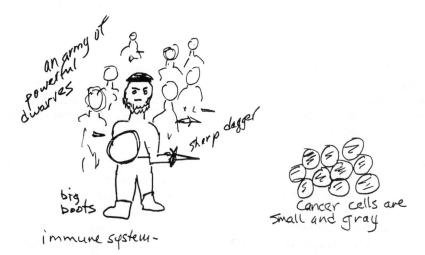

Figure 9.3 Positive Imagery.

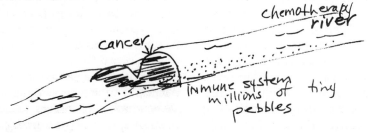

Figure 9.4 Negative Imagery.

system moves passively in a river that flows around a large rock, the cancer.

To determine the relationship between a patient's imagery and prognosis, studies with the Simontons' patients (Achterberg, Lawlis, Simonton, & Simonton, 1977) and with county hospital patients (Achterberg & Lawlis, 1978) were conducted. Each patient drew a picture of the three elements—the cancer, the treatment, and the immune system. The patient described the imagery in detail to the interviewer. The imagery was assessed on several dimensions, including the vividness, movement, and strength of cancer cells; the vividness, movement, number, size, and strength of white blood cells; and the effectiveness of treatment. The researchers found that positive imagery is associated with a positive prognosis, and that imagery is more predictive of status two months after the drawing is made than is a blood chemistry analysis done at the time of the drawing.

Through the research on imagery and cancer prognosis, Achterberg and her colleagues evolved a therapeutic technique that has more than predictive value. It provides a mechanism for helping the patient express emotions and beliefs and opens the door for teaching and the development of healing visualizations and renewed hope.

You have perhaps asked a very important question: What about the negative images that physicians and others accidentally conjure up in their patients? What kind of imagery comes immediately to the patient when told that he has only a few months to live? Does the imagery itself make the prognosis a self-fulfilling prophecy? I (JG) was angered and frustrated when a client's physician told her that a bone scan was necessary because "something might be lurking in there." That accidental image triggered a severe psychological setback. We were able to counter the image, but I wonder how many patients carry catastrophic imagery and how powerful that imagery is in carrying out the physician's prognosis.

The Simontons and their colleagues developed a comprehensive self-help program for cancer patients that includes relaxation, visualization, psychotherapy, family counseling, diet, and exercise counseling. Professionals in private practice and in hospitals across the country began adopting the Simontons' techniques, with results including prolonged life, enhanced well-being and quality of life, and occasionally, remission of cancer. Today most of these successes are known only to the patients, their families, and their therapists. Rarely are cases reported in scientific journals, because the use of imagery and visualization for healing does not lend itself to the kind of scientific study required. The study of visualization has the same difficulties as the study of biofeedback training. There is no single independent variable that can be isolated; in imagery and visualization therapy, many variables interact.

Several books written by patients and therapists describe the procedures and results of this type of self-help therapy. We bring to your attention one book that was written by people we know: *I Choose Life* (Norris & Porter, 1986). This personal story was written by Garrett Porter, who was diagnosed with a brain tumor when he was 9 years old, and by his therapist, Patricia Norris of The Menninger Foundation. When Garrett began working with Pat in 1979, he was not expected to live more than two years; the tumor was growing and he was becoming increasingly handicapped. Yet, after many months of intense visualization work, supported by Garrett's special dedication to life and firm belief that he could choose life, the tumor was gone. *I Choose Life* includes Garrett's own story of his struggle and triumph, which he wrote when he was 12 years old, and it is the discussion of the therapist's work from her perspective.

Garrett's Visualization

As with most children, it was easy for Garrett to believe that imagery and visualization can influence the body, and his success with biofeedback training proved this for him. Garrett's visualization centered on a *Star Trek* theme and space exploration, exciting material for a 10-year-old in 1979. Pat Norris writes:

> In Garrett's visualization, his programming ego (the "self") is portrayed by Blue Leader, the leader of a squadron of fighter planes. His brain is represented by the solar system, and his tumor is an invading planetoid which is entering his solar system and threatening its existence. His white cells and other immune defenses are represented by the lasers and torpedoes with which the squadron of fighter planes is armed.
> (Porter & Norris, 1985, p. 28)

Using this theme, Pat and Garrett made a cassette tape in which Pat, as ground control, and Garrett, as Blue Leader, attack the planetoid and after a very dramatic battle, destroy it. As an aid to visualization, Garrett created sound effects for the battle with an electronic game, punctuating all the strikes and misses. Garrett wanted his tape to be useful for all children fighting cancer. His first line on the tape is: "You are about to experience a method used for fighting tumors and cancer."

Garrett also created a more "organic" visualization in which he took a journey across his brain, walking over the convolutions until he came to the tumor. The tumor looked like a meatball. He saw millions of white cells attacking and destroying the tumor. The white cells were balls with large mouths, sharp teeth, eyes and radar antenna—competent and all-seeing.

Garrett used visualization at home before falling asleep every night for over a year. Then one night he could not find the tumor; he looked again, but it was gone. A victory party was held inside Garrett's brain in his next therapy session with Pat; two months later the CAT scan proved that the tumor was gone.

Garrett's story is fantastic, amazing, heart-warming, and encouraging—but not really mysterious or miraculous. When the *National Enquirer* published the story with the usual sensational headline, including the words "miracle boy," Garrett protested, saying "It was no miracle. I worked very hard to get rid of the tumor." Today Garrett is a senior at Kansas State University.

Garrett is not unique. Other children who have had the great fortune of having wise and supportive and believing parents, teachers, physicians, and therapists have overcome disease. Undoubtedly there are many cases that have not been reported. In Chapter 16 we spotlight the Center for Attitudinal Healing in Tiburon, California, where sick children and their families strive for health using techniques such as visualization in an atmosphere of support and love. Please read Box 9.4 now.

We commented that undoubtedly there are children who have healed themselves, unknown to anyone except their parents and physicians and perhaps unknown even to these people. In Chapter 1 we said that there are probably many unreported Mr. Wrights. The experience of Jeanne Achterberg is true of many others in the field. She writes:

> After each presentation of the material on the imagination and health, a handful of people stop me afterwards, and with a glow on their face, obviously still feeling the wonderment of it all, will tell me the circumstances of their return to health. I hear again and again of self-discovered imagery procedures that were adopted out of

SARA

When Sara was 4 years old, inoperable blood tumors developed behind her left eye. Nothing could be done medically. Sara's physician decided that the only solution was to wait until the eye had protruded enough to be removed and then extricate the tumors.

Finding this solution untenable, Sara's parents sought the help of ophthalmologist Leslie Salov, M.D., director of the Vision and Health Center in Whitewater, Wisconsin. Salov was familiar with alternative healing methods and the use of imagery.

Salov explained to Sara that she could get rid of the tumors with imagery and a prop. Sara had a basting bulb filled with red water. As she squeezed the water out of the bulb she imagined that the blood was flowing out of the tumors. Sara was also taught relaxation skills. In keeping with Salov's "wholistic" approach, the family eliminated processed foods from their diet, and Sara was allowed to be outside as much as possible to increase her exposure to full spectrum natural light. In describing this case, Salov noted the complete acceptance and support of Sara's parents.

Within two months the tumors were gone, and within a year Sara's eyesight was nearly normal.

From Morales, 1981, pp. 63–67

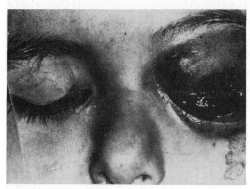

The Blood Tumors behind Sara's Eye Were Not Medically Treatable.
Source: Vision and Health Center, Whitewater, Wisconsin.

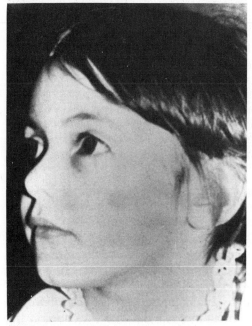

After Several Weeks of Imagery and Other Techniques, the Tumors Are Gone.
Source: Vision and Health Center, Whitewater Wisconsin.

sheer desperation. Fearing the consequences of the disease, or even of proposed treatment, the patients turned inward and began to work intensively with their mind.

(Achterberg, 1985, p. 170)

People who do not accept the power of visualization say, "It would have happened anyway" or "The medical treatment finally worked." Because no one knows the future with absolute certainty, these arguments cannot be refuted. Often, however, the statistics argue strongly against these explanations. Patients who use visualization techniques or who seek non-medical treatments are usually in extreme condition and have a poor prognosis; in fact, their chances of survival may be slight. Very few people are given the opportunity to use relaxation and visualization and positive beliefs to combat disease; but of those who do, and who are dedicated to the work of healing, the success rate, meaning prolonged life and survival, is high. To date, the evidence that we have found indicates that although some patients who follow the treatment program succumb "as expected," many do not.

Accurate assessment of the effects of relaxation and visualization techniques is complicated by the fact that many patients using these techniques also accept conventional medical treatment. The treatment may be toxic to healthy tissue, including the immune system, and not equally beneficial for all patients. I (JG) worked with a cancer patient with a very poor prognosis who was everything a therapist could wish for—a firm believer in his ability to help his immune system through visualization, a successful biofeedback trainee, a patient who practiced daily, and a man whose family supported his work. This man's cancer could not be treated with radiation or chemotherapy, but his progress was surprising. He moved to his retirement home in another state and became a part-time rancher. Yet after many months of regression, the cancer recurred and spread, and his physician decided to try chemotherapy. The patient

was elated, and through several chemotherapy treatments he did extremely well. Finally, however, he began to experience nausea and vomiting, which progressed until the faintest smell of food was unbearable. Although he could not eat and grew extremely weak, he refused tube feeding and died. What had happened? Did the visualization work and then fail? Did the patient, feeling well and involved with his new life, stop using the visualization? Could he have fought off the disease had he not begun chemotherapy? Did the cancer kill him, or did the chemotherapy kill him (or both), or did he die of malnutrition? Does this case prove that visualization is not useful? Would he have died sooner had he not used his skills of relaxation and visualization? Please read Box 9.5 now.

Unfortunately, we have no data from large studies in which top-notch therapists teach relaxation and visualization skills to many patients for comparison with patients who receive conventional treatment and with subjects who receive conventional treatment and a total self-help program.

We think that new disciplines such as behavioral health and behavioral medicine will be a force in three ways: (1) accumulating the data from all sources, including clinical reports and personal reports of patients; (2) establishing treatment protocols (procedures) that make the most of a patient's well-being and struggle for health; and (3) advancing the use of imagery and visualization in all clinical settings as standard elements in medical practice and psychotherapy.

One type of information that we are looking forward to concerns the **mechanisms** of healing through visualization and imagery. Today the physiological mechanisms that enable the immune system to respond to imagery and visualization are unknown. We accept the evidence that this does happen, but until the physiological mechanisms are known, it will be difficult for the scientific community to accept the phenomenon of healing through visualization.

BOX 9.5

OLIVE OIL QUESTIONS:
A RESEARCH ISSUE

You could argue that people who use alternative non-medical therapy such as relaxation and visualization techniques to combat cancer are "self-selected," and therefore the sample is biased. In other words, you could argue that people who use self-help techniques get well not because of the particular technique used, but because they have a particularly strong will to live and will live regardless of the technique used.

It is true that people who seek non-medical adjunctive treatments are unusual simply because such treatments are unusual and often a special effort must be made to find a knowledgeable therapist or program. By definition, a person who seeks self-help treatment believes that the self can help.

In addition, people who seek self-help programs are often ready and able to change diet patterns, exercise patterns, work patterns, and family patterns while participating in relaxation and visualization training and perhaps psychotherapy. This is appropriate self-help treatment, but the effectiveness of a single variable cannot be determined. However, no clinician would suggest that for the sake of scientific research only a single element should be used to study the effectiveness of that element.

Although the relative effectiveness of the many variables in self-help cancer treatment is difficult to assess, in clinical practice all variables are used. It seems clear that our overall goal should be the development of effective "treatment packages," because we are certain that many variables play a role in sickness and health.

SECTION FIVE: MECHANISMS OF HEALING THROUGH VISUALIZATION

This section reviews the few but intriguing studies that demonstrate effects of relaxation and visualization on the immune system. To refresh your memory, reread the section on the immune system in Chapter 4. Evidence for the effect of negative emotions and stress on elements of the immune system is more abundant than the effect of positive emotions, relaxation, and visualization. In Chapter 6 we described research by McClelland and Kirshnit on the effect of exposure to a film on Mother Theresa

and level of IgA, the antibody (immunoglobulin) found predominantly in the respiratory tract. In Chapter 12, we will describe the research by Dillon (1985–1986) on the effect of humor on IgA. Although research about the impact of positive emotions, visualization, and relaxation on the immune system is in its infancy, data are available from research projects that go beyond IgA measurement.

Hypnosis

Hypnotherapists agree that imagery is the medium of hypnosis. Using hypnosis, the therapist may direct the client, suggesting exactly what the client is to imagine, or have the client create the imagery of the desired goal, in which case the technique is usually called self-hypnosis. As with other imagery techniques, hypnosis begins with deep relaxation. Howard Hall of Case Western Reserve University and his colleagues Longo and Dixon (Hall, 1983) studied the effect of self-hypnosis on several elements of the immune system.

Subjects. The subjects were 20 healthy volunteers, age 22–85, male and female.

Procedure. The procedure began with a prehypnosis blood sample, and all subjects took the Stanford Hypnotic Susceptibility Scale. After relaxation was induced, the subjects were asked to visualize and feel their white blood cells increasing in number, and, like powerful sharks, attacking germs; the visualization was maintained for five minutes. The subjects were given instructions in self-hypnosis, using the visualization. The subjects were instructed to practice the self-hypnosis procedure twice a day for one week. Blood samples were taken immediately after the first hypnosis session and one week later. T cells were challenged with mitogen and activity levels were determined.

Results. All subjects had an increase in T cell activity, an effect that was statistically significant only for younger subjects. Total white blood count was elevated for one hour after the hypnosis procedure only for the highly hypnotizable subjects, an effect that was not found one week later.

In a series of experiments with highly hypnotizable and trained subjects, Black and his colleagues demonstrated that through hypnotic suggestion, reactions to various allergens and tuberculin could be inhibited. In the tuberculin experiment (Black, Humphrey, & Niven, 1963), three of four subjects who normally had positive reactions had no reaction after the hypnotic suggestion not to respond, and the fourth had only a mild reaction. Biopsies of the tissue showed that cells of the immune system were at the site of the injection, but that the tissue was not inflamed.

Mental Imagery and Visualization

Research with Healthy Subjects

An unpublished research manuscript by Schneider, Smith, and Whitcher (1988) describes several studies about the impact of specific visualization on specific responses of neutrophils. Neutrophils are the mobile scavengers that fight infection and bacteria through phagocytosis. To do this job, neutrophils in the blood first adhere to the capillary wall and then change shape in order to squeeze out of the capillary into body tissue, where they travel to the site of the infection. The research of Schneider and his colleagues focused on these two functions of neutrophils. In a preliminary study on himself, Schneider found that neutrophil activity could be influenced by several conditions, including relaxation and visualization. The four studies summarized here further explore the effects of relaxation and visualization.

Experiment 1

Subjects. The subjects were nine male and nine female healthy volunteers, with a mean age of 27.4 years. The subjects were informed of the purpose of the experiment and were accepted only if they believed that they would be able to influence neutrophil activity.

Procedure. In the first session, two blood samples were taken 25 minutes apart, and the subjects completed three personality inventories. In the experimental session, blood samples were taken before and after the procedure, which was either 20 minutes of relaxation using the Relaxation Response of Benson, 20 minutes of relaxation training using EMG feedback, or

20 minutes visualizing neutrophils becoming sticky, adhering to the capillary wall, changing shape, and leaving the bloodstream. Cell shape and adherence measures were made on pre- and post-training blood samples.

Results.   No differences were found between pre- and post-experimental conditions in neutrophil function.

Comment.   The experimenters hypothesized that the lack of results in Experiment 1 might have resulted from the stressful environment in which the experiment took place (the Department of Psychiatry) and the failure of the subjects to become relaxed. Furthermore, the subjects were not coached in any way, and it was hypothesized that the visualization was not precise enough. These hunches led to changes in the procedures of the following experiments.

Experiment 2

Subjects.   The subjects were eight females and eight males, mostly medicine and psychology students; they believed in their ability to influence immune functioning.

Procedure.   The subjects were instructed on the nature and function of neutrophils and saw slides of neutrophils changing shape. The subjects were given two hours of relaxation and visualization training before the experiment began, in the environment in which the experiment would take place. They were given an extensive explanation of the purpose of the study and rationale, including a discussion of the Simontons' work, and they drew pictures of their visualization of the neutrophils changing shape and leaving the blood stream. The subjects were encouraged to practice the visualization at home. In the single experimental session, blood was drawn before and after the relaxation/visualization procedure, in which subjects

relaxed and visualized for 20 minutes. After the visualization period, the subjects were asked to describe their visualizations. The reports were rated on several dimensions.

Results.   In the blood sample taken after the relaxation/visualization procedure, the total white blood count was significantly decreased, mostly because of decrease in the neutrophil count of an average of 60 percent; the remaining cells had a significant decrease in adherence and no change in shape. The change in neutrophil count was significant at the $p < .0001$ level.

Comment.   The experimenters hypothesized that the relaxation and visualization enhanced neutrophil activity and that the decrease in adherence and lack of change in shape of the remaining neutrophils occurred because the responsive cells had already left the blood stream. The third experiment was designed to test this possibility.

Experiment 3

Subjects.   An additional 12 subjects were added to the subject population of Experiment 2. The new subjects were trained with the procedures of Experiment 2, and the original subjects were given a two-hour training session in which they created and practiced a visualization of the neutrophils remaining in the blood stream.

Procedure.   The procedures were identical to those in Experiment 2, except that in the visualization the neutrophils remained in the blood stream and were available for the blood sample.

Results.   As expected, there was no change in the total white blood count between the pre- and post-relaxation/visualization blood samples, and a significant increase in adherence occurred (p < .001) in the sample taken after relaxation/visualization.

Comment.   These results substantiate the results of Experiment 2, reinforcing the assumption that the visualization did cause responsive neutrophils to adhere to the capillary wall and move out of the bloodstream. In this experiment the visualization promoted a maintenance of homeostasis. To test the power of visualization further, the experimenters conducted a fourth experiment with an element that is contrary to normal functioning.

Experiment 4

Subjects.   Fourteen medical students who had not participated in previous experiments but met all other subject conditions were used.

Procedure.   The training and testing procedures of Experiment 2 were used, except that subjects were instructed to create visualization of an increase in neutrophil count and a decrease in adherence.

Results.   There was no change in pre- and post-relaxation/visualization white blood count, but there was a slight but significant decrease in adherence (p < .01).

Comment.   It was hypothesized that the white blood count did not increase because relaxation promotes a decrease in white blood cells in the bloodstream, which the visualization counteracted but did not overcome.

The experimenters concluded that visualization can change neutrophil functioning and does so independently of relaxation, but the results varied with the visualization. Please read Box 9.6 now.

On one hand, the results of these experiments seem astonishing. On the other hand, we think, "Of course, mind → body is true for all the cells in the body. The neutrophils are

living cells and have central nervous system input; why shouldn't they respond to the mind?" These experiments may illuminate one of the mechanisms that enable people to reduce and eliminate cancers through positive visualization.

Research with Cancer Patients

Working with cancer patients, a research team from the Medical Illness Counseling Center and George Washington University in Maryland (Gruber, Hall, Hersh, & Dubois, 1988) conducted a one-year study of the effects of visualization and relaxation on the immune system.

Subjects.   The subjects were 10 psychologically well adapted and medically stable patients with metastatic cancer, ages 34–69. The subjects felt that they had adequate social support, and as evaluated on the Rotter scale for locus of control, they were above average on internal locus of control. This sense of internal control and self-responsibility increased over the study.

Procedure.   Two blood samples were taken before the study, and samples were taken once a month during the study. Patients were taught a modified form of progressive relaxation. Instruction on the functions of the immune system were given. Patients were instructed to create a visualization of the immune system acting on the cancer, but no specific guidelines were given. Patients were instructed to see themselves becoming healthier every day. A tape with the relaxation and visualization instructions was made, and the patients were instructed to listen to the tape twice a day, every day. The 10 patients met as a group once a month for relaxation and visualization training; after each meeting they drew pictures of their visualization for later analysis by the research team, but no counseling was given. At six months, a group meeting was held and data

---

BOX 9.6

RESEARCH NOTE

How would you account for the differences in the results of Experiment 1 and Experiment 2 in Schneider's research?

There is a common error in research in procedures such as biofeedback training, hypnosis, visualization, and relaxation techniques that involves learning and physiological change: insufficient training. A recurring pattern is the discovery of a phenomenon in clinical practice, the report of which is called anecdotal, followed by research (sometimes by nonclinicians) designed to find out whether or not the phenomenon actually exists. The research may hinder learning and physiological change (because of insufficient training, poor coaching, or misleading instructions) and may lead to false conclusions.

Schneider, et al. (1988) attempted to overcome these research problems by enhancing the training procedures.

We comment on this issue because it is possible that measurable effects of visualization on immune system functioning take time and a kind of effortless effort that must be learned. And because visualization may be most effective when the imager is deeply relaxed, relaxation must also be learned. The brief, inadequate training of some subjects may not be sufficient to verify clinical results in which patients such as Garrett Porter use relaxation and visualization day after day for months.

We remind you again that in evaluating the results of research on a treatment that involves learning, it is important to carefully examine the training procedures. Unless the subjects are well-trained, it is not possible to evaluate the effectiveness of a treatment that involves learning and use of a skill.

---

from the blood studies were presented; patients also watched a video on healing by Norman Cousins. In the seventh month, half of the group began EMG feedback training for enhancing relaxation skills, and after six sessions the other half received six sessions of EMG feedback training. Ten measures of immune system functioning were made, including lymphocyte response to various challenges; interleukin-2 (interferon) production; serum levels of immunoglobulins IgG, IgM, and IgA; and natural killer cell level. Blood level of cortisol was also measured.

Results. Compared with baseline measurements, several changes in immune system function measures were statistically significant.

Interestingly, most of the effects occurred in the last months of the study. The response of lymphocytes to challenge was significant on two tests, because in the last month surprising increases occurred (Figure 9.5, a and b). The effect seen in Figure 9.5c, the mixed lymphocyte response measures the ability of cytotoxic T8 cells to respond to foreign cells. Increase in natural killer cell activity is seen in Figure 9.5d. Increased production of interleukin-2, which activates T cells, is seen in Figure 9.5e. Over the 13 months of the study, cortisol levels and total white blood count did not change.

Comment. According to the authors, these striking results cannot be accounted for by changes in therapy, season, or normal recovery

visualization for all purposes: Visualize and let it go. This concept was expressed by Elmer Green (Green & Green, 1977) through analogy: When a farmer plants a seed, he does not dig it up to see whether it is growing. Just so when using visualization—plant the image and let it go, with the faith that it will grow; do not fiddle with it or wonder whether it will work. Faith is the key.

The following are principles of visualization for healing:

1. Patients need a sound rationale for the power of imagery and visualization to affect physiology. It is based on knowledge of mind-body interaction, the stress response, advances in psychoneuroimmunology, and so forth.
2. One rationale for relaxation with imagery and visualization is body = classroom and mind = teacher, and the classroom must be quiet to hear the teacher.

FAITH

"Faith can move mountains."

At least faith can get the movers of mountains moving. We suspect that placebos work as well as they do (having no power in themselves to change physiology) because the person taking the placebo has no reason to doubt that the "drug" is real and has been told that it will have certain effects. The person has faith.

In self regulation, faith is essential to get started. This does not have to be absolute faith; it can be based on a hypothesis. The essential aspect is willingness to trust in the process. In the case of visualization, it is important to practice with the faith that it will work.

3. The body's forces for healing must be understood by the patient. They should be visualized vividly and given power and intelligence, as well as mobility when white blood cells are visualized.
4. The visualization should include the desired outcome; the visualization is described as a blueprint (Norris & Porter, 1986).
5. In healing, the visualization must be consistent with the imagers' beliefs about the best way to kill the disease.
6. The disease should be visualized as weak, confused, and immobile.
7. The potentially harmful chemotherapy and radiation treatments for cancer should be visualized as helpers that have little effect on healthy tissue and destroy cancer cells.
8. The visualization should be "planted" with faith and not "dug up."
9. The visualization must be felt inside the body as a sensory experience.
10. The relaxation and visualization must be practiced with great diligence and constancy.
11. Spontaneous changes in imagery should be interpreted as a reflection of psychological or physiological change or both, and the patient should be encouraged to view these changes as useful information.

Critics of imagery and visualization techniques argue that the use of these techniques for healing is premature because there are insufficient research data to warrant its use, and that the placebo effect, not imagery, accounts for positive results. It is further suggested that using imagery and suggesting that the patient can play a role in the disease process gives the patient false hope. The false-hope criticism is never valid. Hope is neither true nor false; hope is hope, and few people today would argue that patients should not have hope.

It is true that research on the ability of humans to affect disease processes in the body through visualization is scarce compared to other treatments. Data are accumulating yearly, however, and clinical cases will grow exponentially as more and more people gain the hope and skills needed to influence the course of disease.

IIII➡ CONCLUSION

We have come a long way in this chapter. We have introduced a variety of imagery and visualization techniques for enhancing health and well-being, and in doing this we have introduced concepts and topics that may appear to be on the cutting edge of health research—such as healing the body through visualization or undoing the past. We cannot imagine a more exciting frontier.

Visualization is a versatile and powerful tool because mind ⟶ body is true. The body tends to follow what the mind suggests, as demonstrated by imagining the taste of sour lemon juice or the touch of your lover, or by imagining that there is a prowler in your house at night as you lie in bed. The body responds to imagery because what is real in the mind is real to the body, and images in the mind are real. That the body responds to positive emotions and to positive imagery and visualization is no surprise. We are not surprised that the mind can have a positive role in healing or that visualization is a medium through which this happens. We expect an increasing use of this tool in clinics and hospitals everywhere.

We also expect years of research before the mechanisms of mind-body interaction are known. In the meantime, we can trust the wisdom of the body and know that the physical being responds to the mind. In discussing mental wart removal, Lewis Thomas marvels at the engineer, chief executive officer, and cell biologist within each of us, saying that if we understood how a wart is thought away, "we would be finding out about a kind of superintelligence that exists in each of us, infinitely smarter and possessed of technical know-how far beyond our present understanding" (Thomas, 1980). However it happens, we seem to be able to direct the cell biologist through imagery and visualization.

Above all, visualization is a medium through which the mind directs the mind. Techniques such as stress inoculation, desensitization training, reliving the past, stress rehearsal, and relaxation training use imagery and visualization for self regulation of the mind itself.

We discussed the stress response and the relaxation response as the result of the mind-body interaction. In this chapter we introduced the idea that people have a wise self, a "higher self," that is a source of insight. Getting in touch with it is a fascinating use of imagery and visualization and has great potential. If people do have a wise self that knows more than the personality or ego knows, then it makes sense to explore ways of getting in touch with this self. Imagery and visualization are media through which this occurs, both as a directed experience such as a dialogue with the inner adviser and as the medium through which the inner self makes itself conscious, as in the creative imagery of such people as the chemist Kekule.

The study of imagery and visualization takes us to the frontiers of health and wellness, and perhaps to the frontiers of the human mind. Through imagery and visualization the mind sees around corners, travels inside the body and direct its activity, relives the past and anticipates the future, and opens the door to creativity. Through imagery and visualization we can explore our inner selves and discover the deeper meaning of things. We can play in fantasy without a thought for reality. We can find peace.

CHAPTER 10

Cognitive and Multicomponent Approaches to Stress Resistance

Memorial Day, 1981. It is a beautiful spring day in the Rocky Mountains. The snowy ridges of the Mummy Range and Longs Peak form a majestic backdrop against the blue sky. We have a beautiful place for a picnic, near a small stream. Yellow wildflowers are everywhere. No one is around except Judy; my children, Mike and Kim; and their friend, Daisy. We spread out the red and white checkered tablecloth on the grass and light the charcoal. The children wade in the cold stream. Soon the charcoals are hot, and I (RS) open a can of "sizzle-links"—vegetarian hot dogs. I feel peaceful. What a perfect day.

Crack! A gunshot shatters the stillness. *Crack!* The shots are very close. *Crack!* I feel a strong flush of anger. Someone is shooting near us. *Crack!* Someone is target-practicing. They can't practice here. They know that. They see our van and smell the charcoals—they know we are here. As I charge up the embankment, suddenly I think, "No one makes you angry. You make yourself angry." These words ring clearly in my mind. For six years I have taught this concept in biofeedback and stress-management classes. Well, I'm furious.

"May I come with you?" I look around, startled. Blue-eyed, golden-haired Daisy follows me. She is only 11 years old. I think for a second.

"Sure. Come along."

As we reach the top of the river embankment, we see a black truck next to our van. Fifty feet away, two people fire into the embankment. *Crack!* They are wearing jackets, boots, and ear protectors. As we get closer, the woman fires a .30–'06 rifle with a telescopic sight. A man near her has a two-handed grip on a pistol. The gun looks like a .45 and makes an ear-splitting sound. We walk up to them.

"Hey!" I shout. "Hey!" I am three feet from the guy. He has a scraggly beard and my build. I wait. I'm sure he heard me.

The man slowly turns and removes the ear protectors.

"Yeah, what do you want?" he replies with a slight sneer.

I think, "This guy's weird. His eyes are lifeless. We're nothing to him, just a nuisance. Keep cool."

"Look, we're having a great picnic. We're by this beautiful stream, and we're just beginning to cook our hot dogs. (I certainly don't tell him we're cooking vegetarian hot dogs out of a can!) Suddenly your guns made a terrific racket."

Angrily, he says, "Well, there just aren't any places to target-practice in Larimer County. They closed up the only target range they had. They don't give a damn about people. All they want to do is sell more land and make more money. Pretty soon all of this will be subdivisions with houses everywhere."

He's mad, too. Keep calm. Listen carefully.

"I can understand that. They should have a place for target shooting. Your shooting makes a lot of noise. The noise sure disturbs our picnic."

"Yeah, but there's no place to target-practice in Larimer County. This embankment is a good place."

"You're right, they should have a place for target practice in Larimer County. I can see this embankment is a good place for target practice. But the noise sure disturbs our picnic."

"Yeah, this is the only place for us to target-practice. Why didn't you go on up to Carter Lake? They have lots of picnic tables there."

"We were planning to when we saw this beautiful place. Nobody was around. At Carter there are too many people. So we were having a great time, and we're just ready to cook our hot dogs when. . . ."

He interrupts me. "You should have gone up to Carter Lake. This is a good place for target practice."

"I can see this is a good place for target practice, but we would like to finish our picnic. Then we'll go to Carter. We need 30 more minutes to finish our picnic, then you can target practice without disturbing us."

"W-e-l-l-l." Suddenly he looks at Daisy and says, "You shouldn't be barefooted out here!"

Puzzled, Daisy looks at him. I look at him, and his friend looks at him, and he looks at us—and then he says, "All right. But we'll be back in 30 minutes."

"Thank you," I say. "We appreciate that!" Whew! Some weird character! He displaced his anger on Daisy.

They get in their truck and spin out. I feel good. "I did that very well," I tell myself. "I stated our needs; I listened to him; I didn't get off track. I didn't back away. I listened. I problem-solved."

We finish our picnic in peace. Then we go to Carter Lake.

Stress is inevitable in human relationships because people have different needs. I dealt effectively with the picnic situation because I have studied rational-emotive therapy and Ray Novaco's stress-inoculation methods and taught stress-management training for many years. Without training in stress management, I might have reacted very differently. My childhood did not foster this approach to conflict.

As a child my personality was deeply influenced by the values and religious framework of my community. This orientation taught "God first, others second, you last." I was taught not to confront people, even when another person's needs were unreasonable. I was taught nonresistance in human relationships. In the past, I would have avoided the confrontation with the target shooters and simply left. I would have simmered, probably elevating my blood pressure for hours, perhaps days. The situation would have been unfinished—I would have remained frustrated and would have gone over and over what I should have done. Sometimes in the past, instead of nonresistance, I overreacted and got angry. When that happened, the stressful situation was still unfinished, and I still was obsessed about what I should have done, and I felt guilty.

Stress-management skills enabled me to transform a stressful situation into a challenge. One of the important characteristics of stress-resistant people is their ability to transform stressful situations into challenges and to have the necessary skills to deal with the situation. The man shooting the .45-caliber pistol looked and acted paranoid. My training in empathy skills and problem-solving gave me a sense of self-efficacy (confidence) in being able to defuse the explosive emotions in the situation so that a compromise could be reached.

Stress is unavoidable. Stressful situations may develop even when you are having a peaceful picnic! Being stress-resistant is an essential dynamic in health and wellness. For this reason, stress-resistant means coping effectively in all areas of life—in the classroom, in the workplace, in the family, and on vacations.

In this chapter, we present several methods for enhancing stress resistance. In Section One, a variety of cognitive restructuring techniques are explored. In Section Two, we examine one of the most effective and extensively researched programs for teaching stress resistance: stress-inoculation training, developed by Donald Meichenbaum. Stress-inoculation training includes relaxation, imagery, cognitive techniques, and role playing. In Section Three, multicomponent programs for helping people cope with anger are discussed. Finally, in Section Four, we examine multicomponent programs that help people cope with the pressures of academic performance. Figure 10.1 summarizes the methods for becoming stress-resistant described in this chapter and in previous chapters.

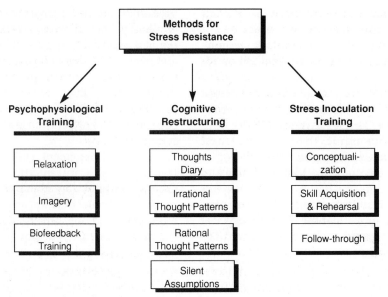

Figure 10.1   Methods for Becoming Stress Resistant.

SECTION ONE: COGNITIVE RESTRUCTURING

Have you ever been unable to sleep because you were worrying about an upcoming date, exam, or interview? Have you ever been agitated by criticism that you could not get out of your mind? Have you boiled with anger because someone treated you unfairly? Chances are that like most people, you have experienced these stressful reactions. The twentieth century has been characterized as the age of anxiety because worry is so pervasive. We wrote this on "Black Monday," October 16, 1987, the day the stock market had its greatest decline in history. Like other Americans, we were beginning to worry. Will the stock market go down further? Are we going to have a depression, as we did in the 1930s? How bad will the recession be?

Numerous coping techniques have been created in recent years to teach people how to be stress-resistant and how to combat worry. Corporations pay large sums of money for stress-management programs. People are taught time-management, relaxation, and biofeedback skills; social skills; meditation; the Quieting Response; and on and on. Like the 31 flavors at Baskin-Robbins, which one do you choose? Which coping skills will get to the heart of the problem?

Many theorists and therapists say that the heart of the problem of stress and worry is negative cognitions—meaning negative thoughts, images, and perceptions—and that therefore stress management must begin with techniques that combat negative cognitions. You are familiar with this idea from your knowledge that stress often is the result of perceptions. By confronting negative thoughts, images, and perceptions, it is possible to counter stress and the stress response, and self-perpetuating worry is stopped. In Chapter 6, we described Viktor Frankl's technique for coping in a concentration camp. Frankl survived the extreme stress by controlling his cognitions. Michael Rosenbaum emphasized that self regulation of cognitions is the first skill necessary for learned resourcefulness.

In the past 30 years, research on cognitive coping skills has proliferated, and effective methods for teaching these skills have been developed. In this section, we described a key method, cognitive restructuring. Cognitive restructuring refers to the process of restructuring negative cognitions (thoughts, self-statements, perceptions, and images) into positive cognitions. Cognitive psychologists Albert Ellis (1975), Aaron Beck (1979), and Donald Meichenbaum (1977) have developed specific methods for restructuring thoughts and attitudes to help people develop healthy coping styles. Four of these methods are (1) keeping a thoughts diary, (2) identifying irrational thought patterns, (3) replacing irrational thought patterns with positive rational thought patterns, and (4) identifying silent assumptions.

A Thoughts Diary

The **thoughts diary** is what the term suggests, a log of thoughts that were triggered by particular events throughout the day. The purpose of the diary is to identify patterns of thinking that are negative or reflect negative perceptions and to identify irrational thoughts. **Irrational thinking** is the term used by Ellis (1975) to describe the fact that people create stress for themselves by thinking irrationally. Some irrational thoughts are negative and irrational, such as "All teenagers are reckless drivers." Some are just irrational, such as "If I love him enough, he will turn into the person that I want him to be."

From a study of the irrational thought patterns of 451 students, Jerry Deffenbacher and colleagues at Colorado State University concluded that in helping a student overcome test, speech, social, and other kinds of anxiety, it is essential to focus on the person's unique irrational thought patterns (Deffenbacher, Zwemer, Whisman, Hill, & Sloan, 1986). To identify irrational thoughts, students keep a daily thoughts diary for at least one week. At the end of each day a student writes down the time, emotion, and thoughts of the main events of the day. The following thought diary entries are of a student, Jane. Jane took our class, Biofeedback and Stress Management II. Some of her entries are shown at the top of page 294.

After keeping a thoughts diary for a week, Jane studied her diary for irrational thought patterns—illogical thoughts that are repeated in many situations.

Irrational Thought Patterns

People have a variety of irrational thought patterns. Consider the following statements: "It's not fair. Life is always doing me a dirty trick." "I did poorly on my SAT scores, so I must not be very smart." "I asked two girls out for a date and they both turned me down. I am not very attractive." "I got fired from my job. I am a failure." People make these statements when faced with stressful situations at school, work, and in interpersonal relationships. Common patterns of irrational thinking (Beck, 1979) are:

1. Overgeneralization. "My last landlord kept my deposit even though the apartment was spotless. All landlords are out to rip you off." A general conclusion is derived from one or two situations.
2. Global labeling. "My neighbor is a real redneck. He only had an eighth-grade education." An illogical leap is made from one characteristic to a general category that includes many characteristics.
3. Mind reading. Jane says, "Jack walked by without saying 'Hi.' In fact, he acted like he didn't see me. He is mad at me." Jane assumes that she knows what Jack is thinking and feeling and why he is behaving the way he is. In fact, Jack was preoccupied with his own problems.
4. Filtering the negative. "My plans are ruined for today. It's raining. What a bummer." Negative details are magni-

Time	Event	Emotion	Automatic Thoughts
7:30	Car breaks down on I-25	Anger, fear	It's not fair. Life is always doing me a dirty trick. What if a dirt-bag comes along? That's all I need, is some creep to come along and hassle me.
8:00	Highway Patrol calls wrecker	Relief	What a nice guy.
9:00	Wrecker comes by	Relief	Great! Only a clogged fuel filter.
10:00	Advanced Writing—C on essay	Anger	What a creep of a teacher. She didn't like my political views. That's why she gave me such a poor grade.
11:00	Anatomy and Physiology—Announcement of exam	Anxiety	I'll never do well on his exams. It is all memorization—how stupid. I'll never have time to memorize everything.
12:00	Biofeedback and Stress Management—Project—Assignment on self-control	Anger	It's none of his business whether I smoke or not. If I want to quit, I'll quit. I don't need to do any thought analysis of my rational or irrational ideas.

fied, and the positive aspects of the situation are ignored.

5. Catastrophizing. "He hasn't called me for a week. I know he hates me. I'll never see him again." The reality of the present situation is ignored and replaced with fantasies about disaster.

6. Blaming. "If you would be more sexually free, we'd have a happier marriage." "You made me angry." "It got so bad in the group that I had to leave." External events and people are perceived as responsible for the person's happiness.

7. Fallacy of fairness. "It's not fair that she received the merit scholarship. My grades are better than hers." The assumption is that life must be fair and people must agree on the standards for fairness.

8. Polarized thinking. "You either like me or you don't." Things are black or white. There is no middle ground.

9. Should. "If you have children, you should stay home with them." "People should always be on time." Rigid rules and expectations are accepted for all conditions.

Once irrational negative thought patterns are identified, they can be replaced with positive and rational thoughts.

Positive and Rational Thought Patterns

Here are several guidelines for replacing each irrational thought pattern discussed above with a rational thought pattern.

1. Replace the language of overgeneralization (*always, never, all, everybody*) with situational language (*sometimes* instead of *always; some people* instead of *everybody; Bill and Jack* instead of *all men*). For example, instead of saying, "I always do badly in performance situations. I am a failure," say "Sometimes I do poorly in performance situations." Substitute "All men are chauvinists" with "Some men are chauvinists."

2. Replace the language of absolute needs (*must* and *have to*) with preferences (*prefer, like,* or *want*). Instead of saying "I just have to get into an Ivy League college," "I must get an A on my history exam," and "You must love me," say "I prefer to get into an Ivy League college," "I would like to get an A on my exam," and "I really want you to love me."

3. Replace the language of helplessness (*can't, that's the way I am*) with the language of responsibility (*I find it difficult, I don't want to,* or *I choose not to*). Replace "I can't stop smoking" with "I find it difficult to stop smoking" or "I choose not to quit smoking." Instead of saying "I can't change," say "I find it difficult to change."

4. Replace the language of external control with the language of internal control. Instead of "You make me angry," think "I make myself angry when you criticize me."

After becoming familiar with irrational thought patterns and the rational alternatives, the next step is to rewrite the automatic thought patterns that contributed to bad feelings. We return to Jane's diary to see how she identified her irrational thought patterns and constructed rational thought patterns.

Cognitive restructuring is a useful method for reducing stress. The key is to become conscious of negative cognitions and irrational patterns and then to change these stress-producing cognitions into stress-reducing cognitions.

Identifying Silent Assumptions

Many people cope with stress in habitual, negative ways: getting angry, depressed, or anxious. Two researchers at the University of Pennsylvania Medical School, Arlene Weissman and Aaron Beck (Weissman, 1979; Weissman & Beck, 1978), have identified a set of basic beliefs that create a predisposition to negative emotional responses. These basic beliefs are called silent assumptions by their colleague, David Burns (1980). The assumptions are silent because people are unaware of them and of their influence on the people's manner of coping with stress. These therapists emphasize the importance of identifying negative silent assumptions and replacing them with positive assumptions.

A variety of techniques can help identify silent assumptions. The first technique is to become aware of the negative assumptions that are common to most people. The following list of beliefs are examples from Arlene Weissman's Dysfunctional Attitude Scale (1979), which she developed from her studies with college students.

1. My moods are primarily created by factors that are beyond my control, such as the past, or body chemistry, or hormone cycles, or biorhythms, or chance, or fate.

2. There is no point in trying to change upsetting emotions, because they are a valid and inevitable part of daily living.

3. I cannot find happiness without being loved by another person.

4. If a person I love does not love me, it means I am unlovable.

Automatic Thoughts	Irrational Pattern	Rational Thought
It's not fair. Life is always doing me a dirty trick.	Extended generalization	This is the first time that my car has broken down.
What if a dirt-bag comes along? That's all I need, is some creep to come along and hassle me.	Filtering	Some jerk might come along, but there are many highway patrol officers on this road. I will wait for a highway patrol.
What a creep of a teacher. She didn't like my political views. That's why she gave me such a poor grade.	Blaming, mind reading	I'm not sure why she gave me a C. I will talk to her to see how I can raise my grade.
I'll never do well on his exams. It is all memorization—how stupid. I'll never have time to memorize everything.	Castastrophizing, extended generalization, blaming	I'll set aside some time each day to memorize the names of the muscles. I'll make some cards and memorize while driving to school in the morning when I am most alert.
I feel so tired. I dread the rest of the day. Life sure feels hopeless.	Filtering	When I feel tired, I tend to look at the worst side of everything. I am getting my work done.
She's a jerk. She's so picky. Who cares if you don't have the commas and periods in the right place on the filing cards?	Blaming, filtering	I'm pretty lucky to have a job. My friend, Mary, had to quit school because she could not find a job and go to school at the same time. And she has two kids to take care of.

5. Being isolated from others is bound to lead to unhappiness.
6. It is best to give up my own interests in order to please other people.
7. I need the approval of other people in order to be happy.
8. If someone important to me asks me to do something, then I really should do it.
9. To be a worthwhile person, I must do something outstanding.
10. A person should do the best at everything he/she undertakes.

After becoming familiar with these dysfunctional attitudes, the next step is to determine their presence in your own life. A useful technique is to keep a weekly thoughts diary and look for patterns of feelings and thoughts. For example, Jane discovered in her diary that her most common negative emotion was depression and discouragement. She then examined the beliefs that were common to her situations of being depressed and discouraged. A characteristic belief was that she was inadequate if she did poorly in her classes, and then people would not like her and she would not have friends.

The vertical-arrow method (Burns, 1980) is another useful technique for identifying assumptions. Using this technique, you explore the meaning of a feeling to its logical conclusion. You do this by identifying the automatic thought embedded in the feeling without challenging its rationality. Instead, you assume the truth of the automatic thought and ask, "Why does it upset me?" Inevitably, another automatic thought emerges for which you ask the same question, until you have a chain of automatic thoughts that leads to the final, fundamental automatic thought. Burns gives the example of a medical student, Art, who was training to be a psychiatrist. Art had become depressed when his supervisor informed him that he made a mistake with a patient and that the patient was upset with Art. Art used the vertical-arrow technique. He identified his first automatic belief and then examined the implication of each automatic belief in turn until he arrived at the final silent assumption.

1. Dr. B probably thinks I am a lousy therapist.
   "If he thinks this, why would it be upsetting to me?"

2. Since Dr. B is an expert, then I must be a lousy therapist.
   "If this is true, what does it mean to me?"

3. This means I am a failure—I am no good. "Why would this be a problem?"

4. Other people might find out, and then my reputation would be ruined. No one would respect me. I would get drummed out of the state medical society and I would have to move to another state.
   "And what would that mean?"

5. I would feel so worthless, I would want to die.

After identifying the chain of negative thoughts, Art then substituted objective positive responses.

The vertical-arrow method, keeping a weekly diary, and becoming familiar with dysfunctional attitudes through the Dysfunctional Attitude Scale are effective ways of identifying silent assumptions that contribute to negative feelings and behaviors.

"But why do we have to identify our negative thoughts and assumptions? Why can't we just use positive self-statements to make ourselves feel better?" These are common questions asked by students and clients. Research studies have attempted to answer these questions. Robert Schwartz (1986) of the University of Pittsburgh School of Medicine found from his research of healthy and unhealthy copers that healthy copers are conscious of both their negative and positive thoughts and use positive thoughts to overcome negative ones. Schwartz found that it is not sufficient to simply say, "I am going to be happy no matter what happens in life." Positive affirmations may result in "Pollyanna" thinking, a denial of the negative realities of life and the negative aspects of thought patterns and attitudes. Therefore, people who fail to confront and change their negative thought patterns may fail to transform behaviors and attitudes that create stress (Schwartz, 1986). Other researchers (Deffenbacher, 1986; Deffenbacher, Zwemer, Whisman, & Sloan, 1986; Kendall & Hollon, 1981; Kendall, Williams, Pechacek, Graham, Shisslack, & Herzoff, 1979) have also found that negative thoughts and assumptions must be disputed and eliminated because negative self-statements foster feelings of guilt and anxiety, poor self-image, and poor social skills. Negative thought patterns distract students during exams, lowering the quality of their performance, and are the major cause of test anxiety (Deffenbacher, 1986). People who learn to reduce anxiety, overcome phobias, or become more socially adept decrease negative thinking more than they increase positive thinking. As Schwartz concludes, "Negative

Dr. B probably thinks I'm a lousy therapist.	Just because Dr. B pointed out my error doesn't follow that he thinks I am a lousy therapist. I'd have to ask him to see what he really thinks, but on many occasions he has praised me and said I had outstanding talent.
Since Dr. B is an expert, then I must be a lousy therapist.	An expert can point out only my specific strengths and weaknesses as a therapist. Any time anyone labels me as lousy they are simply making a global, destructive, useless statement. I have had a lot of success with most of my patients, so it can't be true that I'm lousy, no matter who says it.
This means I am a failure— I am no good.	Overgeneralization. Even if I were relatively unskilled and ineffective as a therapist, it wouldn't mean I was a total failure or no good. I have many other interests, strengths, and desirable qualities that aren't related to my career.
Other people might find out, and then my reputation would be ruined. No one would respect me. I would get drummed out of the state medical society and I would have to move to another state.	This is absurd. If I made a mistake, I can correct it. The word isn't going to spread around the state like wildfire just because I made an error! What are they going to do, publish a headline in the newspaper: "NOTED PSYCHIATRIST MAKES MISTAKE!"?
I would feel so worthless, I would want to die.	Even if everyone in the world disapproves of me or criticizes me, it can't make me worthless because I'm not worthless. I must be quite worthwhile. So what is there to feel miserable about?

thoughts interfere with coping more than positive thoughts facilitate it" (Schwartz, 1986).

Summary

Positive thinking is important, but it needs to be supplemented with methods for identifying and eliminating irrational thought patterns. Because our culture fosters negative and irrational attitudes about health and self-responsibility, people are not aware of the effects of negative thinking. Negative thinking is often automatic and occurs without awareness. Usually, however, people are aware of the results—feeling bad. By applying cognitive restructuring techniques, negative assumptions can be identified and replaced with positive assumptions and

thoughts. People need not be victims of negative thinking and silent assumptions.

SECTION TWO: STRESS-INOCULATION TRAINING

Stress-inoculation training is a program for "inoculating" people against stress. Bacterial inoculation is Donald Meichenbaum's analogy for his concept of stress inoculation. When a person is exposed to a small dose of toxic bacteria, the immune system creates antibodies against the germ to protect the person against future exposure. The idea behind stress-inoculation training is that when exposed to a stressor in small doses, a person develops a tolerance for future stressors by developing psychological antibodies. Psychological antibodies are actually coping skills such as cognitive restructuring, desensitization, behavioral rehearsal, and relaxation.

Meichenbaum first described stress-inoculation training in *Cognitive-Behavior Modification* (1977) and described the refined procedures in *Stress Inoculation Training* (1985). In the past 10 years, studies have demonstrated the effectiveness of stress-inoculation training with athletes, teachers, police officers, probation officers, military recruits, parachutists, drill instructors, scuba divers, children, surgical patients, women on public assistance, students, public speakers, and rape victims (Meichenbaum, 1985). Stress inoculation involves three phases: conceptualization, skills acquisition and rehearsal, and followthrough (see Figure 10.2).

Conceptualization

How would you teach stress resistance? Would you begin with a relaxation technique or a cognitive technique? Stress-inoculation training begins with neither. Imagine that you are leading a stress-management group and begin with autogenic training. During the training, one person thinks, "This won't work. This technique won't make my job better. The reason I am so stressed is because of my rotten boss." Another person is thinking, "I don't have time to practice this technique. My family and my job keep me too busy!" These negative thoughts disrupt the relaxation training.

To learn relaxation or any other stress-management skill, Meichenbaum says that the trainees must have a receptive conceptual framework. The purpose of the conceptualization phase is to provide that framework.

The first step is assessment of the trainee's conceptual framework for understanding stress. Meichenbaum asks people to list stressors and their thoughts and feelings about each stressor. Many people have a concept of stress as something that happens to them that they cannot control. They are not aware that thoughts, perceptions, and behaviors create stress. The second step is to reconceptualize stress as an interaction between the stressor

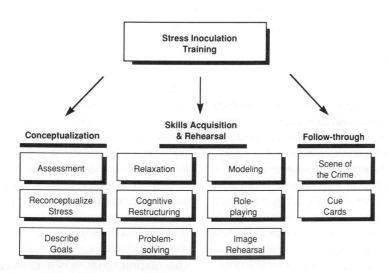

Figure 10.2   Elements of Stress-Inoculation Training.

and the person's thoughts and perceptions. The person learns that cognitions (perceptions and self-talk) increase or decrease stress. Concrete examples are used to illustrate these concepts. If you are taking an examination and have butterflies in your stomach and you worry that you may have diarrhea, the worry will stress your body and increase the possibility of diarrhea. The third step is to describe the goals of stress-inoculation training in concepts that are relevant to the trainee.

If the reconceptualization phase is successful, the trainee will expect stress inoculation training to help. The trainee will also understand how his or her perceptions increase or decrease stress. The trainee is then ready to learn and practice specific skills.

The importance of appropriate conceptualizations as the foundation for skills acquisition and self regulation cannot be understated, whether in sports, teaching, or therapy. In our teaching and therapy, we take time to establish the conceptual foundation for every skill, and we find that sometimes the conceptualizations themselves are therapeutic. That is why we give you a detailed conceptual framework for each topic, as did the team of experts who talked with Mr. Wright.

Skills Acquisition and Rehearsal

To regulate both mind and body, stress-inoculation trainees learn relaxation, cognitive restructuring, and problem-solving skills. The two main relaxation skills are regulation of breathing and progressive relaxation, which are discussed in Chapter 7. Cognitive restructuring includes identifying irrational thought patterns and replacing negative self-statements with positive self-statements, such as, "I did it," "It wasn't as bad as I expected," and "I am getting better at it each time I practice." Problem-solving techniques include the following steps:

Steps	Questions
Problem identification	What is the concern?
Goal selection	What do I want?
Generation of alternatives	What can I do?
Consideration of consequences	What might happen?
Decision-making	What is my decision?
Implementation	Now do it!
Evaluation	Did it work?

Source: From Wasik (1984) cited in Meichenbaum (1985)

After trainees have learned the basic steps of the relaxation, cognitive, and problem-solving skills, they rehearse the skills during simulation of stressful situations and watch films in which people apply the skills in a variety of situations (modeling).

Role-Playing

As part of a stress-inoculation program for police officers, Sarason and colleagues (1979) had the officers play out roles of working with a suicidal woman, settling a landlord-tenant dispute, and responding to a belligerent person involved in a traffic accident. Follow-up results showed that after the stress-inoculation training program, the officers felt less job stress, indicated by lower blood pressure and fewer anger responses than before the training.

Forman (1982) taught urban secondary school teachers how to cope with a variety of school-related stressful situations. Teachers learned to identify spontaneous stress-producing thoughts and then to replace them with stress-reducing thoughts. Then the teachers played roles to help them cope with the stressful situations. For example, Forman simulated a situation in which a belligerent student refused to do classroom assignments. The teachers practiced identifying the stress-producing thoughts and replacing them with stress-reducing thoughts:

Stress-producing	Stress-reducing
How could he say this to me?	I want to know why he said that. I guess I can talk to him about it.
He's getting me really upset.	I can stay calm if I want to because I can control how I feel. I can relax and then I'll be able to solve this problem.

The training resulted in a decrease in the teachers' self-reported anxiety and stress at a six-week follow-up.

Imagery Rehearsal

As the term suggests, imagery rehearsal is the process of rehearsing events in imagery. Just as a play that is well rehearsed is likely to be performed well, so stressful situations that are first rehearsed in role-playing and through visualization are likely to be handled well. The specific steps in imagery rehearsal are to rank stressors from least to most stressful and to imagine using the coping skills in relation to each stressor.

Jack, a ranger employed in a national park, participated in a stress-inoculation program (McKay, Davis, & Fanning, 1981). After learning cognitive and relaxation coping skills, he ranked 20 stressors. The 10 biggest stressors were:

1. Cutting back undergrowth in a poison oak area.
2. Dealing with an auto accident in the park.
3. Car breaking down, major repair necessary. Worrying about money.
4. Wife complains about the isolation and loneliness—she is irritable and withdrawn.
5. Helping a snakebite victim.
6. Fighting a brush fire, digging trenches in intense smoke and heat.
7. Stomach begins to act up. Continual heartburn for several days.
8. Hearing a rattlesnake.
9. Boss ill, temporary supervisor is officious and authoritarian.
10. Wife leaves to spend week with parents because she is unhappy with the isolation of the park. Feeling alone and worried about the marriage.

Jack imagined himself using his coping skills with each stressor. He visualized each stressor for about 30 seconds, and he used deep breathing and progressive relaxation to reduce tension. He also used coping statements such as "I can handle this. I've done it before," and "I can relax rather than get tight." Jack practiced image rehearsal 20 minutes twice a day for one week until he had mastered relaxation while visualizing all 20 stressors. After successfully using the relaxation and coping skills with each stressor, Jack gave himself reinforcing statements such as "I'm getting good at coping under stress," "I can turn off my worry now," and "I did a good job just then."

Jack was successful with the image rehearsal and was able to relax as he thought about each stressful scene. He was now ready for the final stage of stress-inoculation training: followthrough.

Follow-Through

In the final stage of stress-inoculation training, the trainee uses coping skills at the "scene of the crime"—the actual situations on the hierarchy. Jack typed such phrases as "I can relax rather than get tight" on 3 × 5 cards and put the cards in obvious places: the bathroom mirror, his key case, and on the door lock and the dashboard of his truck. With these constant reminders, the coping thoughts and relaxation skills became automatic responses to stressful situations.

Summary

Systematic stress-inoculation training—with its phases of conceptualization, skill acquisition and rehearsal, and follow-through—is an effective program for teaching people to cope with stress. The program includes a variety of coping techniques: relaxation, cognitive restructuring, problem-solving, image rehearsal, role-playing, self-reinforcement, and practicing skills at the scene of the stressor. The inclusion of these techniques into one powerful program has helped people in all walks of life (Dobson, 1988). In the next two sections of this chapter, we will discuss particular applications of stress inoculation and other multicomponent programs to anger and performance stress.

⫸

SECTION THREE: STRESS-INOCULATION TRAINING AND COGNITIVE TECHNIQUES FOR COPING WITH ANGER

In a court hearing for abusing her son, the woman said, "I couldn't stop myself. He gets me so irritated, I just explode."

In response to immediate threat, anger is useful for defense. Anger energizes the body— the stress response is activated to prepare for action. Sometimes anger motivates people to solve problems of injustice, and sometimes anger facilitates thinking and hard work. In general, however, anger is a self-defeating emotion that causes physiological, psychological, and social harm. Parents abuse their children in fits of rage, and partners separate after angry fights. Anger is a precursor of violence and causes or exacerbates many psychosomatic illnesses such as peptic ulcer, colitis, and high blood pressure. Anger and aggression are often a major obstacle to effective interpersonal relationships. Teaching people how to regulate anger is of vital importance to society.

Psychiatrists Aaron Beck (1979) and David Burns (1981) at the Pennsylvania University School of Medicine have studied the causes of anger and have developed techniques for coping effectively with it. Working with police officers, Navy drill instructors, and other professionals, social psychologist Ray Novaco (1975) pioneered stress-inoculation methods for coping with situations that produce anger. In the 1950s, psychologist Albert Ellis developed cognitive approaches to dealing with emotions, including anger. In this section we describe the techniques and methods that have evolved from the work of these and other cognitive therapists and researchers.

Perception and Anger

What makes us angry? Most of the time it is other people. We often hear statements like "She made me upset." "He made me angry." "She got me so mad I couldn't help myself." The core of angry feelings is usually the perception that someone else is at fault and deserves to be punished with angry feelings and aggressive behavior. Imagine that you are riding on a crowded subway and someone jabs you in the back as if trying to push you out of the way. You get angry. You swing around and see a blind man. Your anger instantly disappears. Why? Because you judge the jab to be unintentional. The man was not at fault.

Like stress, anger depends upon perceptions. How one thinks about anger-provoking situations can lead to more anger or less anger. If you believe that people are deliberately attacking you or that you are a victim of injustice, you feed the fires of anger. If you believe that people do not know what they are doing or are confused or disabled, your anger cools.

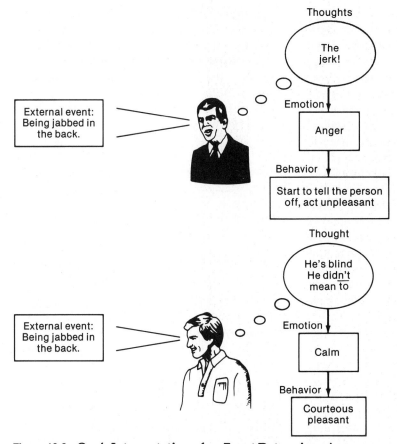

Figure 10.3   One's Interpretation of an Event Determines Anger.

Cognitive psychologists argue that no one makes us angry, we make ourselves angry. People may say things that we do not like, but we choose to react with anger (Beck, 1979). Chronically angry people use irrational statements significantly more often than other people (Lopez & Thurman, 1986).

People typically use five kinds of irrational patterns to fuel their anger (Burns, 1981). The first is **mind-reading**. You do this when you make up motives to explain someone's behavior. In the subway example, you became angry because you assumed a negative motive on the part of the person who jabbed you. When you are angry, you believe that you know the motives of the other person.

The second irrational pattern is **labeling**:

"He is a jerk." "She is a gossip." Through labeling you make yourself feel morally superior to the other person. This moral superiority gives you the justification for being angry and vindictive.

Magnification is a third irrational pattern. To magnify is to exaggerate. People become blind with rage by interpreting a frustrating situation as a calamity.

Making rigid **should** judgments is a fourth irrational pattern. "He should have given me an A. I missed the cutoff between A and B by only one point." Rigid should judgments reflect a narrow view of people and a narrow view of reality. If people do not act and think the way you believe they should, then you feel justified in becoming angry at them.

The fifth and most important irrational pattern is the **perception of unfairness**. Burns believes that the perception of unfairness and injustice is the ultimate cause of almost all angry feelings (Burns, 1980). When people believe that they are treated unfairly, they almost always get angry. But, Burns says, it is important to realize that people have different understandings of fairness. What may seem unfair to one person may seem perfectly fair to another. It is irrational to expect the world to meet your standards of fairness.

Perception of unfairness fuels angry feelings. Is this always bad? To say one should never get angry over unfairness commits the fallacy of overgeneralization. Sometimes it is important to get angry and to take constructive action. Being able to distinguish between appropriate anger and inappropriate anger is crucial to coping effectively with anger.

Coping with Anger

The first step in coping with anger that is not the result of immediate threat of physical harm is to determine whether the anger is useful or self-defeating. This is done by making a list of the advantages and disadvantages of being angry. If anger is useful, then constructive steps are taken to change the stimulus for the anger by using problem-solving techniques, by discussing the problem and seeking advice, and by taking action. If anger is not useful, then several cognitive steps need to be taken to reduce it (Figure 10.4).

The first step in reducing anger is to identify the "hot thoughts" that are fueling the anger. The second step is to replace the "hot thoughts" with "cool thoughts" such as "He may look at it differently" or "He's doing the best he can." The third step is to be empathic, try to understand the person or situation that is the stimulus for anger. As described in Chapter 6, empathy is understanding another's thoughts and feelings. Non-cognitive approaches to reducing anger— physical exercise, relaxation, and play—are also

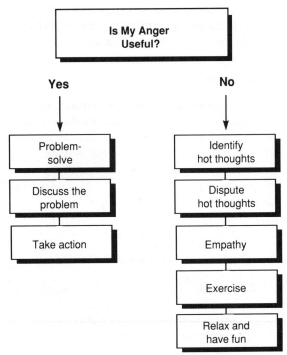

Figure 10.4   Steps in Resolving Anger.

effective. Vigorous exercise and relaxation take the edge off anger by reducing physical arousal, which intensifies anger. And play is diverting.

In many situations, people do not have the luxury of going through a checklist to determine whether anger is useful. For example, police officers are constantly exposed to situations that demand immediate action. Next, we study Ray Novaco's anger-prevention programs for police officers, Navy drill instructors, and other professional groups.

Prevention of Anger

Ray Novaco, a professor in the department of social ecology at the University of California at Irvine, uses stress-inoculation procedures to help people prepare for situations that produce anger. His program (1975) includes (1) assessment, (2) redefining anger, (3) cognitive restructuring, (4) relaxation, (5) empathy training, and

(6) image rehearsal and role-playing. We focus on assessing and redefining anger here. We have already discussed the other steps.

Assessment

To help people become aware of their anger responses, Novaco uses questionnaires and physiological measures of heart rate, blood pressure, and perspiration. The following examples are from Novaco's anger scale. Each item is scored on a scale from 0 to 4: 0 = little annoyance, 1 = irritated, 2 = moderately upset, 3 = quite angry, 4 = very angry.

1. You unpack an appliance you have just bought, plug it in, and discover that it doesn't work. ____
2. You are overcharged by a repairman who has you over a barrel. ____
3. You are singled out for correction, when the actions of others go unnoticed. ____
4. Your car gets stuck in the mud or snow. ____
5. You are talking to someone and they don't answer you. ____
6. Someone pretends to be something they are not. ____
7. You have hung up your clothes, but someone knocks them to the floor and fails to pick them up. ____
8. You are hounded by a salesperson from the moment that you walk into a store. ____
9. You are joked about or teased. ____

From Burns' *Feeling Good* (1980)

The Novaco anger inventory can help you become aware of the situations that are most anger-provoking for you. The next step is to redefine the anger.

Redefining Anger

Novaco teaches people to perceive other people's anger not as a threat but as a problem to be solved. When anger is redefined as a problem, energy and feelings are directed toward problem-solving, and anger does not escalate. To redefine anger, a person must identify the automatic thought patterns that perpetuate anger. Next, negative perceptions and automatic thought patterns must be replaced with reasonable statements, such as "This is a tough situation and I can cope with it" or "It isn't his fault."

Empathy and Role-Playing

Teaching people to empathize with the provoker's behavior is a key element in Novaco's stress-inoculation training. To help police officers develop empathy, Novaco hired actors to act out provocative situations such as taunting or teasing the police officers. After role-playing the provocative situations, the police officers discussed their feelings and thoughts. They learned to stay cool and detached and to use empathic thoughts. Instead of taking derogatory comments personally, the officers were taught to focus on accomplishing the task.

In 1970, at the college where I (RS) worked, confrontations between black and white students were increasingly more violent. I brought the leaders of the groups together to find a way to defuse the conflict. I used role-playing. First, I had the students reverse roles: the blacks walked and talked like the white students, and the white students walked and talked like the black students. Second, I asked them to call each other names: "Look, an Uncle Tom," or, "Hey, Honky, what are you doing here?" Third, they shared what it was like to be called derogatory names. Fourth, they resumed their original roles and called each other derogatory names again, and again shared what it felt like to be called names. Fifth, they role-played situations that provoked anger and discussed alternative ways of dealing with anger. Through role-playing and sharing for eight weeks (two hours each week), the students became tolerant and understanding of each other, and the angry confrontations ceased.

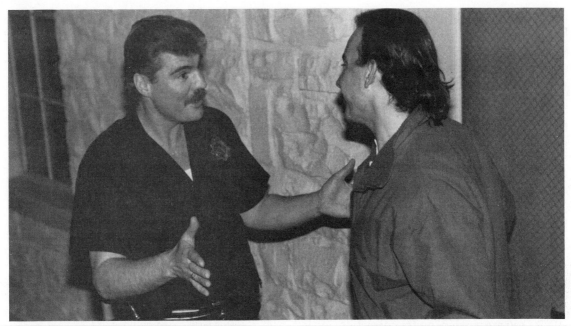

The Policeman Defuses Anger with Empathy.
Source: Gordon Steward, Denver, CO.

Stress-inoculation training for reducing anger has been used in several situations. Schlichter and Horan (1981) trained 38 male inmates in stress-inoculation skills. Compared to a no-treatment control group, the inmates' verbal aggression against one another and against the guards significantly decreased. Nomellini and Katz (1983) substantially reduced abusive behaviors of parents toward their children through stress-inoculation training. Novaco (1975, 1977, 1980) helped police officers, Navy drill instructors, and other professional groups to reduce their anger.

If you cannot participate in a formal program for overcoming anger, there are many things you can do on your own. You can first take the Novaco anger inventory and then use image rehearsal to practice coping with the situations that are most stressful. Imagine an anger-provoking situation, and then imagine yourself using positive self-talk and short relaxation exercises. You can learn to have realistic expectations about the world. David Burns suggests that people learn to "expect craziness" (Burns, 1981, p. 158). Do not expect perfection from your children, friends, and teachers. Expect them to do irrational things at times. Burns lists 10 things to know about anger. Read Box 10.1.

Summary

Cognitive restructuring and stress-inoculation training are powerful methods for teaching people to self regulate strong emotions like anger. The cognitive and stress-inoculation techniques for self regulating anger are also useful for regulating many other emotions such as depression, fear, and anxiety. In the next section, we study cognitive restructuring and stress-inoculation training for managing anxiety and stress to enhance performance in sports and education.

REALISTIC THOUGHTS ABOUT ANGER

1. The events of this world don't make you angry. Your "hot thoughts" create your anger.
2. Most of the time your anger will not help you. It will immobilize you, and you will become frozen in your hostility to no productive purpose.
3. The thoughts that generate anger more often than not will contain distortions. Correcting these distortions will reduce your anger.
4. Ultimately your anger is caused by your belief that someone is acting unfairly or some event is unjust.
5. If you learn to see the world through other people's eyes, you will often be surprised to realize their actions are not unfair from their point of view.
6. Other people usually do not feel they deserve your punishment.
7. A great deal of your anger involves your defense against loss of self-esteem when people criticize you, disagree with you, or fail to behave as you want them to. Such anger is always inappropriate, because only your own negative distorted thoughts can cause you to lose self-esteem.
8. Frustration results from unmet expectations. Since the event that disappointed you was a part of "reality," it was "realistic." Thus, your frustration always results from your unrealistic expectation.
9. It is not just childish pouting to insist you have the right to be angry. Of course you do! Anger is legally permitted in the United States. The crucial issue is—is it to your advantage to feel angry? Will you or the world really benefit from your rage?
10. You rarely need your anger in order to be human. It is not true that you will be an unfeeling robot without it. In fact, when you rid yourself of that sour irritability, you will feel greater zest, joy, peace, and productivity.

Feeling Good (1980), by David Burns

IIII➡

SECTION FOUR: MULTICOMPONENT APPROACHES FOR ENHANCING PERFORMANCE

Millions of television viewers and thousands of people in the audience were in suspense as Greg Louganis approached the springboard for his sixth dive at the 1988 Summer Olympics in Seoul, South Korea. On his previous dive, Louganis hit his head on the springboard; he now had a bandage on the back of his head covering several stitches. The audience wondered whether the accident would ruin the performance by Louganis, a gold medalist in 1984. Could he concentrate? Louganis walked out to the end of the springboard and made a beautiful dive. He continued to dive well, winning gold medals in the springboard and the high platform competitions.

Performing well is important for almost

everyone. Students need to perform well on examinations to succeed in school. Professionals need to perform well on board examinations to succeed in law, medicine, clinical psychology, counseling, social work, nursing, and aviation. Amateur and professional athletes must perform well. Performance situations, however, can be exceedingly stressful, and the stress hinders performance. The preceding chapters described a variety of techniques for helping people overcome stress—biofeedback training, visualization, relaxation, and cognitive restructuring. Earlier in this chapter, we described a multicomponent approach that integrates these techniques into a program for inoculating people against stress. In this section, we describe multicomponent approaches that integrate relaxation, biofeedback training, cognitive restructuring, and visualization for helping people overcome academic stress.

Athletic Performance and Sports

How did Louganis retain his concentration under the pressure of competition, and how did he combat the fear of failure and of serious injury? In Chapter 6, we noted that the key to successful performance is the ability to stay on task and not become preoccupied with fear. By relaxing and visualizing, Louganis stayed focused on diving. From many years of training, Louganis had learned to center himself by focusing on his breathing and visualizing himself successfully performing the dive. Olympic sports psychologist Richard Suinn has pioneered in teaching athletes visualization and relaxation techniques to help them improve performance (Suinn, 1976, 1983).

Visuomotor Behavior Rehearsal

In 1973, Suinn conducted his first experiment with the alpine ski team at Colorado State University. The team was divided into two groups of skiers with equal ability. One group received the usual training, and the other group received the usual training plus a multicomponent program that Suinn calls Visuomotor Behavior Rehearsal (VMBR). VMBR procedures include deep relaxation, EMG monitoring, and image rehearsal. Athletes reach a level of deep relaxation and then rehearse in imagery the athletic event. Suinn calls his procedure visuomotor behavior rehearsal because athletes who achieve deep levels of relaxation and visualize the upcoming event have visual and motor experiences—as though they were actually in the event.

After training for several weeks, the performance of the skiers in the experimental group improved significantly in comparison with the control group. When the final team was chosen for competition, the coach used the entire experimental group and only one skier from the control group.

Suinn's results with alpine skiers stimulated research on the effectiveness of the VMBR method with basketball players, cross-country skiers, archers, shooters, golfers, and divers (Suinn, 1983). Most of the controlled studies found that VMBR procedures enhance an athlete's performance more than when an athlete uses either relaxation or visualization alone. The combination of visualization and deep relaxation produces the best results.

In some VMBR studies, however, significant improvement did not occur (Mahoney & Avener, 1977; Schleser, Meyers, & Montgomery, 1980). Suinn hypothesizes that VMBR was not successful in those studies because athletes may not have reached deep levels of relaxation and thus did not experience the immediacy of the imagery rehearsal. Suinn (1983) calls methods that use image rehearsal without achieving deep levels of relaxation "mental rehearsal." Mental rehearsal techniques fail to achieve the reality of experiencing—as if the event is actually happening (Suinn, 1983).

Suinn hypothesizes that VMBR is effective because an integrated learning occurs when athletes deeply relax and experience the visualization as if it were real. Suinn uses the term "integrated" because emotional, behavioral, sensory, and physiological experiences are integrated, just as they are in "real life."

Suinn (1986) has expanded his training program for athletes to include seven components: relaxation, stress management, positive thought control, self regulation, VMBR, concentration, and energy.

Relaxation training includes progressive relaxation, diaphragmatic breathing, and short relaxation exercises. Diaphragmatic breathing helps the athlete "center." By centering, Suinn means focusing on the breathing process and emptying the mind of negative thoughts and expectations. Centering helps athletes avoid self-preoccupation. Stress management includes identifying stressful situations and using relaxation skills. Positive thought control is identifying negative thoughts and replacing them with positive thoughts. Suinn has an interesting definition of self regulation: "Self-regulation deals with getting psyched up and feeling ready. It involves both that frame of mind of feeling good and for competing as well as having bodily sensations that feel right" (Suinn, 1986, p. 25). To get psyched up, Suinn suggests using music, using conversation, establishing goals, and stretching and walking. Visuomotor behavior rehearsal involves relaxing and visualizing the performance event. Concentration training involves techniques that help the athlete focus on the performance regardless of the situation. Athletes need energy to perform effectively. "The driving force behind speed, endurance, or power is personal energy" (p. 45). Suinn describes many techniques for enhancing energy. In one technique, the athlete visualizes a ray of light energizing the body. "Imagine an energy force attached to your body/arm like a ray of light. . . . Visualize the light extending in the proper direction. . . . (For hurdlers, the light starts at your shoulders drawing you to the tape at the finish.) Repeat the visualization until you know your direction, can see the light, and feel it *pulling* you toward success" (p. 46).

Suinn's seven-step program of enhancing performance integrates the self regulation techniques described in this text. Combining these components into one program will undoubtedly add to the effectiveness of athletic training; so far, the total program has not been evaluated.

The skills for coping with the stress of athletic performance are similar to the skills needed to cope with any performance stress. Suinn's multicomponent program is a prototype of a comprehensive approach that includes specific skills like relaxation and visualization, and draws upon the inner resources of the person.

Academic Performance: Overcoming Test Anxiety

In Chapter 3 we briefly discussed the case of Brick as an example of performance anxiety in school. The ending to his story can now be told.

Brick appeared one morning at my office door dressed in a motorcycle jacket, cap, black leather chaps, and boots. He said, "I hear that you have a biofeedback class that might help me deal with my test anxiety." As we talked, it was clear that Brick was bright but became very nervous at exam time. He blushingly admitted that he had severe diarrhea before taking exams, which made the situation worse. After talking for a while, he decided to enroll in the class.

The biofeedback and learning class taught both concepts and skills. Students met for 30 hours of class time and worked in the biofeedback laboratory twice a week or more, practicing relaxation and stress inoculation.

Concepts

The key concepts taught in the class have been described in this text. Stress is the result of perceptions, and the ability to cope is not something that happens from external sources; people can learn to reduce stress; stress reduction enhances performance; and mind → body. These concepts facilitate a cognitive shift in the student from blaming external, uncontrollable causes, to assuming internal, controllable causes. Research has verified that academic performance is enhanced when students shift from perceiving their performance as a result of external causes to perceiving it as a result of internal causes that they can control (Noel, Forsyth, & Kelley, 1987).

Skills and Image Rehearsal

Brick used the biofeedback laboratory daily to practice relaxation skills. He learned a variety of relaxation techniques and used EMG biofeedback. He also learned cognitive restructuring skills and became adept at identifying negative thought patterns and replacing them with positive thought patterns. Several studies have verified the importance of both relaxation and cognitive skills for enhancing test performance (Deffenbacher, 1986; Hunsley, 1987; Meichenbaum, 1985).

After Brick mastered deep levels of relaxation, he began visualizing that he could stay calm under pressure. He constructed a hierarchy of performance stressors and visualized performing effectively. Electromyograph measures verified his ability.

Follow-Through

Finally, after Brick had desensitized himself to tests in imagery, it was time to use these skills in the real situation. Brick practiced psychology and mathematics exams while receiving EMG feedback. When Brick was able to maintain low arousal of muscle tension while taking exams in the laboratory, he took the regular class exams. He received an A on the psychology exam but panicked on the math exam. Math was difficult for Brick, and it took several months of tutoring and biofeedback training before he passed the math.

Stress inoculation helps students become "unstuck" by replacing negative cognitions with positive cognitions. Students learn skills for coping with stress and practice these skills in image rehearsal and in real life. The steps to success are diagrammed in Figure 10.5.

Several programs for helping students overcome performance anxiety have been successful. Baruch College psychology professor Mary Valdez (1985) has conducted a biofeedback and stress-management class for many years. Students listen to relaxation tapes, use biofeedback training, and learn cognitive restructuring techniques. Valdez compared grades of students who took the class with grades of students on a waiting list. She found that students who took the class significantly improved their grades. These students also reported feeling less anxious and had fewer illnesses in the six months following the class.

At the College of the Mainland in Texas City, Texas, Stout, Thornton, and Russell (1980) conducted a biofeedback and relaxation study

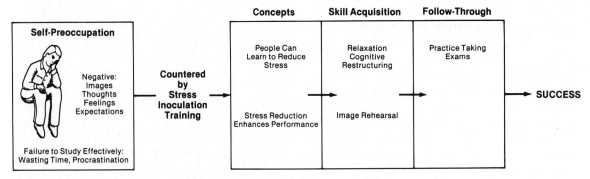

Figure 10.5   Stress-Inoculation Training Can Be Used to Overcome Test Anxiety.

with 45 students. Students were randomly assigned to a biofeedback training group, a progressive relaxation group, or a no-treatment control group. Students in the biofeedback training and progressive relaxation groups significantly improved grades and class attendance in comparison with the control group. The authors concluded that relaxation training helps academic persistence and performance by reducing anxiety.

Summary

In Chapter 3 we described the devastating effects of performance anxiety—blank mind, out-of-control physiology, and inability to perform. The academic manifestation of this stress, test anxiety, can ruin a student's academic career and self-esteem. In this section we described several multicomponent stress-management programs that can help students reduce anxiety and enhance performance. Most colleges and universities have programs for overcoming test anxiety.

||||➡

CONCLUSION

"Stress is like a river with dangerous rapids and whirlpools." Some people are excellent swimmers, and others are drowning in the rapids and whirlpools. Health professionals stand on the bank and pull people out of the rapids and whirlpools. Some people are studying the good swimmers to find out how they survive the rapids and whirlpools. Others are teaching people how to swim. Many people are refusing to learn to swim and simply jumping into the river unprepared.

Antonovsky uses the river analogy to point out that one problem with modern approaches to health is the "downstream focus." Billions of dollars are spent each year as health professionals of all types pull people out of the stream. Few professionals "raise their eyes or minds to inquire upstream, around the bend in the river, about who or what is pushing all these people in" (Antonovsky, 1987, p. 89). We add that few professionals have concentrated on teaching people how to avoid the river or how to swim through the rapids and whirlpools.

The past five chapters examined the dynamics and tools for becoming hardy and stress-resistant—an "upstream focus." We studied hardiness and social support as buffers against stress. We described ways for avoiding the river of stress and for staying afloat if pushed in: relaxation, cognitive restructuring, focusing, problem-solving, biofeedback training, image rehearsal, and stress-inoculation training. Never before have so much knowledge and so many resources been available to a society, and to each person, for becoming hardy and stress-resistant. We return to Suzanne Kobasa's statement.

You don't have to accept a victim's fate. There are ways to change from helpless to hardy.

—Suzanne Kobasa, 1984, p. 64

PART Four

Self Regulation, Lifestyle, and Health Behavior

Self regulation is the dynamics and ingredients of health and wellness put to use. Self regulation is a dynamic itself, without which health and wellness are in jeopardy. Control by forces other than the self is risky.

We devote a part of this textbook to self regulation because for most people, it is the foundation of health and the basis of recovery when health is lost. We included a self regulation expert on Mr. Wright's team because several of the tools needed for his recovery involve self regulation.

As noted in the preface, although the genetic and environmental cards might be stacked against health and wellness, humans have the power to intervene. Self regulation is the intervention, the "change agent." On the other hand, a person might have every genetic and environmental advantage and, lacking self regulation,

lose the advantage entirely through destructive lifestyle habits.

The importance of self regulation applies to all aspects of life—biological, psychological, and social—but has been studied primarily in the context of lifestyle habits. This emphasis reinforces the dual focus of Part Four, self regulation and lifestyle.

Chapter 11, Self Regulation and Health, describes the principles and ingredients of self regulation, often using examples from that aspect of life to which self regulation so aptly applies, lifestyle habits. If self regulation is the cornerstone of health, then lifestyle habits are the mortar that supports or weakens health; this is why our definition of health includes healthy lifestyle habits. In Chapter 12, Healthy Lifestyle, we discuss the essential ingredients of several lifestyle habits that promote health. This single chapter is not meant to be all- inclusive; it is a survey of lifestyle topics. Several of them are familiar to you, and several may be new to you.

Knowledge is one thing, action is another. In Chapter 13, Developing Health Behaviors, a variety of school, clinic, community, and family-based programs are described. These programs foster prevention and modification of unhealthy habits and promote health behaviors.

The challenge for everyone is to make self regulation a way of life, not as a punishment, nor as a necessary evil, but as a delight for health's sake.

CHAPTER *11*

Self Regulation for Health

IIII➡

In previous chapters, self regulation is described as the heart of stress resistance and learned resourcefulness. In Chapter 8, psychophysiological self regulation is described as the goal of biofeedback training. Self regulation training for the treatment and prevention of disease and illness is the hallmark of new approaches such as biofeedback training, that come under the umbrella term "behavioral medicine." Now we add that self regulation also means taking control of one's lifestyle and health behaviors, so that lifestyle is the result of choice and not the result of chance and ignorance. As stated throughout this textbook, self regulation is the cornerstone of health and wellness.

In this chapter we come to grips with self regulation—what it is and why it is a dynamic in health and wellness. Chapter 1 introduced you to a member of Mr. Wright's team of experts, Dr. Self Regulation, who explained to Mr. Wright that although the self regulation needed to give up a destructive habit might feel like punishment, it was better than being controlled by something other than oneself. Recall Mr. Wright's words: "So you are saying that I have more power than I knew to regulate myself, and self regulation is what health is all about. But I have to learn how, and I have to choose to do so."

Self regulation refers to control of physiological and psychological processes gained through internal and external resources and through choice. Self regulation is a central dynamic in health and wellness, because anything else is a risk. Control by circumstances, the environment, peers, habit, or cultural values may promote disease and illness.

The term "self-control" may be used instead of self regulation but may carry a negative connotation, stemming from the command of the parent or teacher to "Control yourself!" Self-control is precisely what people want, however; no one wants to be controlled by others or by disease.

We describe self regulation from the same perspective as stress resistance. Chapters 6 and 10 described the characteristics and development of stress resistance, asking, "How do people stay well?" rather than "How do people get sick?" In this chapter we describe self regulation skills and resources for health, focusing on how people gain self regulation rather than on how they lose it.

We are impressed by the fact that without professional help millions of Americans have quit smoking, and thousands have stopped drinking excessively and abusing narcotics (Robins,1974; Robins, Helzer, Hesselbrock, & Wish, 1980; Schachter, 1982). Columbia University psychologist Stanley Schachter states:

> It does appear that the generally accepted professional and public impression that nicotine addiction, heroin addiction, and obesity are almost hopelessly difficult conditions to correct is flatly wrong. People can and do cure themselves of smoking, obesity, and heroin addiction. They do so in large numbers and for long periods of time, in many cases apparently permanently.
>
> (Schachter, 1982, p. 442)

The ability of so many people to overcome negative habits testifies to the power of human beings to regulate themselves.

Because the study of health and wellness is a recent addition to psychology and medicine, however, knowledge of the dynamics of self regulation is derived mostly from work with people who do not have self regulation. Many of the techniques and skills described in this chapter are based on the creative work of therapists and researchers working with people who lack skills for overcoming symptoms and addictive behaviors and who seek professional help. Consequently, we describe treatment populations and clinical applications of self regulation techniques, often referring to work with smokers. When the Surgeon General's report of 1964 clearly identified smoking as a risk factor in lung cancer and other diseases, programs to help smokers become ex-smokers proliferated, and the literature on these programs is abundant. So, although we discuss many elements of self regulation in the context of overcoming destructive habits, remember that the same elements apply to adopting and maintaining health habits.

The emphasis on lifestyle habits in this chapter arises from the fact that such habits as smoking, excessive drinking, overeating, and lack of exercise can be studied and are clearly linked to disease. The alarm over the increasing medical bill of the American people has been a stimulus to face this fact: Any disorder that results from a destructive lifestyle habit is preventable. Arnold Ardell, a pioneer in the study and promotion of wellness and prevention, refers to destructive habits as "worseness" habits, to be easily contrasted with wellness habits (Ardell, 1979). Prevention means giving up or never adopting worseness habits. Self regulation is the foundation of prevention, in a society in which one can indulge in seemingly unlimited worseness habits.

In this chapter we identify the ingredients of self regulation. The research reported pertains particularly to lifestyle habits, but remember that the ingredients of self regulation apply to all aspects of health and wellness. In Section One we analyze the process of self regulation. In Section Two the discussion continues with a description of the ingredients of self regulation.

Section Three is a summary of skills that enable people to gain self regulation in three domains of health—physiological, cognitive, and behavioral. Keep in mind the focus of this book: the biopsychosocial approach to the dynamics of health and wellness. Like many other dynamics, self regulation is a biopsychosocial phenomenon in which biological, psychological, and social factors play a greater or lesser role, depending upon the context in which self regulation occurs. At the same time, self regulation has biological, psychological, and social effects, depending upon the goal of self regulation.

We hope to leave you with an appreciation of the importance of self regulation as a dynamic in health and wellness, for you personally and in prevention and treatment.

|||➡

SECTION ONE: SELF REGULATION: A CLOSER LOOK

Let the term "self regulation" roll around in your mind for a moment. Wait for the felt sense. Does "self regulation" conjure up a good feeling or a bad feeling, a little of both, or neither? Would anyone claim that self regulation is not a good idea? What exactly does self regulation mean?

Little Tif in the potty story finally gained control and learned to use the potty; that is physiological self regulation. A student uses autogenic training and learns to increase blood flow in her hands—psychophysiological self regulation. One of the authors, RS, consciously remained calm when confronting the shooters— emotional self regulation. Sue, the student using cognitive restructuring, consciously changed a cognition "Some dirt-bag will come along and hassle me!" to "I have never been bothered by anyone"—cognitive self regulation. An easily distracted student forces his mind to focus on a single task—mental self regulation. You study for several hours without eating junk food, an alcoholic consciously breaks the pattern of excessive drinking, the adult child of an abusive parent consciously breaks the pattern of abusing his children—behavioral self regulation. A person learns empathy skills to improve a relationship—social self regulation.

The essence of self regulation, as we are using the term, is conscious, willful, internally directed behavior that promotes health and homeostasis. We would not say that smoking, overeating, or staying angry are examples of self regulation even though they might be conscious and willful acts.

Now imagine a person who inherited perfect genes, had good parents who modeled health behaviors, was raised on a low-fat and low-sugar diet and continued this diet in adulthood, was athletic, was intelligent and "never had to study," was not influenced by peers and advertising, lived in a fairly stress-free environment, was hardy, and was stress-resistant. Is self regulation an important issue to this person? He probably does not even think about it.

Now think of someone who did not have the advantages of our hypothetical person. Imagine a person who came from an impoverished background with angry, impulsive, and abusive parents who had no knowledge of the dynamics of psychological and physical health and wellness, for whom psychological and physical health did not come naturally; who drank, smoked, and was violent just like his peers; who the school system "lost"; and who could not handle stress. Is self regulation an important issue to this person? He probably does not even think about it. Now imagine that this person committed a crime, was put on probation and saw a social worker, you. You might say, "This person is a victim," and you might be right. Now suppose that through your work this victim had a glimmer of a better life. Where would you begin?

What is the essence of "victimness?" Is not the essence of victimness a lack of self regulation, a lack of conscious wise decisions about behavior? People say, "I can't help it, that is just the way I am," or "I am violent because my father was violent" or "My mother and grandmother

have migraines, it is genetic, so there is nothing I can do," or as the Jets said in *West Side Story*, "We're depraved on a'count of we're deprived." Yes, but the kids were depraved on a'count of they did not choose to be any different. You might say they couldn't make choices because they didn't know any other way to be. And even if they had made better choices, they could not have carried them out. So perhaps you would begin by helping your client develop the skills for making better choices and carrying them out. You would end up with a self regulating individual.

As it happens, most people are neither of these extremes. Most people are in-between, with some parts of life that do not demand self regulation and some that do. For anyone in-between, self regulation is important. What makes it possible for the extremes to "escape" self regulation?

In the example, one escapee has a lifestyle that does not conflict with his goals, and the other has no goals to conflict with his lifestyle. For the former, health habits are natural and easy to maintain; for the latter, smoking, violence, and junk food are natural and easy to maintain.

When there is no conflict, or at least no discrepancy between what is and what one would like, then there is no desire to change and no self regulation. Self regulation is necessary for most of us because we have goals to achieve, tasks to perform, health issues to attend to, habits to break, temptations to withstand, and so on. Is it all worth it? That is exactly what the conflict is about.

Imagine that you decide to stop eating meat. You make this decision because you have studied the consequences of high blood cholesterol and you know that meat has cholesterol. Eating meat, however, is part of your lifestyle. You grew up on meat, you order meat at restaurants, you pride yourself on being a good meat cook, you have learned how to buy cheap cuts and know a million ways to cook hamburger, and when you have guests for dinner you serve meat. Not eating meat is also a lifestyle, and the two conflict. Is not eating meat worth the effort to change? When the answer is "yes," many things must change besides food—tastes, social habits, assertive behavior, the way you rear children, the recipe box, your choice of restaurants, perhaps even the people with whom you associate. The backbone of all this change is self regulation.

Self regulation and self-responsibility go hand in hand. Obviously, if you do not think that you are responsible for your health, you will probably not worry about self regulation. And like the need to take responsibility for your health because no one else will, you get to regulate yourself because no one can do it for you. When you are making a lifestyle change, people may sabotage your progress or hope that you succeed, but no one can do the work for you.

Once we are past childhood, few people care what we do in private. Usually. We know two executives who had suffered a heart attack, whose wives took over. These women took over the cooking and the exercise program; they monitored the drinks, the stress, the weight, and the blood pressure. In short, these gentlemen gave up self-responsibility and self regulation to the most responsible person of the pair. From the wife's point of view, one scare was enough! This arrangement is very rare, and it puts a burden on the responsible spouse. Do not count on it ever happening to you—do not even wish for it. And by the same token, attempting to regulate someone else can lead to trouble. For the majority, self regulation is a personal issue that makes sense, because your "self" is with you 24 hours a day, as no other self is.

||||➡

SECTION TWO: THE INGREDIENTS OF SELF REGULATION

People may not be born with the ability to regulate all aspects of life, but they can learn. Self regulation begins early in life, out of fear of punishment, or hope of reward, or for the pure joy of it. As life becomes more complex, with more and more options, temptations, and goals, the need for self regulation grows exponentially, but the ability may not. But we are not lost. We think of self regulation as a skill, and like all skills, self regulation can be learned and becomes easier with practice. There are several basic principles, and there are tools and methods for learning.

The large and growing literature on self regulation comes primarily from the research and clinical experience of people who have developed behavior therapy techniques for helping clients overcome worseness habits and addictions and from research with people who gain self regulation on their own. The combined work of the leaders in the field contributes more than a century of research to the study of self regulation (Bandura, 1986; Janis 1958; Kanfer, 1970; Leventhal, Zimmerman & Gutmann, 1984; Mahoney, 1974; Marlatt & Gordon, 1980; Meichenbaum, 1985; Mischel, 1974; Rosenbaum, 1983; Thoresen & Mahoney, 1974). The ingredients of self regulation that we describe come from these sources.

Before we begin, once again let the term "self regulation" roll around in your mind. Now think of what you would do, and what characteristics you would need, to maintain self regulation long enough to attain a difficult goal.

■ **A NOTE:** If we could write in three dimensions, it would be easier to demonstrate how these ingredients interact. Writing makes concepts seem linear, but they are actually interwoven. Some of these ingredients are synergistic and cannot exist independently. For example, we describe goals and commitment as separate processes, but in fact goals cannot be reached without commitment, and without the success of achieving goals, commitment fades.   ■

Figure 11.1 encapsulates the ingredients described below; please review it before proceeding.

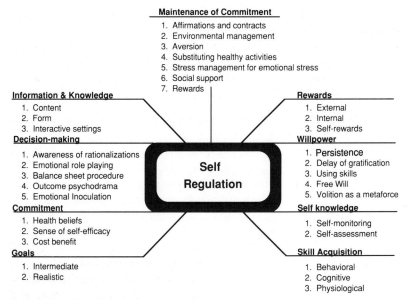

Figure 11.1.   The Ingredients of Self Regulation.

Information and Knowledge

Information & Knowledge
1. Content
2. Form
3. Interactive settings

To get started on the path of self regulation, people must know that the goal of self regulation is important and why (information), and how to proceed (knowledge). When lifestyle is the issue, it is necessary to have information and knowledge about habits that promote health and about those that promote disease and illness. To intelligently regulate lifestyle, people need to be informed about the consequences of their choices. The Surgeon General's 1964 report on the health risks of smoking informed millions of people about the dangers of smoking, and many people quit smoking. Because information helps people develop healthy lifestyles, much attention has been given to determining the best "components of information" and the best way to spread health information.

Content

Suppose that you are a health educator working for a large corporation. Your job is to persuade the employees to stop smoking through an educational program. What material should you use? Would you try to persuade them by showing the advantages of a life free of smoking, or would you try to show the disadvantages of smoking, such as the risk of lung cancer? Or, would you use both approaches? University of Wisconsin psychologist Howard Leventhal would be a valuable consultant. Leventhal has studied the components of information that help people choose healthy lifestyle habits, particularly fear and imagery.

Leventhal and Watts (1966) examined the effectiveness of using fear-producing information to help people stop smoking. In the study, a movie of a painful lung cancer operation was shown to smokers, followed by messages to stop smoking and get a chest X ray. The smokers failed to get an X ray, but many quit smoking. The movie scared people into quitting, but it also scared them out of getting an X ray. Leventhal found that using fearful information to bring about behavioral change may be counterproductive, because some people feel overwhelmed when exposed to the negative consequences of their behavior and may lose confidence in their ability to change. Leventhal found, however, that when clear instructions on how to cope with the problem are included, frightening information is useful (Leventhal, Singer, & Jones, 1965).

In Chapter 9, we described the power of *images* to elicit feelings and behavior change. It is not surprising that informative messages that include concrete images are more effective than word messages in producing change in health behaviors (Leventhal, Meyer, & Gutmann, 1980). Images can elicit strong emotions of fear and joy, thus motivating people to change behaviors. Noted sleep researcher and longtime cigarette smoker William Dement had a vivid dream about his own funeral. In his dream he observed grief-stricken family members parading past his casket. Dement knew that his early death was due to smoking. On waking, Dement resolved never to smoke again (Dement, 1976).

Because imagery elicits strong emotions, fearful images can overwhelm people. Leventhal and colleagues found that people with physical symptoms may not seek medical treatment because they conjure up vivid images of death or surgery. As with word messages, visual information should include positive images of people acting to solve the problem (Leventhal, Meyer, & Gutmann, 1980; Leventhal et al., 1984).

In summary Leventhal found that the content of effective information on lifestyle habits should include:

1. The consequences of a particular behavior, especially negative consequences that elicit fear.
2. Concrete images that elicit strong emotions such as hope or fear.

3. Instructions on how to change the negative behavior.
4. Models that provide vivid visual examples of overcoming negative lifestyle behaviors and replacing them with healthful behaviors.

It is interesting that fear-arousing information and information on how to change is more persuasive than fear information alone. It has always been our impression that people like to regulate themselves; information on how to begin apparently taps into this desire so that people are scared enough to change and encouraged enough to try.

The power of images and models is well known to the advertising industry. Messages about the glamor of destructive habits abound. We discuss this in Chapter 20, Societal and Cultural Forces Against Health and Wellness, but it is worth noting here that one task of wellness information is to counteract the messages used to sell worseness habits.

Take your heart to court.

Or on a bike ride. Or out for a jog. Whatever your sport, vigorous exercise can help keep your heart healthy.

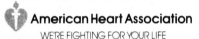

American Heart Association
WE'RE FIGHTING FOR YOUR LIFE

This Ad Provides Positive Instruction and a Helpful Image.
Source: American Heart Association.

Setting

The setting in which information is received is also an important variable in the effect of the information. In some settings in which information is given through television, posters, or lectures, the recipient is passive. In other settings, the recipient interacts with the information giver. Information given in interactive settings such as health fairs, classes in which students can participate, and counseling is more likely to be used for behavioral change than information that is passively received (Farquhar, Maccoby, & Solomon, 1984; Farquhar, 1978; Levine, Green, Deeds, Chalox, Russell, & Finlay, 1979; Petty, Ostrom, & Brock, 1981).

When people are passive recipients, they may feel that they are being coerced or they may discount the information as irrelevant to their unique situation (Janis & Mann, 1977; Leventhal et al., 1980). When people are active participants, they do not feel coerced. Interactive situations also enable individual assessment and application of health information to a person's unique situation. For example, a health counselor can provide information that is directly related to the needs and concerns of the client and can counter rationalizations for maintaining unhealthy habits.

Across the United States, many towns and cities have a yearly health fair, and many corporations have health-assessment programs. Health fairs and health-assessment programs provide a variety of physiological measures, including blood pressure and blood cholesterol, and with lifestyle assessment, including nutrition, exercise, stress level, and Type A behavior. Some fairs and corporations provide a computer printout with a detailed explanation of the person's health risks along with specific instructions for reducing risks. The person meets with a health counselor, who interprets the printout and answers questions.

Today, information is abundant; anyone who wants information on health and health risks can get it. Public services such as the American Heart Association, the National Cancer Institute, and the Government Printing Office provide information on all aspects of health. Health programs are offered by hospitals, community colleges, sports centers, and conditioning spas. Public and commercial television stations broadcast health programs, including exercise and yoga classes, and results of health research and health tips are reported on news broadcasts. Popular books on health have increased manyfold in the past decade, and anyone who has access to a bookstore or library has a ready source of usable information and knowledge. Even the physician's office is becoming a good source for useful information on health. Claiming ignorance as an excuse for maintaining worseness habits is almost impossible.

But none of this information and knowledge will do any good unless people make wise decisions based on it.

Decision-Making

I am my choices.
    Jean-Paul Sartre

Decision-making

1. Awareness of rationalizations
2. Emotional role-playing
3. Balance sheet procedure
4. Outcome psychodrama
5. Emotional Inoculation

Self Regulation

Decisions, decisions, decisions. Life is the result of personal decisions, from the amount of fat clogging one's arteries to the number of children that one gives birth to. The importance of making decisions lies in the simple fact that decisions play a key role in health and wellness and create the future. Also, without wise decision-making, self regulation is meaningless.

People who do not want to make a decision say, "I can't decide" or "It isn't that important to me." Sophisticated people say, "I have no basis for making a decision. The data are insufficient. As soon as the data are definite I will make a decision." In fact, lifestyle decisions are made every day, whether we know it or not. And furthermore, not deciding is a decision. Not making a decision can kill just as surely as making the wrong decision.

A decision to take prohealth action, called "prevention adoption process" and "protective behavior" (Weinstein, 1988; Weinstein, 1987), is based on many interacting variables that include the person's perceived susceptibility ("if I continue to smoke I will get cancer"), perceived severity of the hazard ("cancer could kill me"), perceived effectiveness of the action ("if I quit smoking my lungs will recover quickly"), and perceived costs ("not smoking is very hard; I will feel rotten; I should join a group, but that would cost too much, and I don't have the time anyway"). To estimate the likelihood that a decision will be made, theorists have attempted to put values for these beliefs into algebraic equations that give a cost-benefit ratio, suggesting that decisions to take action occur when benefits exceed costs. Weinstein argues that these models, such as the health belief model (Janz & Becker, 1984) and the reasoned action model (Ajzen & Fishbein, 1980), the most popular and thoroughly researched models of decision-making, do not take into account the complexity and variability of psychological and social variables and circumstances that are involved in making decisions. In "small" decisions, however, people may make an instantaneous cost-benefit estimate and act accordingly.

Anyone who is orchestrating a lifestyle change makes many daily small decisions. Imagine how often a first-day nonsmoker must decide not to smoke. And think of the decisions that the dieter going through the cafeteria line must make! The familiar "one more won't hurt me" rationalization is a quick cost-benefit analysis in which the benefit of not eating a delicious fattening food, is momentarily smaller than the cost; to state it the other way, the benefit of eating the delicious fattening food is suddenly greater than the cost, that is, the weight gain.

In addition to everyday decisions, "big" decisions must also be made: decisions about career and work, where to live, and with whom to share life, whether or not to initiate a lifestyle change. Sometimes apparent "life and death" decisions must be made. Patients with diagnoses of cancer decide whether to have chemotherapy, surgery, radiation, or no medical treatment. Heart patients may have to decide whether to have bypass surgery or to use medications, or to rely on diet and exercise for recovery.

Decision-making can be stressful, and the action that must follow the decision may be stressful, which is why people decide not to decide. Good decision-making can be facilitated, however, and can be learned.

Yale University professor emeritus of psychology Irving L. Janis devoted his professional life to research on decision-making and self regulation. In 1982 he received the Scholarship for Distinguished Scientific Contribution from the American Psychological Association in honor of his work on decision-making and conflict resolution. The citation statement said: "His pioneering work on stress and his continuing interest in self regulation are basic to the emerging field of health psychology" (*American Psychologist,* 1982, p. 37).

Janis focused on decisions about smoking, exercise, diet, and medical treatment. Much of his research was conducted at the counseling center at Yale University. In this section we describe the fundamentals and methods for decision-making that Janis distilled over years of research and clinical experience, described in the monumental book *Decision Making: The Analysis of Conflict, Choice and Commitment* (Janis & Mann, 1977). As the book's title suggests, conflict starts the process rolling, and, as we noted in Section One, conflict makes self regulation an issue. Conflict can be as mild as being healthy and wanting to maximize health, or as severe as having a long tradition with a destructive habit and also believing that the habit is a killer. A sense of conflict is good because it says "pay attention, a decision needs to be made."

Janis found that some people avoid the conflict by ignoring or discounting all information about the risks of a worseness habit. A 50-year-old man continues to smoke, eat high cholesterol foods, and not exercise even after a diagnosis of angina pectoris. He feels no conflict because he ignores information about the dangerous consequences. This is a likely possibility for the "impoverished" person that we created earlier in this chapter.

In a similar vein, people avoid conflict by procrastinating or shifting responsibility to someone else, or they construct wishful rationalizations. A 17-year-old smoker says, "I'll stop when I am 40." The smoker with high blood pressure states, "My doctor said I don't have to stop smoking because it might make me too stressed. He said I should work at not getting stressed."

On the other hand, some people avoid conflict by uncritically adopting whatever course of action is recommended. During a routine medical check-up, a young woman's blood pressure is found to be elevated, and she uncritically accepts medication; another is told that she is having panic attacks and uncritically accepts the diagnosis and medication. These are not examples of self regulation, but they are related to decision-making and health.

Another decision-making style occurs when a person panics and makes an impulsive decision without studying the alternatives and consequences. Health decisions made in this way may backfire, as often happens when a person panics about obesity and chooses a "crash" diet, or when a sedentary person panics about having a heart attack and decides to jog 10 miles every day. Some people cannot make a decision because they are unable to weigh the advantages and the disadvantages of changing.

According to Janis and Mann, the best decision-making occurs when a person examines all the relevant information and alternatives

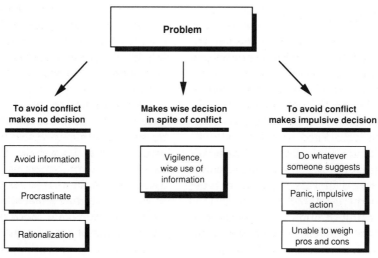

Figure 11.2. Decision-Making Styles.

in an unbiased manner. Janis calls this type of decision-making "vigilance." Vigilance implies staying aware and paying attention to new data that can be used to make good decisions (Janis & Mann, 1977). The crucial task for health psychologists, says Janis, is to teach people how to be vigilant in making decisions. The advantage of vigilance is that a prohealth decision is backed by information.

Decisions to change behavior or to acquire a new behavior for the sake of health and wellness are not easy, whether the behavior is cognitive, like changing a belief, or overt, like exercising. Even when the information supporting the change is accepted as indisputable and the conflict that the information creates is fully felt, it is difficult to make decisions that involve change. When self regulation is a struggle, the decision to initiate self regulation is also a struggle.

To make decision-making easier, Janis and his colleagues created several techniques and tested them in a variety of programs. They found five techniques to be helpful for enhancing decision-making: awareness of rationalizations, emotional role-playing, the balance sheet procedure, outcome psychodrama, and emotional inoculation.

Awareness of Rationalizations

To avoid the conflict of eliminating bad habits, people use rationalizations, which are excuses to avoid changing. "You have to be Type A to get ahead in this world." "I don't drink as much as a lot of people and they are okay." "It will never happen to me." To help people counter their rationalizations, Reed and Janis (1974) developed an "awareness of rationalizations" technique that includes studying a list of common rationalizations and listening to a tape that refutes the rationalizations.

The first step in countering rationalizations is to become aware of them. Reed and Janis created the following list of common rationalizations used by smokers:

1. "It hasn't really been proven that cigarette smoking is a cause of lung cancer."
2. "The only possible health problem caused by cigarettes that one might face is lung cancer."
3. "I have been smoking for a fairly long time now, so it is probably too late to do anything anyway."
4. "If I stop smoking, I will gain too much weight."
5. "Smoking just seems to be an unbreakable habit for me."
6. "I need cigarettes to relax; I will become edgy or irritable without them."
7. "If I prefer to smoke, I am only hurting myself and nobody else."
8. "So smoking may be a risk; big deal! So is most of life! I enjoy smoking too much to give it up."

Janis and Reed gave this list of rationalizations to smokers, who then answered these questions: "Have you ever used these excuses?" "Do you think deep down that this might be at least a reasonable or valid argument?" "Have you ever heard anyone use this excuse?" The final step was to have the subjects listen to a recorded lecture refuting each of the rationalizations.

In a study of 74 people who wanted to quit smoking, Reed and Janis (1974) randomly assigned half the subjects to the awareness of rationalizations procedure and half to a matched control group. The control group watched two antismoking films that presented information on the risk of lung cancer and emphysema. In a three month follow-up, the experimental group expressed greater awareness of susceptibility to lung cancer and emphysema and a stronger belief in the harmfulness of smoking than the control group. The experimental subjects were beginning to refute their rationalizations. The study showed that the taped lecture used to refute rationalizations was more powerful than the information presented on film, although much of the information was identical.

Emotional Role-Playing

Sometimes people fail to make a prohealth decision because they cannot associate the negative consequences of destructive behavior with themselves. A person may know that smoking is implicated in lung cancer, but she does not associate that dire consequence with herself. Therefore, the association of smoking and lung cancer does not contribute to a decision to quit smoking. To help people become aware of the consequences of their behavior, Janis and Mann (1965, 1977) developed a technique called emotional role-playing.

In emotional role-playing, a scenario is created in which the person is a victim of a specific disaster as a result of a decision to maintain a destructive behavior. The person acts out the scenario and the facilitator acts out the role of the physician. Janis describes the case of a young woman who was a heavy smoker. She acted out a scenario in which she is returning to her physician's office to get the results of X ray and other medical tests to identify the cause of a persistent cough. The young woman spontaneously responds as if each scene of the scenario were actually happening to her.

Scene 1. In the waiting room. The woman worries while waiting for the doctor's verdict. She expresses her thoughts out loud: "What if it is cancer?" "What if it is emphysema?" She then tries to decide whether to light a cigarette. "Gosh, I'd like to smoke a cigarette now. But what if I have cancer? That will make it worse."

Scene 2. The woman and doctor converse as the doctor gives the diagnosis.

Doctor: I am going to tell you the whole truth, since that is what you have requested. (He points to the chest X ray.) It's bad news. There is a mass in your right lung. You need immediate surgery.

Woman: I'm shocked. I don't know what to say. (Feeling panicky, she stifles tears.) I want to know everything. What will be the results of the surgery?

Doctor: There is a moderate chance for a successful outcome from surgery for this condition.

Woman: I'm scared. But I guess you're right. I guess I should have surgery.

Scene 3. Soliloquy while the doctor phones for a hospital bed. The young woman expresses her thoughts and feelings aloud while the doctor is telephoning in the next room. "Oh, God! I can't believe this. . . This can't be happening to me. Maybe it's nothing. . . maybe. Oh, God, if it's only just benign, that's all I ask for. One out of three survive! With my luck I'll be one of the fatalities. Why did this ever happen to me. . . cigarettes. . . . . one out of three. . . If I ever asked for anything, I asked for this. I've read all those reports and I just wouldn't believe them. Please, make it be okay. . . . Tomorrow, I'll go into the hospital. . . ."

Scene 4. Conversation with doctor concerning hospitalization.

Doctor: Report to the hospital tomorrow at 8:00 A.M. Bring materials to read and study. Expect to be in the hospital for at least six weeks, because surgery of the chest takes a long time to heal.

Woman: I can't believe this. It feels like a bad dream. It must be a bad dream. Six weeks in the hospital! And, I may still be sick after six weeks.

Scene 5. Conversation with the doctor about smoking as a cause of lung cancer.

Doctor: Are you aware of the connection between smoking and cancer?

Woman: Yes, but I thought it would never happen to me. I am so young.

Doctor: You need to stop smoking immediately. Will you be able to do it?

Woman Yes.

Emotional role-playing made a significant impact on the young woman. She immediately decided to stop smoking.

In a study involving a single role-playing session, significant changes in the attitudes of smokers occurred (Janis & Mann, 1965). When asked what had made the greatest impression on them, participants cited the scene involving immediate threat of hospitalization most often. Similar results with heavy drinkers are described by Toomey (1972).

Emotional role-playing is effective because it involves the whole person—thoughts, feelings, and behaviors. The participant is active, and thus spontaneous feelings, thoughts, and behaviors are brought out, rather than the old excuses for maintaining a bad habit. Emotional role-playing creates fearful images and messages, and it includes instructions for solving the problem.

Balance-Sheet Procedure

As noted above, people avoid making decisions by ignoring the conflict, by rationalizing, and by ignoring information. But sometimes decision-making bogs down because the person cannot weigh the advantages and disadvantages and remains stuck in a quagmire of "buts," "ifs," and "maybes." Janis (1983a) developed the balance-sheet procedure to help students make wise decisions. The balance sheet is a table with columns in which the student enters responses to four possible consequences of a decision: (1) tangible gains and losses for oneself, (2) tangible gains and losses for others, (3) self-approval or self-disapproval, and (4) social approval or disapproval.

Janis used the balance sheet procedure with a group of 36 Yale University seniors who had to decide what to do after graduation. The balance-sheet procedure involved five steps.

The first step was to generate a variety of options for the coming year through brainstorming. Procedures for brainstorming were: (1) think of as many alternatives for next year as possible; (2) be original; (3) do not evaluate while generating alternatives; (4) modify

flawed alternatives; (5) ask other people for suggestions; and (6) daydream about the ideal situation that you would like to be in next year.

The second step was to fill out a balance sheet on the most attractive alternative. The third step was to fill out a balance sheet for the other alternatives that seemed viable. One student's most attractive alternative was going to business school to become an executive in his father's firm on Wall Street. Then he filled out a balance sheet for going to law school, with plans to work in a legal aid clinic or in public interest law.

The fourth step was to compare the balance sheets. The senior compared the balance sheet on being an executive with the balance sheet on being a lawyer. On the executive balance sheet he found no comments on self-approval or self-disapproval, but on the lawyer balance sheet he saw several self-approval comments. He realized that being an executive did not satisfy his desire to help people, and that the comments on self-approval or self-disapproval were more important to him than any of the other comments. He also realized that his plan to major in business was primarily for the approval of his parents.

The fifth step was to answer the following questions: "Is there any more information you need?" "Which alternatives look the best?" "Do you feel ready to commit yourself to the best alternative by allowing others to know your decision?" "Are you prepared for any negative consequences of the alternative you choose?" "What contingency plans do you need to make before starting to implement your decision?" The senior was elated after discovering that he wanted to be a lawyer, but he conscientiously explored the negative consequences of being a lawyer. He noted parental disapproval, relatively low income of legal-aid lawyers, and poor prospects for travel abroad. Although not as elated as before, he nevertheless felt certain about his decision. As Janis states, "This graduate worked out his career plan entirely through the balance-sheet procedure" (Janis, 1983a, p. 174).

The effectiveness of the balance-sheet procedure has been studied with several subject populations. It helps people lose weight (Colten & Janis, 1982) and exercise more (Hoyt & Janis, 1975; Wankle & Thompson, 1977).

The idea of thinking through the pros and cons of a decision is not new. Nevertheless, systematically completing the balance sheet helps people consider gains and losses that they may otherwise overlook. People often overlook issues that involve self-approval or self-disapproval.

When starting a health habit, a person could find added incentive by filling out the self-approval/self-disapproval section of the balance sheet. Even if the person could not find clear objective gains by adopting a health habit, self-approval in itself would be an important gain.

Outcome Psychodrama

This technique helps a person make a wise decision by acting out the consequences of various options. Janis and Mann (1977) developed the procedure with clients who came to the Yale Counseling Center for weight reduction, smoking cessation, and marital counseling, and with college students making career decisions. For example, a college student was trying to decide whether to become a high school teacher or a lawyer. First he acted out what life would be like as a lawyer. He created a variety of vivid scenarios. Most of the scenarios portrayed life as a lawyer as "full of dull routines," "stifling of all creativity," and "ethical problems." In contrast, few negative scenarios developed while role-playing life as a teacher. The student decided to be a high school teacher.

Outcome psychodrama is similar to emotional role-playing. In emotional role-playing, however, a specific scenario is created in which the person confronts a specific consequence of a particular decision, for example, lung cancer as the result of a decision to continue smoking. In outcome psychodrama, no specific scenario or specific consequence is suggested by the facilitator. The person simply imagines and role-plays the consequences of various decisions.

Emotional Inoculation and the "Work of Worrying"

The fifth step in effective decision-making is to prepare for stressors that cause emotional upset. Emotional stress is one of the major reasons that people change their mind after deciding to adopt a healthy habit. In a study of 264 ex-smokers, 71 percent of those who relapsed reported anxiety, anger, or depression as the cause (Shiffman, 1982). This is true for people who are overcoming any addiction, whether cigarettes, food, alcohol, or drugs (Brownell, Marlatt, Lichtenstein, & Wilson, 1986).

Preparation for emotional stress is the "work of worrying," or the process of mentally rehearsing anticipated problems and developing reassuring cognitions to alleviate stress when a crisis is encountered. The work of worrying inoculates people emotionally against stress because they expose themselves to small dosages, in imagery, in order to tolerate large doses in life (Janis, 1958). Like Meichenbaum's stress inoculation training, which was discussed in Chapter 10, emotional inoculation creates "emotional antibodies" for tolerating stress. These emotional antibodies are reassuring thoughts such as "I'll be able to do it," or "If I make a mistake the first time, I can try again." "A slip is not a relapse." As people "worry" about a stressful event, they think of alternative strategies for dealing with it and practice reassuring cognitions. After doing the work of worrying, people are not taken off-guard by events and can apply strategies that were rehearsed. For example, being laid off would be a good excuse for an ex-smoker to begin smoking again. By anticipating stressors and developing coping strategies, the person may not relapse when stressors occur. Coping skills help people maintain prohealth decisions when faced with difficult problems instead of relapsing or becoming overdependent on family, friends, physicians, or professional counselors (Janis, 1983a).

Summary

The techniques developed by Janis are useful in making wise decisions about health and for enhancing self regulation. Emotional role-playing helps a person experience the consequences of negative behaviors, thus enhancing the probability of deciding to change the behaviors. This technique can be used to motivate any kind of behavior change. The consequences of anger, or violence, or a lack of exercise can be explored as easily as the consequences of addictive behaviors.

The "awareness of rationalizations" technique helps people counter rationalizations that sustain destructive habits. The balance-sheet procedure helps a person clarify the gains and losses of decisions. Through outcome psychodrama, the consequences of a variety of possible decisions are experienced. Emotional inoculation through worrying helps a person identify and prepare for stressors that might sabotage a wise decision.

Making wise decisions is essential for health and wellness. Now we come to an important issue: Effective decision-making incorporates a commitment to a goal. This is a truism that must not go unnoticed. When a person says, "I decided to become a schoolteacher," the goal of becoming a teacher is stated by stating the decision. When a person decides to quit smoking, but doesn't have a timetable, there is a lack of commitment to quit. It is unlikely that wise decisions will turn into action unless the person is willing to commit to a goal. Commitment goes hand in hand with the decision to achieve the goal.

Commitment

Commitment

Self Regulation

1. Health beliefs
2. Sense of self-efficacy
3. Cost benefit

Information and knowledge have no value unless they are used to make wise decisions, and a wise decision to achieve a goal has no value unless it is backed by commitment.

When you say that someone is "really committed," what do you mean? You probably mean that the person is willing to put energy and time into accomplishing a certain goal. For most of us, maintaining healthy lifestyle habits takes time and energy, or commitment. For most people, brushing their teeth every day does not take commitment, but exercising every day for cardiovascular health does. The difference is that beyond childhood, few people hate brushing their teeth, the effort is minimal, and the reward is immediate. On the other hand, to exercise every day, a person must schedule the time, overcome inertia, and work hard for a goal called "living longer with good health" that has little immediate meaning or reward. Commitment to exercising is essential if one loathes exercising. People make exercise a part of life when they are committed to it.

Health Beliefs

What enables a person to commit the energy and time needed to eliminate a destructive habit, to exercise, or to take medications for years? The answer is **belief**, based on information and knowledge. People have to believe that a particular health goal is so valuable that it is worth the commitment, even when this means sacrifice of personal comfort, or major change, or pain. Belief, knowledge, decision-making, and commitment are connected.

A colleague, Bill, smoked for 20 years. Bill became committed to not smoking when he finally believed that smoking was causing serious physical damage to him and that if he stopped smoking, the threat of physical damage would be reduced or eliminated. In other words, Bill came to believe that smoking has severe consequences, and that not smoking would reduce the threat and damage already done. As noted in the section on decision-making, the perceptions of severity and efficacy are important beliefs in making a decision and a commitment.

Bill's dramatic change occurred, as it does for many people, after an alarming medical check-up. Bill was told that he had emphysema (damage of the air sacs of the lungs) and that if it progressed, he would be severely handicapped or die. He was told to quit smoking immediately. Suddenly Bill "got commitment" because he had the beliefs necessary for change. Bill believed that smoking seriously affected his own health (perception of severity) and that if he stopped his health would improve (efficacy of treatment). People will engage in "painful" health behaviors only when they believe that there is a significant threat if they do not, and a significant payoff if they do.

A Sense of Self-Efficacy

To quit smoking, Bill must also believe that if he tries hard enough he can quit. In other words, he must have a sense of **personal self-efficacy**, or confidence in his ability to overcome a difficult habit (Bandura, 1986). A person's sense of self-efficacy is a reliable predictor of overcoming addiction to cigarettes, food, or alcohol (O'Leary, 1985). In Bill's case, the most difficult belief to sustain is that he can quit smoking for life. After the diagnosis of emphysema, the severity of the threat was easy to believe in, as was the importance of not smoking. Believing in

his own strength to quit, forever, is not easy, and yet it is essential for making a commitment to not smoke again (Tipton & Riebsame, 1987).

In summary, to be committed to a behavior change or to a particular wellness behavior, a person must believe that the goal is so valuable that the time and energy needed to achieve the goal are worth the sacrifice. In addition, the person must believe that the goal is achievable through personal effort.

Goals

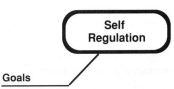

Setting goals sounds simple, but it is not. Appropriate goals can lead to success, and inappropriate goals can lead to failure.

Bandura (1986) found that for successful self regulation, a person's goal must be realistic and achievable through several intermediate goals. People stay committed to change, and to maintaining wellness behavior when the goals of the behavior are specific and attainable. This is why Bandura emphasizes the importance of having intermediate goals that can be achieved. The goal of longer life is vague and far off for most of us and may not bolster commitment at all. However, the intermediate goals of staying in shape, looking good, or having a good treadmill test are attainable, and are in fact their own rewards, and thus are easier to be committed to. As long as people stick with the intermediate goals, the end goal will be achieved.

Bill established many small goals each day, such as not smoking after teaching a class, while eating lunch, and while drinking coffee. Each little success bolstered his confidence and enhanced his commitment.

Bandura's research also showed that it is important to have goals that are consistent with one's abilities. A goal that exceeds one's abilities results in feelings of discouragement, failure, disappointment, and finally rejection of the goal.

A person may do all the right things—gather appropriate information, make a wise decision, create a reasonable goal, feel deeply committed, and act—and still fail in self regulation and never achieve the goal. The hardest part in self regulation is sticking with it.

Maintaining Commitment

Maintenance of Commitment

1. Affirmations and contracts
2. Environmental management
3. Aversion
4. Substituting healthy activities
5. Stress management for emotional stress
6. Social support
7. Rewards

Self Regulation

It seems to be human nature to get excited about a change, stick with it for a while, and then backslide. Health spas, sports centers, and weight-loss programs can attest to this, as can psychotherapists, health counselors, and teachers. The dynamics of backsliding are not well researched, but loss of commitment seems to be an important element.

It might be tempting to tell someone who is trying to maintain a lifestyle change "If you are really committed, you will stick with it." Commitment is not something that we have or do not have, or that we can instantly turn on. Nonetheless, commitment can be enhanced. Imagine that you have just decided to quit smoking, lose weight, quit drinking, or exercise regularly. You would probably need techniques to help you maintain your commitment. The following

techniques have emerged from the research on self regulation and health. Most of the research is based on helping people stop smoking. We begin with simple techniques and progress to more complex.

Affirmations and Contracts

Affirmations and contracts are a way of privately and publicly affirming goals. The typical behavior contract includes a statement of (1) the goal, (2) the consequences of not meeting the goal by a given date, and (3) the rewards when the goal is met. The contract has the signatures of the person making the change and a supporter, usually a friend, family member, teacher, coach, or counselor. Box 11.1 is a generic behavior contract. Research shows that self-imposed goals, rewards, and standards lead to success more frequently than those that are externally imposed (Brownell, Colletti, Ersner-Hershfield, Hershfield, & Wilson, 1977; Bandura, 1986).

In Bill's case, he did not immediately tell his friends and colleagues that he had stopped smoking. He waited until someone noticed, and then with pleasure he said, "I was wondering when you would notice! I made my decision to quit smoking three days ago and have not had a cigarette since." By involving his friends and colleagues in his decision through his public affirmation, Bill enhanced his motivation to maintain his decision to quit. Bill did not make a formal contract with a friend, but he did make an informal contract with his friends by sharing his decision, by talking with them about his plans and strategies, and by describing the techniques that he used.

Contracts and affirmations help people maintain commitments for various reasons. For some people, the involvement of another person is the key element. For others, the specificity of the goals and rewards in the contract helps them concentrate on achieving the goal. Some people find a contract helpful, because for them a contractual obligation is sacred and cannot be

---

BOX 11.1

BEHAVIOR CONTRACT

Goal _____

Specific steps _____

_____

_____

Resources _____

_____

_____

Rewards _____

_____

_____

Consequences
   if not met _____

_____

I will begin my new
   lifestyle behavior on _____

_____   _____
         My signature   Partner's signature

---

broken. For others, the contract symbolizes the challenge of a new goal. For others, the embarrassment of breaking a contract is the main motive for honoring it. Whatever the reason, simple contracts and affirmations are commitment enhancers for many people (Cormier & Cormier, 1979; Janis, 1983a; Kiesler, 1971; McFall & Hammen, 1971).

Environmental Management

Focus on the word *temptation*. What feelings arise? Temptation!

At times you probably will feel a conflict between giving in to momentary pleasure, otherwise known as temptation, and achieving a goal. The word *temptation* may elicit images of a double-layered chocolate cake, greasy french fries, or having a cigarette and watching TV after dinner. These forbidden delights conflict with the goal of following a healthy lifestyle. Succumbing to temptation is a momentary loss of commitment.

One of the easiest ways to avoid yielding to temptation is to remove temptations from the environment. You cannot snack on junk food if there is no junk food nearby. It is amazing how often people stock up on cookies and candy bars, saying, "I buy that stuff because my kids like it," and then succumb to temptation.

Another way to reduce the risk of yielding to temptation is to avoid situations that make it difficult to resist. Bill carefully avoids situations that elicit the desire to smoke. Bill knows that he likes to smoke when drinking coffee, while watching television, or while reading, and so he drinks coffee with friends who do not smoke and reads in the library, where he cannot smoke. When he feels the need to smoke as a break from work, he calls a friend and distracts himself with conversation.

For people overcoming addictions, the most tempting situation is to be with friends who are still addicted (Shiffman, 1984). The easiest approach for most ex-addicts is to avoid these friends. New friends and new social situations may be sought as a way of finding support for the new lifestyle.

Aversion

It is not possible for most people to create or find an environment that eliminates all temptations. People cannot give up their friendships. Parties, business meetings, and conferences are hotbeds of temptations. The ultimate victory, therefore, is to eliminate the desire to eat "bad" food, smoke, or use drugs or alcohol. In the ideal situation, these stimuli would not be temptations, because they would no longer be pleasurable.

Aversion means a strong feeling of dislike, repugnance, or antipathy. The goal of aversion techniques is to help people associate feelings of dislike with formerly pleasurable objects. Instead of anticipating pleasure at the sight of cigarettes, the goal of aversion techniques is to feel repugnance. Aversion techniques pair a negative experience (nausea or pain) with the stimulus that is to be avoided. Drugs that create nausea are paired with a stimulus such as alcohol. In aversion techniques, the pleasurable stimulus is paired with an aversive stimulus.

I (RS) accidentally experienced the power of nausea and vomiting to extinguish a formerly pleasurable stimulus when I was 12 years old. I was given a double-layered box of cream-filled chocolates on Christmas morning. Throughout the day I ate chocolates until they were gone. At midnight I began vomiting and continued until I had the dry heaves. I was weak all the next day and felt miserable. For years after, the thought of chocolates made me feel nauseated. To this day, I do not eat cream-filled chocolates.

Satiation can also lead to repugnance. Rapid smoking is a satiation technique for helping to eliminate the taste for cigarettes. In rapid smoking, a puff is inhaled every six seconds until the person cannot stand to smoke another cigarette.

Covert aversion techniques are also useful. These techniques are also called covert sensitization, a term used by Joseph Cautela for pairing pleasurable stimuli with negative images and thoughts (Cautela, 1967). For example, Dement's dream about his funeral paired death and grief of family members with cigarette smoking. An imagery technique for alcoholism pairs on image of vomiting in the glass with drinking.

The most effective aversion techniques pair the habitual behavior with its negative consequences. Janis' research on emotional role-playing has been effective for many types of addictions. In the example of emotional role-playing, college students paired smoking with the emotional reaction to coughing, lung cancer, seeing a doctor, hospitalization, and surgery. Emotional role-playing solves a major problem with negative lifestyle behaviors such as Type A behavior, smoking, lack of exercise, drinking, and drug addiction. The consequences of the behavior are not immediately experienced, and therefore the negative consequences are not paired with the behaviors. People can smoke or drink for years with apparent impunity. Emotional role-playing eliminates the time gap and pairs the negative consequences with the behavior immediately.

Aversive techniques eliminate the desire

to continue negative habits. For many people, however, eliminating habits can lead to feelings of loss and emptiness. Participation in new activities can be the key to maintaining abstinence.

Substituting Healthy Activities

Substituting prohealth behaviors for destructive behaviors is one of the most important techniques for maintaining commitment and overcoming addictions. In a study of 2,500 runners, 81 percent of the men and 75 percent of the women who had been smokers when they started running quit within one year (Kaplan, Powell, Sikes, Shirely, & Campbell, 1982). In a study of ex-smokers, Shiffman (1984) found that exercise was very effective in preventing relapse. Murphy, Pagono, and Marlatt (1986) found that aerobic exercise was effective for helping heavy drinkers become moderate drinkers.

Meditation, listening to relaxing music, and hobbies can replace addictive behaviors. These activities can be particularly valuable for people who are always on the go.

The increase in YMCAs, health clubs, community recreation centers, and classes at community colleges and universities has increased everyone's opportunity for healthy fun.

Developing Stress-Management Skills

Stress is a major factor in relapse. People who maintain commitments cope with emotional stress better than people who fail (Abrams, Monti, Pinto, Elder, Brown, & Jacobus, 1987; Katz & Singh, 1986; Shiffman, 1982, 1984). Shiffman studied 264 ex-smokers in Los Angeles who called a telephone hot-line service while experiencing a relapse crisis. The sample consisted of 41 percent ex-smokers who relapsed and 59 percent who survived the crisis. Shiffman found that the survivors had a variety of cognitive and behavioral skills that helped them. The behavioral skills were: using

food or physical activity as a substitute for smoking; relaxation; distraction; escaping a tempting situation; delay, or simply waiting for the difficult situation to end; and talking to people. The cognitive skills were: thinking about the positive consequences of not smoking; thinking about the negative consequences of smoking; thinking about negative consequences unrelated to health, such as disapproval by others; using raw willpower without specific coping cognitions; punitive thoughts, such as "you weakling"; distraction by shifting attention to pleasant things or by thinking of other problems; and self-talk, such as "There is really no reason to be upset" or "I don't really want to smoke. I just want to relax."

Several other studies have demonstrated the importance of coping skills for preventing relapse and maintaining commitment. Psychologists Roger Katz and Nirbhay Singh (1986) hypothesized that ex-smokers who avoided relapse would score higher on the Self-Control Schedule than those who quit smoking and then relapsed. The Self-Control Schedule (described in Chapter 6) measures cognitive and problem-solving skills, the sense of self-efficacy, and the ability to delay gratification. Katz and Singh administered the Self-Control Schedule to 52 smokers and 77 ex-smokers. Sixty-three of the ex-smokers were "self-cured." The smokers and ex-smokers had begun smoking at an average age of 16 and had smoked for an average of 18 years. The ex-smokers had not smoked for an average of 6.7 years. Katz and Singh's hypothesis was supported. Ex-smokers scored significantly higher than smokers on the measures of learned resourcefulness, indicating that ex-smokers had better coping skills than those who were unable to quit.

People who learn social, problem-solving, and cognitive skills, and who can maintain these skills, are more likely to maintain commitment to a health behavior than people who do not have these skills (Davis & Glaros, 1986). Stress-management classes and assertiveness-training classes teach people many of these skills and are an important aspect of a lifestyle change program.

Social Support

You are familiar with the relationship of social support and health, discussed in Chapter 6. Here we refer to social support as the support of others for achieving a goal. If you are having a difficult time overcoming addictive behaviors on your own, or if you are having a difficult time maintaining commitment to health behaviors, you may be missing one of the most powerful dynamics for overcoming addictions and developing a healthy lifestyle—social support (Brownell, Marlatt, Lichtenstein, & Wilson, 1986; Coppetilli & Orleans, 1985; Janis, 1983b).

Social support comes in many varieties. One type will remind you of summer camp when you had to have a buddy to go swimming; you and your buddy kept an eye on each other. The buddy system, or the partnership system, as it is often called, was pioneered by Alcoholics Anonymous and is highly effective for weight control, smoking cessation, and overcoming substance abuse. Janis and Hoffman (1982) conducted a 10-year follow-up on 30 heavy smokers, 10 of whom had been assigned to a high-contact partner, 10 to a low-contact partner, and 10 to a control group in the original study. In the original study, the high-contact partners called each other on the phone for 10 minutes every day for three weeks. They praised each other for success, criticized each other for backsliding, and were skeptical about excuses for not improving. The low-contact partners met in the clinic once a week to discuss their progress. The follow-up interviews 10 years later revealed that people in the high-contact partnerships were more successful in maintaining smoking cessation than those in the other two groups.

The results were replicated by Nowell and Janis (1982) at a weight-reduction clinic. The subjects were 48 adult women with an average weight of 165 pounds. Subjects were assigned to high-contact partners and low-contact partners. The high-contact partner group members talked to each other 10 minutes every day for three weeks. Members of the low-contact group met once a week to discuss their progress. The high-contact group lost significantly more weight in the eight-week period than the low-contact group.

Support from a spouse can also help maintain a health habit. In a study of 125 women who quit smoking, partner support was more predictive of continued abstinence than length of years of smoking, number of cigarettes smoked daily, age, education, socio-economic status, sense of self-efficacy, and self-image. Partnership support includes encouragement, minimizing stress by avoiding interpersonal conflict, taking over responsibilities, showing empathy, toleration of moodiness, concern about quitting, and problem-solving assistance (Coppotelli & Orleans, 1985).

Self-help groups are also a valuable source of social support. As the term suggests, self-help groups encourage people to help themselves. In self-help groups, understanding and caring people with common experiences support one another; no one feels alone or unusual, and newcomers find role models with whom they can identify and from whom they learn ways of dealing with problems. Members in self-help groups emphasize the importance of being able to share a feeling with someone else who is like them and having someone say, "I know how you feel. I've been there, too" (Gartner & Riesman, 1984). The Albert Einstein College of Medicine professor, Virginia Goldner, M.D., describes her experience as a member of Overeaters Anonymous.

> A little over 4 years ago I went to my first meeting of Overeaters Anonymous, or O.A. I was 50 pounds overweight, and to put it simply, unable to stop eating. A therapist friend of mine with the same problem had told me about the program, and after procrastinating in the usual ways, I finally took myself, skeptical, contemptuous, and desperate, to a dreary, ramshackle

church where, as I had been told by recorded message, I found a "beginners meeting." That was June 1976. By June 1977, I'd lost all 50 pounds, and in the process, had found I believed a new way of living.

(Goldner, 1984, p. 65)

Goldner is convinced that self-help groups provide a service that cannot be provided by professionals. Professionals, she says, do not have the time nor interest in helping people manage a lifelong disorder. Many people do not have the money to pay professionals for lifelong support. In contrast, members of self-help groups are experts in their disability, and by pooling their knowledge and resources, they provide lifetime support for lifelong disabilities (Goldner, 1984).

We cannot underestimate the value of social support in developing a healthy lifestyle, in coping with serious disease, and in overcoming addictions, including addictive relationships.

Rewards

No one doubts that rewards are powerful motivators for maintaining commitment.

In summary, maintaining a commitment so that a wise decision will continually be manifested in behavior is the core of self regulation. We described six techniques for maintaining commitment: affirmations and contracts; eliminating temptations through managing the environment; eliminating temptations through aversion; fun, rewards, and healthy activities that substitute for negative habits; stress-management skills for coping with emotional stress; and social support. The seventh element in maintaining commitment is reward.

Success and Rewards

"Success is its own reward." Because this statement is true, we discuss these topics together. Little needs to be said about the value of

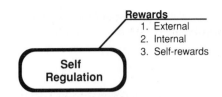

success in maintaining both commitment and behavior, but the importance of success does highlight the need for establishing intermediate goals that are attainable.

The fact that rewards motivate behavior is something every animal trainer, parent, teacher, child, and student knows. Just as meeting short-term goals helps a person pursue a long-term goal, so intermediate, tangible rewards help a person "hang in there" for a reward that is far in the future or is doubtful (Bandura, 1986).

The ability to give oneself rewards may seem like an unusual ingredient in self regulation. The fact is, however, that just as we must assume self-responsibility because no one else will, we must rely on ourselves for tangible rewards; people soon tire of rewarding us for good behavior that has become habitual. Furthermore, to maintain lifelong habits, the habit must be reinforcing and meaningful. Long-lasting change in behavior is usually the result of the initial motives and the development of secondary positive rewards such as improved self-image, positive feelings, "runner's high," or reduction of anxiety and depression (Bandura, 1986; Leventhal, Meyer, & Gutmann, 1980). In a study of 54 ex-smokers that included 20 who quit on their own, 18 who attended an aversion-therapy group, and 16 who attended a behavior-management group, all rated self-liberation from the addiction as the most important factor in quitting. For these people, self-liberation became the reward (DiClemente & Prochaska, 1982).

Most people are good at rewarding themselves, but often the reward promotes worseness instead of wellness, for instance, eating junk food or having a few beers as a reward for finishing a term paper. The ability to establish wise rewards is as important as establishing wise goals. The trick in self regulation is to use wellness rewards, and to be content with experiencing the accomplishment of a goal as the reward.

Our colleague Bill rewards himself for not smoking. During the process of weaning himself from cigarettes, Bill reinforced himself every day. He bought freshly squeezed orange juice and ate his favorite foods. After overcoming an especially difficult time, he rewarded himself with a movie. Today he feels a deep sense of satisfaction and self-efficacy as he grows more confident that he can overcome a habit that he thought would be impossible to change.

The important thing in self regulation is to be conscious of one's need for reward and to know what type of reward is motivating. For some people success is a sufficient reward, while others need to give themselves tangible rewards such as new clothes for losing weight or a trip to the fresh air of the mountains for not smoking, a massage for regular exercise, or an extra hour of play for hard work. Some people stick with wellness behavior for praise from others, and for these people social support is an important element in maintaining commitment. Rewards enhance self-nurture. Self-nurturing is especially important when the rewarded behavior involves self-deprivation such as dieting or giving up an addiction.

In addition to external and internal rewards, overcoming symptoms and feeling good are rewards that motivate many people to adopt new behaviors. Surprisingly, some people are unable to reward themselves or to accept rewards. These people will work for goals because they think that they should, or because they are in physical of psychological pain, but the work lacks delight. They may ultimately give up or seek medical solutions for their discomfort and symptoms.

In clinical practice, after introducing a new skill or goal, and describing the home practice that the client must accomplish, we ask, "How are you going to reward yourself when you have done this work?" Our task is to help the client establish wise rewards that are motivators, that are consistent with the person's goals, and that can be thoroughly enjoyed.

Willpower

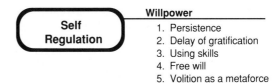

Self Regulation	Willpower
	1. Persistence
	2. Delay of gratification
	3. Using skills
	4. Free will
	5. Volition as a metaforce

The underpinning of self regulation is willpower.

During a breakfast break while writing this section on willpower, we saw the following advertisement on television:

Scene: A young, attractive couple are in bed. The woman gets up, goes to the dresser, and lights a cigarette
Man: Are you going to do that now?
Woman (looking distraught and frustrated): I have to. I guess I just don't have willpower; I just don't have your willpower.
Man (now out of bed, comforting the woman): It isn't willpower. Maybe you have a nicotine addiction. Nicotine addiction is a disorder. See your doctor. Doctors treat disorders. Your doctor has a program that can help; it helped me. See your doctor.
Woman (now studies the cigarette as though it were a curious object, looking hopeful).
White letters on black screen: SEE YOUR DOCTOR
Sponsor for the ad: _____ pharmaceutical company

There are several messages in this scenario, subtle and not subtle. What do you think?

Now think of someone you know who has willpower.

Perhaps you thought of a friend who was told that he would never walk again after a car accident, yet learned to walk during a difficult year of physical therapy and exercise. Or perhaps you thought of someone who is not very bright but studied hard and eventually earned a degree. Or someone who quit smoking, lost weight, or became an outstanding athlete, or someone who stopped using depression as the solution to every problem. What qualities characterize this person? Such people have goals. They do not give up or succumb to discouragement. They are determined, they can work without immediate reward, and they persevere. When these qualities are applied to a difficult task, we say that the person has willpower.

Persistence

People with willpower are persistent in the face of difficulties. They can tolerate stress and persist even when plagued with self-doubt and conflicts. When we reflect on the clients that we have worked with over the years, we note that willpower is one factor that distinguished those who got well from those who did not. Clients with willpower work hard. They practice the skills that enable them to get well. In a study of 77 ex-smokers, the subjects ranked willpower as the most important variable in

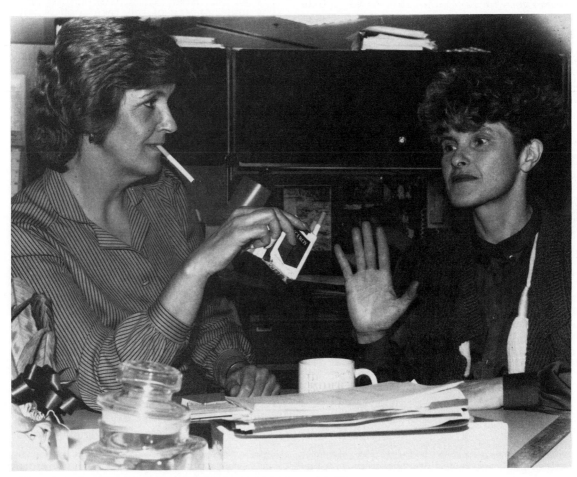

The Ex-Smoker Who Refuses a Cigarette Uses Skills and Willpower.
Source: Gordon Steward, Denver, CO.

quitting. They ranked willpower above social support, professional help, improved self-image, the challenge of quitting, confidence in their ability to quit, and feeling healthier (Katz & Singh, 1986).

Some types of self regulation do not necessitate extraordinary willpower, and others do. The amount of willpower needed for any task depends upon the learner and the particular goal. A person who loves physical exercise would not need great willpower to begin and maintain an exercise program, while a person for whom exercise is a dirty word would need much willpower.

Although many people say things such as "I had to use a lot of willpower,"many psychologists say that the concept is unnecessary for explaining behavior. John Farquhar, director of the Stanford Heart Disease Program, talks about willpower in his book, *The American Way of Life Need not Be Hazardous to Your Health* (1978).

> Within the last few years, we have gathered confirming evidence that skills needed for lifestyle changes can be systematically and readily taught

---

WHEN YOU HAVE WILLPOWER, YOU CAN:

1. Delay gratification.
2. Strive for indeterminate long-term goals.
3. Tolerate frustration and pain while completing a task.
4. Override unpleasant emotions and continue the task.
5. Persevere despite physical discomfort.
6. Persevere despite social criticism.
7. Persevere despite internal conflict and doubt.
8. Concentrate on the goal.

---

and learned and that the individual need not depend upon that mystical and unmeasurable factor called willpower to change deep-rooted habits. It is actually better for our emotions and more productive for our health to forget about willpower, with its Calvinistic connotations, and embrace instead the skills of behavior modification.

> (Farquhar, 1978, p. 38)

Farquhar and others take this stance against willpower because they recognize that it may be quite useless to expect behavior change by demanding change or expecting that the change will come about by sheer willpower. You cannot tell someone to use their willpower and expect instant change, any more than you can tell a stressed person to just relax and expect the person to instantly relax, without skills. Farquhar emphasizes that skills are needed. We include willpower as an ingredient in self regulation and as a dynamic in health and wellness because skills have no power to create change unless they are used, which means using willpower. "Calvinistic connotations" refers to the idea that willpower is a moral good and that a lack of willpower is morally offensive; it also refers to the notion that using willpower should involve suffering, or at least "gritting the teeth and bearing it." These concepts are not included in willpower as we use the term.

Using Skills

A battery of skills facilitates self regulation and reduces the need for sheer willpower. As a simple example, imagine overcoming a candy bar addiction. You could take the sheer willpower route and force yourself to reject candy bars even though they are a part of your everyday environment, or you could take the willpower-plus-skills route. Your skills might include eliciting social support (joining a candy bar crisis support group), imagery rehearsal (seeing yourself rejecting a candy bar in high-risk situations), assertiveness (telling a friend that offers you a candy bar to buzz off), or substituting wellness behaviors when the craving is upon you (jogging or relaxation).

When a person fails to gain or maintain self-control, the behavior therapist refers to insufficient skills and rewards but not usually to insufficient willpower.

We use the word *willpower* because it is commonly used. It is a good description of a faculty that is essential to self regulation and a faculty that people who maintain healthy lifestyles deem essential. Self regulation and willpower go together simply because regulation by oneself does not happen without effort.

Free Will

The experience of willpower has been analyzed by philosophers, theologians, and psychologists for centuries, until this century, when it went the way of the mind with the advent of radical behaviorism. William James included a chapter on the will in *The Principles of Psychology* (1890) and gave the subject considerable importance. James was particularly keen on the concept of free will, because at a time when he was extremely depressed and contemplating suicide (being unable to convince himself that human beings are more than the result of physical mechanisms), he made a leap of faith and decided to believe in free will. He said that his first act of free will was to believe in free will, and to act as though it were a certainty. The depression vanished. **Free will** refers to a human's ability to escape conditioning, to choose one's destiny; willpower is the driving force.

The Italian psychoanalysist Roberto Assogioli kept a light burning for the will in his own therapy and writings. Assogioli, a contemporary of Freud and Jung, created a therapy that he called psychosynthesis (Assagioli, 1965). Psychosynthesis helps the client integrate the many aspects of the self into a healthy being. The integrating force is the will. In his book *The Act of Will*, Assagioli describes the many aspects of the will and the enhancement of willpower. On the importance of the will, he wrote:

Let us realize thoroughly the full meaning and immense value of the discovery of the will. In whatever way it happens, either spontaneously or through conscious action, in a crisis or in the quiet of inner recollection, it constitutes a most important and decisive event in our lives.

The discovery of the will in oneself, and even more the realization that the self and the will are intimately connected, may come as a real revelation which can change, often radically, a person's self-awareness and whole attitude toward himself, other people, and the world. . . . This enhanced awareness, this "awakening" and vision of new, unlimited potentialities of inner expansion and outer action, gives a new feeling of confidence, security, joy—a sense of "wholeness."

(Assagioli, 1973, p. 9)

We hope that every reader has felt the special quality of will that Assagioli is referring to: the extra effort that is put into a task, that moment of certainty that indicates success, the knowledge that we have an inner resource. Sometimes a certain experience of willpower is monumental, staying in memory for years and becoming a referential experience. As to the function of the will, Assagioli wrote:

The true function of the will is not to act against the personality drives to *force* the accomplishment of one's purposes. The will has a *directive* and *regulatory* function; it balances and constructively utilizes all the other activities and energies of the human being without repressing any of them. The function of the will is similar to that performed by the helmsman of a ship.

(Assagioli, 1973, pp. 9–10)

The description of the will as a directing and regulatory function fits well in our skills model of self regulation. James wrote that a strong will is crucial for surviving crises. But as the faculty with which we direct and regulate our lives, willpower is a part of everyday life. Assagioli was convinced that people can consciously enhance willpower through the exercise of the will. Assagioli recommended training the will by performing deliberate actions for that purpose only. This idea was not new to Assagioli, and perhaps at some time in life everyone has been told "Do it because it will strengthen your will." Of this James wrote:

> Keep alive in yourself the faculty of making efforts by means of little useless exercises every day, that is to say, be systematically heroic every day in little unnecessary things; do something every other day for the sole and simple reason that it is difficult and you would prefer not to do it, so that when the cruel hour of danger strikes, you will not be unnerved or unprepared.
>
> (James, 1912, p. 75)

Even more poetically, James wrote of the person who has trained the will:

> When disaster occurs, he will stand firm as a rock even though faced on all sides by ruin, while his companions in distress will be swept aside as the chaff from the sieve.
>
> (James, 1912, p. 76)

With willpower, wise decisions are made and commitments are maintained; skills for self regulation are used instead of being "swept aside as the chaff."

Willpower can be practiced and enhanced, so the use of the will is a skill. Willpower is the effective use of the will to achieve a goal. While it is unlikely that many people actually practice willpower for the purpose of enhancing it, we can think of self regulation as exactly that. People who make behavioral changes of any type are practicing willpower. Using willpower becomes easier with practice; simultaneously, one's sense of self-efficacy increases.

A few psychologists who are interested in self regulation have studied willpower and its enhancement. Stanford University professor Walter Mischel has studied willpower for many years (1961, 1974, 1984). Mischel equates willpower with the ability to achieve goals. "Willpower is the ability of the individual to affect his own outcomes and to influence his personal environment. . . . Always it entails the individual's efforts to modify conditions in the light of particular goals" (Mischel, 1976, p. 437).

Delay of Gratification

Mischel was fascinated by the problem of enhancing willpower, and for him the essence of willpower is the ability to delay gratification. "One especially striking characteristic of human 'will' is that people frequently impose barriers on themselves, interrupting their own behavior and delaying available gratification. . . . It is hard to imagine socialization, or indeed civilization, without such self-imposed delays" (Mischel, 1976, p. 437). The ability to delay gratification is essential for accomplishing goals. For example, suppose that you want to lose weight and are rationing calories. On a particular day you have made special dinner plans, so you plan to have only vegetables for lunch. Unexpectedly, one of the office staff brings in homemade cinnamon rolls for everyone—the wonderful aroma drifts into your office; you are hungry, you feel deprived, but you deny yourself the pleasure of eating a roll because you know that a rich dinner awaits you, that is, you delay gratification.

Most students know the importance of delaying gratification. Throughout academic life students must deny themselves the immediate pleasure of watching television, partying, or just "hanging out," in order to study for exams or complete assignments. Students learn to delay pleasurable activities until after the exam or the term paper is completed.

Mischel began studying delay of gratification with preschoolers, using a simple procedure: The child is presented two rewards. One is obviously preferable, such as one marshmallow versus two marshmallows. The child is told that she can have two marshmallows if she waits until the experimenter returns to the room, but can have the single marshmallow at any time by ringing a bell, which signals the experimenter to return. Mischel and his colleagues found that some children can wait no more than a few seconds, while others waited 15 minutes until the experimenter returned. Children who successfully delayed gratification used a variety of cognitive strategies such as not thinking about marshmallows, distracting themselves, focusing attention elsewhere, or focusing on irrelevant characteristics of the sweets. Some covered their eyes. Mischel reports that by the sixth grade, children who delay gratification understand these strategies and use them consciously. Choosing between one or two marshmallows is not the same as choosing between a negative task now, such as studying, and pleasure now, such as going to a movie, but undoubtedly cognitive strategies are useful for sticking with the task and delaying gratification. What strategies do you use to help yourself study on a beautiful spring day?

Mischel, Shoda, and Peake (1988) reported a 10-year follow-up study of 67 children who were tested in preschool. They found that children who delayed gratification in preschool were more likely to be considered academically, cognitively, and socially competent by their parents than children who were unable to delay gratification. The correlation coefficients between delay time in preschool and characteristics in adolescence are low, however, as is the reliability of the measure of delay time. While these results are interesting and seem to make sense, they are not definitive.

Bandura and Mischel (1965) demonstrated that children can be taught to delay gratification by observing adults who model delay of gratification. Prison inmates who preferred immediate rewards were taught to delay gratification by observing peers who modeled delay of gratification (Stumphauzer, 1972). Conversely, parents who preach self-control while lounging in front of the television model immediate gratification behaviors that children imitate (Mischel & Liebert, 1966).

The ability to delay gratification is the ability to stay on task in the face of pleasant diversion. As important as the delay of gratification is, however, it is only one aspect of willpower.

Deliberate change is a continuing process for those who are not stagnating their way to death. Changing all kinds of habits requires willpower.

Psychophysiological self regulation, by definition, requires willpower. Although the body can maintain homeostasis when it is cared for, willpower is needed when the body is thrown off balance. Willpower is needed for simple processes such as relaxation to counter stress and for complex processes such as daily hand warming with biofeedback instrumentation to prevent migraine headaches.

Volition as a Metaforce

The pioneers of biofeedback training who you met earlier, Elmer and Alyce Green, use the term volition rather than willpower and describe volition as a "metaforce" in psychophysiological functioning (Green & Green, 1976).

Imagine that you live in a house that is heated by a furnace. The furnace is controlled by the thermostat that you set at a certain temperature each day before leaving the house. If you set the thermostat at 60° then the thermostat and the furnace automatically maintain the house temperature at 60°. All day the furnace turns on and off, maintaining temperature homeostasis. Is there volition in this system? Can the thermostat decide that the house is too cold and make the furnace turn on, or can the furnace refuse? There can be no change in this closed system until you come home.

When you get home, you move the thermostat up to 70°. You are a force that comes into the thermostat-furnace system and creates change; you are a metaforce. Now the thermostat and the furnace will keep the house at 70° until you set the thermostat at 60° once again.

The Greens use this metaphor to describe the relationship of volition (or willpower) and physiological processes. The autonomic nervous system runs automatically, like the thermostat and the furnace, even when becoming increasingly diseased. When a person changes the physiological functioning, the person's volition comes into the system like a metaforce, "resetting the thermostats."

The concept of volition as a metaforce highlights the unique nature of being human: the ability to influence physiological processes, to escape the slavery of conditioning and genetics, and to counteract unhealthy homeostasis. As described in Chapter 2, Mind and Body Dynamics, and in Chapter 8, Biofeedback Training, the neurochemical pathways are available; through willpower and skills psychophysiological change and homeostasis are possible.

Willpower is increased by strengthening the other ingredients of self regulation. Mustering the willpower for maintaining a health behavior is easiest when one is committed to it, has a sense of self-responsibility, is committed to the goal, achieves intermediate goals, has internal standards, and is rewarded.

Self-Knowledge

Self Regulation —— Self knowledge

1. Self-monitoring
2. Self-assessment

We described information and knowledge as the first ingredients in self regulation. That discussion referred to information and knowledge about the physical world, including information about lifestyle habits and physical health. Self-knowledge refers to being aware of one's emotional and mental habits. Both types of information and knowledge are essential for self regulation.

Self-knowledge includes awareness of one's motivations, feelings, rationalizations, expectations, goals, self-talk, values, goals, potentials, and scripts (compulsive life patterns). Self-knowledge also refers to understanding how these aspects of the self relate to overt and covert behavior. For example, a Type A person might be motivated to change, but she may have a script that says "burn out, don't rust out," based on feelings of insecurity and a parent

who modeled Type A behavior. Without knowledge of these dynamics, it might be difficult for this person to change. Self-knowledge also means insight into necessary conditions for change, gaining a sense of what will be acceptable to the self. For example, changing deeply entrenched and rewarded Type A behavior may create anxiety. The person must have enough self-knowledge to know the sources of the anxiety and how to change without jeopardizing or neglecting valued aspects of the self. In Chapter 9, we described several imagery techniques for self-exploration, leading to self-knowledge. The imagery and role-playing techniques are important in developing skills for gaining self-knowledge.

This discussion of self-knowledge will remind you of the discussion of the dynamic in self regulation training, that consciousness leads to control. These are similar concepts, and we could say that self-knowledge leads to control. In the chapter on biofeedback training, we said that consciousness is increased through the feedback of information, which is the basis of almost all learning. Self-knowledge is increased through feedback and through many other processes: focusing, introspection, meditation, imagery and visualization, dreams, rational thinking, psychotherapy, self-monitoring, and self-assessment. Self-monitoring and self-assessment are useful tools for initiating and maintaining a behavior change.

Self-Monitoring

Self-monitoring is exactly what the term implies. Carefully attending to all the internal and external variables in behavior change is a valuable skill that has been a part of behavior modification from its inception.

To quit smoking, Bill identified the times when he is most likely to smoke and the situations that stimulate the desire to smoke. Bill likes to smoke after eating, when drinking coffee, and while watching television or reading. Each of these are situations in which he smoked in the past. Self-monitoring enhances Bill's awareness of these stimuli and situations, and it gives him an opportunity to act. As the first step in smoking cessation, one program has smokers wrap a self-monitoring record sheet around the cigarette package so that every time a cigarette is withdrawn, the smoker can easily record the situation, time, and mood (Shiffman, Read, Maltese, Rapkin, & Jarvik, 1985).

Careful self-monitoring also helps Bill identify negative self-talk such as, "I can't enjoy dinner without smoking," or "I can't tolerate the frustration of not smoking" and he identifies the rationalizations that could sabotage his program. In addition, Bill identifies the situations that create emotional stress and tempt him to smoke as a way of coping. Awareness of self-statements that weaken his desire to quit, awareness of the stimuli that have a strong effect on his desire to smoke, and awareness of situations that create emotional stress enable Bill to use skills to counter the forces that would defeat him. A leader in the field of relapse prevention, G. Alan Marlatt of the University of Washington, writes:

> Awareness of choice-points and alternative responses in the addictive behavior sequence may be one of the most significant allies in the client's coping repertoire. Most habitual behaviors, by definition, are characterized by a low level of awareness. Addictive behaviors such as smoking or drinking often represent "automatic" and overlearned responses. Self-monitoring reintroduces conscious awareness into the process and thereby has a profound dehabitualizing effect.
> (Marlatt & Gordon, 1985, p. 55)

In weight loss, self-monitoring includes monitoring calorie intake and weight. In acquiring a "positive addiction" such as regular exercise, self-monitoring promotes awareness of situations that lead to not exercising, like eating a big meal with the intention of jogging afterward, and rationalizations. After the high-risk situations are identified, the serious potential jogger restructures her day to place exercise at a time when she isn't likely to feel lazy.

Self-Assessment

Throughout this text you have had opportunities to assess aspects of your behavior and personality. Self-assessment is an important element in self regulation for the simple reason that by knowing where you stand you have a better sense of where you need to go. When combined with information and skills, self-assessment is a useful tool.

People do not always want to assess themselves because ignorance feels like bliss. If a person does not know that his blood cholesterol is high, then he cannot feel too guilty about not trying to lower it. We use several self-assessment questionnaires in our classes and with clients, as tools for enhancing self-directed change. Self-assessment is needed for self regulation. Today, many self-help books, and nearly all textbooks on health, include self-assessment questionnaires.

Another type of self-assessment that is important in relapse prevention is assessment of **relapse risk**. This includes assessing relapse history, sense of self-efficacy, high-risk situations, beliefs about relapse, and need for other lifestyle change (Shiffman et al., 1985). As Marlatt says, "Forewarned is forearmed" (Marlatt & Gordon, 1985).

Once a person has honestly assessed the likelihood and conditions of relapse, the next step is to assess coping skills. Box 11.2 is an example of coping responses assessment for an ex-smoker, created by Shiffman et al. (1985).

Self-knowledge sounds as if it might come with the territory of being human, but it does not. People seem to be more or less in touch with themselves—their needs, goals, motives, memories, conditioning, habits, and on and on. Because self-knowledge is important for self regulation, it is fortunate that self-knowledge can be gained through the techniques described in this text.

BOX 11.2

COPING RESPONSES

THINGS YOU MIGHT THINK:

1. Thinking about the positive benefits of not smoking (health, pride, etc.).
2. Thinking about the negative effects of smoking (bad taste, expense, etc.).
3. Giving yourself commands ('Don't do it!'; "Stop!").
4. Encouraging yourself ("C'mon, you can do it.").
5. Reminding yourself how hard it was to quit in the first place.
6. Telling yourself, "I really don't want to smoke."
7. Imagining something relaxing, like a favorite spot.
8. Imagining the bad effects of smoking (black lungs, etc.).
9. Imagining yourself as a successful ex-smoker.
10. Distracting yourself by thinking about other things.
11. Going over your reasons for quitting.

12. Telling yourself, "I just need to get through the next few days."
13. Recognizing the difficulty of quitting.
14. Imagining your friends' or families' reactions if you were to smoke.

THINGS YOU MIGHT DO:

1. Have something to eat or drink.
2. Physical exercise.
3. Slow deep breathing to relax.
4. Distract yourself by doing something else like going for a walk or occupying your hands with something.
5. Avoid high-risk situations (e.g. other smokers, parties).
6. Delay, put off having a cigarette.
7. Get support from others.
8. Treat yourself with rewarding or comforting activities.

Shiffman et al. (1985, p. 492)

Skill Acquisition and Application

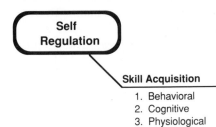

Self Regulation

Skill Acquisition
1. Behavioral
2. Cognitive
3. Physiological

At the beginning of this chapter we said that self regulation is a skill. In fact, self regulation is the result of using skills that are described throughout this text. Previously we described cognitive and behavioral self regulation skills pertaining to stress management, stress resistance, and learned resourcefulness. We have also described relaxation skills. In this chapter we discuss self regulation skills that are particularly related to behavior change and lifestyle—self regulation is the key to healthy lifestyle habits.

Like the other ingredients of self regulation, skills are valuable only when they are used. It is of little value to have stress-management skills and then fail to use them. It is also true that when striving for a health goal, the more skills and strategies a person knows, the greater the chance of achieving the goal (Bandura, 1986).

To quit smoking and prevent relapse, Bill uses skills he knew before quitting, as well as some he had to learn. We have described most of these techniques: relaxation, environmental restructuring, assertiveness, rationalization awareness and countering techniques, self-monitoring, and self-reward. Bill uses self-statements to counter negative thoughts. To make his environment more compatible with his new goals, he drinks coffee with friends who do not smoke, and he reads in the library, where he cannot smoke. When he feels the need to smoke as a break from work, he calls a friend. Bill also carries a carton of orange juice because the tartness lessens his desire to smoke. These may not seem like very impressive activities, but they all reflect a self regulation skill. Bill is also using the four strategies that are described by Shiffman and colleagues (1985) as "so broad that they are nearly universal and constitute a first line of defense in almost any situation": avoidance, escape, distraction, and delay. The total package, backed by willpower, has led to success. Bill is an ex-smoker.

Here is an obvious fact: Our goals do not seek us. We seek them, through skills. Learning and using skills, however, does much more than get us to our goals. Skills also enhance self-efficacy. If you have ever seen a toddler throw a tantrum because someone tried to help him put on his jacket when he wanted to do it himself, or if you have ever comforted a tearful 4-year-old because she could not get her shoelaces into a bow, or if you remember when you were that way, then you know the drive that human beings have to gain a sense of self-efficacy.

To our knowledge, the need for a sense of self-efficacy is never outgrown or lost. Like success, a sense of self-efficacy encourages continued effort and use of skills, which in turn enhance self-efficacy. Self-efficacy enhances self regulation, which enhances self-efficacy, which enhances self regulation, and so forth. Self-efficacy and self regulation counteract helplessness and "victimness." In the realm of lifestyle habits, self-efficacy takes on a different flavor from the shoe-tying sense. Rather than the feeling of self-efficacy that comes from doing something "in the world," the sense of self-efficacy must come from doing something for one's self that may not be praised. In both cases, self-efficacy results from doing something by oneself, using a skill and accomplishing a goal. Jogging another block, controlling anger or appetite, seeking information—all health-oriented activities give one a sense of self-efficacy. If you are engaging in a health habit, you already know this.

SECTION THREE: THE TREE OF SELF REGULATION

We begin this chapter's concluding section by sharing with you the history of the chapter. Self Regulation for Health began as a section of Chapter 14, Introduction to Behavioral Medicine. As we were writing the final draft of that chapter, a persistent unease finally leapt into consciousness. We were writing about the dynamics of health and wellness in a chapter that begins with models of disease and illness and focuses on treatment. This was because, as we noted at the outset of this chapter, most of the literature on self regulation and the techniques for enhancing self regulation come from working with people who do not have self regulation and who seek treatment.

Our discomfort finally crystallized as a reconfirmation of our fundamental orientation: The ingredients of health are everyone's

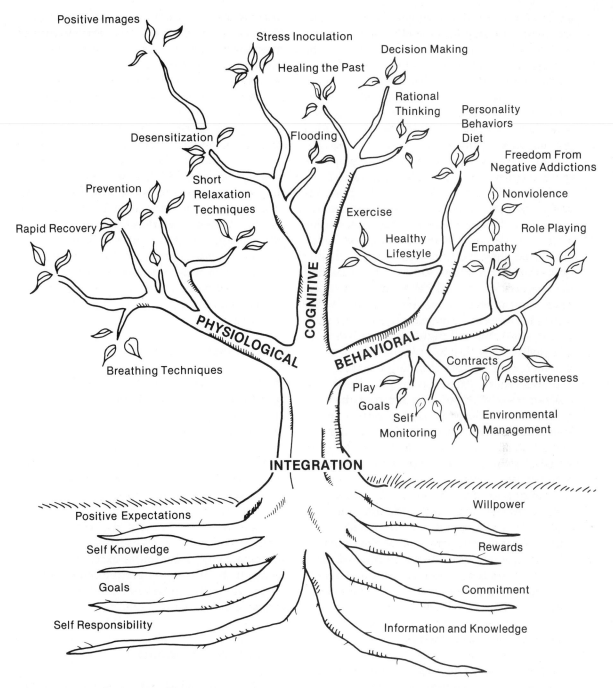

Positive Images
Stress Inoculation
Decision Making
Healing the Past
Rational Thinking
Desensitization
Flooding
Personality Behaviors Diet
Freedom From Negative Addictions
Prevention
Short Relaxation Techniques
Nonviolence
Rapid Recovery
Exercise
Role Playing
Healthy Lifestyle
Empathy
PHYSIOLOGICAL
COGNITIVE
BEHAVIORAL
Breathing Techniques
Contracts
Assertiveness
Play
Goals
Self Monitoring
Environmental Management
INTEGRATION
Positive Expectations
Willpower
Self Knowledge
Rewards
Goals
Commitment
Self Responsibility
Information and Knowledge

Figure 11.3.   The Tree of Self Regulation with Physiological, Cognitive, and Behavioral Branches.

natural heritage and should be described in the context of health and wellness, not in the context of illness and treatment.

Self regulation became a topic to address independently of its importance for overcoming illness and worseness habits, and we were free to give self regulation its proper place as a dynamic of health and wellness, as the foundation of healthy living.

We have created a visual summary of the elements of self regulation, Figure 11.3, The Tree of Self Regulation Skills. We conceptualize self regulation as a tree with many roots, branches, and leaves. A tree is a useful metaphor, because, like self regulation, trees grow, and they grow in a particular terrain, with roots that nourish growth and branches that spread into leaves. Models of dynamic, interacting processes, however, cannot accurately be described on paper; the branches and leaves of the self regulation tree are continuously interacting to promote wellness. In this metaphor, the branches are the three domains of health, the leaves are the skills and tools of healthy living, and the roots are the essential characteristics that a person must have if the tree is to grow. This is not a perfect metaphor, but we hope that it will serve as a useful review for you. The tree is a summary of the ingredients of health described throughout this text, including the elements of healthy lifestyle that are described in the next chapter. As you review the tree of self regulation, remember that the branches are not separate; for example, a healthy lifestyle promotes physiological homeostasis, and relaxation skills could be on the behavioral branch.

The Physiological Branch

The bottom line of physical health is healthy homeostasis achieved through balance in all the branches; unhealthy behavior and cognitions can disrupt homeostasis. For the physiological branch, the most appropriate leaves are the skills of relaxation: deep relaxation, quick relaxation during stress and to prevent the build-up of stress, and proper breathing.

In Chapter 7, Relaxation, we described the relaxation response as the flip side of the stress response, and we described relaxation as the process that brings the body back to homeostasis. We cannot underestimate the power of relaxation for regaining and maintaining homeostasis. Maintaining homeostasis by preventing and counteracting the stress response is prevention. Relaxation skills are part of stress-inoculation training and desensitization training, because relaxation is incompatible with panic and stress. In addition, relaxation of mind and body is an important first step in using imagery techniques, particularly for healing.

The Behavioral Branch

For the behavioral branch, we focus on behaviors that are part of a person's repertoire of healthy coping skills and on lifestyle behaviors that promote health.

Social skills are behaviors for interacting with others. These skills, such as empathy, can be learned. Effective social skills facilitate social support, an invaluable resource in self regulation.

The behavior branch also includes personality behaviors such as Type A behaviors. It emphasizes overcoming excessive Type A behavior by turning anger into empathy, lecturing into listening, and competition into compromise.

The Cognitive Branch

At this point, you are well aware of the power of cognitions to influence behavior and health. You understand the physiological effect of stepping on the garden hose and thinking that it is a snake, you know something about the power of irrational thinking and how to combat it, you know that your feeling of stress is often the result of your perceptions, you know that goals and purpose in life pull people through difficult times, and you know that belief in a placebo is the force behind the effect. In Chapter 6 you learned about hardiness, resourcefulness, and cognitive skills that promote health. Chapter 9 described other important cognitive skills: imagery and visualization for stress management, self-exploration, healing, and overcoming the past. In Chapter 10 you studied the techniques and applications of stress-inoculation training and cognitive restructuring.

The cognitive branch is the central branch of the self regulation tree because cognitions are the foundation of self-directed change. Learning relaxation skills to promote homeostasis involves cognitions, just as changing poor health habits does. The cognitive branch itself has to do with using cognitions to change cognitions, learning particular skills such as decision-making, and using cognitions as the driving force behind psychological and physiological healing.

The leaves of the cognitive branch illustrate the diversity of cognitive skills that can be used to combat stress, to become stress-resistant, and to promote healing and a healthy lifestyle.

The Roots

This chapter is primarily about the roots of the self regulation tree. Just as a tree needs strong roots to grow and weather storms, so masterful self regulation needs strong roots. And just as the roots and the branches begin small and take time to grow, so the roots and branches of self regulation may begin weak but will grow.

Take a minute: Without looking at the roots of the self regulation tree, review the ingredients of self regulation; there are nine. If you cannot recall them, then answer this question: "If you were initiating a new behavior, what would you need to achieve your goal?"

Do It Now.

We hope that you recalled the major ingredients of self regulation because they make sense and not simply because they might be on the next exam.

The roots of self regulation are all equally important and cannot be ranked; in fact, they may seem like different ways of talking about the same thing. Like the branches of the tree, the roots are interacting and mutually supporting, and like success, they create more of the same. A person may begin self regulation with shallow and puny roots, but the roots grow, and nourish the branches and leaves. Our tree metaphor fails on this point: Real trees depend upon nourishment from outside agents, humans, or nature, but people must ultimately rely on themselves for growth.

Now you might be thinking, "How is all this related to self regulation? This tree is just a skills tree." The use of physiological, behavioral, and cognitive skills for health *is* self regulation. To be a self regulating person, rather than a victim of circumstances and bad habits, people must develop certain skills, beliefs, and characteristics that will guide them through difficult times.

Self regulation is a two-edged sword. On one edge, self regulation brings liberation from control by external forces and the misery of poor decisions and ill health; on the other edge, self regulation demands information and knowledge, wise decision-making, commitment, maintenance of commitment, goals, rewards, self-knowledge, skill acquisition, and willpower. Self regulation is work, until physiological, cognitive, and behavioral health habits become a way of life. So while self regulation is the essence of health and wellness, many people choose not to develop it.

We have examined nine ingredients of self regulation, and all are a complex interaction of psychological and social variables. Goals and rewards, decision-making and maintenance of commitment, and information and knowledge are all heavily influenced by social values and customs. At the same time, a person's self regulation behavior is in continual interaction with the social environment. Self regulation itself can occur in the three domains of the biopsychosocial approach to health and wellness: lifestyle habits and stress management for physical health; mental and emotional processes for psychological health; and social behaviors such as empathy, assertiveness, and other interpersonal skills for social health. The tree of self regulation, with physiological, cognitive, and behavioral branches, could have been drawn with biological, psychological, and social branches instead.

Self Regulation as a Way of Life

The ingredients of self regulation described throughout this text apply to overcoming addictive behaviors, to complex psychophysiological processes, and to emotional and cognitive processes. The role of self regulation in life cannot be overemphasized. For most of us, self regulation is simply what it takes to get to where we want to go, while maintaining physiological and psychological health.

If you think of the misery that comes from the opposite of self regulation—regulation by circumstances, by other people, or by bad habits—then you will immediately appreciate the joy of self regulation.

Healthy Lifestyle

IIII➡

I lost a friend yesterday. Death set upon him like a monster, gripping him with pain and fear, overwhelming him with fatigue, and finally shaking him loose, lifeless. Gone is a husband, gone a father, gone a brother. In my grief, I am angry. Death came early, uninvited; it was not a welcome release at the end of a fulfilled life. It came as an interloper, seizing a man at the center of his time.

(Farquhar, 1978, p. 1).

This is the dramatic first passage of *The American Way of Life Need Not Be Hazardous to Your Health,* quite a gripping way to begin a book on adopting health habits. John Farquhar, a cardiologist and director of the Stanford Heart Disease Prevention Program (who emphasized skills, not willpower), is writing about his patient Roger, who died at age 45, five months after his first heart attack. As Farquhar says, the records tell when and how Roger died, but not of what he died. Roger died of obesity, of smoking, of hypertension, of stress, and of a lack of exercise; in other words, his lifestyle killed him. The coroner wrote *myocardial infarct*, not *lifestyle* as the cause of death on the death certificate, although both were true.

Where did Roger go wrong? Your answer: "Roger failed to take responsibility for his health, and he did not gain self regulation of his lifestyle habits." That is right.

Roger's lifestyle killed him. Because lifestyle is a factor in health and wellness, we cannot write a textbook on the dynamics of health and wellness without discussing the basics of lifestyle habits that promote health. Anyone interested in personal health and in the health of others must know the basics.

Take a minute: Mentally list the elements of a healthy lifestyle.

Do It Now.

The Other Guy. Drawing by Mankoff; © 1985, *The New Yorker* Magazine, Inc.

YOU AS MODEL

If you plan to become a health professional, plan now to be a good model. It will not do for health professionals to have worseness habits.

If you are a parent or plan to have children, plan now to be a good model. Whether they like it or not, parents are the most important models for children, more than advertising and even peer pressure. When parents model wellness behaviors, children learn wellness behaviors.

You probably thought: regular exercise, good diet, no smoking, no drug abuse, moderate alcohol use, stress management, and maybe using a seat belt. These are typically described as the essentials of a healthy lifestyle because they promote health. Lifestyle, then, refers to habits that make up the way that we live. We include three additional ingredients of lifestyle that are health behaviors and are part of a healthy style of living, but that are not usually considered: assertiveness, nonviolence, and play. The second section of this chapter covers these important ingredients.

Of all the dynamics of health and wellness, lifestyle is most clearly related to social factors. Habits begun in the family are supported or changed by the peer group and may be encouraged by society. Even something as simple as shopping for groceries reflects these variables at every turn of the shopping cart and every choice the buyer makes. The choice not to shop at all—to order out or eat out—is a given in our society. Lifestyle is a biopsychosocial phenomenon with biopsychosocial effects.

SECTION ONE: HEALTHY LIFESTYLE—THE USUALLY INCLUDED

Lifestyle does not sneak up on people and hit them over the head. Roger killed himself.

We do not know about Mr. Wright, but had he been our client, we would have taken a long, hard look at his lifestyle habits. We do not mean the way he dressed, the type of car he drove, or the neighborhood in which he lived. We mean the daily habits that affect health and wellness. This is the new meaning of **lifestyle.** It has taken many decades of research to determine the relative risks of various factors such as smoking, obesity, and hypertension. Determining the risks associated with particular behaviors takes time because lifestyle risks do not

have immediately perceivable effects on the body, and not all people who have a health risk develop symptoms or die as a result. That is why a destructive habit is called a risk and not a certainty.

Typical to the study of health, knowledge of lifestyle habits that promote health comes primarily from studying disease and illness. By studying people such as Roger, the "do nots" of healthy living become apparent: Do not smoke, do not drink alcohol excessively (perhaps not even moderately), do not eat too much fat, do not lead a totally sedentary lifestyle, do not become obese, do not have excessive Type A behaviors, and do not suffer excessive stress.

When these "do nots" are translated into "do's" for guiding health behavior, the question "how much?" immediately arises. How much fat in the diet is safe? How much exercise is good? How many pounds over ideal body weight is okay? How much alcohol, how much stress, how much Type A behavior can the mind and body tolerate without ill effects? Because the factors that affect health are on a continuum, the exact amount that is optimum for any individual is uncertain. For this reason guidelines are created for the general population, meaning people who do not already have health problems. The guidelines for health habits, and the guidelines for physiological parameters such as blood pressure and blood cholesterol, are changed as data accumulate. Please read Box 12.1 now.

This textbook provides guidelines that are accepted today for the major lifestyle components. When the guidelines are followed, the likelihood of a long, disease-free life increases. No one can guarantee a disease-free life, because the guidelines are based on group data and statistics. However, as we tell our students and clients: "You do not know who you are; you do not know whether or not you can have poor health habits and live and die exactly as you wish. And since you do not know, it makes sense to gamble on the side of health."

BOX 12.1

BLOOD CHOLESTEROL AND OTHER FATS

Our grandparents had blood cholesterol but did not know it; no one knew it. They also had globules of high-density lipoproteins, low-density lipoproteins, and very-low-density lipoproteins floating in their blood and did not know that, either. Today most people have at least heard of cholesterol and know that too much fat in the blood is risky; many have their blood fat levels measured routinely.

This impressive advance in medical and public knowledge results from the effort to understand coronary heart disease. The first step was to link the fatty substance found in arteries at autopsy to fat that is carried in the blood. Simultaneously a way of measuring blood fat was developed. Next, the link between dietary fat and blood fat was established. Through laboratory animal and human research, these associations have been made. At the same time, research on the molecular structure of dietary fat, blood fat, and the fat that clogs arteries revealed that there are many types of fat, including cholesterol, which is a component of the fatty plaques that clog and damage the artery walls. It was also important to determine how the body manufactures and metabolizes fat.

Once it was established that coronary heart disease results from clogged and damaged arteries, that cholesterol is a component in plaques, and that cholesterol can be measured, then the question of how much blood cholesterol is harmful arose.

Fifteen years ago blood cholesterol level was not a routine measure. When it was measured, the patient was rarely given the result unless it was above 300 mg/ml, because at that time the "normal" range went as high as 300 mgs for a 45-year-old man. When one of the authors (RS) had a cardiovascular checkup after his father's early death, he was given neither his blood pressure nor blood cholesterol levels and was simply told that he was healthy. It was several years later that RS, having informed himself about these physiological parameters, asked for his records and discovered that both were high according to the data at that time.

Today blood cholesterol level guidelines adopted by the National Heart, Lung, and Blood Institute and the American Heart Association are: high risk, 240 mg/dl or above; borderline-high, 200–239 mg/dl; desirable, 200 mg/dl or lower.

Nutrition

Rarely will you find co-authors with such divergent nutritional childhoods. RS ate meat three times a day, savored crispy chicken skin, dunked bread in whatever grease there was, poured gravy over everything, and ate dessert every night. I, JG, was born into the original health food family. First the knowledgeable and creative grandparents became vegetarians, then the parents, and then the children, somewhat unwillingly. The grown-ups in the family were thrilled by the virtues of sunflower seed and millet patties. They served up fried soybeans, put powdered yeast in tomato juice as a snack, and marveled at the technological advances that produced powdered milk, which in those days was lumpy and blue, and was made barely tolerable with black-strap molasses, also a favorite. "Dessert" was how I misspelled the dry place where cacti grow. In grade school I volunteered as many times as possible for cafeteria monitor so that I could eat the cafeteria food. Home cooking was that bad (at least to a nine-year-old).

Now I am glad. I have been nutritionally conscious for a long time. After his father died, RS became nutritionally conscious, and together we have become more knowledgeable. If you let your diet be determined by your friends, fast-food chains, convenience stores, the kitchen cupboard, the refrigerator, or habit, you may be victimizing your body, the innocent bystander. Your body never forces you to eat anything. Everything you eat is the result of a decision.

Guidelines are created to help people make wise choices. The Human Nutrition Information Service of the United States Department of Agriculture (1985) has published seven general nutrition guidelines for Americans:

Eat a variety of foods.
Maintain a desirable weight.
Avoid too much fat, saturated fat, and cholesterol.
Eat foods with adequate starch and fiber.
Avoid too much sugar.
Avoid too much sodium.
If you drink alcoholic beverages, do so in moderation.

Sometimes guidelines are stated more specifically. For example, Nathan Pritikin, founder of the Pritikin Longevity Centers and Pritikin foods, created stringent guidelines for the consumption of protein, carbohydrate, fat, and cholesterol because he worked primarily with people who were at risk for cardiovascular disease or who were already sick. The American Heart Association has published less stringent guidelines. Table 12.1 shows the guidelines of Pritikin (1979), the American Heart Association (1988), and what the average American actually eats.

These guidelines are of little value without information. To follow them one must know what "too much" means, and what one's "desirable" weight is, and what "moderation" in drinking refers to. Specifically, one must know:

1. The number of calories consumed daily.
2. The number of calories needed to maintain ideal weight, if you do not exercise.
3. The foods that are primarily fat, protein, or carbohydrate.
4. The amount of fat, protein, and carbohydrate in the foods you eat.
5. The meanings of saturated, monounsaturated, and polyunsaturated fats and the foods that contain them.
6. The milligrams of cholesterol in the food you eat.
7. The milligrams of sodium in the food you eat.

Table 12.1   American Heart Association and Pritikin Guidelines

	Percent of Total Calories		
	Average American	Pritikin	American Heart Association
Protein	12	10	12
Carbohydrate	46	80	58
Pure sugar	18		10
Fat	42	10	30
Monounsaturated	19		10
Saturated	16		10
Polyunsaturated	7		10

In addition, you should know:

1. What your ideal weight is, and what you weigh now.
2. What your blood fats and cholesterol should be, and what they are now.
3. What your blood pressure should be, and what it is now.

As a start, we provide little lessons. To be fully informed and the best guardian of your health, you need to research these issues on your own. Fortunately, this is easy. Bookstores, the federal government, and organizations such as the American Heart Association provide all the information that you need to understand your diet and to modify it if necessary.

Little Lessons

The body must have six ingredients: water, vitamins, minerals, carbohydrates, fats, and proteins. Some nutritionists say that taking vitamin and mineral supplements is unnecessary for people who eat a balanced diet with lots of fresh vegetables, fruits, and whole grains. Unfortunately, many people do not eat balanced meals. These little lessons will focus on the "macronutrients": carbohydrates, fats, and proteins.

Carbohydrates

You may have heard that some carbohydrates are complex and some are simple. **Simple** carbohydrates are called sugar, the simplest being sucrose, of which table sugar is a variety. Fruits

contain a simple carbohydrate called fructose. The simplest sugar molecule looks like this: $C_6H_{12}O_6$. **Complex** carbohydrate molecules have the same atoms—carbon, hydrogen, and oxygen—but the sugar molecules are arranged into much more complex structures. Some complex carbohydrates are starch, and others are fiber. The starches in rice, potatoes, beans, all the grains, nuts, corn, and other vegetables have different arrangements of the molecules. Glucose, which is blood sugar, is the primary energy molecule of the body and is the only source of energy for the brain. For this reason the body is a master at absorbing sugar and breaking down complex carbohydrates into glucose. The body stores any extra glucose as fat.

So what is wrong with living on Twinkies? Do this: mold two Twinkies into one form about the size of a baking potato. Now compare your "Twinkie potato" with a real potato, as shown in Table 12.2.

In other words, foods loaded with sugar and fat such as pastries, pies, and cakes are nutrient-poor for their calories; foods that are primarily complex carbohydrates such as pasta, breads and cereals, vegetables, and grains are nutrient-rich for their calories. Go for the real potato unless it is turned into potato chips or french fries in which case you are eating one potato plus three tablespoons of fat, or one potato plus two tablespoons of fat.

Complex carbohydrates (which are not refined of nutrients and bran, as white flour and white rice are) are good sources of protein and **fiber** and are low in fat. As a bonus, plant carbohydrates have **no** cholesterol because plants do not make cholesterol. One type of

Table 12.2

	Calories	Fat	Carbohydrates	Protein	Sodium	Cholesterol
Twinkie potato (approximate)	239	14.9 gm	22.9 gm	3.8 gm	141 mg	23.6
Real potato	115	.1 gm	26.7 gm	2.5 gm	12 mg	0

fiber provides the bulk that the gastrointestinal tract needs (wheat bran is a good source), and the other carries cholesterol out of the system (oat bran and the fiber in apples are good sources).

Fats (Lipids)

Fat molecules are made of carbon, hydrogen, and oxygen atoms, allowing the body to store sugar in a convenient package and convert the package back into sugar as needed. Enzymes convert glucose into fat and fat into glucose. The most common dietary fat molecule, triglyceride, is made up of three fatty acids, which are chains of carbon atoms with hydrogen attached, connected to a glycerol body. About 95 percent of all dietary and body fats are triglycerides; the rest is mainly cholesterol. Triglycerides are either saturated, monounsaturated, or polyunsaturated. **Saturated** fats have hydrogen atoms connected to every carbon atom in the fatty acid chains; these fats are solid at room temperature and are the bad guys. Most animal fats are saturated and become quite solid on your dinner plate or in the frying pan when it cools. Most of the fat that Americans eat comes from animals and is saturated. Saturated fat raises blood cholesterol. "Better" fat, which is not naturally saturated and is liquid at room temperature, can be saturated by adding hydrogen atoms, a process called hydrogenation. Some margarines are made of liquid vegetable oil that has been hydrogenated so that the stick of margarine will stay firm through dinner on a warm summer evening. Saturated fats are used in processing food, such as making potato chips, because they have a longer shelf life then polyunsaturated fats. (Your shelf life goes down but the shelf life of the potato chip goes up when saturated fats are used in processing.)

The monounsaturated fats (coconut and olive oils) and the polyunsaturated fats (corn, safflower, and peanut oils) are liquid at room temperature and below. Although olive oil has recently been given a better report card, the best oils are the polyunsaturated. Nevertheless, the best advice is to eat less fat of all types. The number one killer of Americans is heart disease, and the fatty American diet is partly responsible.

The body needs only one tablespoon of fat per day, but the average American adult body gets about six tablespoons; what is not burned or carried out of the body is stored as fat. Obesity is a hazard to the cardiovascular system. It is associated with diabetes and possibly certain cancers, and it is a strain on joints. But obesity is only one side effect of too much dietary fat; the other is clogged arteries. The fat that clogs arteries and may result in a heart attack or stroke is the fat that travels in blood after processing in the liver.

To travel in blood, fat must be packaged. The protein packages are of three types: **high-density lipoproteins** (HDLs), **low-density lipoproteins** (LDLs), and **very-low-density lipoproteins** (VLDLs). When blood fat is measured, values for these lipoproteins may be given. Research indicates that a high level of HDLs is good, because HDL carries cholesterol out of the blood into the liver. LDLs carry cholesterol into the blood. This is a simplified story; in fact, there are different types of HDL and LDL, called fractions. The fractions have varying beneficial or harmful effects.

Protein

If all the water were taken out of your body, you would be mostly protein, which is the building block of bones, teeth, hair, enzymes, antibodies, blood, tendons, and much more. Proteins contain carbon, hydrogen, oxygen, and nitrogen atoms. Proteins are complex structures that are made up of simpler structures called amino acids. Some proteins are made up of as many as 300 amino acids. The body combines 21 basic amino acids to form all the proteins in the body. It constructs 13 amino acids from carbohydrates and fats. The eight other amino acids must be part of the diet because the body cannot manufacture them; these are called the essential amino acids because it is essential that we provide them in the diet.

A generation ago it was thought that eating a lot of protein was good. Now we know that we need very little protein, as long as we get the essential amino acids. The problem with eating a lot of protein is not that protein itself is bad for health as much as the fat that comes with it is, particularly saturated fat, because the main source of protein in this country comes from meat and dairy products. Plants are also a good source of protein.

Sodium

Sodium is part of table salt. The body needs 200–500 mg of sodium daily; the average American consumes more than 6,000. Look at this:

chicken dinner (fast food)	=	2,243 mg
processed cheese (1 oz)	=	337
canned green beans (1cup)	=	326
tomato juice (1 cup)	=	878
cottage cheese (4 oz.)	=	457
Bran Chex (2/3 cup)	=	262
chicken soup (canned)	=	1,107
pancake mix (1 cup)	=	2,036

People on a restricted-sodium diet try to consume only 1,000–2,000 mg a day. You could have a wholesome lunch—chicken soup, cottage cheese, and tomato juice—and consume 2,442 mg of sodium without touching the salt shaker. The primary sources of sodium are processed foods, table salt, and preservatives. The taste for salt is acquired and begins in childhood with processed baby foods.

If you do not have the time or inclination to create a nutritional program for yourself, but are nutritionally conscious enough to know that you are probably not on target with the guidelines, then follow the suggestions in Box 12.2.

People who are near ideal weight, feel great, and are never sick might think the guidelines do not apply to them. They are wrong. The guidelines are for today, for the simple reason that what people do now sets up the future, and a string of todays is the future. Good nutrition today prevents nutrition-related disorders in the future and is an important factor in preventing obesity, a health risk in many disorders.

When you eat more unrefined carbohydrates and fresh vegetables and less fat, meat, and processed foods, you will get several bonuses: less sodium, less sugar, fewer preservatives, and more fiber. You can be as creative or as simple as you like. If your schedule is

---

BOX 12.2

TIPS FOR BETTER NUTRITION

Fat: Cut back all types of fat and especially animal fat found in red meat, chicken skin, whole and 2 percent milk, cheese, french fries, chips, and deep fried food.

Carbohydrates: Cut back on all sugar-type carbohydrates, including candy bars, pastries, and sodas, as well as some cereals and sauces. Eat complex carbohydrates such as potatoes, pasta, all grains, and whole wheat breads. Eat vegetables and fresh fruits.

Protein: If you are a vegetarian, combine plant proteins to get all the essential amino acids. When you cut back on animal products, you will automatically cut back on protein, which is good.

Cholesterol: Cut back on high-cholesterol foods—eggs, meat, dairy products, and shellfish—so that you get no more than 300 mg a day.

Sodium: Cut back on foods that contain high amounts of sodium, such as pickles, lunch meats, processed foods, canned vegetables, cheeses, sauces, cocoa, tomato juice, and instant pudding. Increasingly, manufacturers are producing processed foods with less sodium, including corn chips, soy sauce, canned vegetables, cottage cheese, and margarine.

LABELS ARE THERE TO READ

There was never a chance that the body could evolve as fast as the food industry. That is why the best diet is "back to basics." The human body evolved on a diet of low meat, low sodium, low sugar, low fat, and low preservatives. It was not designed to handle the luxuries of modern life. The typical American diet is excessive in everything except the foods that are best for the body. Take a good look at your diet, waistline, and blood fats before you decide that you have nothing to worry about.

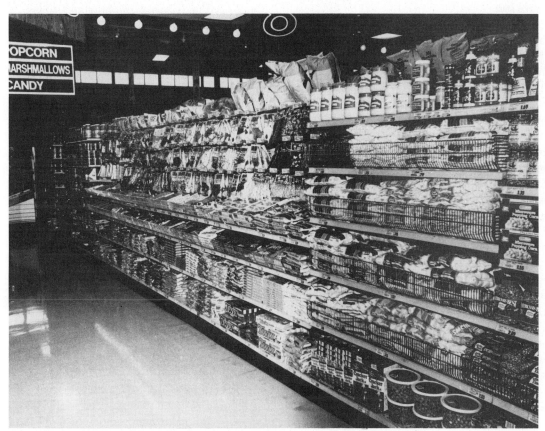

The Selection of Non-Nutritious Food is Staggering.
Source: Mike Shellenberger, Greeley, CO.

tight, simplicity is the answer—not the simplicity of a TV dinner, but the simplicity of a bowl of tofu and stir-fried vegetables, or boiled potatoes and greens covered with salsa. Keep a couple of quarts of cooked brown rice ready to heat; make a large salad and serve it as supper.

It is unlikely that you will be required to take a nutrition class to graduate, get married, or parent a child. You will probably have to become nutritionally conscious and knowledgeable on your own. This is what self regulation is all about.

Exercise

The cardiovascular system, muscles, ligaments, tendons, and bones were born to be used. Only since the Industrial Revolution, city dwelling, desk work, and mechanized farming has a sedentary lifestyle become the norm. Today, we must create exercise programs and consciously make physical exercise a part of daily life. If we do not get organized, we will not get exercised.

The amount of exercise you get should not be at the mercy of friends, circumstances, habits, or the weather. Making exercise a part of your lifestyle, however, may be just as hard as making good nutrition a part of your lifestyle. If you are starting from scratch, putting together a cardiovascular fitness program may be easier than putting together an eating program. Like the billiard balls that we all studied in physics, human bodies have inertia. Or is it the human mind? If you have the habit of not exercising or do not have an "athletic person" as part of your self-image, then getting started may be your biggest hurdle. Please read Box 12.3 now.

Once you decide to get serious about exercising, you have only to decide what activity you can do that will meet the FIT guidelines for frequency, intensity, and time. Based on extensive research on cardiovascular fitness, the American

---

BOX 12.3

TIPS FOR GETTING STARTED

1. Join something: a gym class, jogging club, YMCA, or sports center.
2. Invest some money in your program.
3. Be around people who are getting started.
4. Watch *Chariots of Fire*.
5. If exercising is not its own reward for you, figure out good rewards.
6. Say to yourself a thousand times, "I am a person who exercises."
7. Think of someone who is sedentary and sickly, or a victim of heart disease, and muster your determination not to be like that.
8. Reread the sections on decision-making, commitment, and maintaining commitment.
9. Think of your 20-year high school reunion and how you want to look.
10. Visualize yourself doing your activity with your best qualities shining through the sweat: grace, determination, speed, humor, endurance, and a go-for-the-gold side of you that even you did not know about.

College of Sports Medicine (1980) suggests the following guidelines for aerobic training:

Frequency: 3–5 times a week; every other day is good. Some sports physiologists recommend a minimum of 4 periods of exercise a week for cardiovascular fitness (Getchell, 1987).

Intensity: Begin at 70 percent of maximum heart rate and work up to 85 percent.

Time: 20–30 minutes for continuous exercises such as jogging; 40–50 minutes for stop-and-go exercises such as tennis.

These guidelines are meaningless unless you know:

1. Which exercises are aerobic.
2. How to calculate your target heart rate.

You probably know that aerobic means *with oxygen*, and aerobic exercises are those that cause the body to burn oxygen. Aerobic exercises put a demand on the lungs and cardiovascular system to deliver the oxygen efficiently. Aerobic exercises include running, jogging, walking, biking, skiing, swimming, racket sports, rowing, and skipping rope.

You also need to know the basics of the warm-up and cool-down stretches with which you should begin and end every exercise session. You might also like to know your fitness level at this time. You can take a stress test, which involves running on a treadmill or riding a stationary bicycle while your heart rate, blood pressure, and ECG are monitored. Or you can take the field test developed by the father of aerobic exercise, Dr. Kenneth Cooper. Using Cooper's test (1982), you measure how far you can walk or run in 12 minutes. We

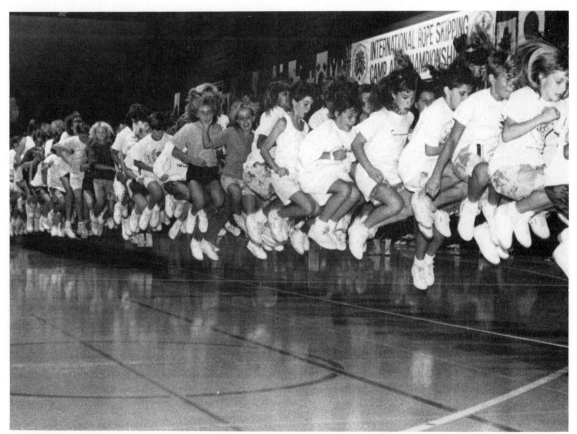

Exercise Could Be a Societal Norm. Unfortunately, Many of These Young People Will Become Obese Adults.
Source: Gordon Steward, Denver, CO.

recommend a look at Cooper's point system described in *Aerobics* (Cooper, 1968). The goal is to earn 30 points a week. Points are earned by amount of time and type of exercise. Twelve minutes of jogging in place is equal to 20 minutes of moderate swimming. If you think that 12 minutes of jogging in place is nothing, get up and try it.

Following are some basic principles of aerobic exercise to help guide you in determining your program.

1. If you have been sedentary, begin slowly.
2. Your exercise must involve the large muscles of the body, particular the leg muscles.
3. Let your body be your guide; do not push it when it hurts.
4. It takes effort to get in shape; staying in shape takes less effort.
5. If you have an injury or think that you might have a heart condition, consult a physician before beginning your exercise program.
6. Your intensity level should not be greater than a level at which you can carry on a conversation.
7. Design a program that will help you meet your personal goals.
8. Make it fun.

Once you get into a regular exercise program you can expect these benefits: lower blood pressure; more efficient heart and lungs; increased stamina; more collateral blood vessels to the heart; stronger bones; a slower heart rate; larger stroke volume; less peripheral resistance; an increase in HDL and a decrease in LDL; less body fat; less depression; more self-esteem; and much, much more.

If regular exercise simply cannot be a part of your lifestyle now, then at least walk a little faster; park your car a couple of blocks farther from work; use the stairs; take a stairs break instead of a coffee break; bend over twice to pick up something; stand up when you talk on the phone; and do a few stretching exercises while waiting for the teapot to come to a boil.

Smoking

Guideline: Never. Cigarette smoking is the most important preventable cause of death in the United States. A study conducted by the California Department of Health Services for a single year, 1985, estimated that in California smoking was directly responsible for 31,289 deaths; 310,018 years of potential life lost; 313,065 hospital admissions in which the person lived; $4.1 billion in-hospital and other medical-care costs; and more than $7.1 billion in total costs, including health-care and other costs in the state (Centers for Disease Control, 1989). These data for a single state are representative of the United States.

Alcohol Consumption

Alcohol is the most abused drug in the United States. It is responsible for more highway and other deaths, highway and other injuries, disease, and violence than any other drug. The cost of alcohol abuse in deaths, lost productivity, crime, incarceration, alcoholism treatment, and medical treatment is over $100 billion each year. Yet drinking is a social institution in this country, and alcohol products are extensively advertised. This contradiction arises in part because drinking in moderation has not been associated with physical or social harm, and even drunkenness and driving while drunk have been tolerated behaviors. In the 1980s, social and legal pressure against alcohol abuse intensified. Organizations such as Mothers Against Drunk Driving (MADD) and Students Against Drunk Driving (SADD) have been important in increasing public awareness of the problem and in raising and enforcing the legal penalties for alcohol abuse, particularly driving while intoxicated. At the same time, treatment centers for alcoholism have proliferated, and most colleges have counseling for problem drinkers on campus.

Before considering guidelines for alcohol use, remember these facts: Alcohol is a sugar and adds empty calories to your diet; alcohol affects the brain and reduces coordination, reaction time, and judgment; chronic and heavy use of alcohol may damage the brain, liver, heart, vascular system, and gastrointestinal tract; moderate to heavy alcohol use may affect unborn children; alcohol interacts with other drugs and may be dangerous or fatal when combined; and no two people have the same

tolerance for alcohol, and the amount that is safe for you cannot be determined by the amount that your friends drink.

Guideline: The most common guideline is slight to moderate alcohol consumption for healthy people without central nervous system, liver, cardiovascular, or gastrointestinal disorders, who are not taking medications that might interact with alcohol, and who are not pregnant. Moderate drinking is defined as drinking at least once a week with small amounts (one drink) per occasion, or 3–4 times a month with moderate amounts (2–4 drinks) per occasion, or no more than once a month with large amounts

Table 12.3

Body Weight (Pounds)	100	120	140	160	180	200	220	240
Number of Drinks in 1 Hour								
1	.03	.03	.02	.02	.02	.01	.01	—
2	.06	.05	.04	.04	.03	.03	.03	.02
3	.10	.08	.07	.06	.05	.05	.04	.04
4	.13	.10	.09	.08	.07	.06	.06	.05
5	.16	.13	.11	.10	.09	.08	.07	.07
6	.19	.16	.13	.12	.11	.10	.09	.08
7	.23	.19	.16	.14	.13	.11	.10	.09
8	.26	.22	.18	.16	.14	.13	.12	.11
Number of Drinks in 2 Hours								
1	.01	.01	—	—	—	—	—	—
2	.04	.03	.02	.01	.01	.01	—	—
3	.08	.06	.04	.03	.03	.02	.02	.01
4	.11	.09	.07	.06	.05	.04	.03	.03
5	.15	.12	.10	.08	.07	.06	.05	.04
6	.18	.14	.12	.10	.09	.08	.07	.06
7	.22	.18	.15	.12	.11	.09	.08	.07
8	.25	.20	.17	.15	.13	.11	.10	.09

Source: National Institute on Drug Abuse, Rockville, Maryland.

(5 or more drinks). A "drink" is 12 ounces of beer, 4 ounces of wine, or 1 ounce of distilled spirits.

Guideline for drinking and driving: One guideline for driving and drinking is simple—if you drink, don't drive. If you are drinking in a group, choose a designated driver who will not drink and who will be responsible for driving the drinkers home; otherwise, take a cab or call a friend. In fact, many people who drink also drive. Because it is illegal (and obviously dangerous) to drive while intoxicated, a way of determining intoxication has been established, based on the level of alcohol in the blood. The amount of alcohol in blood depends upon several factors: (1) body weight; (2) amount of alcohol consumed in a given time; (3) amount of food in the stomach; and (4) body chemistry.

In most states, intoxication is defined as 0.1 percent blood alcohol, but central nervous system changes can occur with as little as 0.05 percent. Table 12.3 gives approximate blood alcohol levels for given body weight and number of drinks consumed. If you consider using the data in the table as a guideline for your drinking, remember that you are unique and that a table may not be accurate for you. You are the best judge of your response to alcohol and the

ARE YOU A PROBLEM DRINKER?

Section One: Yes   No

1. Do you occasionally drink heavily after a disappointment, a quarrel, or when the boss gives you a hard time?
2. When you have trouble or feel under pressure, do you always drink more heavily than usual?
3. Have you noticed that you are able to handle more liquor than you did when you were first drinking?
4. Did you ever wake up on the morning after and discover that you could not remember part of the evening before, even though your friends tell you that you did not pass out?
5. When drinking with other people, do you try to have a few extra drinks when others will not know about it?
6. Are there certain occasions when you feel uncomfortable if alcohol is not available?
7. Have you recently noticed that when you begin drinking you are in more of a hurry to get the first drink than you used to be?
8. Do you sometimes feel guilty about your drinking?

Section Two:

9. Are you secretly irritated when your family or friends discuss your drinking?
10. Have you recently noticed an increase in the frequency of your memory blackouts?
11. Do you often wish to continue drinking after your friends say that they have had enough?

Yes   **No**

12. Do you usually have a reason for the occasions when you drink heavily?

13. When you are sober, do you often regret things you have done or said while drinking?

14. Have you tried switching brands or following different plans for controlling your drinking?

15. Have you often failed to keep the promises you have made to yourself about controlling or cutting down on your drinking?

16. Have you ever tried to control your drinking by making a change in jobs or moving to a new location?

17. Do you try to avoid family or close friends while you are drinking?

18. Are you having an increasing number of financial and work problems?

19. Do more people seem to be treating you unfairly without good reason?

20. Do you eat very little or irregularly when you are drinking?

21. Do you sometimes have the shakes in the morning and find that it helps to have a little drink?

Section Three:

22. Have you recently noticed that you cannot drink as much as you once did?

23. Do you sometimes stay drunk for several days at a time?

24. Do you sometimes feel very depressed and wonder whether life is worth living?

25. Sometimes after periods of drinking, do you see or hear things that aren't there?

26. Do you get terribly frightened after you have been drinking heavily?

If you answered "yes" to two or more of the questions in the above sections, the National Council on Alcoholism suggests that you reevaluate your drinking behaviors.

Section One (Questions 1 to 8):   Early stage—drinking is a regular part of your life.

Section Two (Questions 9–21):   Middle stage—you are having trouble controlling when, where, and how much you drink.

Section Three (Questions 22–26):   Final stage—you can no longer control your desire to drink.

Source: National Council on Alcoholism

only person who is responsible for limiting your drinking.

Seat Belts

Guideline: Use seat belts, and add child restraints for your children. Thousands of traffic deaths and serious injuries are prevented each year by the use of seat belts and child restraints.

Stress Management

Guideline: Always.

Now that chronic stress is known to be deleterious to health, stress management is given the status of a component of healthy lifestyle.

In Chapter 3, Stress, you assessed three areas in which stress is manifested—physical, emotional and behavioral—and you know whether you are a victim of paper-clip stress. You have calculated your level of daily hassles and major life events, and you know that perceptions play a major role in stress. You know that unmet needs create stress, and that needs, as described by Maslow, are complex. You understand hardiness, stress resistance, and learned resourcefulness; you know that social support and social skills are important in resisting stress. Your stress-management style comprises your hardiness, stress resistance, and learned resourcefulness, combined with stress-management skills. You are familiar with stress inoculation, long and short relaxation techniques, autogenic feedback training, two-stage breathing, imagery and visualization for relaxation, self-exploration, and rehearsal. Other stress-management skills are time management, assertiveness, decision-making, and problem-solving.

The essence of good stress management is reducing stress through internal processes such as relaxation, imagery, stress inoculation, and cognitive restructuring. The term also means "managing" in the sense of "doing something about," and that refers to the external environment. Restructuring the external environment to reduce stress is an extremely important aspect of stress management. This includes simple changes such as getting a brighter reading lamp or having your own tube of toothpaste that you can squeeze any way you want, and more complex changes such as getting dormmates to honor the quiet time or getting your children and spouse to do their own laundry, or the city to repair the streets. Getting one's needs met, including environmental restructuring, necessitates assertiveness, and that is why we include assertiveness as a component of healthy lifestyle.

The effect of stress on physical and psychological well-being cannot be underestimated, and therefore the importance of stress management cannot be underestimated. Stress management must be a part of everyone's lifestyle. When everyone handles stress better, there is less stress to handle.

IIII➡

SECTION TWO: THE USUALLY NOT INCLUDED

Assertiveness

Guideline: Be assertive when you have an important need or want that is not being met.

Assertiveness is the skill of looking out for one's needs and wants with clarity, tact, and a sense of compromise. Interpersonal conflict—conflict with parents, spouse, children, boss, or employees—is a major stressor and is usually the result of unmet or threatened needs and wants. In Chapters 6 and 10, social skills such as friendliness and empathy were discussed as resources for coping with stress. Assertiveness skills are also important for coping with stress because these skills are the key to getting one's needs met.

Many clients that we see in our private

practice are unassertive. For example, one unassertive client, Mrs. Smith, says that she does not have time to practice relaxation skills because, after working an eight-hour day, she must fix dinner for her family, clean up, do the wash, and make the childrens' lunches. After that, she is exhausted and falls asleep while doing the training. When asked why she does not change this routine by enlisting her husband and children, she replies that she can't. She has a hundred reasons, including failure in her previous attempts to change the routine. Mrs. Smith is not assertive; she can become angry or depressed, but she does not know how to be assertive.

Joseph Wolpe (1958) defined assertiveness as "expressing personal rights and feelings." In working with patients who have psychophysiological disorders, a discussion of reasonable rights is important. It became important for Mrs. Smith to believe that she had a right to take time to practice relaxation training. This meant that she had a right *not* to do all the cooking and cleaning. She had a right to expect her husband and children to share the work.

Consider the following "Bill of Personal Rights":

You have a right to make mistakes.
You have a right to change your mind or decide on a different course of action.
You have a right to protest unfair treatment or criticism.
You have a right to put yourself first, sometimes.
You have a right to your own opinions and convictions.
You have a right to negotiate for change.
You have a right to ask for help or emotional support.
You have a right to ignore the advice of others.
You have a right to say "no."
You have a right not to take responsibility for someone else's problem.

Your Perfect Right,
Alberti & Emmons (1970)

Assertiveness training is often stereotyped as aggression training. The belief is that people become irritable, manipulative, and aggressive after assertiveness training. In reality, the purpose of assertiveness training is to teach people how to be more relaxed in interpersonal situations so that they can express needs and feelings in appropriate ways and avoid both aggressive and passive modes of communication.

After Mrs. Smith was convinced that she had a right to practice relaxation training, she role-played inappropriate and appropriate ways of expressing her needs.

Inappropriate Communications: Aggressive

Mrs. Smith to family: "I'm tired of being your slave! I can't believe how selfish all of you are. You don't care whether I'm sick or healthy as long as your dinner is on the table. You've become irresponsible brats including you, Dick [to husband]! From now on, I'm doing my relaxation exercises every day when I get home whether you like it or not."

Inappropriate Communications: Passive

Mrs. Smith to family: "My therapist says I need to practice my relaxation training five times a week. I'm wondering if you would be willing to share in some of the cooking and cleaning so I'm not so tired when I do my relaxation exercises."

Appropriate Communications: Assertive

Mrs. Smith to family: "In order to learn the necessary skills for getting over my high blood pressure, I need to practice relaxation training five times a week. The best time for me to do this is when I come home after work. After dinner I am too tired and fall asleep, and I am not really learning to relax.

"I would like us to take turns fixing the evening meal. There are five of us, so we can each fix one dinner a week. On the sixth night, we will go out for dinner, and the seventh night we will each fix our own dinner. This will enable me to come home after work and practice for 30 minutes five times a week."

Mrs. Smith role-played a variety of situations and possible responses from each family member. She replied first from the aggressive stance, then the passive, and finally the assertive. She then used her assertiveness skills with the family. The family was surprised at first but understood her need to practice relaxation training. Life at home became more pleasant, and she felt much better about her children and husband, who took responsibility for chores. Of equal importance, the family members gained awareness and respect for one another's needs, an important benefit of assertiveness. The tricky element in the right to be assertive is that the right belongs to everyone. When people feel that their needs are worth being assertive about, then compromise—involving empathy and problem-solving—must be a companion skill.

Assertiveness must be a part of everyone's lifestyle until the day comes when everyone anticipates and honors everyone else's needs.

Nonviolence

Guideline: Always be nonviolent, except in self-defense, unless one is practicing *ahimsa*, described below, in which case not even then.

We live in a violent society. The United States has a homicide rate 50 times higher than New Zealand. Hong Kong is far more densely populated than the city of Detroit, yet the citizens of Hong Kong suffer far less violence. Child abuse is virtually nonexistent in China (Stevenson, 1974). In the United States each year 200,000 children are physically abused, another 100,000 are sexually abused, and 800,000 are neglected (American Humane Association, 1981).

In this country, violence is glorified and condoned as viciousness, justified retribution, self-defense, and entertainment. As viciousness, violence is punished at the same time as it is "glorified" in the media as being newsworthy. As retribution or as self-defense, violence is condoned. As entertainment, violence is a box-office hit. As a way of life, physical and psychological violence against children, women, and minorities has gone unnoticed or accepted in this society for decades (Archer & Gartner, 1985).

Violence destroys, damages, perpetuates fear and anxiety, alienates, prevents normal psychological development, and begets more violence. Ninety percent of adults who abuse their children were abused as children (Macklin & Rubin, 1983). People who lash out verbally or physically, who justify violence, and who trap others in a snare of spoken or unspoken threats have a violent lifestyle. When family members must "walk on eggs" in fear of triggering violence, the family has accepted a violent lifestyle, even if overt violence is rare.

The type of violence seen in newspaper headlines is uncommon compared to the insidious and sometimes subtle "put-downs," insults, shouting matches, slaps, threats, and angry outbursts that punctuate life in some families and relationships. In Chapter 20, Societal and Cultural Forces Against Health and Wellness, we discuss violence further. Our purpose here is to introduce nonviolence as an essential dynamic in a healthy lifestyle. We include nonviolence as a component of healthy lifestyle because nonviolence is good for everyone's health and wellness. Nonviolence perpetuates an atmosphere of love and caring in which people can grow to their full potential of physical, psychological, and spiritual well-being.

Principles of Nonviolence

Throughout history violence has had great champions, but so has nonviolence: the Buddha, Jesus, St. Francis of Assisi, Gandhi, and Martin

Luther King, Jr. Today nonviolence is usually associated with nonviolent political action, but these champions practiced and taught nonviolence as a way of life, not merely as a political tool. While domestic and societal violence are slowly becoming issues of public concern, methods for preventing violence and interest in adopting nonviolence as the cultural norm are sorely lacking. The great champions of nonviolence, many who died by violence, have had little impact: Christians ignore the Sermon on the Mount, Hindus ignore the extensive Hindu scriptures on nonviolence. On the earth today no society is devoted to nonviolence. As a way of life, nonviolence is practiced only in isolated religious communities, perhaps the largest of which is the Jains in India. In the West, religious groups such as the Amish, Mennonites, and Quakers practice nonviolence as a way of life. The Quakers especially have focused on nonviolence as a viable way of life for society, beyond its religious connotations and the religious community.

What does "nonviolent lifestyle" mean? When we look for the best sources on nonviolence, we find that they are religions. Although most religions contain doctrine on nonviolence, Jainism, Hinduism, and Buddhism have the most extensive texts and the longest tradition of teaching nonviolence. It was from these traditions, and from his study of the Sermon on the Mount, that India's leader of nonviolent change during the struggle for independence from Great Britain, Mahatma Gandhi, fashioned his philosophy that guided every aspect of his life (Sheehan, 1987). The Hindi word for violence is **himsa,** and **ahimsa** means nonviolence.

The principles of *ahimsa* that are common to all teachings are these:

> (1) Not only nonviolence, noninjury in one's thoughts, words, and actions which may be directly committed, commissioned or consented to, but also love in one's thoughts, words, actions and intentions; (2) truthfulness; (3) nonstealing; (4) detachment; (5) control of the senses (passions); (6) not only nonanger, but love; (7) not only nongreed, but generosity; (8) desire for the welfare of all beings; (9) treating all equally; (10) simplicity; (11) peace of mind; (12) compassion; (13) forgiveness.
>
> (Sheehan, 1987, p. 95)

In addition, the major teachings emphasize the fact that violence begins in the mind, as does nonviolence, and that we can blame no one for our violence; we alone are responsible for our thoughts, words, and actions.

We see that the practice of nonviolence does not mean merely noninjury to others, for it includes the positive, that is, love, generosity, equality, and so forth. To be nonviolent, one must do more than merely eliminate injurious negative thoughts, words, and actions; one must actively practice positive thoughts, words, and actions. The Judeo-Christian Golden Rule—Do unto others as you would have them do unto you— encapsulates *ahimsa* as it is practiced in daily life. And the essence of the Golden Rule is love.

The doctrine of love—manifesting love in thoughts, words, and actions—is common to all major religious teachings and is in many ways the hallmark of Christianity. Love is the heart of nonviolence, because love dispels violence. Love and violence cannot coexist in the same thought, word, or action. If you know anyone who is truly loving, you will notice that the person is also nonviolent.

For people who live in a violent society and do not practice nonviolence as part of a religious tradition, the practice of nonviolence in daily life is probably as hard as getting the proverbial camel through the eye of the needle.

Conflict seems inevitable. People have different needs and backgrounds, and power struggles occur, particularly in families. In families, there are two natural periods in which power struggles are likely: when a child, about age 2, develops a budding sense of self as separate from parent, and says "no" as a demonstration of individual power; and in adolescence, when the identity of the self as a separate individual, with ideas and values different from parents, must be completed. The manner in which the early power struggle is handled can set the pattern for the family, and there are many unhealthy styles, such as passive, pleading, coercing, or violent. In violent relationships, conflicts are solved through physical and psychological abuse.

Nonviolence in the Family

Gandhi taught that the place to begin the practice of *ahimsa* is in the home, and only when mastered at home can it be practiced as a tool for righting social inequality. Similarly, child psychologists emphasize that the key to developing healthy people is a healthy home, and healthy means nonviolent. Children learn empathy and understanding from their parents; children have difficulty learning to be empathetic when they have no empathetic role models or their role models are dictatorial. Parents can model problem-solving through negotiations, or they can model violence and rigidity.

Unfortunately, the adage "Spare the rod and spoil the child" is deeply rooted in many families; many people believe the only way to solve problems is through spanking, hitting, or beating children or spouses. Children and other members of families in which problems are solved through violence often learn to resolve conflict through aggression or withdrawal, they become aggressive or passive. It is amazing to us how often an adult who was beaten as a child condones the violence, saying "I deserved it" or "It straightened me out." Perhaps this is a protective mechanism that Freud called "identification with the aggressor"; in any case, such people usually condone their own violence, because someone deserved it, or needed to be straightened out, or it was for their own good—and the violence continues.

The structure of families is similar to the structure of a society: authoritarian, laissez faire, or a constitutional democracy. Laissez

THE PERILS OF CHILDHOOD

German child psychiatrist Alice Miller has written extensively about the perils of childhood in her books, *For Your Own Good: Hidden Cruelty in Child-Rearing and the Roots of Violence* (1984); *Prisoners of Childhood* (1981); and *Thou Shalt Not Be Aware: Society's Betrayal of the Child* (1984). Miller describes the hidden violence in families that is supported by authoritarian parenting (particularly prominent in German child-rearing) and the child's psychological need to hide the truth. The combination of violence and obedience in childhood leads to passive powerless adults or adults who are angry and violent. Miller notes that Hitler was severely abused as a child but learned never to cry. In *Thou Shalt Not Be Aware*, Miller criticizes psychoanalysis in particular and society in general for either subtly blaming the child when he or she is abused or looking the other way.

faire and authoritarian families do not produce healthy people. Laissez faire families produce spoiled children who lack a sense of self-responsibility or respect for others, and authoritarian families produce aggressive or passive children who lack a sense of self-responsibility and self-respect. Generally these patterns continue into adulthood. Families that function like a constitutional democracy tend to produce healthy people. Such families honor a "Bill of Rights," giving each member equality and respect, which are important aspects of nonviolence. Family meetings, like town hall meetings, occur regularly, and family members learn how to listen, communicate, solve problems, and compromise on basic issues that are important to the health and welfare of each member of the family. The enforcement of the "constitution" (agreed-upon rules and procedures) is fair and is based upon discipline rather than violence. Does this sound like the average American family? Perhaps not, but nonviolence in the family can be learned.

Discipline by Logical and Natural Consequences. In healthy, nonviolent families, discipline follows the principles of **natural and logical consequences** (Dreikurs & Stoltz, 1964): (1) With privileges come responsibilities; for example, with the privilege of using the family car comes the responsibility of driving carefully and paying for the gas. (2) Failure to be responsible results in loss of privileges, not in violence. (3) Natural consequences follow the laws of nature; for example, when dinner is served at 6:00 P.M. and someone shows up to eat at 6:30 P.M., dinner is cold. That is the natural consequence of being late—no violence is needed to make the point that being late is bad. (4) Logical consequences follow the action; for example, if television is not used properly, the logical consequence is losing the privilege of watching television. Failure to pick up toys in a family space means losing the privilege of playing with the toys for a while. A person who does not share the cooking does not share the eating, unless the family has agreed that the privilege of eating will be compensated for by something else. Logical consequences do not happen naturally and must be agreed upon by family members as reasonable and fair. The parent and child must agree that toys left around cannot be used and that clothes on the floor do not get washed.

The concept and methods of discipline by logical and natural consequences was created by Dreikurs and described in his book, *Children the Challenge*. Dreikurs hoped to counteract two child-rearing practices: (1) discipline by physical violence and its obvious damage to the child; and (2) lack of discipline, which fosters a lack of responsibility in children. When children are allowed to suffer the logical and natural consequences of their actions, and are not continually "bailed out" or abused, they develop self-responsibility and a sense of self-efficacy and self-esteem, the opposites of the effects of violence.

The differences between an enforcement system that operates according to discipline rather than punishment are:

Punishment	Discipline
1. Consequences follow from the arbitrary power of a particular person.	1. Consequences follow from the power of the laws of nature (natural consequences) and the laws of society (logical consequences).
2. Uses moral judgments: "You bad boy."	2. Moral judgments are not made.
3. The emotional tone of people administering punishment is anger and guilt.	3. Neutrality and calmness characterizes the emotional quality of people administering consequences.
4. The focus is on the past and future: "Just wait until your father comes home."	4. The focus is on the present: Consequences follow immediately after the behavior.
5. Results: passivity, aggressiveness, and lack of self-responsibility.	5. Results: self-responsibility and respect for others' needs.

Ideally, discipline by logical and natural consequences fosters nonviolence. It frees the parent from taking either the authoritarian, punitive role of the bad parent or the role of the patsy parent who has no power at all. However, discipline by logical and natural consequences is easier to write about than carry out. The system breaks down when the child refuses to "suffer" the consequences and the parent resorts to violence or capitulation. Administering consequences with compassion and nonviolence requires self-discipline and assertiveness on the part of parents.

Many parents feel liberated by the Dreikurs/Sheehan system because they have steps for being nonviolent and effective in discipline, and children gain self-responsibility and respect for others. Some parents, however, will not give up the authoritarian, punitive role because they need it to justify their violence. Some parents maintain power struggles so that they can abuse their children and "win". On the other hand, some parents are unable to enforce logical consequences or allow their children to suffer natural consequences, because for these parents, it is easier to continually rescue the child and avoid conflict. This approach is nonviolent, but the parents become doormats and model a lack of assertiveness and a lack of self-respect.

We have focused on the family because nonviolence must begin at home. Love, generosity, peace, protection, equality, and physical and psychological safety should be part of everyone's home life. Gandhi believed, however, that *ahimsa* should be followed in all institutions—family, schools, businesses, governments, churches—and in all circumstances.

In a nonviolent lifestyle, conflicts are solved through problem-solving and negotiation. Harvard University psychologist David McClelland founded a business consulting firm that studies conflict resolution in corporations, schools, labor unions, and the federal government. The firm found that the most important skill in conflict resolution is **objective empathy**. Objective empathy is the ability to understand several conflicting viewpoints simultaneously. All alternatives are examined objectively and understood. For example, I (RS) can understand my 16-year-old son's desire to borrow the car to go skiing, his mother's objections, and my own feelings.

We have emphasized the importance of empathy. As discussed in Chapters 6 and 10, empathy helps people reduce anger and aggression and is crucial for effective social support. Empathy also helps people resolve conflict effectively. In short, empathy is at the core of a nonviolent lifestyle and is a dynamic of health and wellness.

How many people actually practice empathy? How many people know that escalation of conflict and frustration (which lead to violence) can be stopped by saying, "Okay, let me see if I understand what you are saying . . . you are saying that . . ." and then giving the person the right to respond without being lambasted or cut short? After the conflict is clarified, reason and logic can be used to solve it.

Using reason and logic to achieve goals and reach agreements and compromises is another important skill in nonviolent conflict resolution. For example, it is not enough for me (RS) to understand the viewpoints of my son, his mother, and myself. We must be able to clearly evaluate each position and come to a logical and reasonable resolution of the conflict.

Psychologists Stuart Schmidt and David Kipnis at Temple University (1987) have studied blue-collar and clerical workers, supervisors, sales representatives, and chief executive officers of several hundred businesses and corporations. The most successful people in all positions are those who use reason and logic to achieve their goals. Schmidt and Kipnis call these people "tacticians." The most unsuccessful people, called "shotguns," were those who used any means possible to achieve their goals. The shotguns, say Schmidt and Kipnis, have the highest levels of job tension and personal stress.

How many people in an escalating conflict

use reason and logic? A precursor of violence is rigidity. In violent families there is no recourse to reason and logic; the person in power (usually an adult, but sometimes a child) determines what is right by whimsy, tradition, selfishness, ignorance, or viciousness, and no one is allowed to differ. In such families the person in power justifies violence whenever "the law" is questioned or violated. (Remember that violence is injury done by thought, words, and actions.) In such families "laws" are violated primarily because no one has the nerve to suggest that the law is wrong and needs to be changed. The power people then commit violence in the name of justified punishment for wrong-doing and "willfully disobeying" and the cycle of conflict and violence is maintained.

Take a minute: Can you imagine nonviolence in thought, word, and action—and the expression of love in thought, word, and action—becoming a way of life in this country? Imagine a nonviolent society. Would you like to live in such a society? If you would, then examine your lifestyle and determine how you can more closely follow the path of nonviolence. If not, ask yourself how you condone violence and whether it is a choice that you really wish to make.

Do It Now.

Today violence is part of the American way of life that is hazardous to your health. We look forward to the day when nonviolence is the American way of life, along with good nutrition, exercise, seat belts, and all the other ingredients of a healthy lifestyle.

Play

Fun and Humor

A cheerful heart is good medicine, but a downcast spirit dries up the bones.

Proverbs 17:22, *The Bible*

News Alert! Play, fun, and humor are essential to health!

Stockholm, Sweden. The Swedish government passes the Play Law. Play must be provided for all children in hospitals.

New England Journal of Medicine (Cousins, 1976). Writer, editor, and statesman Norman Cousins recovers from a degenerative illness, ankylosing spondylitis. Cousins, former editor of the *Saturday Review of Literature*, had only a 1–in–500 chance of recovering when he instituted his special brand of therapy: **laughter therapy** and vitamin C. Every day Cousins watched *Candid Camera* shows and Marx Brothers movies. His sedimentation rate dropped by five points during laughter (sedimentation rate is an indicator of severity of inflammation or infection), and Cousins says that 10 minutes of belly laughter gave him two hours of pain-free sleep without medication.

Houston, Texas. Oncologist John Stehlman of St. Joseph Hospital requires a joke a day from all cancer patients. Joke books and magazines are provided for cancer patients unable to come up with their own jokes. The hospital provides a living room with a large television so that cancer patients can watch funny movies and TV programs (Justice, 1987 p. 271).

International Journal of Psychiatry in Medicine (Dillon et al., 1985–86). Humor increases S-IgA antibodies. S-IgA antibodies help the body fight off colds, flus, and respiratory infections. In a study of the effect of laughter on S-IgA levels, subjects in the laughter group who watched *Candid Camera* clips had significantly higher S-IgA levels than the no-treatment control group subjects.

Santa Barbara, California. The Laughter Research Project at the University of California at Santa Barbara finds that laughter stimulates beta-endorphins. Beta-endorphins produce natural highs in humans.

Chicago, Illinois (Dubow, Huesmann, &

Eron, 1987). Playing card games and board games is more effective than behavior or cognitive therapy in reducing aggression in elementary school boys (N = 104). Researchers at the University of Illinois were startled when they found that children in an attention/play control group significantly decreased aggressive behavior, in contrast to children .in three experimental groups: cognitive training, behavioral training, and combined cognitive/behavioral training.

Waterloo, Ontario, Canada (Martin & Lefcourt, 1983). Humor is shown to counter the effects of stress. In three studies using a humor scale, a humor coping scale, and a challenge to respond with humor to a stressful situation, researchers found that students who score high on these scales have fewer mood disturbances such as depression and anger during and after stressful events than less humorous students.

Schenectady, New York. "Laughter is good medicine," says Lenore Reinhard, coordinator of the new humor program at Sunnyview Hospital and Rehabilitation Center. Last week [1987], Sunnyview had the grand opening of its humor room, which is in the third-floor lounge. The program, the first of its kind in a capital district hospital, was made possible by a generous grant from William and Estelle Golub. The room, a humor resource center, is decorated with posters and jokes and equipped with audio- and videotapes, puppets, and games. The purpose of the program is to get the patients, their families, and the staff back in touch with laughter, because humor plays a vital role in being healthy. (Humor Project, Saratoga Springs, New York.)

Nurses for Laughter (1984). Debbie Lieber, instructor at the School of Nursing, Oregon Health Sciences University, founds Nurses for Laughter, an educational organization devoted to the promotion of laughter in health care.

Conference Announcement (1988). The Institute for the Advancement of Human Behavior announces the sixth annual conference, western region, *The Power of Laughter and Play —Applications in Health, Business, Education, Relationships, and Lifestyle,* to be held at the Disneyland Hotel. Presentation highlights include:

> Stress Management and Humor: S/He Who Laughs Last, Lasts
> Growing Young: The Functions of Laughter and Play
> Putting Play to Work: The Power of Humor in the Work Environment
> Laugh Your Way to Health
> A Lighthearted Approach to a Healthy Heart: The Practical Physiology of Laughter and Play
> The Magic of Humor: A Ho-Ho Holistic View
> Humor and the Health Professions

Laughter is Good Exercise. William Fry, Jr., a California psychiatrist, says that laughter is good exercise, similar to stationary jogging; during a good belly laugh, blood pressure increases and the heart rate may double.

The story of Norman Cousins' miraculous recovery from ankylosing spondylitis and his unusual treatment is well known. Cousins began to recover after checking out of the hospital and into a hotel where he could take large doses of laughter and Vitamin C (Cousins, 1981). Cousins was so impressed that he changed the focus of his career and began to study the effects of the positive emotions on health. Today Cousins is a statesman for the role of the mind in health and illness.

Unlike Cousins, Joel Goodman was not sick when he became interested in the power of humor, but his father was. Goodman, founder and director of the Humor Project in Saratoga Springs, New York, "got into" humor in a shuttle van between his hotel and the hospital in which his father was recuperating from heart surgery. The van driver was a natural wit and kept the passengers in stitches. The stress relief was so intriguing that Goodman decided to study humor. Today Goodman coordinates programs for the Humor Project, is the editor of the Humor Project publication *Laughing Matters* and carries his message on the practical advantages and health benefits of humor to businesses, hospitals, and professional organizations across the United States.

Laughter, play, and humor are becoming serious business in health. And this makes sense. If negative emotions have negative physiological consequences, then surely positive emotions have positive effects. Laughter, like love, heals.

Balancing Work and Play

In the days before entertainment became big business, before mechanization and time-saving devices, people worked 10 hours a day, six days a week, and believed in moderation in all things except work. Hard work was thought to do good things for people, keep them out of trouble, give them a "stiff spine," make them honest, and make their dreams come true. The work ethic was especially good for bosses. It took unionization to combat the cruelty of overwork in the adult world and laws to combat the cruelty of child labor. Today many people still work too much, either of choice or of necessity. Probably the most overworked population is mothers who work away from home, and whose work in the home, as the saying goes, is never done.

Humans can handle chronic stress by using a few stress breakers, and fun is one. Having fun should be part of everyone's daily stress-management program, but fun does not sneak up and tickle people from behind. Fun must be planned, created, experienced spontaneously, bought, found, sought, and noticed. Stress-management fun, which takes the edge off stress throughout the day, must also be brief, repeatable, diverting, and thoroughly enjoyable. It should not be a destructive habit, and it *must be experienced as a treat for the self*.

This latter point is highlighted because people who feel pressured all day long and feel that they are depriving themselves have the best rationalization for indulging in a worseness habit: "I deserve it." People will talk themselves into all sorts of worseness habits on behalf of themselves, with the help of clever advertising and a culture that supports immediate gratification. Rarely will you hear, "I am going jogging. I worked hard all day and I deserve it."

FUN ON THE RUN

Coast around the store on your shopping cart. Chew an entire pack of chewing gum, one stick after another. Make little bubbles come out of the top of the dishwashing soap container before you put it away. People-watch. Put a furry stuffed toy with a big smile in your work area and smile at it a lot, even hug it. Draw a heart for yourself in the steam on the bathroom mirror. Get a good joke book and read a few jokes every day. Take your shoes off a lot. Get a bubble pipe and blow bubbles as often as possible. Eavesdrop while waiting in line and create an instant novel on what you hear. Make up a fantasy trip while at the red light. Psychoanalyze the recording while you are on hold on the phone. Put something on the back of your pants and conduct a sociological study on how people tell you about it.

THE SITCOM

Have you ever caught yourself watching a stupid sitcom on television and wondering why you keep watching? You keep watching because humans have eternal hope for one more funny line. Laughter feels that good.

HUMOR HASH

Ingredients: Nonthreatening environment, funny bone, laughter, timing, receptive audience, positive feedback, puns, jokes, humor, exaggeration, surprise.

Directions: Use a playful pan. Grease well with laughter. Flower lightly with humor. Add 1/4 cup of exaggeration, a pinch of puns, a jigger of jokes, 2 tsp of fun flavoring. Season with surprise. Bake in a nonthreatening environment. Serve to a receptive audience.

Laughing Matters, Vol. 1, no. 1

The importance of balancing work and play to avoid the "I deserve it" mentality is described by Alan Marlatt at the University of Washington, who pioneered treatment for addictive behaviors. Marlatt found that when work and taking care of "shoulds" far outweighs taking care of "wants", then a high-risk situation is created that is a set-up for self-indulgence justified by self-deprivation. Marlatt writes:

> My experience in working with a variety of addictive behavior problems suggests that the degree of balance in a person's daily lifestyle has a significant impact on the desire for indulgence or immediate gratification. Here, *balance* is defined as the degree of equilibrium that exists in one's daily life between those activities perceived as external "hassles" or demands (the "shoulds"), and those perceived as pleasures or self-fulfillment (the "wants").
>
> (Marlatt & Gordon, 1985, p. 48)

A balance of doing our "shoulds" and getting our "wants" is important for maintaining a healthy lifestyle. Fun of all types promotes health by turning on the positive emotions and turning off the need to indulge.

Perhaps the ancient Greeks were too serious to create a god of play; in any case, we cannot find one. Yet Western civilization should have created a god of play so that adults would have permission to play like children.

CONCLUSION

In *The American Way of Life Need Not Be Hazardous to Your Health,* John Farquhar says, "People live as though their habits don't count." A person will say, "It's just a habit of mine," while guzzling the tenth soft drink of the day, and feel okay because habits don't count. But lifestyle is no more then habits combined, and lifestyle counts.

Your greatgrandparents, and even your grandparents, may have had little choice about lifestyle habits. Today the opportunity for choosing poor lifestyle habits is overwhelming. If you choose not to exercise, you can make it through a day without taking more than a hundred steps outside of your house or workplace. If you choose not to prepare a nutritious meal at home, you can pick up a burger, drink, and fries at a fast-food dealer without getting out of the car. If you choose to eat at home, you can order out or throw a highly-processed TV dinner into the microwave. If you choose to smoke, you are rarely more than a mile from a cigarette machine. If you choose to drink, use drugs, or pick a fight, you can find what you want with little trouble.

Your greatgrandparents, and even your grandparents, had little knowledge of the hazards of poor lifestyle habits. Today knowledge is beginning to keep pace with the opportunities for poor choices. If you have not paid much attention to lifestyle habits, then you know more now. Using what you know is your choice.

We have included this chapter on lifestyle habits because there are many ingredients to health and wellness, and none can be neglected with impunity. It would be foolish to know a great deal about the psychosocial dimensions of health and nothing about the lifestyle dimensions. It would never do for a therapist to know about the importance of purpose in life and not know about the importance of fiber in the diet.

And the ultimate irony would be for a health professional to die of a lifestyle disease while teaching about the value of hardiness, imagery, and relaxation.

We think of lifestyle as the word suggests— the style in which life is lived. Because mind and body interact and are never separate, lifestyle is a mind-body enterprise. In that sense, all the habits that promote psychological health are part of a healthy lifestyle. We include assertiveness, nonviolence (not just the lack of violence, but love), and play as important ingredients in healthy lifestyle for this reason. You can probably think of many other wellness ingredients.

This chapter on lifestyle immediately follows the self regulation chapter because for most of us, a healthy lifestyle and self regulation go hand in hand. When people make lifestyle changes or try to maintain health habits, they have adopted self regulation as a way of life. We conclude with a thought from the previous chapter: When self regulation becomes a way of life, it no longer feels like regulation of the self. It just feels like the self.

CHAPTER 13

Development of Health Behaviors

Paul: "I was raised on a small Indian reservation in one of our Western states, and my life was influenced by the good and the bad of both cultures. My first drunk was in the summer of my 12th year, when I ventured to town with some friends. We purchased a jug and found a place to drink it. I got drunk, blacked out, and got sick, and we went back to get some more. The accepted attitude was: When you take a drink, you're supposed to get drunk.

"When I was 16, I left the reservation and joined the Navy. While home on boot leave, I had my first experience of being jailed as a result of drinking. My drinking increased. I had more money, and it seemed everyone drank. When I drank, there was no fun, none of the benefits of a relaxing, sociable evening with friends. When I drank, there was always trouble. I developed feelings of guilt and loss of self-respect. I became afraid of people, of being alone, of everything around me.

"One night when I was on Canal Street in Chicago, the man in the cage next to mine died in D.T.'s and convulsions. I remember thinking he should have had more sense than to drink that much. . . ."

From *Do You Think You're Different?*
(Alcoholics Anonymous, 1980)

Carmen: "As a 17-year-old-senior in high school, I had a 'model daughter' image and lived up to it by winning a four-year college scholarship. Still I entered college with a full-blown case of rebellion against all school authority and any other authority. Primarily I was drinking only at parties and on weekends at that time. I was elected to several student-body and organizational offices. But because of low grades and having been caught drinking on a university-sponsored trip, I was removed from most of these honors. And by the end of my freshman year, I had lost my scholarship, too.

"That summer, when I was 18, my parents decided I needed a vacation. My dad and I had fought over his heavy drinking and my engagement to a guy in the black-leather-jacket set; so, to restore family peace, I went to Atlanta, Georgia. There I began daily drinking, sitting around a country-club swimming pool with other vacationing students. In this atmosphere, drinking at 10 a.m. all day, and into the night seemed to me nothing but 'social drinking.'

"My sophomore year saw alcoholic drinking take over my life. If I drank before class, I was embarrassed and ashamed to attend. But after living awhile with these fears, I started drinking in order to attend class, in order to date, to go to games or parties."

From *Young People and A. A.*
(Alcoholics Anonymous, 1981)

Richard: "I am 5'10" and I weighed 320 pounds. I didn't think I was an overeater. My wife pleaded with me to go on a diet. She fixed low-calorie foods and I all but threw them on the floor demanding that she give a decent meal to a hard working man—ha! I was a bus driver. Although it was hard work, it hardly used up the calories I ate. Often after dinner I would go out to buy junk food and eat it in front of her—just to show her who was boss.

"One evening I collapsed. My wife called the paramedics and I was rushed to the hospital. The diagnosis: a coronary. This time my doctor didn't say as he had for years. 'I think it would a good idea if you lost weight.' He said, 'Lose weight or die. I suggest you call Overeaters Anonymous'."

From *To the Man Who Wants to Stop Compulsive Overeating, Welcome*
(Overeaters Anonymous, 1980)

The stories of Paul, Carmen, and Richard may seem unrelated to your life. But for most people, at one time or another, the words of St. Paul are true: "What I would not do, I do; what I would do, I do not." Many people know what they should do to be healthy, and yet they do the opposite. Think of yourself: you know the key ingredients of a healthy lifestyle, as discussed in Chapter 12, and you know the key principles and techniques of self regulation, as discussed in Chapter 11. But knowledge is not action. Will you follow through on developing a healthy lifestyle?

In the past decade, millions of Americans have made significant improvements in lifestyle. More Americans are exercising, smoking less, and maintaining a healthy diet. Nevertheless, 54 million Americans still smoke, and 24 percent of adult men and 27 percent of adult women are overweight (Najjar & Rowland, 1987).

Chemical addiction continues to be a major problem in the United States. From 1982–1987, the number of people admitted to emergency rooms for cocaine use increased fivefold, for heroin use threefold, and for alcohol use twofold (Adams, Blanken, Gfroerer, & Ferguson, 1988; National Institute on Drug Abuse, 1987). The Drug Abuse Warning Network found that from January to June of 1987, the drugs most frequently involved in death were alcohol, 37 percent; heroin, 32.44 percent; and cocaine, 31.88 percent (National Institute on Drug Abuse, 1988). One out of 10 adult Americans is an alcoholic, and adolescent alcoholism is increasing (National Center for Health Statistics, 1986). Please read Box 13.1 now.

Designing and implementing programs to help people make significant and lasting lifestyle change is a continuing challenge for health professionals. This chapter spotlights model behavior change programs. In Section One, we examine school health-education programs that promote a healthy lifestyle and freedom from addictive behaviors in children and adolescents. Section Two begins with an overview of many techniques and approaches

---

BOX 13.1

PRESCRIPTION DRUGS AND DRUG ABUSE

The largest number of admissions to emergency rooms and the largest number of chemically related deaths are from prescription drugs. The major abused prescription drugs are Valium (diazepam), codeine, Xanax (alprazolam), Ibuprofen, and amitriptyline. Prescription drugs are identified in almost 60 percent of all drug-related emergency visits and 70 percent of all drug-related emergency room deaths (National Institute on Drug Abuse, 1988).

---

that have been used to modify problem behaviors and adoption of health behaviors. We next describe clinical and community programs for behavior change.

The introduction to Part Four said that self regulation is the cornerstone of health and wellness, and lifestyle behaviors are the mortar that can enhance or hinder health and wellness. For this reason we devote a chapter to the problem of preventing, modifying, and eliminating destructive lifestyle behaviors and adopting health behaviors.

The focus of this chapter is health-promotion programs in family, classroom, clinic, and community settings. If you read between the lines, you will gain invaluable information, perhaps insight, about yourself.

Take a minute: Ask yourself, "Do I have destructive lifestyle habits that I should change?" Be honest.

Do It Now.

IIII➡

SECTION ONE: HEALTH EDUCATION PROGRAMS

Prevention of Smoking and Promotion of Health Behaviors

Recall the health-education class that you took in junior high or high school. Did you learn about the risk factors for heart disease, cancer, and stroke? Did you learn about high blood pressure, high fat diet, the effects of lack of exercise, and the consequences of smoking? Did you change your lifestyle?

A team of health-education researchers at the United States Center for Health Promotion and Education in Atlanta, Georgia, were curious about the impact of health education in schools. They designed a study to find out how effective health classes really are. The health classes that were evaluated are described below.

School Health Education Evaluation

Over a three-year period, 30,000 students in grades four to seven, in 1,000 classrooms in 20 states, were assessed on their health knowledge and health behaviors (Connell, Turner, & Mason, 1985). Three groups were compared: (1) students who did not have health-education classes, (2) students who participated in the School Health Curriculum Project, and (3) students in Ohio, Oregon, and Georgia who participated in special health-education programs. Each program is briefly described.

School Health Curriculum Project.   The School Health Curriculum Project was developed by the U.S. Public Health Service in the 1970s to prevent smoking and alcohol and substance abuse among students. This is the most widely used health-education curriculum in the United States. The goal of the program is to influence attitudes and behavior by teaching children in elementary school how to enhance health and prevent disease in four physiological systems: (1) digestive, taught in grade four, (2) respiratory, taught in grade five, (3) cardiovascular, taught in grade six, and (4) central nervous system, taught in grade seven. The project includes a variety of learning strategies such as peer-led discussions, movies, experiments, projects, and plays.

Health Education Curriculum Guide, Canton, Ohio.   In 1973, community leaders, educators, and parents in Canton, Ohio, organized a committee to create a health-education program in the elementary schools. The goals of the program were to promote positive health behaviors and attitudes, and to teach decision-making skills concerning health behaviors. The curriculum covered six areas: nutrition, family life, substance abuse (tobacco, alcohol, and so on), safety, human development, and mental and environmental health. These topics were integrated into language arts, reading, sciences, mathematics, and social studies.

Project Prevention, Dallas, Oregon.   In 1975, educators developed a health curriculum to foster healthy lifestyle, beginning with elementary school children. The curriculum included mental health, safety and first aid, social relationships, human development, death and dying, and community health and resources. A nine-week unit was created for each grade.

High Blood Pressure Prevention, Georgia.   In conjunction with the American Heart Association, schools throughout Georgia developed programs for sixth-graders on high blood pressure and how to prevent it. Five class sessions were devoted to risk factors, the circulatory system and blood pressure, and choices for a healthy lifestyle.

The children took a one-hour pencil-paper health inventory before the program and at one and two years after beginning the program. Students were measured on health knowledge, attitudes, and behaviors. Items on health behaviors concerned smoking, alcohol, and drug use.

Results.   The team at the Center for Health Promotion and Education found that the results of these programs varied with the goals of each program and with the amount of money invested in the program. The School Health Curriculum Project received the largest grant and had the best results. The more extensive the intervention, the better the results. Also, the more health-education training the teachers had, the better the results. The Health Education Curriculum Guide focused on general knowledge, and students demonstrated overall knowledge of health. Few changes were reported on health attitudes and health behaviors. The High Blood Pressure Intervention project succeeded in teaching children about blood pressure but had little impact on behaviors like smoking. The goal of Project Prevention was to improve decision-making skills, and students demonstrated knowledge about decision-making, but they made no change in concrete behaviors such as smoking.

The overall results of these programs showed that students learned about health, but that little change occurred in health attitudes and behaviors, with the exception of the School Health Curriculum Project. Twelve percent of the children were smoking in the other programs in the seventh grade, while only 8 percent of the children in the School Health Curriculum Project were smoking in the seventh grade (Connell, Turner, & Mason, 1985).

Peer-Based Programs

If you were designing a school-based smoking and drug-abuse prevention program for adolescents, what would you include? Using material from Chapter 11 on the ingredients of self regulation, and using your own experience in

school, what principles and techniques would you incorporate in the program? Would you capitalize on the importance of peers? Peers are the most influential factor in adolescents' decisions about smoking and drug use (Hawkins, Lishner, Catalano, & Howard, 1985).

One of the first studies to incorporate peer influence was conducted by University of Houston psychologist Richard Evans (Evans, 1976; Evans, Rozelle, Mittelmark, Hansen, Bane, & Havis, 1978). Evans used films in which adolescents were given information about smoking and role-played scenes in which peers used social pressure to get a friend to smoke. The films also included instructions on how to resist social pressure from friends and how to counter advertising. Students in the films modeled coping strategies for resisting peers. After watching the films, peer leaders led discussions that reinforced not smoking.

Using self-reports to determine smoking behavior in adolescents is always suspect. To enhance the validity of self-reports, Evans told the students that nicotine use would be measured by a spectrometric analysis of saliva in a random sample of students. This "threat" encouraged accurate self-report data; the spectrometric analysis on a random sample of students verified the self-report data.

Evans (1988) conducted a three-year follow-up in 13 junior high schools and found that 8 percent fewer students were smoking in the prevention groups than in the control group. This difference was statistically significant, although from a health standpoint, 8 percent is not very substantial. Eight percent fewer smokers is good, but not good enough to offset the health hazard and medical cost of smoking in this country.

One critic of school intervention programs, Guy Parcel, professor of pediatrics at the University of Texas at Galveston, contends that in order to maintain lasting changes, health-education programs must focus on the entire community rather than the individual child;

too often programs set up conflicts between what is taught in the classroom and what is emphasized in the peer group or at home, or reinforced in the community (Parcel, 1985). Parcel believes that health-promotion programs should be conducted in the context of the family and the community. The Minnesota Health Heart Program is a prototype of such a program.

Minnesota Heart Health Program

The Minnesota Heart Health Program is an ideal health program for young people that concentrates on both the family and the community. The program is a community-based health-education program devoted to reducing cardiovascular disease and promoting health by teaching health behaviors to children, adolescents, and adults. The director of the youth branch of the Heart Health Program, Cheryl Perry, and co-workers (Perry, Klepp, Sillers, 1989) are conducting a 10-year longitudinal study of health behaviors of two groups of students. To date, 871 children are in a control group, and 1,100 have participated in the health-education program that includes (1) changing peer group values, (2) identifying with healthy role models, (3) learning social skills to resist pressures to adopt worseness behaviors, and (4) developing health-enhancing behaviors.

The first stage is the Lunch Bag program. Sixth grade students have a one-hour session on how to fix a nutritious lunch (low-fat, low-salt, and complex carbohydrates), and each child receives a healthy lunch. Students then create a newspaper about healthy diets called *Get Ready for the 21st Century.*

The second stage is the Keep It Clean program, a six-session smoking-prevention program for seventh-grade students, taught by peers. Through small group discussion, brainstorming, and role-playing, students learn social skills to resist social pressure to smoke,

and cognitive skills to resist advertisements to smoke, and they learn about the immediate and future consequences of smoking (bad breath, getting into trouble, and poor health).

In the Health Olympics Program, seventh- and eighth-grade students write greeting cards expressing their views on physical exercise and smoking to seventh- and eighth-grade students in Sweden, Norway, and Australia. Students from those countries respond with greeting cards expressing their views on health.

FM 250 introduces eighth-grade students to heart rate monitoring, aerobic exercise, and safety procedures. Each week groups compete with each other to log the most exercise miles. The winning group receives gift certificates from a local sports store.

Shifting Gears is a six-session smoking and alcohol-abuse prevention program taught by peer leaders for ninth graders. Students learn social skills for resisting social pressure to use tobacco and alcohol, and they learn how to critique and resist advertising messages promoting smoking and drinking. The students produce videotapes that are edited professionally and are shown to other ninth-grade classrooms.

In the tenth grade, the Slice of Life Program uses peer leaders and teachers to teach decision-making skills for developing a healthy lifestyle. Students practice making nutritious meals and make videos about healthy lifestyle.

The Minnesota school-based program takes place in the context of community emphasis on health promotion. With funds from the National Heart, Lung, and Blood Institute, Minnesota established community health programs that include media ads, classes for adults, and health assessments. In addition, local merchants set up rewards for students who quit smoking. If students quit for at least a month, they are able to draw for a trip to Walt Disney World. Four prizes are given. Smokers who quit also receive congratulatory telephone calls, and their names are published in the local

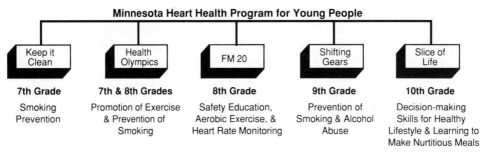

Figure 13.1.   The Minnesota Heart Program for Young People. From Perry, Klepp and Sillers (1989). *Health Education Research, Vol. 4, 87–101.* **Adapted with Permission.**

newspaper. Student representatives from elementary and junior high schools participate on a Student Health Council. The Student Health Council and local representatives from the Health Heart Program design projects that foster health in the schools. Students on the Student Health Council publish a health newspaper and co-teach health classes.

Results.   The only data reported at this point are on smoking rates. Smoking rates were determined by self-report and by saliva thiocyanate tests (thiocyanate is a byproduct of

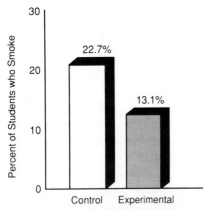

Figure 13.2.   Reduction in Smoking Rate for Students in the Minnesota Healthy Heart Program. From Perry, Klepp and Sillers (1989). *Health Education Research, Vol. 4, 87–101.* **Adapted with Permission.**

smoking tobacco that can be measured in saliva). Students in the Heart Health Program had smoking rates 40 percent less than those in the control group—13 percent were smokers in 1987, compared with 22.7 percent in the control group. The average number of cigarettes smoked per week in 1987 was 6.2 in the Heart Health Program, compared with 16.9 in the control group (Perry, Klepp, & Sillers, 1989).

Unlike other smoking-prevention programs, the benefits of the Heart Health Program increased over time. Perry believes that the program was relatively successful because it used peer leaders and because the youth prevention program is part of a larger community-oriented program, the Minnesota Heart Health Program. Other community-based prevention programs have had similar results. A comprehensive community health program in North Karelia County in Finland, described in the next section, reduced the incidence of smoking by 30 percent (Vartiainen et al., 1986).

Prevention of Substance Abuse

Illicit drug use in the United States is the highest of all industrial nations (Adams, et al., 1988). For the past 20 years, prevention programs have failed to reduce the overall incidence of illicit drug use, and today drug use is most frequent among 18- to 25-year-olds.

Fifty-seven percent of seniors in high school have tried an illicit drug (Adams, et al., 1988). The pattern for alcohol use is similar. In 1987, 92 percent of high school seniors had used alcohol, 66 percent were current users, and 37 percent were heavy drinkers, the same rates as in 1975 (National Institute on Drug Abuse, 1987). The School Health Education Evaluation survey showed that school-based health-education programs had no impact on prevention of substance abuse.

The highest incidence of illicit drug use is in New York City (Johnston, O'Malley, & Bachman, 1988). Gilbert Botvin, professor in the Department of Public Health at Cornell University Medical College, has pioneered in substance-abuse prevention programs in city schools (Botvin, Baker, Renick, Filazzola, & Botvin, 1984; Botvin & Wills, 1985). Botvin's program is similar to the Minnesota Heart Health Program, with an added emphasis on the development of personal and social competence to enhance positive self-image. Extensive experience in the field of prevention of substance abuse and longitudinal data on substance abuse (Demone, 1973; Jessor & Jessor, 1977; Kaplan, 1975) convinced Botvin that children who are the most susceptible to

substance abuse have low self-esteem, low self-confidence, low self-satisfaction, a low sense of personal control, and a need for social approval. Botvin theorized that a successful substance-abuse prevention program would need to enhance self-esteem in addition to providing knowledge and skills for combating substance abuse. Botvin designed the Life Skills Training (LST) program with these ideas in mind.

To test the Life Skills Training program, Botvin conducted three studies with adolescents for prevention of smoking (Botvin & Eng, 1980; Botvin & Eng, 1982; Botvin, Renick, & Baker, 1983). The results were quite significant, with 58 percent fewer new smokers among students in the Life Skills Training after one year than among students in a control group. Following this success, Botvin began a series of prevention program studies for alcohol, marijuana, and cigarette use. Eventually, over 25,000 students from 100 schools participated in the program. The results are significant: After nine months, 73 percent fewer LST students report "heavy" drinking compared to students in control groups, 54 percent fewer LST students were drinking, and 71 percent fewer students smoked marijuana compared to control students (Botvin & Dusenbury, 1988). The program received the New York Governor's Certificate of Merit Award and was designated an exemplarary program by the national Centers for Disease Control.

The Life Skills Training program begins in the seventh grade. Twenty class periods include the following components:

1. **Information.** Students are made aware of the immediate negative consequences of substance abuse, such as financial cost, social consequences (rejection by others), and addiction. Many adolescent youth believe that they are invulnerable to the addictive qualities of substances and that they will be able to stop at any time. To counter this belief, facts about

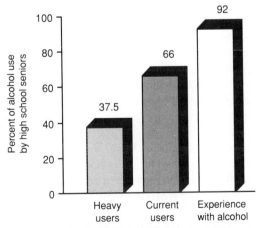

Figure 13.3. Alcohol Use among High School Seniors Is High. (Adapted from Johnston, O'Malley and Bachman, 1988).

the addictive qualities of substances are presented through discussion and film interviews with high-status peers and famous people. In films, high-status peers and famous people reject opportunities to use drugs. Biofeedback instruments are used to show the immediate physiological effects of various substances. Information is presented in an interactive setting in which students can interact with peers and teachers about the issues presented.

2. **Development of self-esteem through self-directed behavior change.** Class sessions focus on the importance of self-image and how self-image can be improved through self-improvement projects. Students discuss perceptions of themselves and share personal strengths and ways in which they would like to enhance self-image. A self-improvement plan is developed for each student, to be completed by the end of the 10-week session. Students work with one another and receive support and encouragement from peers and Life Skills Training leaders. (Note that the self-improvement technique is similar to compensatory self-improvement taught by Maddi and Kobasa to enhance hardiness, Chapter 10.)

3. **Decision-making.** Students discuss the importance of decision-making and the decision-making process. Strategies are practiced, and students learn to identify peer tactics and advertising tactics that may influence decisions. Students learn to resist harmful advertising by identifying the emotional appeals, and they formulate counterarguments. Students learn to think critically.

4. **Coping with anxiety.** Students learn to identify the symptoms of anxiety and the most common situations that produce anxiety, and they learn techniques for coping with anxiety. Students practice diaphragmatic breathing, hand-warming, mental rehearsal, guided imagery, and progressive relaxation.

5. **Social skills.** Students learn to be assertive and to say "no" to peers; they learn to express feelings and beliefs, they acquire conversational skills, and they learn how to initiate social interactions. Skills for overcoming shyness, enhancing boy-girl relationships, and asking someone for a date are practiced through role-playing exercises.

In the eighth grade, 10 sessions are devoted to reviewing the knowledge and skills gained in the seventh grade. In the ninth grade, five sessions are devoted to reviewing the acquired skills. The main emphasis in the eighth and ninth grades is demonstration of decision-making, problem-solving, stress-management, assertiveness, and social skills.

Assessing the acquisition of skills through role-playing is a strength of Life Skills Training. In role-play situations, students demonstrate social skills and ability to resist peer pressure to smoke, drink, or use substances. The focus on improving self-image is another strength of the program. As noted previously, adolescents who are most susceptible to substance abuse have low self-esteem. Substance use is often a way for these adolescents to boost self-esteem, by becoming part of a group. The life skills program provides alternative ways for adolescents to bolster self-esteem and to become part of a social group whose identity is not based on substance use.

Botvin's programs have been conducted primarily with white middle-class youth. Currently, he is conducting one study with 3,000 urban black students in New Jersey and another with 5,000 Hispanic students living in New York City. The efficacy of these programs is still being determined (Botvin & Dusenbury, 1988).

Prevention of Teen Pregnancy

In this country, 1 out of 10 teenage girls will become pregnant, and the rate is even higher in minority groups. The United States has the highest teenage pregnancy rates of Western industrialized countries (Figure 13.4).

Many teen mothers are drug users. In one chemical-abuse intervention study, 50 percent of the teen mothers who abuse drugs were themselves offspring of a teen mother (Griswold-Ezekoye, 1985).

At a time when other communities were seeing an increase in teen pregnancies, a community intervention program in South Carolina reduced pregnancies by 60 percent. Schools, churches, the media, and families were involved in establishing a teen pregnancy prevention program.

The targeted community in South Carolina was 58 percent black and 42 percent white and had one of the highest teen pregnancy rates in South Carolina. With funds from the U.S. Public Health Service, Murray Vincent and colleagues (Vincent, Clearie, & Schluchter, 1987) at the University of South Carolina developed an intervention program. The intervention program focused on (1) decision-

SEXUAL ACTIVITY AMONG TEENAGERS

Sexual activity among girls increased by two-thirds between 1970 and 1980, and this increase was accounted for almost entirely by unmarried white teenagers.

Twelve million American teens are sexually active—7 million males and 5 million females. About 11 million are unmarried.

Fifteen million teens are not sexually active, but half of those will begin to have sex before their 20th birthday.

Teens become sexually active at an average age of 16. One out of every five 15-year-old girls and one out of every three 15-year-old boys are sexually active.

Building Health Programs for Teenagers, Adolescent Pregnancy Prevention Clearinghouse, 1988.

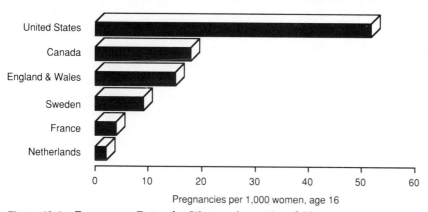

Figure 13.4. Pregnancy Rates for Women Ages 16 and 19.
Source: E. F. Jones, et al., "Teenage Pregnancy in Developed Countries: Determinants and Policy Implications," *Family Planning Perspectives, Vol. 17, No. 2,* (March, April 1985), p. 55, Fig. 3. © The Alan Guttmacher Institute.

making skills; (2) developing interpersonal communication skills; (3) enhancing self-esteem; (4) integrating personal values with those of the family, church, and community; and (5) teaching the anatomy of reproduction and methods of contraception. To implement the program, teachers took classes in sex education instruction. The teachers then taught sex education in all grades (kindergarten through high school). Rather than being taught as a separate class, sex education was integrated into units of biology, science, and social studies. Parents, community leaders, and the clergy also took minicourses in sex education. Many churches offered special classes and programs for youth to enhance personal values and decision-making skills.

Local newspapers and radio stations discussed wise decision-making in the context of prohealth choices. Faculty from the University of South Carolina were available to address community organizations. Students wrote newspaper articles and appeared on television to promote responsible decision-making. A "national family sexuality education week" included programs and workshops on sex education. The community was saturated with pregnancy-prevention messages.

The program worked. After one year, the teen pregnancy rate had dropped by 60 percent. In a second-year follow-up, teen pregnancy was maintained at the same low rate, in contrast to other counties in South Carolina, in which teen pregnancies increased (Vincent, et al., 1987).

Teen pregnancy-prevention programs have been established in major cities throughout the United States, based on the South Carolina model (Adolescent Pregnancy Prevention Clearinghouse, 1986). The Catholic Family and Children Services has established family-centered programs in sexuality education throughout the United States. The Teen Outreach Program began through the collaborative efforts of the St. Louis public schools,

the Danforth Foundation, and the Junior League of Women. Teen Outreach Programs are located in community high schools. The focus is on enhancing the self-image of teenagers and providing information about sexuality. The programs have been carefully evaluated, using matched control groups. Teens participating in the programs are less likely than matched controls to become pregnant.

Many teens have little knowledge about adaptive ways of meeting their needs, and they lack skills and knowledge for making wise decisions about sexual activity and pregnancy. Through teen pregnancy-prevention programs that provide information, decision-making skills, and social support, teens learn to make wise decisions.

Summary

Health education programs that rely on information alone have not worked in preventing smoking, substance abuse, and teen pregnancy. Multicomponent programs, which use peers and focus on development of life skills and self-esteem, are more successful. These multicomponent programs apply the key principles and techniques of self regulation: information, decision-making, enhancing self-esteem, contracts, social support, self-monitoring, rewards, and the development of cognitive-behavioral skills. Except for the teen pregnancy program in South Carolina, the effectiveness of prevention programs for minority youths has not been established. The Life Skills Training approach is now being applied to substance abuse with minorities. Results from these studies will provide valuable information on preventing problem behaviors in minority youths.

We cannot overestimate the importance of starting early. The refrain "if only I had never started" is testimony to the importance of preventing destructive behaviors at an early age. It seems logical, and people say that it is harder to quit than it is to not start a worseness habit. This is undoubtedly true, but the fact is that not starting is not easy. The need to belong, to have an identity, to rebel, to overcome loneliness and anxiety, to be independent, and to feel the bravado of youth ("It could never happen to me") are forces that make it easy to adopt problem behaviors and hard not to.

IIIII➡

SECTION TWO: MODIFYING PROBLEM BEHAVIORS

Millions of teens and adults are overweight, smoke, are sedentary, or abuse drugs. Programs abound for behavior change: non-profit programs in hospitals, for-profit and non-profit clinical programs, commercial programs, and self-help programs. Researchers and clinicians in the field of health behavior note that high drop-out and relapse rates are common to all of these programs. Dropping out and relapse are ongoing problems that are being tackled through self regulation techniques and social support. We begin this section with an overview of methods and programs for modifying problem behaviors, and we then describe model programs and the ingredients that contribute to successful behavior change.

Overview of Behavior-Modification Techniques

Many people change behaviors on their own, without help. Many people cannot modify their own behaviors, however, and seek help. Table 13.1 summarizes techniques and approaches that have been used to help people change problem behavior, and examples are given in the text. On the Table, "yes" means that the approach has been applied in the particular problem area.

Surgery

Surgery to reduce stomach size, and thus food intake, and to reduce absorption of food through intestine bypass is used to help morbidly obese people lose weight. "Morbid" obesity is defined as 100 percent above ideal body weight, or a gain of 100 pounds. Although the safety and effectiveness of surgery are not clearly established, an analysis of data from many studies found that through surgery 85 percent of patients lost at least 50 percent of excess weight when the surgery was combined with behavior modification (Diagnostic and Therapeutic Technology Assessment, 1989).

Pharmacology

Pharmacologic interventions to counteract destructive habits have been widely used, with diet pills being the most popular. Nicotine gum for smoking cessation has a bitter taste that reduces the craving to smoke. To counteract heroin addiction, drugs such as methadone are used. The use of drugs can lead to dependence, and the relapse rate may be as high as 99 percent unless used in conjunction with a behavioral program (Brownell & Wadden, 1986). A recently reported study compared the effectiveness of nicotine gum (N = 210) and placebo gum (N = 105) for smoking cessation. All subjects received 30 minutes of instruction and reading material on nicotine gum and smoking cessation. At one week, cessation rates were 75 percent for both groups, and at one year approximately 70 percent of subjects in both groups were smoking again (Hughes, Gust, Keenan, Fenwick, & Healey, 1989).

Mechanical Devices

In a recently developed weight-control procedure, a plastic balloon is inserted into the stomach through the mouth to create the sensation of fullness. After the person loses a significant amount of weight, the balloon is removed.

Table 13.1   Techniques for Modifying Behavior

Approach	Eating	Smoking	Substance Abuse	Comments
Surgery	Yes			55 percent weight loss, but liver disease develops in some cases
Pharmacologic	Fenfluramine, amphetamines	Nicotine gum	Methadone, emetics	Reduces craving but can lead to addiction; 50–100 percent relapse rate
Mechanical	Plastic balloon in stomach	Fading with filters		High relapse rate used alone but effective when combined with self-management methods
Hypnosis	Yes	Yes	Yes	Short term success—50–100 percent relapse rate
Aversion	Covert sensitization	Rapid smoking	Emetics, electric shock	Initial success but 50–100 percent relapse rate
Exercise	Yes	Yes	Yes	Results are good for people who follow the program—50 to 80 percent fail to maintain the exercise program
Diet regimens	Yes			Varies with diet and program
Behavior modification	Yes	Yes	Yes	Initial success but 50–90 percent relapse rate
Self regulation and relapse prevention, social support, exercise	Yes	Yes	Yes	Initial success with good maintenance. Long-term studies have not been completed
Behavioral change programs—clinical, non-profit, commercial, etc.	Yes	Yes	Yes	Varies with program
Self-help groups	Yes	Yes	Yes	Varies from group to group to group—some have high success and some low
Community programs	Yes	Yes	Yes	High success rate maintained

People who have the balloon inserted are required to participate in a self-management program. Relapse data are not available.

Aversion Techniques and Hypnosis

Electric shock, rapid smoking to nausea, nauseating drugs, and visualizing nausea have been paired with problem behaviors to eliminate the craving for cigarettes or chemical substances. Aversive techniques and hypnosis have had short-term positive results but have not helped people maintain health behaviors (Brownell, et al., 1986). Without an alternative behavior, the old pattern is likely to return (Marlatt, 1983). To overcome the relapse problem, Marlatt and other health professionals teach self regulation techniques to help people maintain health behaviors for a lifetime.

Exercise

Exercise enhances the maintenance of many health behaviors. Exercise is one of the few factors correlated with long-term weight loss (Graham, et al., 1983). Exercise is also an important tool in long-term maintenance of cessation of smoking and substance-abuse behaviors (Brownell, Marlatt, Lichtenstein, & Wilson, 1986; Shiffman, 1984). For many people, exercise is a way of coping with stress, and it is a healthy alternative to problem behaviors. Maintaining an exercise program also enhances self-efficacy.

Diet Regimens

Scores of diets are available to help people lose weight. Some diets are fads and some are actually harmful, but some are valuable and allow healthful weight loss at a safe rate. The Weight Watchers diet follows the guidelines of the American Dietetic Association, with a low-fat, high-fiber diet of complex carbohydrates, including fruits, grains, and vegetables. People who stay with programs such as Weight Watchers or Take off Pounds Sensibly (TOPS) are often quite successful, but the dropout rate is high (Brownell & Wadden, 1986; Stuart & Mitchell, 1980).

Behavior Modification

Traditional behavior-modification techniques include self-monitoring, stimulus control (the person avoids or eliminates stimuli that are associated with the habit), and contracts with rewards. Aversion techniques are sometimes used. The relapse rates for behavior-modification programs, however, are fairly high, varying from 50 percent to 90 percent (Brownell, et al., 1986).

Self Regulation and Relapse Prevention

To reduce relapse, Marlatt and Gordon (1985) proposed a Relapse Prevention Model that includes social support, exercise, and a variety of self regulation techniques such as decision-making, cognitive-restructuring, and stress-management skills for modifying any problem behavior. Participants in programs that include these elements learn techniques for identifying and coping with high-risk situations that lead to relapses. Exercise and self-help groups are used to maintain health behaviors.

Behavioral-Change Programs

Programs abound for smoking cessation and weight control. Non-profit organizations such as the American Heart Association sponsor programs, and commercial organizations such as Weight Watchers and SmokeEnders have centers across the United States. Hospitals, churches, colleges, private clinics, and therapists in private practice have group programs. Some of these programs have short-term success, but many have high dropout and relapse rates. However, organizations such as Weight Watchers are inexpensive and are continually available; people can enter and leave the program repeatedly.

Self-Help Groups

Self-help groups serve people around the world. Alcoholics Anonymous is the largest of the self-help groups, with millions of members in 110 countries. The purpose of Alcoholics Anonymous is to provide a supportive environment in which people can accept themselves and tackle alcoholism. AA members meet weekly and follow a 12-point program for self-improvement. The program and the weekly support groups are the foundation of other groups: Narcotics Anonymous, Smokers Anonymous, Overeaters Anonymous, Al-Anon (adult family members of substance abusers), Alateen (teenage children of substance abusers and teenage substance abusers), ACOA (adult children of alcoholics), and co-dependency groups.

AA and other self-help groups have helped millions of people. Two studies indicate that 70 percent of those actively involved in AA for a year or more remain sober, an impressive success rate (Leach & Norris, 1977; Robinson, 1979). Like other self-help groups, however, AA has a high drop-out rate; the participants in these studies were clearly unusual.

There are over 8 million alcoholics in the United States who do not belong to AA and are not participating in modification programs. To significantly affect these people, broad-based community approaches may help.

Community Approaches

Programs that focus on modifying the behaviors of an entire community are effective. The Minnesota Heart Health Program is an example of a community approach. Community programs use mass media, business and professional groups, educational groups, and community institutions to influence people to eliminate problem behaviors and develop health behaviors. Community approaches have helped entire communities adopt and maintain health behaviors for a lifetime.

We summarize this overview with two observations: Resources are available for people who wish to make lifestyle changes, and programs that foster self regulation skills and social support are more successful than programs that do not. Methods, gimmicks, and programs for behavior change are on a continuum from a complete lack of self regulation and relapse skills, such as the use of drugs for weight loss, to the development of these skills for lasting behavior change and adoption of health behaviors. The results are in proportion to the development of these skills. For this reason, an evolution from quick-fix solutions to multicomponent maintenance programs is occurring. In the remainder of this chapter, we describe several multicomponent programs.

A Model Program for Weight Loss

Being overweight is a serious health risk among the moderately to severely obese, and it is a constant source of psychological and social discomfort for many. Obese people suffer self-denigration as they try and fail to lose weight, and they experience social isolation and prejudice. The roots of obesity are a combination of biological, psychological, and social factors; in other words, obesity is a complex biopsychosocial problem. Obesity is increasing in the United States, as is overweight. As seen in Figure 13.5, childhood obesity increased significantly between 1976 and 1980. In the National Health Examination Survey, obesity was defined as a triceps skinfold greater than or equal to the 85th percentile for children of the same age and sex; superobesity was defined as a triceps skinfold greater than or equal to the 95th percentile (Gortmaker, 1988).

As obesity has increased in this country, and as both the medical and psychosocial problems associated with obesity are understood, behavior-modification programs, techniques, and gimmicks for weight loss have also increased. As noted above, a characteristic of all approaches is high drop-out and relapse rate after initial success. Building on the successes and failures of

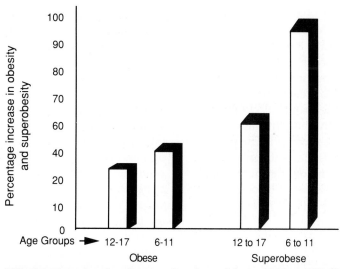

Figure 13.5. National Health Examination Survey Conducted from 1966 to 1970 (Period One) and 1976 to 1980 (Period Two) Showed Significant Increases in Obesity and Superobesity among Children Ages 12–17 and 6–11. Adapted from Gortmaker, (1988). Increasing Pediatric Obesity in the United States. *American Journal of Disorders of Children, 141,* **535–540. Copyright 1987, American Medical Association.**

behavior-modification and dietary approaches to weight loss, and on using evidence of the value of exercise for weight loss and maintenance of weight loss, Kelly Brownell (Brownell & Foreyt, 1985; Brownell & Wadden, 1986) and colleagues at the University of Pennsylvania School of Medicine in Philadelphia and Baylor College of Medicine Diet Modification Clinic in Houston, Texas, created a weight-loss program with five factors: behavior-modification techniques, exercise, cognitive restructuring, social support, and nutrition. Within this framework, the individual needs of each participant determine the exact format of the 16-week program and follow-up sessions. The guiding principle is that obesity is a complex problem and requires a multicomponent program for weight loss and maintenance that emphasizes self-management and relapse prevention.

Behavioral Techniques

The program uses traditional behavior-modification techniques such as self-monitoring,

stimulus control, changing eating habits, and contracts with rewards.

Exercise

The development of enjoyable exercise, emphasizing an increase in daily activity rather than strenuous aerobic exercise, is an integral part of the program, and activity is monitored and reinforced. Exercise has been shown to be a significant factor in maintaining weight loss.

Cognitive Change

The cognitive component of the program is integrated into every other component, from initial screening to relapse prevention, and includes developing positive attitudes and optimism for maintenance of weight loss, goal-setting, problem-solving, and motivation. Careful attention is paid to self-defeating attitudes and goals. Attention is also paid to an external locus of control in which the client hopes that the program will magically produce weight loss, in contrast to an internal locus of control in which the client knows that success comes from learning skills and personal effort. The screening procedure is a measure of motivation; prospective participants must lose a pound a week for two weeks and maintain a food diary. Once in the program, clients must keep a diary in which thoughts about food and eating behavior are recorded. The program therapists review the diaries and provide specific strategies. Problem-solving must become a skill that the client can use without help. To facilitate this, Mahoney's (1977) Personal Science procedure is taught.

> **S**pecify the general problem.
> **C**ollect information on it.
> **I**dentify the causes.
> **E**xamine potential options.
> **N**arrow the options and try one of them.
> **C**ompare the results.
> **E**xtend the strategy, revise or replace it.

Mahoney's system helps the client gain a sense of personal control when problems arise. Having a procedure to follow is an important ingredient in preventing a relapse. Although formal stress management is not part of this program, problem-solving is an important stress-management technique.

Social Support

The program is particularly sensitive to social and family factors. In addition to detecting family sabotage, participants are taught how to evaluate their social environment and elicit support. Spouses are involved in the program to facilitate long-term weight loss and maintenance. Clients participate in group or individual weekly sessions in which problems and successes are discussed.

Nutrition

For mildly obese people (less than 30 percent to 40 percent overweight), the program provides nutritional counseling and shopping, cooking, and eating behavior guidelines, and participants create an adequate diet with guidance from the program staff. Moderately and severely obese people (40 percent to 100 percent, and greater than 100 percent overweight), are placed on a very-low-calorie diet to facilitate substantial initial weight loss. This diet is essentially a fast (300–600 calories a day), but it prevents the loss of muscle protein by allowing small amounts of protein-containing foods. The diet is maintained for 8 to 12 weeks under careful supervision, and then the client is introduced to a maintenance diet. Weight loss may be as much as 40 to 50 pounds and is an important step for people who have a great deal to lose.

The details of the Pennsylvania/Baylor program are described in a large manual that each participant receives for continual reference. Although the content of the program can be specified, Brownell and Foreyt (1985) emphasize the importance of flexibility and empathy in dealing with the specific biological, psychological, and social needs of each client.

The Pennsylvania/Baylor program was designed by experts after extensive study of weight-loss research and other weight-loss programs, and through clinical experience. The effort was intended to facilitate greater weight loss and counteract the high drop-out and relapse rates of other programs. The program incorporates many of the ingredients of self regulation described in Chapter 11, such as information and knowledge, decision-making, commitment and maintenance of commitment, goal-setting, and skills acquisition. In addition, a sense of self-esteem and personal control are fostered, characteristics that the obese person may lack but that are important for successful weight loss.

The multicomponent Pennsylvania/Baylor program appears to have the ingredients for success, but results of the comprehensive program have not been published to date. Data on aspects of the program are available. For example, 17 women with an average weight of 238

GUIDELINES FOR SELECTING AN OBESITY PROGRAM

1. Is the program preceded by medical and behavioral assessments? For example, assessment of eating and exercise behaviors is important for treatment of obesity, because obesity may be maintained more by lack of exercise than overeating.
2. Does the program offer state-of-the-art treatment? Behavioral programs are the treatment of choice for people needing to lose less than 40 pounds. People needing to lose more than 40 pounds may need to follow a stringent low-calorie diet. These diets are powerful and some are potentially dangerous. Close medical supervision is necessary for many low-calorie diets.
3. Is the program structured to facilitate long-term change? The program must last long enough to help the individual change eating and exercise patterns into a permanent lifestyle pattern. For most people it takes at least a year for these changes to become part of a permanent lifestyle.
4. What is the clinic's success rate? Clinics should give the prospective client data regarding drop-out rate, average post-treatment weight losses, and average weight losses at least one year after treatment.

Brownell & Foreyt, 1985

pounds participated in a six-month program combining diet, exercise, and behavioral modification techniques. The diet regime began with a two-month period on 1,000 calories, followed by two months on the very-low-calorie diet, followed by two months on the 1,000-calorie diet. Subjects lost an average of 45 pounds and after one year had regained only 4 pounds (Brownell & Wadden, 1986). Compared to other programs, these results are impressive.

We are still a long way from understanding obesity, short-term weight loss, long-term weight loss, maintenance of weight loss, and relapse. As programs improve, the amount of the weight loss increases and maintenance improves. However, very obese people must continue to lose weight for one or two years, and as the study of 17 women demonstrates, maintenance is not enough. At the one-year follow-up, these women were still obese because they had failed to continue to lose weight when the program ended.

Clearly, long-term self regulation is a complex problem, and the challenge for health professionals is to better understand the factors that hinder and enhance self regulation.

A Model Program for Alcohol Abuse

Les walked into the Problem Drinkers' Project thinking, "Here I am, 36 years old and in an alcoholism program. I've never needed anything like this before. All I need to do is not drink. What's the big deal?" It was 9:00 a.m. on a Thursday morning. Les had just spent 4 days in detoxification, and he was going to go home that evening, after completing his last day in the program. As he walked into the Day Hospital, a staff member met him and walked him down a hall to a room with a closed door. She said that the first group had just begun and that the group was "goal setting." His palms were sweaty and his stomach felt queasy as he thought, "Goal setting—I've never done that in my life."

As she opened the door, Les walked in and saw familiar faces of people he had met during detoxification. "Hi, Les, glad you're here." He was also greeted by a staff member who had talked with him about the program earlier in the week. The others in the room introduced themselves as well but the names were quickly forgotten and the faces became a blur. He decided, "I'll give this a day, but I probably won't be back. I'm just here to stop my wife from nagging me."

Les watched as everyone blew into a machine, and was told that the machine tested whether people had been drinking or not. He noticed that when one person had a positive reading nobody criticized him. The staff member said, "We'll help you look at what happened that you drank, and how you could have handled it without alcohol." Les was amazed.

As Les sat back, he watched a staff person write on a large white wallboard, using colored markers. Group members were talking about things like "triggers, feelings, thoughts, and alternatives." He became curious and tried to listen. It was still hard to concentrate these days, but the writing on the board seemed to make it easier. People were talking about things they planned to do over the next few days. This seemed to be "setting goals." One man said he was going to call his wife and ask her to come in to a couples group later in the day. Les thought, "Good grief, my wife and I haven't any problems when I'm not drinking. Why should she get involved? She's been through enough." However, he agreed to ask his wife to come in, since the other clients' spouses were coming in for group. After an hour, the group was over, and one of the clients offered to show him around the unit.

McCrady, Dean, Dubreuil, & Swanson (1985), "The Problem Drinkers' Project" in Marlatt & Gordon (Eds.), *Relapse Prevention*, 351–406. Copyright by Guilford Press. Reprinted by permission.

Les is about to participate in The Problem Drinkers' Project (McCrady, et al., 1985). The Problem Drinkers' Project has a 75 percent success rate with alcoholics who have had drinking-related problems for an average of 15 years (Longabaugh, et al., 1983). The participants enter the program after 4 to 21 days of detoxification.

The Problem Drinkers' Project, located at Butler Hospital in Providence, Rhode Island, is a three-week program that includes daily group and individual sessions. A team of nurses, social workers, mental health workers, occupational therapists, psychologists, and physicians conducts a program that combines a self-management approach with the relapse-prevention model.

The general goals of the Problem Drinkers' Project are:

1. To help participants identify the function that alcohol serves for them—how they fulfill basic needs through alcohol.
2. To help participants develop ways of fulfilling needs that lead to positive rather than destructive consequences.

Films and lectures help the drinker understand drinking as a process with six consecutive steps: (1) a trigger, (2) thoughts about the trigger, (3) feelings about the trigger, (4) decision to drink, (5) positive consequences of drinking, and (6) negative consequences of drinking. The **trigger**, such as an argument with a friend, leads to a **cognitive** response, "I'll show her," and to a **feeling** such as anger. The behavioral response, **drinking**, is a response to anger. Drinking has **positive consequences**, such as a pleasant mood and the social support of the people at the bar. It also has **negative consequences**, such as violence or being arrested for drunken driving. Understanding this process is an important step in recovery.

For the participants, the specific goals of the Problem Drinkers' Program are to:

1. Identify the antecedents and triggers to drinking.
2. Become aware of the power of positive consequences and establish realistic goals.
3. Develop skills for implementing alternative behaviors to drinking.
4. Decrease shame and guilt.
5. Develop support systems.
6. Cope with relapses.

The Problem Drinkers' Project uses a variety of methods to achieve these specific goals.

Identify Antecedents and Triggers to Drinking

The goal of this component of the program is to help the drinker become aware of the environmental, cognitive, and emotional triggers for drinking. Most participants are aware of the environmental triggers that set off drinking binges, but most are not aware of the cognitive and emotional triggers. Negative self-statements, irrational ideas, unrealistic expectations of oneself and of others, and unrealistic expectations of life in general, are powerful triggers for drinking. Anger, anxiety, depression, guilt, and shame are also triggers for drinking. An inability to express negative feelings or to cope with feelings positively is the focus of the group work.

Become Aware of the Power of Positive Consequences and Establish Realistic Goals

The drinker examines the positive and negative consequences of drinking and establishes realistic goals. The power of the positive consequences of drinking is emphasized. Positive consequences of drinking set up positive expectations about alcohol: "I will be able to sleep better if I have a couple drinks," or "Alcohol loosens me up," or "I am funny when I drink." The expectation of a positive consequence leads to the decision to drink. The relationship between the expectations of positive consequences and the decision to drink is examined by each group member. Initially, many participants have difficulty acknowledging the positive consequences of alcohol. Through group discussion and feedback, participants discover that in deciding to drink, like deciding to engage in any worseness habit, only the positive consequences are considered and the negative consequences are ignored.

When the participant is fully aware of the connection between the expectation of positive consequences and the decision to drink, the negative consequences are discussed and realistic goals are established. An unrealistic goal would be "I will never drink again the rest of my life." Unrealistic goals can be triggers for drinking. A realistic goal would be "I will stay sober the first week of the program and then establish new goals." Goal sheets are used to record each goal, methods for achieving the goal, and the date for accomplishing the goal.

Develop Skills for Implementing Alternative Behaviors to Drinking

The participants practice cognitive, behavioral, social, and stress-management skills so that they can meet their needs in positive ways and not through drinking. Because irrational thinking is often a precursor to drinking, a five-step procedure for rational thinking is taught: (1) STOP—be aware of negative feelings like anger or depression as signals for self-examination instead of triggers to drink; (2) AWARE—become aware of the thoughts related to the negative feelings; (3) DISPUTE—dispute the irrational ideas related to the negative feelings; (4) TEST—determine the validity of your thoughts; and (5) POSITIVE—think positively.

After acquiring these skills, each participant brainstorms about alternative behaviors to drinking and how alternative behaviors can fulfill his needs.

> Les was sitting with his group during the last meeting of the day on a Friday afternoon. Each group member was planning out the weekend, identifying potentially difficult times and situations, trying to decide how to handle them. Les appeared restless, was tapping his feet and wiping his hands on his jeans. He said he was having a strong desire for a drink as he listened to others make weekend plans (STOP). He mentioned that he was accustomed to drinking after work on Friday afternoons, and that he did not think he would be able to drive past his favorite bar on his way home without having a drink

(AWARE). He said, "I'm so uptight I feel like I'm going to jump out of my skin!"

Immediately, the group members let Les know that they understood how difficult it was to feel the way he was feeling. Someone mentioned that he had a choice about whether he drank or not, and asked him if he wanted to give up how good he was feeling for a hangover, facing his wife, and maybe having a fight at the bar. The group also helped him recognize that it was natural to feel the way he was feeling. Les talked about how much calmer he would feel if he drank, but recognized that although he would feel better temporarily, it was probably not worth the risk (DISPUTE). He decided to take a different route home, bypassing the bar. He planned to play catch with his two boys after dinner, and agreed to meet one of the fellow group members at a nearby AA meeting at 7:30 that evening. He said he would ask his wife to come as well (alternative behavior). The group wished him luck and said that they would see him on Monday morning.

On Monday, Les said that he had managed to avoid the bar, played with his kids, and went to AA as planned. He, his wife, and some AA friends stopped for ice cream sundaes on the way.home. He said that he felt proud of himself (POSITIVE) for getting through a day when he would usually have done a lot of heavy drinking.
(McCrady, Dean, Dubreuil, & Swanson (1985), "The Problem Drinkers' Project" in Marlatt & Gordon (Eds.), *Relapse Prevention*, 351–406. Copyright by Guilford Press. Reprinted by permission.

Instead of going to the bar, Les was able to follow through on several positive alternatives that fulfilled his needs for sociability and fun. Playing ball with his kids, going to an AA meeting with his wife, and going out with AA friends after the meeting fulfilled his needs and gave him a new sense of satisfaction and pride.

Decrease Shame and Guilt

Most substance abusers experience underlying feelings of shame and guilt. They feel guilty over the harm that they have done to themselves, friends, and family members. Shame is the feeling and belief that "something is fundamentally wrong with me." Feelings of guilt trigger shame, and a cognitive-emotional leap is made from "I made a mistake" to "I am no good." Shame is nonacceptance of self: it is despair. In his book, *the Sickness unto Death,* the Danish philosopher Soren Kierkegaard (1954) described the "ultimate sickness unto death" as despair, the feeling of a basic flaw inside that cannot be changed. Shame is the ultimate despair. It is the feeling and belief that there is no way out because the flaw is inside. "Shame is a kind of soul murder" (Bradshaw, 1988).

Some people will do almost anything to avoid experiencing shame. Numbing oneself through alcohol and drugs and with denial and rationalizations are common solutions. When Les joined the Problem Drinkers' Project he felt guilty and defensive. To protect himself from entering the cycle of guilt ⟶ shame ⟶ despair, he immediately minimized his drinking problem and denied relationship problems with his wife.

To examine his life and find new ways of coping with life, a drinker must feel secure enough to move beyond defensiveness and rationalizations. The first task for the Problem Drinkers' Project staff is to provide an environment of emotional and cognitive support. They do this by establishing a nonjudgmental supportive atmosphere and by providing a cognitive framework for understanding alcoholism.

Develop Support Systems

Alcoholics Anonymous meetings are held at the project to introduce the participants to AA members and to the 12-step program. Couples groups are formed to help the participants learn to interact effectively with their spouses. Social skills are practiced, and participants learn to give and receive support from other people.

Cope with Relapses

Participants discuss the problem of relapse and how to cope with relapses. Each participant answers two questions: "What do I do if a slip occurs?" and "What must happen in order for me to realize that a slip is about to occur?" (McCrady, et al., 1985, p. 457). The group explores effective ways for coping when a slip does occur. Suggestions include "A drink is not a failure—I can still choose not to drink"; "I will visit with a supportive friend"; and "I will go to an AA meeting." Considerable discussion is devoted to identifying the patterns that lead to slips, such as not attending AA, not sharing feelings with spouse or friends, and going to bars. Participants identify the triggers that lead to slips. Feeling lonely is a common trigger. The group brainstorms positive ways to fulfill the need for companionship.

After leaving the Problem Drinkers' Project, Les remained abstinent for six months. His relationship with his wife and family improved. His work situation improved and he was feeling really good about himself. Then Les stopped going to AA because he felt too busy at work. It was the Christmas season and Les's wife

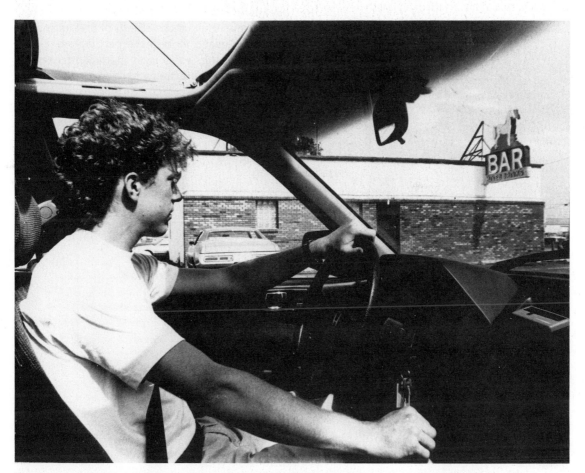

The Problem Drinker Is Tempted, but Drives Past the Bar. Relapse Prevention Is an Important Element in Overcoming a Worseness Habit.
Source: Mike Shellenberger, Greeley, CO.

was very busy getting presents and decorating the house. She and Les were not talking to each other very much. Les began to "bottle up" his feelings and began to slip back into his old habits. Nevertheless, at the company's Christmas party he drank only two beers and felt really good about himself. Then, one day after work Les joined several friends at the club. He planned to have two beers and go home, but he started playing pool and drank ten beers during the game. Les got home late, dinner was over and his family had gone out. Les had several mixed drinks and went to bed drunk. The next morning Les felt sick and stayed home from work. While lying in bed, he remembered how much better his relationship with his family had been in the last six months. He also remembered that his boss wanted him at work as long as he remained abstinent.

Having previously rehearsed "slip procedures," Les reminded himself that a slip is not a defeat, and he called a staff member at the Problem Drinkers' Project to discuss the slip

and the consequences of what had happened. While talking, he decided to remain abstinent and made specific plans for the rest of the day and evening. He took his wife to dinner and shared with her his renewed decision not to drink and discussed the steps that he could take to prevent a slip in the future.

(McCrady, Dean, Dubreuil, & Swanson 1985)

A summary of steps to overcoming problem drinking is presented in Figure 13.6.

The Problem Drinkers' Project is an excellent example of the integration of the ingredients of self regulation and relapse prevention. Realistic goals, self-knowledge, social support, skill acquisition, and methods of preventing relapses are used to help the participants eliminate drinking behaviors and acquire health behaviors. The staff members create a supportive atmosphere and provide a cognitive framework to help alcoholics move from denial and

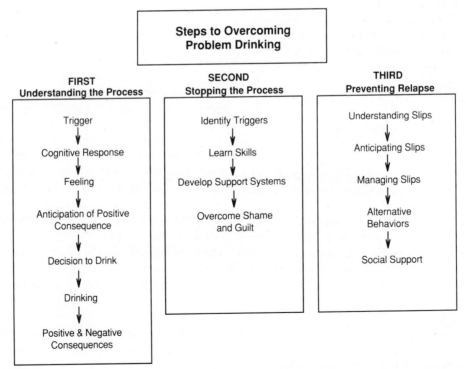

Figure 13.6. Summary of Steps to Overcoming Problem Drinking.

rationalizations to freedom from guilt, shame, and despair. Participants develop and practice healthy ways for getting needs met.

> The best antidotes to addiction are joy and competence—joy as the capacity to take pleasure in the people, activities, and things that are available to us; competence as the ability to master relevant parts of the environment and the confidence that our actions make a difference for ourselves and others.
>
> (Peele, 1985)

In programs such as AA and Problem Drinkers' Project, "communities" are formed; people feel connected, "like family." For many people, the experience of giving and receiving support in a group is invaluable for achieving and maintaining difficult behavior change. Next we describe a program designed for a person's first group, the family, and then we move to programs that encompass larger communities. Programs in the communities— North Karelia County in Finland; Addison Terrace in Pittsburgh, a housing project; and Alkali Lake, a band of Native Peoples living on a reservation in Canada—illustrate the power of community effort to create positive change for many people.

Community Programs for Modifying Problem Behaviors

Families can be the key to preventing disease and illness and promoting health and wellness, and they can also be the key to physical and psychological worseness, disease, and death. Several programs have been developed for families, ranging from improvement of dietary and exercise habits to helping dysfunctional families.

The Minnesota Heart Health Program and Families

In Section One we described the component within the Minnesota Heart Health Program that focused on children and adolescents. Here we describe the family component of this extensive community program. Cheryl Perry, director of the youth wellness team of the Minnesota Heart Health Program, and her coworkers, are convinced that parents must be involved in health-education programs for children. But what must be done to get parents involved? Perry and coworkers (1988b) conducted a telephone survey of 208 parents of elementary school children. Seventy-five percent of the parents preferred behavioral tip sheets, 67 percent preferred worksheets that required parent-child interaction, 42 percent liked informational brochures, 39 percent liked phone calls, and 15 percent preferred parent education, night classes.

Based on the survey results, Perry and coworkers designed a "home-team" five-week correspondence course for third graders and their parents. The goal was to develop healthy nutrition habits. A packet was mailed to each third grader's home each week. The packets included nutritional information, recipes, stories of baseball players who have healthy diets, team hats, and a variety of stickers for labeling good and bad foods. If the packets were completed, the family could draw for a grand prize, which was a trip for four to Walt Disney World.

To assess the effectiveness of the home-team approach, Perry and colleagues (1988b) conducted a two-year study (N = 2,250) comparing this approach to a school-based approach, a school-based and home-team approach combined, and a control group of students who received no instruction. All participants were third graders and were predominantly from middle-class white families. The school-based program lasted five weeks and was similar in content to the home-team approach, but without the family games and family exercises.

Height, weight, and skinfold thickness were measured, and a variety of questionnaires were given to children and parents. In addition, a sample of students from each group received urine tests for sodium. Another sample from each group was selected to receive home visits by a research team member to assess healthy and unhealthy food in the kitchen.

Seventy-one percent of the parents in the home-team program and in the combined home-team and school-based program completed all five packets. All students had at least one parent participate in home-based activities. The fat intake was lower for children in the home-team program and combined home-team and school-based programs than for the control group or school-based program. Healthier foods were found in the kitchens of the home-team and combined groups than in the kitchens of children in the control and school-based programs. Children in home-team groups had more health behaviors than the control children and school-based children. This innovative program, using home packets and parental participation, helped children and their families understand and adopt health behaviors.

North Karelia

Inhabitants of North Karelia County (population 180,000) were alarmed because more and more men and women in their 40s and 50s were dying of heart attacks and being crippled by strokes. In a community effort, the citizens circulated a petition requesting help from the government to counter the epidemic of cardiovascular disease. The response was immediate. The Finnish health authorities and the World Health Organization established a comprehensive community program to combat cardiovascular disease (Vartiainen, McAlister, Puska, Viri, Tossavainen, Niskanen, & Pallonen, 1986).

As a population, Finns have high blood cholesterol and blood pressure, and a high percentage of smokers. The goal of the intervention project was to reduce blood cholesterol, blood pressure, and smoking by changing the North Karelians' lifestyle. The project had six components:

1. **Information.** The risk factors of cardiovascular disease were described on television and radio and in newspapers.
2. **Persuasion.** A sense of community pride was created, and everyone was asked to join the intervention program, even those with no cardiovascular risk, as support for people who were at risk. Leaders called on North Karelians to succeed because the success of the project would be important for all Finnish people and for the whole world.
3. **Training.** Groups were formed to help smokers quit and to help everyone develop new dietary habits. More than 300 cooking clubs were started, teaching low-fat and low-salt cooking. Peer-led smoking-prevention programs and diet classes were provided for all adolescents 13 years and older, through the schools.
4. **Community changes.** Local dairies and a sausage factory cooperated with the intervention program by creating low-fat products. Smoking restrictions were introduced in businesses and community organizations. Antismoking signs were placed throughout the county. Nutritionists, who visited homes of children with high cholesterol and high blood pressure, helped the families establish new dietary habits. The local food industry was persuaded to reduce the salt content of school cafeteria food, and school lunches were modified to reduce saturated fat and salt intake.
5. **Social support.** Family members, doctors, nurses, and friends supported citizens who quit smoking. Exercise groups, smoking cessation groups, and dietary groups fostered a sense of comraderie and mutual support.
6. **Community organization.** The intervention program involved the entire county. Program leaders traveled throughout the county recruiting

ministers, doctors, and politicians; people in business and media services were used to encourage promotion of the program.

After five years, North Karelians reduced cardiovascular disease by 22 percent compared with national norms. Disability payments related to cardiovascular diseases were reduced 15 percent, a savings of $4 million. Psychophysiological disorders were also reduced. Thirty percent fewer students in the prevention programs smoked, compared with students in another county. Residents of the entire county felt a greater sense of health and well-being. A 10-year follow-up study found that these results were maintained (Vartiainen, et al., 1986).

Community intervention programs being conducted in Australia, Switzerland, West Germany, Rhode Island, Minnesota, Pennsylvania, and California have results similar to the North Karelia program (Farquhar, Maccoby, & Solomon, 1984).

The Addison Terrace Learning Center

The highest incidence of illicit drug use is among youths who have dropped out of school and are unemployed or who work for minimal wages. An extensive drug subculture invites youths to earn money through trafficking. Seventy percent of poor black youths are unemployed (Children's Defense Fund, 1988), and for some the trafficking of illegal drugs fulfills an economic need. A survey of drug users in Pittsburgh found that the primary reason for drug use was the frustration of unemployment (Griswold-Ezekoye, 1985).

To make a significant impact on drug use, intervention programs must radically change the drug subcultures by providing meaningful employment and meaningful education to drug users and potential users. Stephanie Griswold-Ezekoye, director of the Addison Terrace Learning Center in Pittsburgh

advocates a multicultural community approach to prevention of substance abuse.

The Addison Terrace Learning Center is an outgrowth of a public housing community, Addison Terrace. In l982, the Center evolved from the efforts of community leaders to stop chemical abuse, the major threat to youths in the housing project. They realized that to make an impact, the total community environment must change. The first step was to create an advisory board of six community residents: a business representative, a religious representative, a health representative, a social service agency representative, a youth representative, and a senior citizen representative.

The advisory board created programs targeting five areas: the individual, the family, the community at large, community organizations, and society at large. In Chapter 1 we said that the biopsychosocial approach is a systems approach; the Addison Terrace project is an excellent example of a systems approach to a complex biopsychosocial problem, as depicted in Figure 13.7. The advisory board members understood that there was no simple solution to the drug problem because the drug problem involved many interacting systems. The board itself represented key systems inside and outside the immediate community of Addison Terrace. To bring these systems into play, the board created several projects that individually might have had little impact but as a united effort has had greater impact.

1. **The single parent/toddler program.** A teen mother was paired with an adult mother, and together they met in a support group where they worked on common life problems. The adult mother was also paired with a female senior citizen for ongoing support. The toddlers participated in an enrichment day-care program four hours a day, five days a week.

2. **The prevention agency group.** A group of leaders from health and service

agencies met to identify youths and families in trouble, and it designed activities to help them out of trouble.

3. **The school group.** Teachers, parents, and administrators formed a group to identify students with chemical-abuse problems, to intervene, and to design school prevention activities.

4. **A youth council.** Adolescents between 14 and 18 counseled peers with chemical-abuse problems.

5. **Auxiliary group.** Representatives from churches, businesses, and the police department supported the activities of the other groups.

Preliminary reports show that positive changes have taken place as a result of this intensive community program. Future reports on the results of the Addison Terrace Learning Center are expected to provide valuable data on ways to prevent substance abuse in poor minority communities, and to solve other problems through a systems approach that involves the key elements, or subsystems, within the larger system. Meanwhile, there is a model program with Native Peoples that significantly modified problem behaviors, focusing on alcoholism.

Alcoholism is a major problem for 75 percent of Native American youth (Owan, Palmer, & Quintana, 1987). Through the U.S. Indian Health Service, 264 communities serving 44,000 people have implemented substance-abuse programs. The programs in the schools begin with Head Start and continue through high school. The programs focus on self-esteem and cultural identity, decision-making skills, countering peer pressure, values clarification, assertiveness, and family enrichment. Local tribal leaders, parents, school staff, the media, and public and private agencies are all used. Evaluations of the effectiveness of these prevention programs have not been completed.

We can describe the results of a program in a community that is an inspiration to many people, Alkali Lake.

Alkali Lake

Alkali Lake lies 250 miles due north of Calgary, Alberta. It is a small community of Native People who have lived in that area for decades in relative peace and health. That began to change in the mid-1940s. The Lake Alkali Band can pinpoint the beginning of change—the day a local merchant gave three trappers whiskey while he examined their furs. By 1970 Alkali Lake had an alcoholism rate of 100 percent; every adult in the community of 300, even the white priest, was an alcoholic. This reservation community was disintegrating. Alcohol-related deaths from suicide, automobile accidents, cirrhosis, and homicide were frequent; children were neglected and malnourished as wages and government social-assistance money went for high-priced illegal liquor; and unemployment was high. The Catholic Church sent a representative from Alcoholics Anonymous, who tried unsuccessfully to help. The complete destruction of the community seemed inevitable.

Then, in 1972 the 6-year-old daughter of Phyliss Chelsea refused to come home. As Phyliss tells her story in a documentary film made by the band several years later, this was a turning point. In tears, Phyliss poured out all the alcohol in her home. She joined an

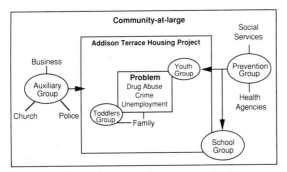

Figure 13.7. A Systems Approach to Combating Substance Abuse in Addison Terrace Housing Project.

Alcoholics Anonymous group in a neighboring town. The leader of the group was a great support to Phyliss. For one year Phyliss was the only sober adult in the community. Phyliss was quiet about this change, and she did not pressure her husband, Andy. Andy decided to become sober one year later, on the day that he walked past the school and really saw the neglect and abuse of the children. He also joined the neighboring Alcoholics Anonymous group. For another year Phyliss and Andy were the only sober adults in Alkali Lake. At Christmas they organized a no-alcohol party in the community center. Only children came, until the last moment when another woman joined the group and started on the road to sobriety.

In 1973 Andy was elected chief. Over the next years he and Phyliss and the small but growing group of sober citizens began to create change. With the help of the local banker, social-assistance money was replaced with vouchers so that money could not be used to buy alcohol; they stopped the flow of alcohol into the community and worked with the sheriff to stop bootlegging by the residents. Getting no help from the priest, they made him leave the reservation. Phyliss and a friend started a grocery store; when community members decided to become sober and left for a six-week treatment program, their homes were repaired and painted; when people returned to the community from treatment they were invited to attend the Alcoholics Anonymous group meetings, which became the town meeting; and a job-training program was started. Another change brought the community more strongly together—a rebirth of traditional ways. Medicine man Albert Lightning was asked to come to Alkali Lake to teach the native traditions; he introduced the sacred pipe ceremony and the sweat lodge, and he taught the meaning of the medicine wheel. The medicine wheel symbolizes the unity of the four worlds of human development: physical, mental, emotional,

and spiritual. The Alkali Lake Band sought to heal and enrich each "world" as they worked for a sober community.

Phyliss and Andy evolved into leaders, not without tribulation and uncertainty, but also not without knowing that they were becoming community leaders and needed help. They enrolled in human-potential and leadership seminars in Seattle. As new members of the band became sober and took leadership roles, they too received training. By 1985, the Alkali Lake community had reduced alcoholism to less than 5 percent (Bopp, 1985). The community that was thought to be unsalvageable had saved itself.

More happened in Alkali Lake than sobriety. Out of the long struggle and years of slow change, a program developed. In 1985 the Alkali Lake community sponsored its first conference, bringing Native Peoples and others from Canada and the United States to Alkali Lake to learn about the process of community change. A dramatic documentary film was made in which the entire community reenacted the years of alcoholism and struggle for sobriety. The film, *The Honour of All* and its theme—"the pain of one is the pain of all, the honor of one is the honor of all"—is a testimonial to the potential for community healing. Today the Alkali Lake community sponsors workshops, training programs and community programs throughout North America.

The success of the Alkali Lake program highlights the essential ingredients in community change:

Leadership: Phyliss and Andy Chelsea evolved into excellent leaders as did many others. They modeled a healthy lifestyle, improved their leadership skills, and helped other community members become effective leaders.

Change in the social environment: Delivery of alcohol was stopped, the voucher system was instituted, sobriety was strongly reinforced, and social pressure was exerted on those who remained alcoholic to enter treatment.

Social support: People helped each other, friendships deepened among community members; the leader of the local Alcoholic Anonymous group provided support and guidance.

Religious renewal: Albert Lightning brought the native traditions to the community and taught the meaning of the medicine wheel.

Community health programs are powerful because they target all sectors of a community and draw upon businesses, schools, churches, government, and the individual citizen. They foster social support and reinforcement of health behaviors, and they instill a sense of unity and common goals that give the individual an added incentive for change. The model programs in North Karelia and Alkali Lake are examples of ways in which communities can help citizens eliminate destructive habits and adopt health behaviors.

IIII➡

CONCLUSION

Paul: I stood at the doors of Alcoholics Anonymous full of fear, guilt, remorse, confusion, and defeat. Those doors were open to me, and I was welcomed in. As my mind clears and I recall the teachings of my ancestors, I believe I have found the best the red man has to offer. Today, I have the fellowship and program of Alcoholics Anonymous and my wonderful wife. I feel that I have found the best the white man has to offer.

Carmen: My new way of life began just the week before I was 21. It made possible a return to my university and a reentrance into campus activities. After a year on the AA program, I was elected a student-body officer—again. After two years, I received two degrees and acceptance for graduate school.

Richard: When I got out of the hospital I called Overeaters Anonymous and went to a meeting. I was unprepared for what I saw. The people were smiling. They seemed to be happy. They looked relaxed. They didn't look like they were fighting food. During the meeting I heard words like "turning it over," "willingness," "one day at a time," and "letting go."

I've lost 134 pounds but, best of all, the compulsion has been lifted. I no longer have cravings. My doctor said, "You see, you did it."

I shook my head, "No, OA and I did it." People without the compulsion, even doctors, do not understand, but there are plenty of people who do. I found them in OA.

People can change, and many people make significant lifestyle change without help. This chapter is about helping people change health behaviors. On two fronts the task is complex and demanding: preventing new problem behaviors and modifying existing problem behaviors. The task is difficult because many worseness habits—smoking, overeating and underexercising, and drug abuse—are complex problems with biological, psychological, and social causes and consequences.

We described 15 programs in this chapter. Some are for preventing worseness habits in children and adolescents, others for helping people change destructive behaviors and adopt healthy behaviors. In general we find that simple, short-term programs with few components are not effective. The evolution from simple to complex approaches, and the shift from external regulation to self regulation, has brought greater success. We can discover several ingredients that are common to the best programs. These ingredients are: self regulation skills, including decision-making, problem-solving, and cognitive restructuring; development of self-esteem and a sense of self-efficacy; social support; information; relapse prevention; and long-term help.

An adolescent has to make a wise decision about sex, an alcoholic about to "slip" must problem-solve and find an alternative to drinking, and a compulsive eater about to binge must apply cognitive restructuring skills. The development of self-esteem, social skills, and assertiveness skills help young people counter peer pressure. People who have severe behavioral problems such as obesity or drug addiction may need years of support, as provided by programs such as Overeaters Anonymous and Alcoholics Anonymous. Social support is the dynamic that provides the staying power for many people, the force that enables people to reject worseness behaviors and maintain health behaviors in the face of stress, social pressure, and daily temptations. The founders of AA were convinced that the key to abstinence is giving support to other alcoholics, and giving and receiving social support is clearly a principle factor in AA's success.

We are impressed by the programs that we have described, and yet, these programs are not enough. What will happen when the programs end? Will the people in North Karelia, South Carolina, New York, Minnesota, and Pennsylvania forget? Will whole communities relapse, or will society make a commitment to carry on, to change the societal values and conditions that promote destructive behaviors?

We are impressed by what is known about the ingredients of self regulation and behavior change. We know that modeling is important, that role-playing is effective, that knowledge and skills are essential, and yet, what is known is not enough. Even the best programs lose people. What are the missing elements? Perhaps purpose in life or spiritual values must be cultivated. The experience of the Lake Alkali Band provides a clue. The band returned to the traditional values of Native Peoples, values that brought meaning to life, values that are antithetical to alcoholism. Perhaps "internalization" of values is the answer, so that people make health choices based on inner values rather than on the values of the group or culture. Perhaps development of willpower is the answer, so that even when social support and rewards are gone, people have the personal strength to maintain health behaviors.

These questions will intrigue health professionals for years. We hope that they intrigue you.

The Dynamics of Health and Treatment

Part Five describes the dynamics, ingredients, and tools of health and wellness in action, as treatment. This topic is dear to our hearts because we are therapists and teachers, and as therapists we teach. In many ways, helping people regain physiological and psychological homeostasis and wellness is the same as teaching healthy people how to stay healthy; many of the ingredients of prevention and wellness are the ingredients of successful treatment.

Part Five concerns a particular type of treatment for which an appropriate motto might be "Skills, not pills." The skills orientation implies self regulation, and for that reason skills-oriented therapy can also be called self regulation therapy. A self regulation treatment approach implies a particular understanding of disease and illness. In Chapter 14, Introduction to Behavioral Medicine: Treatment

Protocols, we introduce the biopsychosocial model of disease and illness and its counterpart, a biopsychosocial approach to treatment. Many of the disorders for which self regulation therapy is appropriate have lifestyle behavior, cognitive behavior, or physiological behavior as a cause or contributing factor. Behavioral medicine is a new discipline that emphasizes behavior as a core element in these disorders and behavior change as a central aspect of treatment. Chapter 14 introduces behavioral medicine, presents a treatment protocol as an exercise for you, and describes the special characteristics of a self regulation therapist. Chapter 14 is an introduction for the following chapters in Part Five.

Chapter 15, Behavioral Medicine: Applications with Adults, presents treatment protocols and research on a variety of disorders ranging from clearly stress-related to organic. Chapter 16, Behavioral Medicine: Applications with Children, covers the same range of disorders and the use of behavioral techniques for helping children cope with hospitalization and with painful and traumatic medical procedures.

We are excited about Part Five because we are excited about health and wellness. Treatment is the process of eliciting the client's innate health and wellness and of facilitating self regulation skills through teaching and guidance. From the perspective of the dynamics of health and wellness, we are impressed, but not surprised, by the breadth and success of behavioral treatments. We are impressed, but not surprised, by the ability of humans to regain health, becoming weller than well.

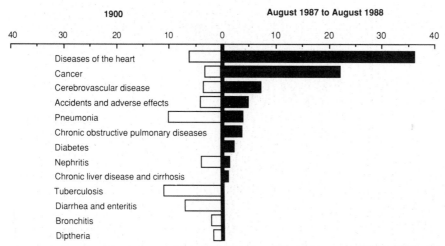

Figure 14.1.   Leading Causes of Death in 1900 and from August 1987 to 1988. Source for 1900 Data is the U.S. Department of Health and Human Services, Health United States 1987, and Source for 1987–1988 Data is the *Monthly Vital Statistics Report, Volume 37*, December 27, 1988.

disease: stress, lifestyle (smoking, diet, lack of exercise), high blood cholesterol, Type A behavior, and so forth. Most of these variables do not fit the medical model of disease, particularly stress, lifestyle, and Type A behavior, because they are not clear physical causes of disease. These are risk factors, and they do not operate like bacteria and viruses.

The greater problem however, concerns treatment. How do you treat a risk factor? Here the medical model has no answer within the scope of traditional medicine.

To summarize so far: (1) The biomedical model of disease cannot account for many modern diseases, such as heart disease, in which no single physical cause can be determined; (2) the medical model fails to acknowledge the multicausal nature of many diseases and illnesses; and (3) the types of treatments that the medical model generates do not apply to lifestyle problems. There is no medical treatment for Type A personality or smoking or failure to express emotions (although the pharmaceutical companies are working hard to create drug treatments for lifestyle problems such as obesity, high blood cholesterol, and stress). As the medical and behavioral

research described in this text painted a clearer picture of the complex variables involved in disease and illness, the inadequacies of the biomedical model became apparent.

Disenchantment with the medical model also comes from another source: the rising cost of medical care. In 1987 health costs accounted for 11.2 percent of the gross national product. Total health costs rose 8.9 percent in 1987 from the 1986 level to an estimated $498.9 billion (Francis, 1988, p. 1). Figure 14.2 illustrates the increasing expenditures for medical care; the inset shows the average cost of coronary bypass surgery.

The rising cost of diagnosis and treatment, and the inability of medical research and treatments to stop the spiral, has stimulated a careful analysis of the nature and causes of the diseases that account for the greatest expenditure. As Figure 14.1 shows, heart disease and cancer are the primary culprits. And, as Roger illustrates, the major killer is often related to poor health habits, habits that have no treatment in the traditional medical sense.

A more inclusive model was needed that would account for the new data, generate appropriate treatments, and guide research.

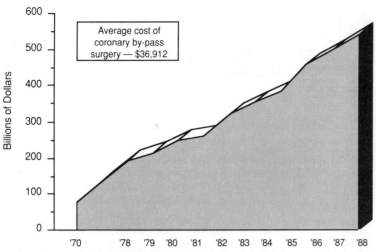

Figure 14.2. Medical Costs Have Skyrocketed in the Last Decade. Cost of Coronary Bypass Surgery from Health Care Financing Administration (1989) and Medical Expenditures from Francis (1988) U.S. Industrial Outlook, 1988, in *Medical Benefits*, pp. 1–2. Adapted with Permission of Kelly Communications.

The Biopsychosocial Model

Summarizing his often-cited article, "The Need for a New Medical Model: A Challenge for Biomedicine," George Engel, professor of psychiatry and medicine at the University of Rochester School of Medicine, writes:

> The dominant model of disease today is biomedical, and it leaves no room within its framework for the social, psychological, and behavioral dimensions of illness. A biopsychosocial model is proposed that provides a blueprint for research, a framework for teaching, and a design for action in the real world of health care.
>
> (Engel, 1977, p. 135)

Like the biopsychosocial approach to health and wellness, the biopsychosocial approach to disease and illness can be simply stated, but it represents complex variables and reflects the interactive nature of these variables.

To understand and treat people such as Roger who have a complex lifestyle disease, the model of disease must point the way to a treatment and prevention approach that includes all the biological, psychological, and social variables that are assumed to play a role in the development of disease and illness. In other words, following the biopsychosocial approach, treatments must include psychological and social factors as well as biological factors, and like the treatments generated by the biomedical model for infectious diseases, biopsychosocial treatments must get at the cause of the problem.

So we return to the question of what caused Roger's death? The infarct that killed enough myocardium to kill the man was the immediate cause of death, but the infarct was merely the final outcome of more complicated causes.

A Hierarchy of Causes

The advantage of the biopsychosocial model over the biomedical model of disease and illness is that it emphasizes the multicausal nature of the diseases and illnesses that plague modern life. Using the example of Roger, we can map out these causes as a kind of hierarchy that led to infarct, the final cause of death (Figure 14.3).

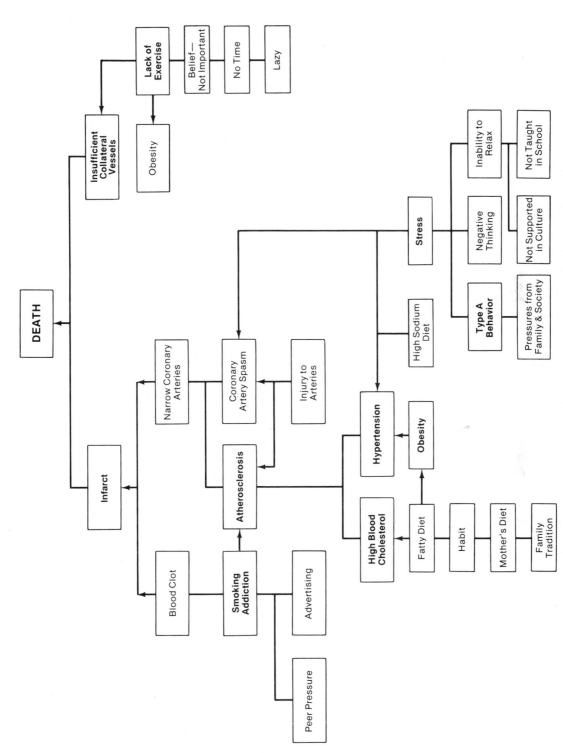

Figure 14.3. The Hierarchy of Causes Leading to Roger's Death. The Major Risk Factors for Heart Attack are Highlighted. These Risk Factors are Primarily Related to Behavior.

Having examined the probable causes of Roger's death, we can see that the simple answer is "infarct." But that does not explain his death, because the causes were many and complex. Yet behind each risk factor—obesity, smoking, hypertension, and stress—we see a common, obvious factor, behavior. Roger's behavior killed him. The coroner could have written on the death certificate "infarct," or "obesity/smoking/hypertension/stress," or "lifestyle," or "behavior."

We began this section by saying that the biopsychosocial model must generate treatments that are relevant to the causes of disease and illness. If Roger had changed a number of behaviors he might not have had the first heart attack, or he might have survived the second. Used in this context, the word *behavior* has a broad definition, including perceptions, beliefs, and overt actions such as overeating, smoking, and Type A behavior. The chronic diseases and illnesses that are handicapping and killing people are disorders of behavior.

Having settled on the fact that behavior plays a key role in disease and illness, we can now introduce the new discipline that focuses on solutions to behavioral problems, behavioral medicine.

Behavioral Medicine

Think for a moment about the term *behavioral medicine*. When the term first became popular some psychologists objected because they feared that "behavior" implied overt behavior or radical behaviorism, omitting the realms of the mind, and that "medicine" implied external treatment given to a passive recipient. As you will learn, "behavior" in the context of behavioral medicine has the broad meaning described in the previous section that includes covert behaviors such as thoughts and images, and "medicine" refers to the science of restoring and preserving health and does not refer to treatments given to a passive recipient.

Examine again the diagram of the hierarchy of causes. Which of these causes are changeable behaviors? Nothing can be done about Roger's childhood habits and childhood obesity, nor his mother's assumptions about good nutrition, nor his genetic structure. All other causes are changeable. Treatments must focus on the behaviors that are changeable.

Behavioral Medicine and Psychosomatic Medicine

Behavioral medicine was formally created in 1977 at a conference sponsored by Yale University and the National Heart, Lung, and Blood Institute, as described in Chapter 1. In 1977 the Society for Behavioral Medicine was formed, and in 1980 *The Journal of Behavioral Medicine* was created. The definition of behavioral medicine most often cited emerged from a second conference in 1978. Behavioral medicine was defined as "the interdisciplinary field concerned with the development and integration of behavioral and biomedical science, knowledge and techniques relevant to health and illness and the application of this knowledge and these techniques to prevention, diagnosis, treatment and rehabilitation" (Schwartz & Weiss, 1978, p. 250). This definition emphasizes the interdisciplinary nature of the field, in keeping with the biopsychosocial model of health and disease.

Doyle Gentry (1984), professor of psychology at the University of Virginia Medical School and the first editor of the *Journal of Behavioral Medicine*, says that behavioral medicine is unique because its research has an interdisciplinary focus. Critics of this position argue that the interdisciplinary focus of behavioral medicine, while important, is not unique (West & Stein, 1982). These critics argue that behavioral medicine is merely "reinventing the wheel" because the field of psychosomatic medicine has the identical purpose and is interdisciplinary.

In 1939 the Society for Psychosomatic Medicine was formed and the *Journal of Psychosomatic Medicine* was created. The purpose of the society was to study the "interrelation of the psychological and physiological aspects of all normal and abnormal bodily functions and to integrate somatic therapy and psycho-therapy" (Dunbar, 1939). In the 1950s, considerable excitement was generated at society meetings by the stress research of Harold Wolff, Lawrence Hinkle, George Engel, Hans Selye, and Ray Rosenman, one of the pioneers of Type A behavior (Wittkower, 1977). In fact, topics discussed in the *Journal of Psychosomatic Medicine* are similar to those in the *Journal of Behavioral Medicine.*

Behavioral medicine and psychosomatic medicine are different, however, in origin and in treatment focus. Psychosomatic medicine was founded by psychiatrists who tried to explain certain illness patterns psychoanalytically, that is, as the result of emotional conflicts in childhood. Naturally, primary treatment for these illnesses was psychoanalysis and medication. Even though psychosomatic medicine moved beyond its psychoanalytic origins to include broader explanations of illness, it has not provided treatments for chronic disorders such as coronary heart disease and cancer, primarily because these are not thought of as psychosomatic. Because they are "lifestyle diseases," the traditional methods of insight-oriented psychotherapies are not necessarily appropriate.

Behavioral medicine is unique because it emphasizes behavioral change through skills, as the treatment. The term itself however, was not the creation of the Yale conference. The term was originally used to describe biofeedback training.

In 1973 former Harvard professor Lee Birk (1973) gathered together in one volume the leading papers on biofeedback training for treatment of tension headache, migraine headache, essential hypertension, Raynaud's disease, epilepsy, and cardiac arrhythmia. Birk titled the book *Biofeedback: Behavioral Medicine,* and he is credited with the first use of the term behavioral medicine. Birk was struck by the fact that biofeedback training is a treatment tool for combating disease and illness, and as such is the domain of medicine. Yet unlike traditional medicine, it enables the patient to change behavior. Therefore, he referred to biofeedback training as behavioral medicine.

In the conclusion to the book, Birk suggests that biofeedback training heralds a new frontier in medicine because the patient is active in the treatment. Birk realized that the participation of the patient is an important aspect of biofeedback training and that the new concept of behavioral medicine emphasizes the patient as active participant in treatment rather than passive recipient. You know from Chapter 8, Biofeedback Training, that this is correct, because the instrumentation has no power to affect physiology and symptoms; only the person using the instrumentation has the power to control psychophysiological processes, and therefore does participate in her or his own treatment.

Becoming actively involved in one's health is not restricted to biofeedback training. In their book *Behavioral Medicine: Theory and Practice,* Pomerleau and Brady (1979) include both behavioral **self-management strategies** and biofeedback training as cornerstones of behavioral medicine. They note that many self-management strategies such as contingency management, self-monitoring, desensitization, self-reinforcement, and behavioral rehearsal are used in behavior therapy to help people control and eliminate destructive habits, which contribute to the development of chronic disorders. As described in Chapter 11, Self Regulation for Health and Wellness, the essence of these self-management strategies is self regulation. Biofeedback therapists and behavior therapists independently developed self regulation strategies that enable people to take control in order to live a disease-free and healthy life. The growth of self-management strategies in behavior therapy and biofeed-back training was a response to the realization that the prevention and treatment of chronic disease and illness must involve behavioral self regulation.

The emphasis on self regulation and the development of methods for teaching self regulation skills distinguishes behavioral medicine from psychosomatic and traditional medicine. In previous chapters we said that self regulation is the heart of stress resistance and health and that it is the essence of biofeedback training and self-management training. Self regulation training for the treatment of disease and illness, for prevention and for high-level wellness, is the hallmark of all the new approaches that come under the umbrella term behavioral medicine.

IIII➡

SECTION TWO: TREATMENT PROTOCOLS

If you were a therapist, stress-management counselor, or lifestyle counselor, what skills would you teach? If you had been the head of the team of experts, how would you have treated Mr. Wright? How would you treat Roger?

You have studied the dynamics of health and wellness, and you are familiar with many tools for promoting health and wellness. Notice that we did not say, "Having studied the dynamics of illness in the previous chapters." The focus on health arises from our conviction that sick people get well by virtue of their innate wellness and their ability to create health and wellness. To help people become healthy, the health professional must understand the dynamics of health and wellness and must know how to facilitate these dynamics in people.

For review, we return to the key ideas of the experts working with Mr. Wright.

General Principles
1. Biological, psychological, and social factors play roles in health and sickness.

2. The resources for health and wellness can be learned.

Psychophysiology
1. Mind ⟶ body.
2. Because mind ⟶ body, stress—often the result of perceptions (including negative and irrational cognitions)—adversely affects the body. It is manifested as the stress response. It is estimated that most visits to a physician are for stress-related complaints.
3. Positive perceptions and emotions, and relaxation, bring mind and body back to healthy homeostasis.

Psychoneuroimmunology
1. Psychosocial stress weakens the immune system.
2. Relaxation and positive moods, imagery, and expectations strengthen the immune system.

Cognitive Psychology
1. Certain behavioral patterns, such as Type A, may predispose a person to illness and disease.
2. Stress-resistant people have particular behaviors and attitudes, such as hardiness and a sense of self-efficacy.
3. Through cognitive restructuring, decision-making, and stress inoculation, and by using role-playing and imagery rehearsal, people learn to confront stressful situations and become stress-resistant.

Relaxation
1. Relaxation promotes physiological and psychological homeostasis.
2. Effective relaxation techniques include autogenic training, progressive relaxation, the quieting response, self-hypnosis, and meditation.
3. Relaxation skills can be improved with biofeedback training.

Biofeedback
1. Through biofeedback training, people gain self regulation of psychophysiological processes, thus countering the effects of stress, overcoming psycho-

somatic illness, and in some cases, overcoming organic disease.

2. Feedback from biofeedback instruments verifies the effectiveness of self regulation strategies for relaxing or for controlling the physiological response being monitored.

Imagery

1. Imagery is the language of mind and body. Images evoke emotional reactions that produce physiological responses.

2. Imagery and visualization techniques help people overcome the stress of past events.

3. Imagery and visualization evoke specific changes in natural killer cell activity, neutrophils, and other immune system functions.

4. Imagery and visualization are effective tools for stress management, relaxation, biofeedback training, self-exploration, and healing.

Lifestyle

1. Health behaviors include proper exercise, diet, relaxation, stress management, assertiveness, a nonviolent lifestyle, and play. Health behaviors promote health.

2. Maintenance of health behaviors is facilitated by appropriate goals and self-rewards, and by environmental management, willpower, self-knowledge, and behavioral and cognitive skills. Social support is an invaluable ingredient in behavior therapy and in health and wellness in general.

Self Regulation

1. The essence of learned resourcefulness is self regulation.

2. Self regulation involves physiological, psychological, and social behavior.

3. Self regulation is the cornerstone of health and wellness.

In addition to these dynamics and ingredients of health and wellness, you are familiar with the basic skills and ingredients of self regulation described in Chapter 11, Self Regulation and Health. The self regulation skills learned in treatment are the skills for healthy living. As a reminder, please review Figures 11.1, the Ingredients of Self Regulation, and 11.3, the Tree of Self Regulation. You also know that many diseases and illnesses, especially the chronic diseases and illnesses of modern life, may have many causes, as seen in Figure 14.3. Review now the characteristics of hardiness in Chapter 6, Figure 6.2, the characteristics of stress-resistant people in Chapter 10, Figure 10.7, and the personal stress signs and stressor inventories in Chapter 3.

Now we can proceed with the exercise of creating a treatment protocol. We choose this format as a device for encouraging you to think about the dynamics of health and wellness in treatment and to challenge your knowledge, not your skill as a therapist. To help in this exercise, we introduce Lea, a 19-year-old woman with a simple stress-related disorder, tension headache. The simplicity of this exercise may be deceiving, and we emphasize that people and their problems are rarely simple and that treatment plans are not rigid but are adapted to the needs of each client. Nonetheless, we invite you to create a treatment plan for Lea, and we describe a typical protocol. Please read Box 14.1 now.

The procedure is this: You create a treatment plan for the first session, following the format; write short phrases (not the details) for the four categories. Set up your worksheet as shown below, putting this information across the top of the worksheet:

Session One

Ideas Taught	Skills Taught	Therapist Tasks	Client Tasks

BOX 14.1

LEA

Lea is a 19-year-old college student who is unemployed and is temporarily living at home. Lea was doing well in school until last quarter, when she lost a good part-time job and had to move home. Lea says that to avoid being with her parents she spends a lot of time partying with friends, and she received two poor grades. Lea's main stressors are school, trying to find a job, living at home, and procrastination.

Lea comes to the Counseling Center for treatment of chronic headache, referred by her physician, who thinks that the headaches are stress-related. She reports that she has three or four bad headaches a week that begin in her neck and gradually encompass her head; they last several hours. Lea has always had headaches, but recently they are worse. The headaches seem to be related to fights with her parents and boyfriend, and they can be severe enough to cause her to cancel a job interview, which she fails to follow up.

Lea vacillates from being apathetic to interested in therapy, and her posture reminds you of a deflated balloon, although you notice that her jaw is tight. She is not overweight and does not smoke, and she does not exercise.

Lea says such things as "My parents make me so angry" and "My boyfriend really stresses me."

After you have created your plan, read the session overview and protocol for the session. Remember that the purpose of this exercise is not to turn you into an instant therapist; the purpose is to encourage you to think through the dynamics of health and wellness and the tools for self regulation from a treatment perspective.

You may find that your first inclination is to teach everything you know and begin biofeedback training and imagery in the first session, which would last about 10 hours! Create your first session protocol with these ideas in mind:

1. You need a history of Lea's headache pattern, and you need to begin to assess psychological (stress-related) and physiological (posture-related) causes of her headaches.

2. Lea needs information about probable physiological and psychological causes of her headaches. She also needs to know how the treatment will help her alleviate the headaches.

3. You need to know what Lea's goals are for therapy.

4. Lea needs to know how these goals will be met, and she must have positive expectations based on knowledge. She must also understand that the success of therapy depends upon her willingness to work.

No two therapists are alike, and probably none have the same protocol for the first session. After the initial history of the symptom and discussion of goals, which are part of everyone's protocol, some therapists conduct a stress profile (described in Chapter 5, Research); some immediately begin a treatment modality such as biofeedback training; and others begin by teaching the principles of self regulation and the basic physiology of the symptom, and by reviewing the overall treatment plan. A first session protocol for Lea would be:

Session One

Overview: Take history of symptom and assess main stressors; set goals for the treatment; introduce assessment questionnaires and rationale for each; describe the principles of self regulation training; teach first stress management technique, two-stage breathing.

Ideas taught:

1. Good therapy is good teaching; knowledge is power.
2. Principles of self regulation training: mind-body, homeostasis, consciousness leads to control (and feedback leads to consciousness), self-responsibility.
3. Stress pushes the body off balance, relaxation brings it back.
4. Our perceptions play a key role in our experience of stress (relate to Lea's perceptions of school and parents).
5. Personality patterns play a role in health and illness.
6. The work involves training both mind and body.
7. Brief description of the physiology of the stress response and the symptom, tension headaches, and how the training is related to the symptom.

Skills taught:

1. Correct breathing; two-stage breathing.
2. Basic cognitive restructuring if needed immediately.

Therapist tasks:

1. Use appropriate assessment tools and explain their importance (Type A questionnaire, assertiveness questionnaire, stress inventories).
2. Help the client establish appropriate goals.

Client tasks:

1. Complete the assessment questionnaires by Session Two.
2. Practice deep breathing as suggested.
3. Pay attention to negative or stress-producing self-talk; keep a stress diary, if suggested.

This first session protocol lays the cognitive groundwork for the training and provides a concrete exercise (two-stage breathing) that can be used immediately for stress reduction and relaxation. It also ensures that the client will perceive herself as an active participant who is expected to take self-responsibility for self regulation and headache reduction.

We give the client reading material related to the symptom and the training, three assessment questionnaires, and a symptom chart for recording the symptom and medications used during the week between sessions. These materials are brought to the second session. This is our standard first-session protocol for the treatment of simple stress-related disorders. The protocol differs for children, cancer patients, and clients with physical problems such as whiplash; in these cases we usually begin biofeedback training or imagery in the first session. And sometimes the entire protocol is temporarily abandoned when the client is in a crisis or needs to share pent-up feelings and thoughts.

Now you create a protocol for the second session, using the same format.

Session Two

Overview: Discuss key responses on the assessment questionnaires; review breathing technique; review the stress response and importance of relaxation training; teach autogenic training; introduce biofeedback training homework based on autogenic training and temperature feedback.

Ideas taught:

1. Review basic principles; answer questions from the reading.
2. Review the physiology of the stress response with focus on blood flow.
3. History of autogenic training and basic principles.
4. Introduce relaxation into daily life to "undo" body habit (headaches).

Skills taught:

1. Autogenic training.
2. Using a temperature feedback device for home training in conjunction with autogenic training; keeping home training records.
3. Simple stress-management techniques such as stopping for yellow lights and enjoying the short relaxation break.
4. Simple stretching exercises for neck and shoulders.
5. Techniques for avoiding a power struggle with parents.

Therapist tasks:

1. Assessment of major stressors.
2. Discuss dynamics of power struggle with parents and methods for avoiding the power struggle.
3. Knowledge of autogenic training.
4. Good coaching.
5. Demonstrate hand-warming using autogenic phrases and temperature feedback.

Client tasks:

1. Begin using stress-management techniques.
2. Practice autogenic feedback training at home 15–20 minutes a day.
3. Use stretching exercises regularly.
4. Practice methods for avoiding the power struggle.

In our standard protocol, autogenic training is taught in the second session. We feel that it is important to involve the client in home training for deep relaxation immediately, and autogenic feedback training is easy to learn. Using an inexpensive weather thermometer taped to a finger, the client receives feedback for finger temperature (blood flow) and records temperature at the beginning and end of each session. Many therapists provide cassette tapes of relaxation procedures, and listening to the tape is the primary homework assignment.

Now you create your protocol for the third session.

Session Three

In this session Lea reports that she has found a job in the accounting office of the college; she has had a continuous headache since starting because the job is very stressful; she enters data into a computer and files records.

Overview: Continue discussion of assessment questionnaires; review use of stress-management techniques; review home training records and symptom chart; five minutes to increase finger temperature on command; introduce short relaxation techniques and give colored dots as reminders, to be placed in Lea's work environment and at home; ask Lea to become conscious of her posture and head position as she works and explain the importance of balancing the head.

Ideas Taught:

1. Short relaxation techniques are the cornerstone of the training and must become automatic. Prevention of stress, the stress response, and thus headaches is the key to good training.
2. No one has the power to make us angry or stress us—we do it to ourselves.

Skills taught:

1. Short relaxation techniques emphasizing head and shoulder rolls while sitting at the computer; mini progressive relaxation.

2. Cognitive skills for destressing.
3. Study skills with rewards for hard work.
4. Body-scan relaxation procedure is taught to augment or replace autogenic training.
5. Recognizing and countering negative self-talk.

Therapist tasks:
1. Provide materials on study skills.
2. Share personal use of short relaxation techniques.
3. If necessary, help Lea problem-solve failure to do homework.

Client tasks:
1. Continue daily relaxation practice.
2. Continue stretching exercises.
3. Practice short relaxation techniques and cognitive destressing throughout the day.
4. Practice problem-solving with parents to defuse power struggles.
5. Begin to counteract negative self-talk.

By the third session many biofeedback therapists would have introduced EMG feedback training. Our approach with Lea emphasizes the prevention of headache by countering the stress response throughout the day. We introduce the short relaxation techniques in the third session so that she can begin incorporating the techniques into daily life. If Lea had not found a job and was not particularly stressed, we might have introduced EMG in the third session and perhaps even in the second.

Now you create your protocol for the fourth session.

Session Four

Overview: Follow up on use of short relaxation techniques and dots; review homework and symptom charts; problem-solve obstacles to training; five minutes of hand-warming on command; introduce basic concepts of assertiveness with parents and boyfriend; introduce EMG training and train on forehead muscle; review posture during work.

Ideas taught:
1. Difference between assertiveness and aggression.
2. Simple physiology of muscles and anatomy of facial, neck, and back muscles.
3. Basics of EMG feedback.

Skills taught:
1. Basics of assertive behavior, taught with role-playing.
2. To feel tension in facial muscles, particularly masseter, and to relax these muscles.
3. To generalize relaxation to the entire body.

Therapist tasks:
1. Provide material on assertiveness.
2. Model assertive behavior.
3. Role-play assertive behavior.

Client tasks:
1. Continue daily practice of stress management, relaxation, and stretching exercises.
2. Practice assertive behaviors.

We usually begin EMG feedback training with electrodes on the forehead muscle; this provides feedback for all the muscles of the face and is a good way to begin relaxation training for jaw tension.

Now you create your protocol for the fifth session.

Session Five

By session five, Lea is doing very well with relaxation training at home and can relax and increase peripheral blood flow on command. In this session it is time to test her mastery of this skill with the challenge of increasing and decreasing hand temperature repeatedly. She reports that she no longer "lets her parents get to her" and that she is using her assertiveness skills and cognitive stress-management skills at work. Her headaches are decreasing.

Overview: Follow up on all techniques taught to date, and problem-solve any obstacles to the training; introduce EMG feedback training on trapezius muscles; discuss exercise program; test mastery of relaxation and hand-warming with stress tape.

Ideas taught:

1. The head is like a 10-pound watermelon that must be balanced on the vertebra of the neck to allow neck muscles to relax; when the head is off balance, neck muscles must be used to hold it up.
2. The head must be balanced on the spine while working on the computer, and posture should be improved in general to reduce headaches.
3. Strong and flexible muscles that are regularly exercised can withstand stress better than weak muscles.

Skills taught:

1. Feeling the delicate balance point of the head on the spine.
2. Maintaining better posture.
3. Relaxing the trapezius muscles while working on the computer and studying.

Therapist tasks:

1. Model good posture.
2. Provide diagrams of muscles and good posture.

Client tasks:

1. Continue short relaxation techniques throughout the day and practice longer and deeper relaxation only three to four times a week.
2. Continue to improve study skills.
3. Look into exercise programs on campus and sign up for an aerobic exercise class.

Lea's therapy would continue for a few more sessions until she felt confident that she could continue practicing and applying her new skills on her own. After that, she would be invited to return to therapy for follow-up sessions as needed.

Obviously we created an ideal case; in reality, therapy rarely progresses in such an organized fashion. Although some people have uncomplicated stress-related disorders, many do not. A person may enter therapy with a simple goal of reducing headaches, for example, and during the course of therapy may reveal many past and current life situations that contribute to the symptom and must be resolved. For this reason, therapists are highly trained or work in close supervision with a therapist who has extensive clinical experience. In Lea's case, her relationship with her parents might become the focus of therapy, or procrastination might be related to deep-seated self-image issues that must be resolved.

From this brief and rather simple example of treatment protocols for five sessions, we can discern several essential elements in therapy:

1. Client education. The client must understand the dynamics that underly self regulation training; the client needs information about the psychophysiology of the symptom; the client needs to know how the skills learned in therapy will affect the symptom; the client must understand the nature of stress and be able to assess stress and stressors.
2. Assessment. Symptom stressors, personality, and lifestyle habits are assessed and goals are established.
3. Acquisition and mastery of physiological, cognitive, and behavioral skills for self regulation.
   1. physiological skills:
      deep relaxation
      breathing
      recovery from stress
      prevention of stress response
   2. cognitive skills:
      positive self-talk

identify and counter irrational
  perceptions
positive imagery
3. behavioral skills:
  assertiveness
  adopting healthy lifestyle habits
4. Home training. Practicing and perfecting skills out of the clinic.
5. Good coaching. Modeling skills and encouraging the client to practice; providing support and praise.

Clients with stress-related disorders are taught basic skills such as deep relaxation, proper breathing, and short relaxation techniques; problem-solving skills and skills for changing lifelong behavior patterns are taught. We emphasize again that (1) self regulation is the central theme in all behavioral therapies and that (2) self regulation is gained through

skills. Self regulation skills must be taught, and that is why good teaching is such an important aspect of behavior therapies. Skills must be practiced, which is why the client must be an active participant and must have a healthy sense of self-responsibility.

Although some elements of the treatment protocol are the same for all clients, the therapist must be able to draw upon a large repertoire of techniques and ideas to helping clients handle the variety of life events and conditions that befall people. This makes behavioral therapies always challenging. Because no two clients are the same, there can never be a set treatment protocol; treatment must be tailored to the needs of the person. Remember this point, because it will come up again when we talk about the difficulties of clinical research in Chapter 15. Please read Box 14.2 now.

BOX 14.2

TRAINING TO MASTERY

The word *skill* appears repeatedly throughout this text. There are relaxation skills, biofeedback skills, cognitive skills, imagery skills, interpersonal skills, assertiveness skills, and decision-making skills. These behavioral skills are learned, through practice and coaching. Guidelines and training criteria are needed to determine whether or not a skill is adequately learned. Training criteria are needed when a certain level of proficiency is needed. For example, a typist intending to get a job as a secretary needs to be able to type at a certain speed with a certain level of accuracy. These criteria are standardized, and typists train until they reach these levels of proficiency.

In the working world, training criteria are important for guaranteeing proficiency at a task. In skills-oriented treatment, training criteria are needed to ensure learning of self

regulations skills. In addition, data indicate that for many clients symptoms are ameliorated only after the client has achieved a particular level of self regulation. For example, criteria are now established for sufficient cardiovascular exercise based on heart rate, called the target heart rate. Target heart rate is based on age and the percent of maximum heart rate that a person wants to reach during training. When we jog we carry a heart-rate monitor so that we can run hard enough to stay at the training criterion that we have set for ourselves.

In biofeedback training, finger and toe temperature-training criteria have been established for reducing blood pressure. The data indicate that the best temperature-training criteria are 95° F to 97° on hands and 91° to 93° on feet (Fahrion, et al., 1987; Libo & Arnold, 1983).

Training criteria have many purposes: (1)

they give the client a clear goal to work toward, (2) they provide a scale by which progress can be measured, and (3) they provide a scientific standard for verifying sufficient physiological change. We have found that clients can make significant change without reaching these criteria. However, when there is no reduction in the symptom and the client has not reached training criteria, then it is likely that more training is necessary.

In addition to training to criteria, we emphasize the need for **mastery**. A skill is mastered when it can be demonstrated under adverse conditions. In academics, exams test mastery; in sports, competition tests mastery. Mastery of behavioral skills is demonstrated by mastery tasks, such as warming one hand while the other is immersed in cold water, or by reducing muscle tension while calculating difficult math problems, or by keeping blood pressure within a normal range while playing a video game. Measurement of physiological processes with biofeedback instrumentation verifies physiological mastery. For other behavioral skills such as assertiveness training, mastery is equated with success. For example, in stress-inoculation training the stressor is confronted "in real life" and handled, or the ex-smoker is offered a cigarette and does not accept it. These successes indicate masterful self regulation.

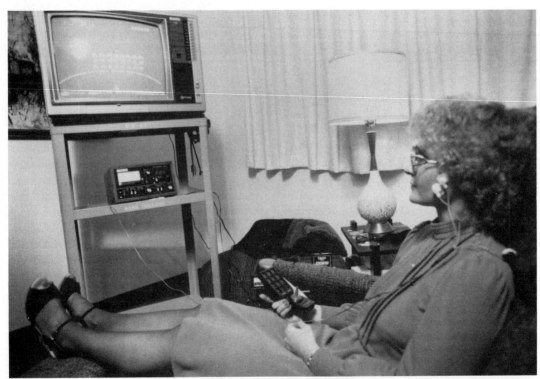

The Trainee Demonstrates Mastery of Jaw Relaxation While Engaging in a Stressful Task—a Video Game. Biofeedback Equipment is Useful for Feedback and Verification of Success.

IIII➡

SECTION THREE: THE SKILLS OF THE THERAPIST

By now you realize that the type of therapy that we call self regulation training, behavioral therapy, or skills-oriented therapy, is not a traditional "talk therapy." It demands work of both therapist and client. The skills-oriented therapist must have a large bag of tricks and a variety of skills. We conclude this introduction to behavioral medicine and treatment with a brief discussion of the skills of the therapist.

Most people learn self regulation skills on their own, but sometimes people need help. Just as a good coach can enhance an athlete's motivation and performance, so a good therapist can enhance motivation and acquisition of self regulation skills.

Before describing the skills-oriented therapist, we must describe the tasks of the therapist. Because behavior includes both overt and covert behaviors, because behavior is at the heart of the disorders that therapists are consulted for, and because behaviors are changeable through knowledge and skills, the therapist must have:

1. All the skills of a good therapist (empathy, active listening, drawing out the resistance, establishing positive rapport).
2. All the skills of a good teacher (explanations appropriate to the interests and intellectual level of the client, good examples and stories, provides teaching materials, encourages questions).
3. Extensive knowledge of mind-body interaction and of how personality plays a role in illness.
4. Extensive knowledge of stress and the stress response, including the physiology of symptoms.
5. Knowledge of the primary classes of medications and their side effects.

6. Extensive knowledge of stress-management techniques (relaxation techniques, time management, decision-making, assertiveness, desensitization, and cognitive restructuring), as well as skill in role-playing techniques, problem-solving, guided imagery, and behavior-modification techniques.
7. Basic knowledge of nutrition and exercise.
8. Knowledge of the basic treatment protocols for many psychosomatic illnesses.
9. Knowledge of good self-help books and community programs available for the client to augment therapy.
10. The ability to assess the strengths and the deficiencies in the client's roots and know how to help the client amend deficiencies.
11. Be a model of the skills and health practices that are taught.

Obviously, these are not easy tasks. In addition, the therapist is knowledgeable about therapeutic techniques that are not on the self regulation tree such as rolfing, acupuncture, and massage therapy, and must assess new behavioral techniques as they arise.

Over many years of teaching biofeedback therapists, we have identified several abilities that are needed by a skills-oriented therapist, a therapist who teaches skills for behavioral change as the primary mode of therapy.

Counseling Skills and Positive Rapport

Anyone who works with people in a helping role must have basic skills and qualities that facilitate rapport. Establishing positive rapport is the first requirement in the art of helping. Positive rapport results from empathy and caring.

Rapport literally means "relation" and refers to a relationship of understanding, warmth, and

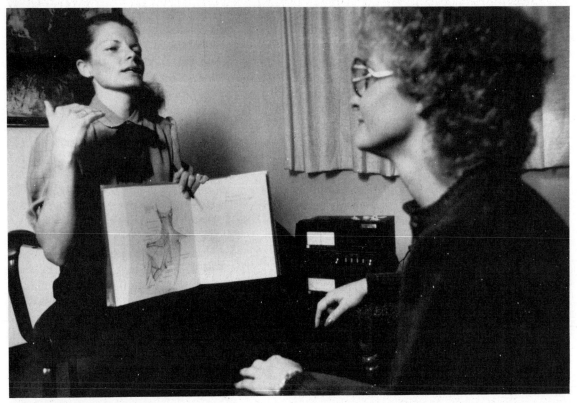

Therapists are Good Teachers.

trust between therapist and client, coach and athlete, doctor and patient, student and teacher, parent and child, or leader and group. Research in psychology, education, and sports has demonstrated the importance of positive rapport. When a therapist is warm and caring, the client is more likely to follow a treatment program longer and with more success than when the therapist is cold, angry, or impatient (McGoldrick & Pearce, 1981; Rubenstein, 1986; Strupp & Binder, 1984). Clients, students, and athletes learn faster and more thoroughly with professionals who are warm and positive than with professionals who are cold and distant (Carkhuff & Berenson, 1976; Taub, 1977; Smoll & Smith, 1984). In a study of 59 clients, the single factor that predicted success was the therapist's warmth and understanding (Free, Green, Grace, Chernus, & Whitman, 1985).

Other basic counseling skills include attending to and observing the client, taking a thorough history, problem-solving, goal-setting, rewarding positive change, feedback, and informative self-disclosure.

Teaching Ideas and Skills

"Knowledge is power." This is our rationale to the client as we teach the material that we think the client needs to knows. To therapists we say, "Good teaching is good therapy."

Good teaching involves clear, jargon-free explanations and a rationale for every idea and procedure taught. Noncompliance with treatments is often traced to the fact that the patient does not understand the treatment program. When procedures and instructions are clear and written down, clients are likely to comply with the program (DiMatteo & DiNicola, 1982).

A good therapist also has the ability to stimulate positive expectations and enthusiasm in the client through teaching.

Assessment

Assessment means measurement. Assessment is an ongoing process in skills-oriented therapies and includes measurement of (1) the cause and history of the disorder; (2) the client's coping style (strengths and weaknesses, assertive behavior, Type A behavior, or secondary gain such as worker's compensation for loss of work because of illness); (3) the client's beliefs about health and illness; (4) physiological responses such as muscle tension, blood pressure, vasoconstriction, breathing pattern, and heart rate; (5) acquisition of skills; and (6) symptom status and well-being.

Therapists use a variety of assessment tools, including standardized questionnaires, homework sheets, symptom charts, physiological measures via biofeedback instruments, weekly self-reports, mastery exercises that challenge the client to demonstrate the learned skills under pressure, and intuition and experience.

Feedback

Good therapists are good observers and are good at giving feedback in a helpful way. A good therapist can detect and understand the client's cognitive and overt behaviors that need to be changed. Like a good coach, a good therapist can give accurate and precise feedback, backed by information about how to make the needed change.

Self-Training and Self-Knowledge

"Practice what you preach" is a perfectly accurate statement of an important dictum for therapists who specialize in helping clients practice wellness behaviors and give up worseness behaviors. Practicing what is preached is essential because modeling is teaching and because failure to model wellness behavior jeopardizes therapy. In order to practice what they preach, therapists must train themselves in the techniques that they teach. This has two advantages. As we practice and model the skills that we teach (including following good diet and exercise programs), we promote our own health and equally importantly, we gain personal experience that is invaluable for teaching. We are good teachers partly because we use our personal experiences as a guide for the client.

Self-knowledge is as important to therapists as it is to clients. Freud insisted that to correctly analyze patients, the psychoanalyst must undergo analysis first. This was to ensure enough self-knowledge so that the analyst would not interpret the client in terms of her own psychological makeup. We do not recommend such a strenuous route, but the basic idea is sound. More importantly, the therapist can guide the client best where the therapist has already been.

Summary

Therapists who teach self regulation skills as the primary treatment must be prepared to work with their clients on every level of human functioning. This seemingly enormous requirement arises from the fact that disease, illness, and discomfort result from complex interactions of mind and body and lifestyle. Those three elements are in themselves extremely complex.

We have discussed the key elements of good therapy and the essential characteristics of the therapist. These elements cannot be ranked, are equally important, and are interacting.

CONCLUSION

This chapter introduced the basic ingredients of self regulation therapy. Chronic disease and illness are often related to behavior. When this is the case, behavior change is the goal of treatment, which is change that occurs through learning and practicing self regulation skills. There simply is no quick fix, a medication or an operation for preventing and curing modern disease and illness. This is illustrated by the fact that after bypass heart surgery, arteries become clogged again in 60 percent of patients. The mandate of behavioral medicine, as a discipline, is to advance our understanding of illness behaviors and the way such behaviors can be changed through treatment.

This textbook began with a discussion of the biopsychosocial approach to health and wellness, noting that health and wellness involve biological, psychological, and social variables in interaction. In this chapter we described the shift from the biomedical model to the biopsychosocial model of disease and illness, a model that recognizes the multicausal nature of many disorders. The biopsychosocial model is a "whole person" approach, a theme that was first expressed by the great modern physician, William Osler: "It is more important to know about the person who has the disease than to know about the disease itself" (1921). In the age of medical specialization, however, it is easy to overlook the fact that the diseased body part or function exists within a person who has mental and emotional responses that influence physiological functioning and who lives in a social system that determines lifestyle and that can influence both psychological and physiological processes.

Behavioral medicine treatments for disorders with biological, psychological, and social components necessarily address these components, treating the whole person. Through multicomponent therapy, people learn physiological, cognitive, and social skills that are necessary for the prevention and treatment of chronic disease and illness.

CHAPTER *15*

Behavioral Medicine: Applications with Adults

Think of Chapter 14 as the introduction to this chapter. We noted at the conclusion of the previous chapter that behavioral therapies take into account the complexity of symptoms, recognizing that the chronic diseases and illnesses of modern life usually result from many factors that cannot be neglected if treatment is to be successful and lasting. Mr. Wright, Roger, and Lea illustrate the diversity of causes of disease and illness as well as the diversity of disorders that may be amenable to behavioral treatments. Section One examines symptom etiology more closely, emphasizing the importance of multicomponent therapy, and Section Two presents treatment protocols and research on many of the disorders that are successfully treated with behavioral techniques.

SECTION ONE: ETIOLOGY OF SYMPTOMS

Where do symptoms come from? By now you have a good idea of how to answer this question. You would say "behavior," meaning lifestyle, cognitive, personality, and stress behaviors and the stress response. You would understand that a symptom may have many causes—a hierarchy of causes.

The hierarchy of causes of a symptom may be simple or complex. So far we have discussed fairly simple causes. Some causes, however, are not easily identified and may be unknown to the client or identifiable and understood but complex. Complex causes include traumatic experiences such as the death of a spouse, abuse as a child, unloving or schizophrenic parents who did not provide good parenting, and all other conditions that stunt the development of a positive self-image and a sense of self-efficacy. Another complex cause is a family pattern that fosters sickness as a way of coping with life.

To fully understand a symptom, we must understand both the cause and the reasons the symptom continues. Some symptoms are maintained simply out of habit or from lack of knowledge, or because the body has been structurally damaged and cannot recover. Sometimes, however, symptom maintenance is more complex, because the symptom fulfills a need. When the symptom serves a useful purpose, a goal of therapy is to help the client understand the underlying need that the symptom fulfills or helps fulfill. "Secondary gain" is the term commonly used to describe the advantage of maintaining a symptom, but the term is somewhat misleading because the gain from maintaining a symptom can be primary. An obvious example is the wife who develops a migraine headache whenever her husband brings home his buddies from work. Without doubt the headaches could be stress-related as she anticipates a rowdy bunch of people who drink too much and tear up the house. But at the same time a headache is an excellent excuse to avoid the situation and could even end it, so the headaches may be useful.

Some symptoms are easily understood, particularly stress-related symptoms when stressors are obvious and changeable. We call these **simple psychosomatic symptoms**. For example, a muscle-contraction headache caused by poor posture at work and time pressure is simple, as is an ulcer caused by a feeling of impossible demands and smoking. Simple symptoms are maintained by habit and lack of knowledge, and they are alleviated quite quickly with the methods of behavioral medicine. On the other hand, **complex psychosomatic symptoms** are not easily changed because they are maintained by habit, a lack of knowledge, and many psychological factors, in addition to stress. Often people with complex symptoms have complex lives with many conflicts.

Figure 15.1 describes factors that promote and reduce symptoms from the biopsychosocial perspective, emphasizing the role of many factors in symptom development and reduction.

You can understand why the treatment of clients such as Mr. Wright, Roger, and Lea is referred to as **multicomponent**. When a disorder has many causes, or contributing factors, therapy must address at least the primary causes.

Such therapy is multicomponent, meaning that many therapeutic components are used. Mr. Wright would benefit from a variety of therapeutic tools, including imagery. Roger's therapy would have included diet and exercise counseling, and Lea would be taught the standard procedures of stress management and relaxation training. Clients with complex symptoms also receive extensive psychotherapy that might include techniques for overcoming the past.

Clinical treatment may be relatively simple and short term (10–15 sessions) or complex and lengthy; the length and complexity of the therapy depend on the complexity of both the client and the symptom. With these ideas in mind, we describe treatment protocols and clinical research on a variety of disorders.

IIII➡

SECTION TWO: TREATMENT APPLICATIONS

This section describes treatment for a variety of disorders, including problems that are (1) clearly stress-related, such as tension headache; (2) disorders that are not clearly stress-related nor clearly organic in origin, such as Raynaud's disease; (3) organic disorders such as epilepsy that may be exacerbated by stress; (4) neuromuscular disorders that result from injury; (5) symptoms caused by organic disorders such as a reduction of blood flow in the feet caused by diabetes; and (6) purely organic disease. An organic disease has a clear physical cause, such as accident or birth defect, and does not have a psychological or stress component as a primary cause; stress can exacerbate most symptoms, however, regardless of the cause. This section also includes the important contribution of behavioral techniques to reduction of the side effects of cancer treatment.

Successful clinical protocols include the basic ingredients described in Chapter 14, and we do not repeat these ingredients except in the description of Patel's work on the

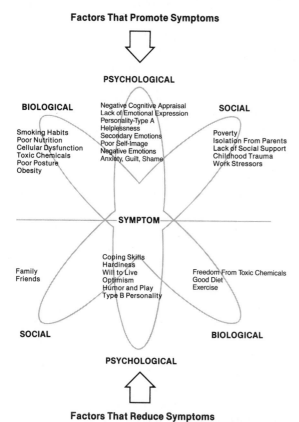

Figure 15.1. Biological, Psychological, and Social Factors that Promote or Reduce Symptoms.

treatment of hypertension and Schneider's work on the treatment of irritable bowel syndrome. We include these as examples of clinical protocols that have been researched. Throughout this section we cite the best research on the disorders discussed. We use the term *best research* to refer to research with the best methodology and results. We do not report research with poor methodology and poor results that have been critiqued elsewhere (Green & Shellenberger, 1986a, 1986b; Shellenberger & Green, 1986, 1987; Steiner & Dince, 1981, 1983). You might correctly ask: "What about clinical research that follows the best clinical methods and also has poor results?" The answer is that after an extensive review of the clinical research literature, we can find no well-conducted studies in which significant reduction of symptoms did not occur. This does not mean that all trainees do equally well or that all reduce their symptoms. For various reasons, the techniques of self regulation training do not benefit all people, sometimes because the techniques are not learned, or used, or both. Group data, however, are very encouraging.

Behavioral medicine research is difficult because, like clinical treatment, it must be multicomponent and must not attempt to isolate the effects of a single independent variable. The importance of multicomponent research has recently been clearly described by experimental psychologists (Sheridan, 1980; Neff & Blanchard, 1987). Clinical procedures used in clinical treatment settings should be the experimental procedures of clinical research, but the complexity of treatment is often difficult to duplicate in a research setting. It is rare that the results of research equal the results of clinical practice because research generally does not allow the kind of personalized treatment that is part of good clinical practice (Andrasik & Blanchard, 1987; Adler & Adler, 1983; Libo & Arnold, 1983a, 1983b).

This section cannot cover all the important and interesting applications of behavioral methods, but it does give you enough detail to

understand the basics of behavioral treatments and to appreciate the variety of disorders that people can overcome when given knowledge and skills.

Hypertension

Please read the section on hypertension in Chapter 4.

Essential hypertension is called the "silent killer" because most people with high blood pressure have no symptoms. Hypertension is a major risk factor in cardiovascular disease and stroke, kidney failure, and congestive heart failure. It is estimated that one out of every five adult Americans has high blood pressure, and yet many do not know that they do (U.S. Department of Health, 1984). Obesity, stress, and atherosclerosis contribute to the development of essential hypertension. The most commonly prescribed drugs in America today are for hypertension, but 50 percent of hypertensives stop taking their medications within one year after diagnosis (Haynes, Mattson, & Engebretson, 1982). This is due in part to the side effects of the antihypertensive medications. Diuretics (drugs that decrease blood volume and peripheral resistance) decrease potassium levels and increase uric acid and sugar in blood, increasing the risk of lethargy, nausea, gout, dizziness, and headaches. The side effects of beta-adrenergic blockers (drugs that lower the heart rate) include impotence, diarrhea, Raynaud's phenomenon, skin disorders, lethargy, nausea, dizziness, headaches, and depression. Vasodilators (drugs that decrease peripheral resistance) increase the risk of heart palpitation, edema, rapid heartbeat, and drug-induced lupus erythematosus. Unlike pharmacological treatments, behavioral methods have no negative side effects (Fischer-Williams, Nigl, & Sovine, 1981).

One of the most successful and carefully researched nondrug multicomponent treatments for essential hypertension was developed by

London physician Chandra Patel. Over a 15-year period, Patel conducted several carefully controlled studies validating the effectiveness of a multicomponent treatment program for reducing blood pressure (Patel, 1973; Patel, 1975a, 1975b; Patel & North, 1975; Patel, Marmot, & Terry, 1981; Patel, Marmot, Terry, Carruthers, Hunt, & Patel 1985). At a time when many biomedical model researchers were studying the efficacy of single-component treatment for essential hypertension, such as direct blood pressure feedback with no coaching or other therapeutic components (Schwartz & Shapiro, 1973; Surwit, Shapiro, & Good, 1978; Miller, 1975/1976; Elder & Eustis, 1975), Patel created a multicomponent treatment that included patient education, biofeedback training, meditation, diaphragmatic breathing, home practice, behavioral monitoring, and good coaching. Patel based the protocol on her clinical experience and knowledge of hypertension.

Clinical Protocol

We highlight Patel's research protocol because it has the important ingredients of a multicomponent treatment for blood pressure reduction.

Patient Education, Treatment Goals, and Assessment. Patel's treatment program begins with group meetings. Films and slides about high blood pressure are presented, the treatment goals and training procedures are explained, and patients are encouraged to ask questions. These meetings with Patel and coworkers establish positive rapport and group support. Lifestyle (exercise, smoking, diet) and personality patterns of nonassertiveness and Type A behavior are assessed. Blood pressure and EDR (electrodermal response) measures are recorded in the clinic. Subjects learn to monitor blood pressures at home using inexpensive blood-pressure cuffs.

Acquisition and Mastery of Skills. In Patel's program, patients use biofeedback to help them learn systematic relaxation skills, beginning with diaphragmatic breathing. Next they learn deep muscle relaxation using a yoga exercise similar to the body scan described in Chapter 7, Relaxation. Muscle tension and electrodermal feedback is used to facilitate deep relaxation training. Meditation, the third skill, is taught after the patient has learned deep relaxation. Meditation training teaches the patient how to focus the mind (Patel, 1984). The meditation technique is adapted to the patient. Some patients prefer to focus on an object, and others prefer to repeat a word such as *one* to quiet and focus the mind. Others focus on the breath, or the imagined sound of a waterfall, or the buzzing of bees, or cars going by. Others use prayer as their quieting meditation.

Patel's program includes a cognitive and behavioral stress-management component (Patel, Marmot, & Terry, 1981). Patients learn to identify stressful events and practice using positive thoughts, positive imagery, and short relaxation techniques to counter the stress of these events. Patients are instructed to practice their skills at every red traffic light by saying, "Great. A red light. Now I can relax for a minute," and then taking deep breaths and relaxing. The patient is given colored dots to place on his wristwatch or telephone as a reminder to use a short relaxation technique (Patel, 1984).

Patients are encouraged to adopt healthy lifestyle habits such as regular exercise, a diet with low fat and sodium, and Type B behavior (the opposite of Type A). They are also encouraged to stop smoking.

Patients meet in groups once a week to discuss their progress.

Homework is essential to mastery of the techniques being learned. Patients are instructed to practice relaxation and meditation twice a day for 15 to 20 minutes and to practice short relaxation and stress-management techniques throughout the day. At the end of training, patients demonstrate their skills during stressors, like putting a hand in a bucket of ice water. Mastery is demonstrated if there is no undue elevation of blood pressure when one hand is in ice water and if blood pressure returns to normal within 10 minutes after the hand is removed from the water (Patel, 1975a).

Coaching and Training Goals. Realistic goals are established for the patients so that they can succeed. "A sense of success is necessary for one's self-esteem and the therapist should keep this in mind when setting goals with biofeedback instruments" (Patel, 1984, p. 36). Patel knows that an effective therapist is a good coach who encourages and rewards patients for acquisition of skills.

Results. In Patel's early studies (Patel, 1975a, 1975b; Patel & North, 1975), patients in the treatment group significantly reduced their blood pressure and medications, in contrast to the no-treatment control groups who were on medications only. Systolic blood pressure reductions averaged 26 mm and diastolic reductions averaged 15 mm, while the no-treatment control group reduced systolic blood pressure by 9 mm and diastolic by 4 mm (Figure 15.2). In contrast to the control group, the treatment groups' subjects also significantly lowered

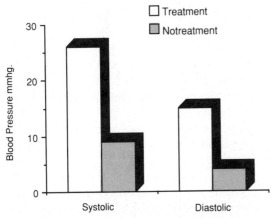

Figure 15.2.   Treatment Group and No-Treatment Group Reductions in Systolic and Diastolic Blood Pressure. From Patel and North (1975). Randomized Controlled Trial of Yoga and Biofeedback in Management of Hypertension. *Lancet 2,* **93–95. Reprinted with Permission of the Author and Publisher.**

serum cholesterol, triglycerides, fatty acids, and medications. At the 12-month follow-up, the treatment group patients had maintained reductions in blood pressure, serum cholesterol, triglycerides, fatty acids, and medications (Patel, 1975b).

Other studies have demonstrated the effectiveness of multicomponent treatment protocols for lowering blood pressure (Blanchard, McCoy, Musso, Gerardi, Pallmeyer, Gerardi, Cotch, Siracusa, & Andrasik, 1986; Fahrion, et al., 1987; Goebel, Viol, Lorenz, & Clemente, 1980; McGrady, Woerner, Bernal, & Higgins, 1987).

Refinements. The major refinement to Patel's multicomponent treatment program was introduced by Green, Green, & Norris (1980), described in Chapter 8, Biofeedback Training. They found that hand-warming and foot-warming are important ingredients in treatment, and patients who achieved temperature training criterion on hands (95 + °F) and feet (92 + °F) significantly lowered blood pressures compared with those who did not meet the criteria. These results have been replicated by Fahrion and coworkers, who treated 42 hypertensives. A 33-month post-treatment follow-up showed that 32 of the 42 patients had reduced blood pressure by 15/10 mmhg (p < .0001) and significantly reduced medications (Fahrion et al., 1987).

Recall the garden hose analogy for blood pressure and the formula for blood pressure (blood pressure = heartrate × stroke-volume × peripheral resistance), and answer this question: "Why is hand- and feet-warming important for treatment of essential hypertension?" If you said, "Because increased hand and feet temperature is the result of increased vasodilation, and vasodilation reduces peripheral resistance, and reduced peripheral resistance reduces blood pressure," you are correct.

Behavioral treatment for essential hypertension helps people who are willing to learn and use deep-relaxation and stress-management skills, and who are willing to make necessary

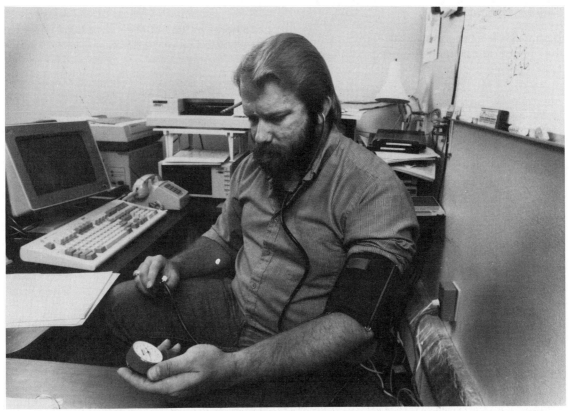

Using Stress Management Skills and Monitoring Blood Pressure at the "Scene of the Crime," in This Case, Work, are Important Elements in Treatment for Hypertension.
Source: Robert Waltman, Aims Community College, Greeley, CO.

lifestyle changes. The clinical protocol developed by Patel and refined by Green, Green, and Norris provides systematic guidelines for the treatment of high blood pressure.

Headache

Please read the section on headache in Chapter 4.

Almost everyone has headaches. Harold Wolff (1948) writes, "Since the human animal prides himself on 'using his head' it is ironic that his head should be the source of so much discomfort" (p. ix). Chronic headache afflicts 40 percent of the adult population (Ziegler, Hassanein, & Couch, 1977) and accounts for

18.3 million physician visits each year (National Center for Health Statistics, 1986). The most common headaches result from muscles abused by poor posture or chronic tightening. Muscle-tension headaches account for 70 percent of all headaches, and migraine for 25 percent (Feuerstein & Gainer, 1982; Feuerstein, Bush, & Corbisiero, 1982). The Ad Hoc Committee on Classification of Headache for the American Medical Association describes 15 types of headaches varying from stress-related to those caused by brain tumors. Behavioral therapies, particularly biofeedback therapy, are potentially beneficial for millions of people with migraine, tension, or mixed headaches who do not want to use medications.

Tension Headache

Perhaps you have a headache right now. You may feel a dull generalized head pain coming from knotted muscles in your neck, shoulders, or head. As you read this book, your 10-pound head may be too far forward, causing your neck and shoulder muscles to contract. Headache relief will begin when you thoroughly relax those muscles by improving your posture and by using a relaxation technique and easy neck and shoulder stretches.

Effective clinical protocols for tension headache include teaching people how to prevent chronic tightening of muscles and how to relax muscles.

Protocol for Prevention and Treatment of Muscle Contraction Headaches.

The first step in prevention and treatment of tension headaches is to identify behaviors that contribute to misuse, underuse, or overuse of muscles. Misuse of muscles includes poor posture while working, driving a car, studying, reading, and doing hobbies such as knitting, sewing, and crocheting. Emotional stress also contributes to misuse through chronic muscle-tightening. Many people chronically tighten the jaw during stress. Underused muscles become weak, inflexible, and more susceptible to emotional and physical stress. Overuse of muscles from overexertion or failure to warm up before exercise and cool down afterward can lead to muscle spasm.

Adopting behaviors such as good posture, stretching, and exercising, and learning techniques for coping with stress is a second step in prevention and treatment of tension headaches. A third step is learning to relax the whole body

and specific muscles. Most of the research on behavioral treatment of tension headaches has concentrated on relaxation techniques alone.

Research on Treatment of Muscle Tension Headaches.

University of Colorado researcher Tom Budzynski and his colleague Johann Stoyva, whom you met in Chapter 8, pioneered in behavioral methods for treatment of tension headache. In his early research, Budzynski (1973) compared three groups of headache patients: a no-treatment control group (n = 6), a false feedback control group that received signals from an EMG instrument that were not related to muscle tension (n = 6), and an EMG biofeedback training group (n = 6). By the end of the treatment, four of the six subjects in the treatment group had significantly fewer headaches. In the false feedback group, one of the six subjects significantly reduced headaches, and in the no-treatment control group no subjects had fewer headaches. Medications were significantly reduced in the treatment group but remained the same or increased in the false feedback and no-treatment control groups. After a three-month follow-up, biofeedback training was offered to patients in the control groups. Eight of the control subjects volunteered for training. After 16 sessions, six of the eight subjects had significantly reduced headaches and medications.

From this first tension headache study, the importance of training to criteria was discovered. Budzynski found a .90 correlation between achieving a criterion of 3.0 μ V (p-p) on forehead and significant headache reduction. In other words, subjects who attained deep

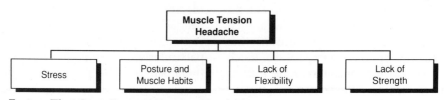

Figure 15.3. Factors That Contribute to Tension Headache.

levels of muscle relaxation had a significant reduction in headaches.

Budzynski described this early work as bare-bones biofeedback because the treatment included only one component, EMG biofeedback. Later, he developed a multicomponent training program that included temperature and EDR feedback, relaxation tapes, short relaxation exercises, desensitization, and stress-inoculation training (Budzynski, 1979). Budzynski also pioneered the use of stressors to help the client gain psychophysiological mastery, a technique that he called "recovery training" after discovering that chronic headache clients fail to return to homeostasis after a stressful event. They do not turn off the stress response, and over time symptoms develop. Budzynski added recovery training to the protocol for treatment of psychophysiological disorders such as tension headache, migraine headache, high blood pressure, and irritable bowel syndrome. Recovery is conscious return to homeostasis after a stressful event. To enhance recovery skills, Budzynski challenges the client with a variety of stressors such as startling noises and mathematical problems that have to be solved in a limited amount of time while listening to a tape of distracting noises. With the help of feedback from biofeedback instruments, clients learn to recover rapidly after confronting a stressor. Figure 15.4 shows EMG data before, during, and after a math stressor. This subject recovered rapidly.

Many clinical researchers have demonstrated the success of multicomponent treatment of tension headache; some examples are Andrasik, Blanchard, Neff, and Rodichok (1984); Andrasik and Holroyd (1983), Blanchard, Andrasik, Guarnieri, Neff, and Rodichok (1987); Hudzinski (1983), and Reich (1989). Ed Blanchard and coworkers at the State University of New York at Albany are conducting long-term follow-up studies of headache patients. Subjects learn diaphragmatic breathing, progressive muscle relaxation, and temperature and EMG biofeedback skills. Of 33 tension headache patients, 73 percent significantly improved by the end of treatment and at four-year follow-up were still improved (Blanchard, Andrasik, et al., 1987).

Migraine Headache

The serendipitous discovery by Elmer and Alyce Green that hand-warming, aided by thermal feedback, could ameliorate migraine headache (see Chapter 8) led to many studies with a variety of behavioral training techniques: autogenic training, progressive relaxation, EMG training, temperature feedback training, and autogenic feedback training.

Migraine headache is primarily a vascular problem beginning with vasoconstriction in the extracranial (*extra* = outside, *cranial* = skull) and cerebral (brain) arteries followed by rebound vasodilation, which causes pain. The exact mechanisms of migraine headache are not clear, but there is general agreement that the culprit is a "hyperactive" vascular system that reacts to stress, muscle tension, certain chemicals in foods, and in some cases changes in the weather (a drop in barometric pressure).

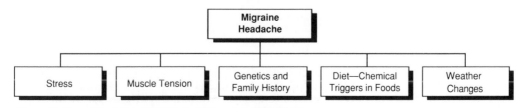

Figure 15.4. Factors That Contribute to Migraine Headache.

Prevention and Treatment of Migraine Headaches. Identification of the conditions that trigger the cycle of vasoconstriction and vasodilation is an important element in prevention and treatment of migraine headache. Questionnaires and diaries help clients identify triggers, including stressors, muscle tension, and foods that contain tyramine, a vasoconstrictor. Through self-monitoring, a person may also become aware of an aura during the vasoconstriction phase before the head pain begins. Migraine patients who sense an aura before a headache may have time to use behavioral skills to prevent rebound vasodilation, and thus may avoid the headache.

The primary element in biofeedback therapy for migraine headache is control of peripheral blood flow through autogenic training and peripheral blood flow (temperature) feedback. Learning to relax the vasculature through hand-warming facilitates homeostasis in extracranial vessels so that extreme constriction and rebound vasodilation do not occur (Fahrion, 1978). Learning to cope with stress and learning deep muscle relaxation are also important skills in migraine treatment. The expression of anger through assertiveness training and changing perfectionistic attitudes may also help.

Research on Treatment of Migraine Headache. Blanchard and colleagues (1980) conducted a meta-analysis (statistical analysis of many studies) of relaxation techniques for treatment of migraine. The results, shown in Figure 15.5, were: (1) Of 146 patients who used thermal feedback with autogenic training, 65.1 percent reduced the number and severity of headaches; (2) of 41 patients using thermal feedback alone, 51.8 percent reduced the number and severity of headaches; (3) of 159 patients using relaxation training alone (progressive relaxation or the relaxation response of Benson), 52.7 percent reduced the number and severity of headaches; and (4) of 234 patients given placebos, 16.5 percent reduced the number and severity of headaches.

From this meta-analysis it is clear that autogenic training using temperature feedback is a successful technique for treating migraine headache. The success rate increases when other components are added, such as training to criterion on hand temperature and muscle relaxation. Fahrion (1978) showed a 71 percent success rate at a six-month follow-up for 21 migraineurs who reached the criterion of 95°F on hands using autogenic feedback techniques. A long-term follow-up study by

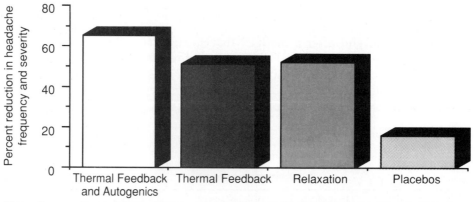

Figure 15.5. Comparison of Three Treatment Methods on Reduction of Severity and Frequency of Headaches. From Blanchard, Andrasik, Ahles, Teders, and O'Keefe (1980). Migraine and Tension Headache: A Meta-Analytic Review. *Behavior Therapy, 11,* 613–631. Copyright 1980 by the Association for Advancement of Behavior Therapy. Reprinted by Permission of the Publisher and the Author.

Libo and Arnold (1983a, 1983b) showed a 100 percent success rate with migraineurs who achieved training criteria of 95° on hands and 3 microvolt readings (peak-to-peak) on forehead during EMG feedback training.

Learning to cope with negative emotions through cognitive and behavioral skills is also an important ingredient in treating migraine headache. In a 10-year follow-up of migraine patients, those who learned relaxation skills, hand-warming to 95°, and skills for coping with anger and other negative emotions had an average decrease in headaches from 35 to 5.8 per year and significant reductions in medications. In contrast, patients who learned hand-warming but no cognitive skills had an average decrease of headache frequency from 35 to 23 per year, and medications were not significantly decreased (Adler & Adler, 1983).

The long history of treatment for migraine headache reveals the effectiveness of a multicomponent protocol that includes deep muscle relaxation, autogenic feedback training, home training, training to criteria, defusing and removing stress triggers, and stress inoculation. Recent examples of multicomponent programs

---

BOX 15.1

CLUSTER HEADACHE: CASE REPORT

Cluster headache is extremely painful. Patients describe the pain as an icepick being driven through an eye. The cause of cluster headache is unknown. Strong medications are only moderately successful in preventing the headaches.

King and Arena (1984) successfully treated a 69-year-old man who had cluster headaches for 37 years. In addition to biofeedback training, a contingency management program was created. "Contingency management" means giving appropriate rewards for desired behaviors and punishments for undesired behaviors. A common reward is attention, and a common punishment is withholding attention.

King and Arena were convinced that the patient's headaches had been "conditioned" by the love and support that he received from his wife every time he had a headache. Consequently, they instituted the following program: (1) the patient agreed not to tell his wife when he was having a headache or to talk about the pain with her (that is, he would no longer elicit a reward); (2) he agreed to treat the headache himself by setting the alarm when he wanted to get up after a headache instead of asking his wife to get him up; (3) his wife agreed to ignore ("punish") her husband when he appeared to be having a headache; and (4) they both agreed to spend at least 16 to 30 minutes a day talking together about positive events or topics when he did not have a headache (reward).

The results of the contingency management program and biofeedback training were spectacular. Before the treatment the patient averaged one cluster headache a day for 20 years and used medications daily. At an eighteen-month follow-up he had four to six days a week without a headache. The pain severity decreased from 7 to an average of 2.3 on a scale of 1 to 7. All medications were eliminated.

are: Blanchard, Andrasik, et al. (1987); Blanchard, Appelbaum, Guarnieri, Neff, Andrasik, Jaccard, and Barron (1988); and Reich (1989). Please read Box 15.1 now.

Irritable Bowel Syndrome

Please read the section on gastrointestinal disorders in Chapter 4.

Irritable bowel syndrome is the most common gastrointestinal disorder in the United States. It is estimated that every year 14 percent of healthy American adults suffer irritable bowel syndrome and that 50 percent of a gastroenterologist's practice is devoted to its treatment (Thompson & Heaton, 1980). Irritable bowel symptom includes pain in the gut, diarrhea or constipation (or both), "bloating," and gas. High-fiber diets, tranquilizers, and muscle relaxants have been used with minimal results (Drossman, Powell, & Sessions, 1977; Hillman, Stace, & Pomare, 1984).

University of Colorado psychologist Carol Schneider pioneered the development of an effective multicomponent procedure treatment for irritable bowel syndrome. Schneider's patients were students who came for treatment at the Student Health Center. Most patients had difficulty in interpersonal relationships with friends, family, or spouse. Most were overdependent on their family, friends, or spouse. They also tended to be unassertive, and 90 percent said that they kept their feelings to themselves. Of 58 students, 73 percent became symptom-free or were greatly improved by the end of treatment and at the one-year follow-up (Schneider, 1983).

Clinical Protocol

Patient Education and Assessment. Clients are given information about normal gastrointestinal functioning and the relationship of stress to disturbances of normal functioning. The importance of healthy lifestyle habits, including a high-fiber diet and exercise, are discussed. Handouts on stress and irritable bowel syndrome are used for instruction. Personality tests, a one-hour interview, and a stress profile using temperature, EMG, and GSR measures are conducted.

Acquisition and Mastery of Skills. Clients are taught diaphragmatic breathing, progressive relaxation, and autogenic training with feedback from EMG and temperature feedback instruments. EDR measurement is also used to assess relaxation skills. If the EDR measures are not normal, then EDR feedback training is used to ensure that the client has learned relaxation.

Our only refinement to this part of the protocol is the addition of foot temperature training. Learning to increase blood flow in the feet facilitates deeper relaxation than hand-warming, and we speculate that the training also increases vasodilation and muscle relaxation in the gut.

Homework training, short relaxation exercises, desensitization, and colored dot relaxation reminders are used. Symptom charting helps the client identify stressors that trigger the symptom and aids the evaluation of progress. Assertiveness and other social skills are taught, and clients learn to define their self-worth internally rather than externally. Patients are also taught thought-stopping techniques, guided imagery, and cognitive-restructuring skills.

Research Results

For his doctoral dissertation at the University of Colorado, Steve Giles (1978) conducted a controlled study of Schneider's treatment protocol for irritable bowel syndrome. He randomly assigned 40 subjects to one of four conditions: (1) forehead EMG biofeedback training alone; (2) psychotherapy alone (social skills and stress-management training); (3) combined biofeedback and psychotherapy; and (4) no-treatment control. Subjects in the three treatment conditions received 15 treatment sessions. The combined psychotherapy and biofeedback training was the most effective treatment, with 90 percent of subjects reporting less diarrhea at the end of treatment ($p < .05$). At the eight-month follow-up, 73 percent of these subjects reported less diarrhea ($p < .05$) and less anxiety ($p < .01$), depression ($p < .05$), and worry ($p < .01$). They also reported feeling more relaxed ($p < .01$), more assertive ($p < .01$), and independent ($p < .01$). The psychotherapy group significantly improved, and the EMG feedback group moderately improved. There were no significant improvements in the no-treatment control group.

The Stress Disorders Clinic at the State University of New York at Albany has conducted several studies on treatment of irritable bowel syndrome (Blanchard & Schwarz, 1987; Neff & Blanchard, 1987). In one study, 10 subjects were assigned to a multicomponent treatment group and nine were assigned to a symptom-monitoring group (daily monitoring of symptoms for 12 weeks). The 10 treatment subjects received 12 one-hour sessions that included progressive relaxation, temperature feedback, and stress-coping strategies (identifying stressors that contribute to the symptom and using positive self-talk and short relaxation techniques to cope more effectively with the stressors). Of the 10 subjects who received treatment, six significantly decreased symptoms of abdominal pain, diarrhea, constipation, and flatulence, while only one subject moderately improved in the symptom-monitoring group (Neff & Blanchard, 1987).

In a two-year follow-up study of 17 patients who were treated for irritable bowel syndrome at the Stress Disorders Clinic, 12 patients had significantly decreased all symptoms (pain, diarrhea, constipation, and flatulence), three reported no change, and two were worse (Blanchard, Schwarz, & Neff, 1988). In addition to reducing irritable bowel syndrome symptoms, the 12 successful subjects also reported improvement in well-being—less anxiety, less depression, and less psychosomatic distress.

Raynaud's Disease

In 1864, Paris physician Maurice Raynaud described a symptom that is characterized by vasospasm in the hands or feet, causing pain and in severe cases, causing tissue damage, chronic sores on the tips of the fingers, or gangrene. Raynaud's disease has been called the "red, white, and blue disease" because digits become white with vasospasm, then blue from anoxia, and finally red from rebound vasodilation. Cold temperatures and stress may trigger the vasospasm.

Although Raynaud's disease is not life-threatening, it is uncomfortable and can be handicapping when fingers or toes are chronically irritated. Raynaud's patients often must wear gloves, even in the summer, and cannot tolerate exposure to cold in everyday activities such as selecting food from the freezer section at the grocery store.

The most common medical treatments for Raynaud's disease are surgery (sympathectomy, or cutting the sympathetic nerves that innervate the vasculature of hands or feet, thus preventing vasoconstriction) and medications such as vasodilators. The results of these treatments are unreliable and usually help for only a short time.

Severe vasospasm in hands or feet can be triggered by exposure to cold or stress. A behavioral treatment technique would include temperature feedback training, desensitization to cold, and stress management. Treatment of Raynaud's with temperature (blood flow) feedback is obvious, because Raynaud's is a blood flow problem, and increasing hand temperature directly counters the spasm. Furthermore, with training, the tendency of the vasculature to overreact decreases.

Clinicians have used thermal feedback combined with desensitization and stress management with Raynaud's clients for many years. Research, with the limitations noted in this text, has been less successful in general, but the studies by Freedman, Ianni, and Wenig (1983, 1985) have been quite successful. In the 1983 study four procedures were compared: (1) finger temperature feedback, (2) finger temperature feedback under cold stress (the finger with the temperature sensor was placed on a cold surface), (3) autogenic training, and (4) forehead EMG feedback training. Each patient did home training, completed 10 training sessions, and received cognitive stress-management training 10 minutes before and after each clinic training session. Frequency of symptoms was reduced by 92.5 percent for subjects receiving the temperature biofeedback under cold stress, by 66.8 percent for the temperature biofeedback group, by 32.6 percent for the autogenic training group, and by 17.0 percent for the EMG training group. Figure 15.6 shows the results of training for each group.

This study is unique because a challenge was incorporated in the training: learning to increase hand temperature in spite of exposure to a cold surface, which the subject felt as increasingly colder as hand temperature increased. The fact that subjects with the cold challenge did significantly better than others in reducing vasospasm attacks highlights the importance of including challenge as an integral part of the training. These results validate the concept that training should be thorough, for the better the training, the better the results will be.

Raynaud's disease has a cousin called Raynaud's phenomenon. Raynaud's phenomenon has the symptoms of Raynaud's disease, but by definition it is secondary to an organic disorder that affects peripheral vasculature. Diseases that affect connective tissue may produce Raynaud's phenomenon. I (JG) have worked with two clients who had Raynaud's phenomenon, and both were able to reverse the peripheral vascular effects of the underlying disorder. The youngest, SA, a 16-year-old boy with scleroderma, rapidly learned to raise his hand temperature on command and could do so outside in a cool breeze or with a cold cloth draped

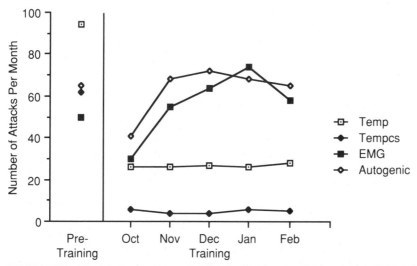

Figure 15.6. Comparison of Treatments for Raynaud's Disease. From Freedman, Ianni, and Wenig (1983). **Behavioral Treatment of Raynaud's Disease: Long-Term Follow-Up.** *Journal of Consulting and Clinical Psychology, 51,* 539–540, **Copyright by the American Psychological Association. Adapted by Permission.**

across his hands. The sores on his knuckles and fingertips slowly healed, and the swelling in his fingers decreased. We had an unusual measure of improvement—the development of wrinkles around SA's knuckles. In addition, the tissue under the skin of his arms began to soften, a change that was noticeable after about three months of training. To aid the body in this task, we created a visualization in which SA moved through the stiff fibrous collagen strands with an army of wire cutters.

My second client, RL, was diagnosed with "mixed connective tissue disease." Her fingertips were tender and were very sensitive to cold. This unusually persistent client used thermal feedback at home at least five times a week for several months. Her home training data are presented in Figure 15.7. After many weeks of training, her starting hand temperature began

to increase, indicating that her vasculature was recovering. Toward the end of the training, which included desensitization to cold, RL was able to take items from her refrigerator freezer without gloves, and she even made ice cream.

Reversal of the organic processes in these cases was medically unexpected. But these reversals were anticipated from a perspective of mind-body interaction and the dynamics of health.

Diabetes

Diabetes is a complicated disease that can be simply described as the failure of the pancreas to produce insulin or the failure of cells to respond to insulin and absorb glucose. Insulin is essential for life because it is the only substance

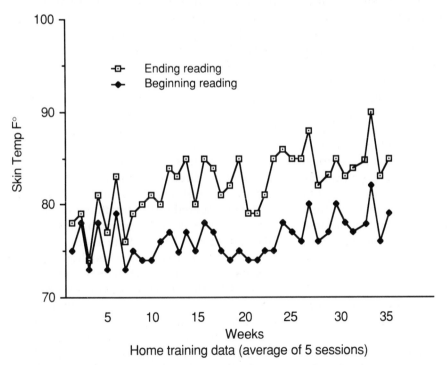

Figure 15.7. A Patient with Raynaud's Phenomenon, Secondary to Connective Tissue Disorder, Gradually Learns to Increase Blood Flow in Her Fingers and Start Temperature Increases, Indicating that Blood Flow is Improving.

inactive and dependent on other people. In some cases, recovery is complicated by financial incentives for staying in pain, such as worker's compensation for disability or a lucrative court settlement for injury and chronic pain.

Chronic pain and treatment of chronic pain are topics in themselves. This section concentrates only on the treatment of low back pain.

Like all chronic pain syndromes, low back pain is complex, and multicomponent procedures are the most successful. The best programs include physiological, cognitive, and behavioral training (Keefe & Hoelscher, 1987; Newman, Seres, Yospe, & Garlington, 1978).

Physiological Procedures

Pain patients are caught in a cycle of pain ⟶ tensing ⟶ muscle spasm ⟶ increased pain ⟶ increased tensing ⟶ increased muscle spasm ⟶ increased pain. Biofeedback-assisted relaxation techniques are valuable in helping patients break the cycle of pain and tension (Flor, Haag, & Turk, 1986; Keefe & Hoelscher, 1987). Three procedures are particularly useful:

1. Progressive relaxation assisted by EMG feedback from the forehead and upper back for generalized relaxation. After patients learn deep relaxation, they are encouraged to practice these relaxation skills during everyday activities.
2. Relaxation in sitting, standing, and lying positions while receiving EMG feedback from the lower back muscles.
3. EMG feedback from the lower back muscles during flexing, rotating, and stretching.

Abnormal muscle activity often occurs only during these activities.

Cognitive Procedures

Hypnosis, imagery, and stress inoculation help people in chronic pain.

Hypnosis. An effective technique for hypnotizable pain patients involves hand anesthesia, tested with a pinprick, followed by hypnotically induced anesthesia of the painful area of the back. About 1 out of 10 people can be deeply hypnotized and can achieve pain anesthesia (Hilgard & Hilgard, 1983). For people who are hypnotizable, hypnosis alleviates pain better than medications such as morphine and Valium and is more effective than acupuncture (Stern, Brown, Ulett, & Sleten, 1977). Please read Box 15.3 now.

T. X. Barber, a pioneer in medical hypnosis, believes that the hypnotic state is not a special state and that people can reduce pain just as well through cognitive and imagery techniques. Analyses of hypnotized patients show that they use cognitive strategies such as distraction or pleasant imagery to modify pain (Chaves & Barber, 1974). Fortunately, people who are unsusceptible to hypnosis can learn cognitive and imagery techniques for coping with pain (Turk, Meichenbaum, & Genest, 1983).

Beliefs, Imagery, and Self-Talk. The power of belief has been demonstrated repeatedly in drug research. The effectiveness of a drug is always measured in relation to a placebo. These studies show a substantial reduction in pain from the placebo effect. When the injection is believed to be morphine, expectation of pain relief can reduce severe pain by 40 percent to 50 percent. Grevert and Goldstein (1985) have demonstrated that people increase their pain tolerance when given placebos and that endogenous opioids are one mechanism by which beliefs reduce pain.

Some pain patients do not believe that they can influence the experience of pain. To overcome this resistance, psychologists Perry London and David Engstrom (1982) designed an ingenious experiment. Using the Rotter locus-of-personal-control test (described in Chapter 6), they identified 32 pain patients who were high on external locus of control,

BOX 15.3

SELF-HYPNOSIS TECHNIQUES FOR LOW BACK PAIN

1. For deep relaxation use a self-guided relaxation induction. Make a tape of your own to guide yourself into a deep state of relaxation. On the tape include suggestions for deep breathing, systematically relaxing your body (autogenics or guided imagery), with phrases such as "going deeper into a state of deep relaxation." Create an image of descending in an elevator or walking down a staircase, or count backwards from 10 to 1.

   Practice induction techniques when you are relatively pain-free. Practice ending the hypnotic session with techniques for returning to your normal waking state, such as counting from 1 to 10, or imagining that you are climbing stairs or riding up an elevator.

2. Create numbness in your hand by repeating the phrase "My hand is beginning to feel cool and numb," or by imagining that you are rubbing Novocain on your hand, which becomes heavy and numb, or imagine that your hand is falling asleep, or that you are wearing a heavy leather glove. Now imagine pinching your gloved hand—feel the dullness and the thickness. Imagine a thick sheath over your hand as you lightly pinch it. Pinch your hand four times, and each time feel a thicker and thicker sheath surrounding your hand.

   After anesthetizing your hand, move to the area of pain in your back. Feel your back getting heavy and cool. Imagine Novocain being rubbed on your back. You feel no pain because your nerves have been deadened. All you feel is a heaviness and thickness.

3. Focus your attention on your back. Relax the muscles around the painful area. Feel these muscles relax and imagine the sore area beginning to relax and become cool. The inflamed area is becoming cool, cool, cool. Feel the discomfort drain out of your back and right out of your body. Feel it drain away. Feel cool sensations, such as cool water flowing over your back. The cool water flows over the area, washing away discomfort, washing discomfort completely away. It soothes your back; you feel relief, relaxation, and comfort. Your back feels soft and flexible.

4. Give your pain a shape—a ball of energy, a red ball. Watch this red ball of energy become smaller and smaller. Imagine the color of the ball beginning to lighten, beginning to change to a soft pink and becoming smaller and smaller. The ball grows smaller, and you feel less and less discomfort; you begin to feel better and better, you feel better as you watch the ball become smaller. Now watch the pale pink ball become tiny, tiny, smaller and smaller; watch the color change from faint pink to pale blue. It is now becoming a small blue dot, small blue dot, and now just watch it disappear, and when it disappears you feel much, much better. You feel better, more comfortable, you feel better, more comfortable, very comfortable. You feel completely comfortable.

5. Give yourself a permanent suggestion: "From now on, my subconscious will keep my back relaxed and stress-free."

Hadley & Staudacher, 1985

meaning that they perceived their life to be controlled by external forces. London and Engstrom told these patients that they would receive either sugar pills or morphine. In fact, all 32 received sugar pills, and all patients reported a significant reduction in pain. After three weeks, London and Engstrom told 16 of the 32 patients that they had been taking sugar pills and offered them the opportunity to learn cognitive coping skills for continued reduction of pain. All 16 accepted the opportunity and learned the skills. At the end of the 10-week training period, all subjects in the treatment group reported decreased pain, and the 16 patients who continued to take sugar pills reported increased pain.

The 16 treatment-group patients learned stress inoculation using visualization, positive self-talk, and positive reinforcement. First, they developed pleasurable mental imagery such as floating in a warm pool and listening to peaceful music. Next they associated the pleasurable scene with pain, so that whenever they began to feel pain they could immediately visualize the pleasurable scene. Third, the patients learned to use positive self-talk such as "I reduced my pain before through my belief that I was taking morphine, so now I can do it again with my beliefs" and "I can think of pleasant scenes to reduce my pain." Fourth, the patients were taught to reward themselves and seek reward from others when they reduced pain, by talking about their success and complimenting themselves.

The effectiveness of cognitive techniques for reducing pain has been demonstrated in a number of studies (Turk, Meichenbaum, & Genest, 1983; Turk & Flor, 1984).

Behavioral Techniques.   University of Washington psychologist Wilbur Fordyce was a pioneer in the use of contingency-management techniques for controlling pain (Fordyce, 1976). Fordyce was one of the first pain specialists to study pain behaviors. Pain behaviors are responses that pain patients unnecessarily adopt, such as moaning, limping, or complaining about

pain as the time for medication approaches. Fordyce has filmed pain patients walking down the hospital corridor toward the nurses' station. As they approach the station, they stoop more and more and go past the nurses appearing to be in excruciating pain. Once past the nurses, they slowly straighten up again.

Fordyce realized that pain behaviors increase the experience of pain and that they are learned. This insight led to the immediate realization that pain behaviors can be unlearned and that consequently, the experience of pain can be reduced. In his first study of 36 hospitalized patients, Fordyce used social incentives to help people control pain by reducing pain behaviors. Family members and medical staff were instructed to reinforce healthy behaviors by ignoring patients' complaints about pain and their pain behaviors. Fordyce also set up a program in which patients received pain medications every four to six hours rather than upon request. The medications were given in a "pain cocktail." The medications in the cocktail were gradually reduced. During the treatment program, patients increased physical activity, decreased pain ratings, and decreased medication. Twenty-two months after discharge from the hospital, patients continued to exercise, used minimal medication, and experienced pain relief (Fordyce, 1976). Other studies have reported similar results using similar techniques (Cairns, Thomas, Mooney, & Pace, 1975).

Pain clinics are found in cities throughout the United States, all using a variety of behavioral techniques. The Portland Pain Center and the Medical School of the University of South Carolina have reported successful results using a combination of physiological, cognitive, and behavioral techniques. The Portland Pain Center reported successful results with 100 low back pain patients. At the 18-month follow-up, patients had maintained reductions in medications, increased exercise, and reduced pain (Newman, Seres, Yospe, & Garlington, 1978; Seres & Newman, 1976). At the Medical University of South Carolina, there was an 80 percent

TRAINED PAIN

Our colleague and biofeedback pioneer Tom Budzynski tells this story:

"I was in the hospital recovering from surgery and I was in a lot of pain. The pain medications were delivered every four hours, and I noticed that my pain increased in intensity right up to the delivery of the medications and then subsided for about 2 hours and then the pain began again. The medications were a tremendous relief, and as the day for leaving the hospital approached, I began to worry. I was told that I would not have Demerol when I left the hospital, but I was still in pain every four hours.

Finally the day came—I left the hospital dreading the usual increase in pain. At home I nervously watched the clock, knowing that this time there would be no medications to knock out the pain. At three hours after the last medication I felt no pain, at 3 1/2 hours no pain, at 3 3/4 hours still no pain. At four hours, pain free, I started to laugh, realizing that in the hospital I had unconsciously increased my own pain."

Budzynski had unconsciously trained himself to feel pain around medication time, and the expectation of pain was always fulfilled. When he understood cognitively that the reward/relief would not be forthcoming, the experience of pain ceased, in spite of his expectation. One cognition counteracted another. The experience of pain is complex and rarely dies so readily, but this is a fascinating example of pain behavior, in which the anticipation of pain and medication increased the experience of pain. This example may also illustrate a precursor of addiction to pain medication. The experience of pain is genuine, and the sufferer is not aware that the pain is conditioned to the anticipation of medication.

Pain-management programs help patients discover and counteract unconscious conditioning of this type.

---

success rate with 15 older patients, ages 55 to 78, and a 68 percent success rate with 19 younger patients, ages 29 to 48 (Middaugh, Kee, & Barchiesi, 1987).

Chronic pain is devastating. Experiencing pain every day strains psychological balance, threatens relationships, and can lead to addiction to medications. The cost of treating chronic pain is high. For example, disability payments from worker's compensation average $7,000 per patient per year. Patients participating in a multicomponent pain-treatment program that includes biofeedback and cognitive training reduced medical costs by 44 percent and disability payments by 50 percent in the first year after treatment. See Figure 15.9.

Coping with Medical Procedures

Treatment of Nausea and Vomiting Caused by Chemotherapy

Nausea and vomiting are extremely disagreeable side effects of chemotherapy suffered by about 50 percent of cancer patients. Antinausea drugs are often not effective, and patients begin to dread treatment and are often severely distressed by the treatment. Some patients stop treatment rather than suffer the side effects of chemotherapy and radiation. After two or three chemotherapy sessions, patients may become conditioned to smells, sights, or thoughts that are associated with the treatment setting. One patient saw her chemotherapy nurse in a

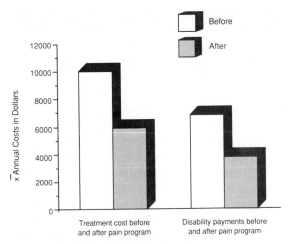

Figure 15.9.   Cost of Pain Treatment and Disability Payment before and after Participation in a Multicomponent Pain Treatment Program. From Steig, R. L., and Williams, R. C., in *Seminars in Neurology, Volume 3*, No. 4, New York, 1983, Thieme Medical Publishers, Inc. Reprinted by Permission.

department store and immediately vomited. Another patient went to a new restaurant and noticed an odor that reminded him of the odor of the hospital's cleaning solution. He rushed to the restroom and vomited (Redd, 1984). You may recall our description of this phenomenon in Chapter 2, in which we described the response as classical conditioning. This devastating effect of chemotherapy can make it hard for even the toughest patient to maintain a fighting spirit. Nausea and vomiting (and other side effects, such as hair loss) are psychologically and physiologically draining. We are not surprised when the will to live begins to fade in a patient with a severe reaction to treatment.

Behavioral training for reducing and coping with the side effects of chemotherapy and radiation is an important addition to cancer therapy. Increasingly, treatment centers across the country are incorporating programs for helping the patient with the psychological and physiological effects of treatment. One of the most effective techniques focuses on the conditioning element in the nausea and vomiting response—desensitization training, with its important ingredient, relaxation. The superiority of desensitization training was demonstrated by Gary Morrow (1986) of the University of Rochester School of Medicine, who compared the effectiveness of three therapeutic techniques in reducing both anticipatory nausea (conditioning) and nausea that is the immediate effect of the chemicals. The subjects were divided into four groups: (1) systematic desensitization (progressive relaxation and hierarchy of nausea producing scenes) , (2) progressive relaxation only, (3) Rogerian counseling, and (4) no-treatment control (subjects completed evaluation forms and were paid for participating in the research) . Twenty-three cancer patients participated in each group. Results of treatment for **anticipatory nausea** were: (1) systematic desensitization, 88 percent improvement; (2) progressive relaxation only, 66 percent; (3) Rogerian counseling, 45 percent; and (4) no-treatment control, 35 percent. Results for **posttreatment nausea** were (1) systematic desensitization, 54 percent improvement; (2) progressive relaxation, 61 percent; (3) Rogerian counseling, 35 percent; and (4) no-treatment control, 50 percent. Patients in the systematic desensitization group significantly lowered their anxiety levels compared to the other groups. Results are shown in Figure 15.10.

Morrow's research confirms the findings of other studies demonstrating that relaxation and desensitization techniques reduce nausea and vomiting in patients undergoing chemotherapy (Lyles, Burish, Krozely, & Oldham, 1982; Redd & Andrykowski, 1982). Desensitization is a counterconditioning procedure and is helpful for that reason. At the same time, we cannot overemphasize the importance to patients of receiving help and of having a skill or technique to use when needed. Anything that reduces feelings of helplessness and loss of control is beneficial, an important aspect of behavioral treatments for all disorders.

Attentive professionals have noted a connection between the cancer treatment center itself and the incidence and severity of nausea and vomiting among cancer patients receiving

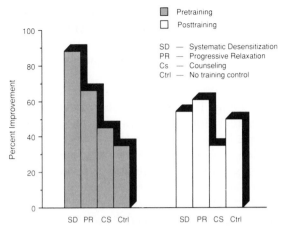

Figure 15.10.   Comparison of Three Procedures and No-Training on Anticipatory Nausea. A Graph Based on Data from Morrow, G. (1986), Effect of Cognitive Hierarchy in the Systematic Desensitization Treatment of Anticipatory Nausea in Cancer Patients: A Component Comparison with Relaxation Only, Counseling, and No Treatment. *Cognitive Therapy and Research,* **10,** **421–446. Plenum Publishing Corporation. Reprinted by Permission of Author and Publisher.**

chemotherapy. The patient's reaction to chemotherapy can be affected by the physical environment, the attitudes of the staff, and the availability of friends and family during lengthy injections (sometimes lasting several hours); access to radio, television, and magazines; and even the comfort of the recliner chair (Cohen, Blanchard, Ruckdeschel, & Smolen, 1986). A pleasant and personal environment reduces nausea and vomiting in patients receiving radiation or chemotherapy.

Summary

The variety and depth of behavioral techniques and applications cannot be covered in a single chapter. In this section we introduced the main disorders for which behavioral medicine techniques have been beneficial. Many other disorders have been treated—as demonstrated through controlled studies—such as

generalized anxiety, asthma, insomnia, motion sickness, urinary incontinence (loss of bladder control), bruxism (grinding the teeth), and temporomandibular joint pain. Other disorders have been treated but not extensively researched. These include: stuttering, tinnitus (ringing in the ear), sickle-cell anemia, esophageal spasm, cold limb in postpolio patients, dysmenorrhea, chronic eye closure, stress-induced syncope (fainting), and visual disorders, If you are interested in articles describing the treatment of these disorders, they are referred to in a summary article (Shellenberger, Amar, Schneider, & Stewart, 1989). We have emphasized the fact that behavioral treatments are multicomponent because, as the biopsychosocial model of disease and illness suggests, many disorders are complex. The treatment protocols focus on the development of behavioral, physiological, and cognitive skills, practice to mastery, and incorporating new behavior into lifestyle.

The clinical research that we describe and cite in this section is also multicomponent, unlike early research that attempted to study a single treatment variable, an approach that was often ineffective. Today the best research uses the key elements of the clinical protocols.

We have described the application of behavioral methods to a variety of disorders to illustrate the great versatility of the treatment procedures, and of humans. We are impressed by the versatility of creative therapists who have developed comprehensive training protocols and who maintain the flexibility needed to treat the whole person. Given the opportunity to learn self regulation skills, people can change the course of illness and disease.

||||▶

CONCLUSION

With knowledge of the dynamics and ingredients of health and wellness, with knowledge of the principles of self regulation therapy and self regulation techniques and tools such as biofeedback training, with knowledge of mind $\longrightarrow$ body and homeostasis, with knowledge of the extensive role of behavior in illness and disease, the success of behavioral medicine treatments is understandable. People can develop the skills of health and wellness, and the body follows.

The treatment protocol that you studied in Chapter 14 and the protocols and applications described in this chapter have common denominators and themes. One theme is learned **self regulation**, and the common denominators are: (1) the acquisition of physiological, cognitive, and behavioral skills, (2) acquired with the help of a skilled therapist, (3) through consistent practice and perseverance, supported by (4) a healthy sense of self-responsibility.

A second theme is **empowerment**. When self regulation skills are used to combat disorders of any type, the patient gains an invaluable sense of control and personal power. People need not be victims of emotional and behavioral conditioning, lifestyle habits, disease and illness, or genetics.

A third theme is **choice**. There is nothing coercive about behavioral treatments. Clients choose the relaxation, visualization, stress-management, and desensitization techniques that are best for them, and they determine their own goals. Clients choose to work or not to work. Unlike traditional medical treatments, the procedures of behavioral medicine do nothing for the person unless the person uses them. As therapists we like that, although the necessity of being a good teacher is everpresent.

The therapist's task is to be a good guide and teacher, but must the therapist be superhuman? Certainly the knowledge and skills of the therapist must be broad enough to facilitate learning and behavior change in all clients, whose lives and disorders may be simple or complex. We anticipate that the need for teamwork will grow as traditional medicine accepts the broad biopsychosocial approach to illness and treatment. As treatments broaden and encompass a great hierarchy of causes, a team of experts such as our fictitious team that worked with Mr. Wright will work together to facilitate health and wellness in patients.

Partnership is a fourth theme in self regulation therapy. The advent of behavioral medicine brings to fruition the partnership of healer and patient. The responsibility for recovery and prevention is shifted from the health professional to the patient, and a partnership is established. Above all, partnership fosters a sense of self-responsibility and mutual respect. It is easy to become complacent about health, but when people choose to be noncomplacent about disease and illness and the struggle for health begins, then the role of the therapist as partner and health advocate is invaluable.

The fifth theme is stated perfectly in Hippocrate's dictim: **Primum non nochare**, "First, do no harm." An advantage of self regulation therapy is the harmlessness of the treatment. The treatment techniques that we have described throughout this text facilitate healthy homeostasis by working with the body's natural ability to heal, and they do not work against it. Similarly, these techniques promote healthy psychological homeostasis and volition. The protocols outlined in this chapter provide a path for people who are noncomplacent and seek nonpharmacological and nonsurgical methods for overcoming illness and disease.

The sixth theme in this chapter is summarized in a saying that is striking for its obvious wisdom:

Give a man a fish and he eats for a day.
Teach a man to fish, and he eats every day.

We would put it this way:

Give a man a pill, and he feels well for a day.
Teach a man skills, and he feels well every day.

CHAPTER 16

Behavioral Medicine: Applications with Children

Carl's mother says that she is mad because he was so good in my office.

"How often do you hug him?" I (JG) ask.

"Hug him? Why would I hug him?" Carl's mother does not like him; for one thing, he made her leave high school, because she was pregnant with him. Carl's parents know about punishment, but they do not know much about love and nothing about reward for good behavior. Carl is either neglected or punished, and he acts out frequently.

Carl's teacher says that she is quite certain that his IQ is more than 79, as tested at school. But Carl's family has a myth. The family believes that Carl is retarded and hyperactive because he ate a bottle of baby aspirin when he was 2 years old, and the aspirin burned his brain. Carl is not going to rock the boat; he does not tell anyone that he is not retarded. He believes however, that he is destined to fail. Carl is 10 years old and working at a second-grade level in school; he is in a classroom for learning-disabled children.

Carl takes 30 mg of Ritalin a day, increased from 10 mg in kindergarten. The school wants him on Ritalin because he is hyperactive. In school, Carl is not hyperactive; in fact, he often stares into space; sometimes he rips holes in his worksheets.

Carl is like thousands of other children with behavior problems who take drugs to control their behavior.

Jessica was diagnosed with asthma when she was 1 year old. By age 11 she is on three medications, receives a weekly allergy shot, and uses an inhalant as needed; she is allergic to pollens, molds, dust, animal hair, and dander. Occasionally she requires a shot of adrenaline to stop an asthma attack.

Jessica cannot play strenuously with her friends without wheezing, but she hates to stop playing. The family cannot have pets, and vacations are punctuated with visits to the nearest hospital for an adrenaline shot.

A continuing battle simmers between Jessica and her mother over medications. Her mother feels caught between Jessica, who complains about the medications and does not want to take them, and the allergist, who insists that the medications be taken. In addition, Jessica was adopted before two other children were born to her adoptive parents, and she holds some anger toward her parents, feeling that she should have been their only child.

Jessica is like thousands of other children with asthma who are limited in their activities and need continual medications and occasional hospitalization, and whose parents often feel helpless and caught in a web of overprotection and disease.

At age 9 Teri began having severe migraine headaches with vomiting, and she is unable to go to school many days each month. She is taking four medications and has been seen by two neurologists, a chiropractor, and a psychologist. The headaches are so frequent that Teri is essentially homebound.

Although the severity of Teri's headaches is unusual, she is like thousands of other children who suffer from tension or migraine headache. Children and adolescents with migraine headache take various medications, miss school, and fear the next headache.

In one month Belle will have extensive surgery to straighten the bones of her right leg. She is frightened because this is her second operation and she knows that it will be painful.

People will not tell her what is going to happen, and no one can understand what it is like. Normally brave and cheerful, Belle now feels frustrated and discouraged. She will have weeks of recovery, she might not be able to walk better, and she will always be handicapped. Belle's parents are also frustrated. Her dad thinks that Belle is being a baby, but her mother tries to understand, and worries.

Belle is like thousands of other children who must undergo medical procedures that are traumatic and painful, and who must suffer treatments that have severe side effects. And Belle is like thousands of other children who have handicaps, chronic diseases, or life-threatening diseases.

In this chapter you will meet these children. You have already met Garret and Sara, children who used visualization to overcome disease, described in Chapter 9, Imagery for Health and Wellness. In Section One we describe the basic ingredients of teaching self regulation skills to children. To illustrate the work in more detail, we focus on the treatment of Carl, Jessica, Teri, and Belle who were the clients of your author, JG. Carl, Jessica, and Teri are like many other children suffering from chronic difficulties such as asthma, maladaptive behavior, learning disorders, and stress-related disorders. We describe research on self regulation therapy for these problems and mention the work of other therapists who have developed special techniques for children. Section Two introduces an area that deserves great attention and yet has been slow to develop: helping children deal with hospitalization, with the trauma and pain of medical procedures, and with chronic disease. Belle and many other children are the stars of this section. In Section Three we discuss the caregivers for children, focusing on the health professionals who have closest contact with children, nurses. We also introduce the Center for Attitudinal Healing, an innovative program for children with life-threatening disease and injury.

All children benefit from knowledge of mind-body interaction, and all children can use self regulation skills such as stress management, relaxation training, cognitive restructuring, and visualization.

The importance of working with children is self-evident. Prevention must begin in childhood. A lifestyle of sickness can begin in childhood. Therapists, nurses, teachers, and parents can take advantage of the flexibility, courage, and optimism of children to shape a healthy future for children in need.

||||▶

SECTION ONE: TREATMENT PROTOCOLS AND APPLICATIONS

Children are psychophysiological self regulation geniuses. Perhaps this is because children are believers—they believe in mind-body interaction; they believe that they have power to help themselves; they believe that they can help the body heal, or take away pain, or stop asthma, or prevent a headache—when a grown-up or peer shows them how to overcome problems. And children love self-responsibility. A child may not carry out the garbage, but he will work for a sense of self-control and self-efficacy that comes from self-responsibility. Children can relax, visualize, and do home training and keep records; they can change their perceptions and self-talk; and they can generalize training from clinic to school and home. Like many therapists who use self regulation methods with children, we find that children can learn all the things that adults learn, in less time, and with faster relief of symptoms. Self regulation training for children is a natural.

It will not surprise you to learn that you know the basic ingredients of self regulation therapy with children: a clear description of the mind-body team and how mind and body work together; rationale for the treatment and the importance of training the whole team, mind and body; breathing exercises and self-hypnosis, biofeedback training with a variety of relaxation techniques; visualization techniques including desensitization; cognitive restructuring; and home training. As with adults, the treatment of children is adapted to the needs and goals of the child.

We begin with the biofeedback therapy protocol for children, described by Judith Green, one of the first therapists to use biofeedback training with children (Green, 1983).

Procedures

Biofeedback Therapy

I am not a family therapist, and my work is primarily with the child individually. I work with any child who would benefit from self regulation training. The entire family is invited to attend the first treatment session so that everyone in the family understands mind-body interaction and biofeedback training, and all participate in the first exercise, autogenic feedback training and deep breathing. The session gives me a chance to observe family interaction and support. If needed, the family is referred to family therapy.

I introduce myself as a biofeedback teacher. I explain that I teach ideas and skills, and that like all teachers, I ask questions and like to be asked questions. The ideas that I teach in the first session are the foundation of the training, and vary according to the problem. For stress-related symptoms, these ideas are: (1) Mind and body are a team, and we train the whole team; (2) stress gets into the body; (3) the symptom is a stress response (simple physiology of the symptom is described); (4) relaxation is the opposite of stress; (5) blood flow in the body changes during stress and relaxation, and hands

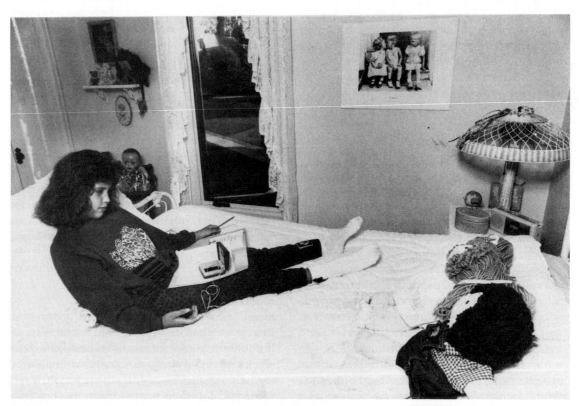

Children, Like Other Clients, Practice Biofeedback Training at Home and Keep Records.

get colder with stress and warmer with relaxation; (6) the feedback of hand temperature can help us learn to relax; this kind of feedback is called biofeedback; (7) the symptom is a bad habit, and teaching mind and body a new healthy habit takes practice.

After these ideas are clear to the child (I know this because I ask the child to explain them), breathing and autogenic feedback training are taught, and the child goes home with a temperature feedback trainer, a set of autogenic training phrases for children, homework sheets for recording each practice session, and a symptom chart. In general the child is totally responsible for doing the home training, without parent help or coercion. Only young children who cannot read or write have the help of a parent. The exceptions to this are described below.

In my practice, all children begin therapy with autogenic feedback training regardless of the problem. I begin with hand-warming because it is easy to learn and because inexpensive temperature feedback units are available for home use. For most children, learning to relax and increase hand temperature is self regulation training of the fun type. Because a child cannot fail at hand-warming, the training leads to success, with increased self-esteem and sense of self-efficacy. To add to the experience of success and as a motivator, the child picks a prize out of my prize bag when she reaches 96°F at home or in my office. A prize is also given for consistent home training regardless of temperature increase. Prizes are also given for other achievements such as lowering muscle tension significantly or reaching a goal of therapy.

Visualization is the child's forte, and all children learn to use imagery and visualization for relaxation and reducing symptoms, for enhancing performance, and for self-exploration.

All children help me make a personal cassette tape for home training. The tape includes the breathing exercises, the child's favorite phrases, special visualization, and anything else that is important to the child.

Children learn a variety of short relaxation techniques and use colored dots as reminders to relax. Our quick relaxation techniques for children are shown in Box 16.1.

Children develop negative cognitions as readily as adults, and they are just as likely to be victims of negative thinking. Children, quick to understand this, are helped to change cognitions by succeeding in training and through coaching. Children create mottos and special phrases that reinforce positive self-image, self-direction and reduction of symptoms. Cultivation of positive beliefs and expectations are continual throughout training.

Mastery tasks are important for children, and mastery of relaxation and stress management is demonstrated through challenges such as increasing hand temperature on command or maintaining hand temperature while performing stressful activities. A variety of computer programs have been created to help children master psychophysiologic self regulation, and video games can be used for mastery training. An ingenious EMG feedback device helps hyperactive children learn to relax and control motor activity. The EMG instrument controls a toy helicopter that flies only when the child lowers the EMG level, a paradoxical task for a child with difficulty controlling activity.

The therapist who works with children needs all the skills of an adult therapist, and also needs to be able to involve the family and the school in the child's training program. We believe that the therapist also needs to be in touch with her or his own inner child.

These are the basic ingredients of self regulation therapy in our work with children. Other therapists have other techniques for teaching self regulation.

Hypnotherapy

Hypnotherapy is another procedure that is effective with children. Today hypnotherapy and self-hypnosis are recognized as valuable tools in behavioral medicine, with the same applications

---

BOX 16.1

RELAXATION QUICKIES

You can't force yourself to relax—just let it happen.

1. Breathing: In two-step breathing, fill the bottom of your lungs first, then add the top; as you breathe out slowly through your nose, *feel the tension flowing out.*
2. Tense-relax muscles: Tighten the muscle that you want to relax—*feel the tension;* now let the muscle become loose and limp—*feel the relaxation.*
3. Body scan: With your mind briefly scan every muscle in your body from the tips of your toes to the top of your head. *If you sense a tight muscle, just let it become limp.*
4. Limp rag doll: Do the two-step breath two times. Imagine that you are a limp rag doll; *feel your mind and body become limp and relaxed*—you may use whatever image you like best.
5. Mind-quieting: To quiet your mind, *focus on your breathing.* As you breathe in say slowly to yourself *"I am,"* and as you breathe out, say slowly to yourself "calm." When your mind feels calm, you may focus only on your breathing, *with no thoughts at all.*
6. Shoulders, arms, and hands heavy and warm: Put your mind into your shoulders, arms and hands—*feel them becoming heavy, relaxed, and warm.*

---

as relaxation and visualization techniques for treatment of psychosomatic illness and aspects of organic disease (Brown & Fromm, 1987). In fact, there is little difference between hypnotic techniques and relaxation/visualization—both induce an "altered state" in which awareness of external stimuli decreases and attention is focused on the internal experience of the visualization and imagery.

The natural ability of children to relax and imagine, and the child's readiness to establish a relationship of trust with adults, makes hypnotherapy a powerful tool in working with children.

Pediatrician Karen Olness, formerly of the Minneapolis Children's Medical Center, now professor of pediatrics at Case Western Reserve University Hospital, has used hypnotherapy with children for many years. Olness describes hypnosis as "an altered state of awareness in which the person is able to accept suggestions which allow him/her to use his/her mental and physical skills in an optimal fashion" (Olness, 1986, p. 96). Hypnotherapy is the use of therapeutic procedures while the patient is in the induced state of hypnosis. Olness continues, "Hypnotherapy is useful in pediatrics both as primary and as adjunctive therapy. It can be used as primary therapy in children who are 6 or more years old with nocturnal enuresis that is not of organic origin, in those with juvenile migraine that has been carefully evaluated, and in those with warts, certain types of habitual tics, or various undesirable habits (e.g. hair pulling). As adjunctive therapy, hypnotherapy is useful in many chronic conditions such as diabetes, hemophilia, malignancies, juvenile rheumatoid arthritis, or any other condition that requires frequent hospitalizations or uncomfortable procedures" (Olness, 1986, p. 97).

Like biofeedback therapy with children, hypnotherapy begins with a clear description of the process appropriate to the child's under-standing; the child explains the problem and determines the goals of therapy; the therapist emphasizes self-mastery and practice of the procedure until mastery is gained. When the child is comfortable and ready, the induction procedure begins. "Induction" is the term used by hypnotherapists to describe the process of becoming relaxed and achieving the altered state of awareness associated with hypnosis. Pediatric psychologist, Jerry Dash, describes a technique that begins

> Now I am going to teach you a very easy and interesting way to control your discomfort. I'd like you to look at my watch, and keep looking at it as I move it slowly above your eyes. As I move it away, just take a nice deep breath, and hold it. Now as the watch moves down, keep looking at it, and let your breath out slowly. When you can't see my watch any more, just close your eyes, and keep them closed until I ask you to open them again. Now, take three more nice deep breaths, and let yourself get more relaxed with each breath. In a moment, I'm going to touch you on the shoulder, and when you feel my hand touch your shoulder, just let all of your muscles go real loose and floppy, just like cooked spaghetti.
>
> (Dash, 1980, p. 223)

This instruction is followed by the image of standing at the top of a flight of stairs, and slowly beginning to descend the 15 steps. At the bottom of the steps is an easy chair, in front of the chair is a television set. The child relaxes in the chair and watches his favorite television show.

Child psychologist Gail Gardner and Karen Olness (1981) describe a variety of induction techniques that help the child move easily into the use of imagery and enhance the child's sense of personal control: imagining a favorite place, playing with animals, being in a flower garden, watching clouds turn different colors, hearing a favorite song, or flying on a blanket. The technique that is used depends upon the age of the child and the child's special interests.

Following the induction, the therapist guides the child through the visualization of the desired behavior or goal. Box 16.2 is the description by Gardner and Olness of their procedure with children who have enuresis (bed-wetting). In surveys of children ages 4 to 14, 15 percent report episodes of bed-wetting (Walker, Milling, & Bonner, 1988). The problem is most common in younger children, and boys are more likely to have enuresis than girls.

As you see from the description of hyp-notherapy for bed-wetting, the key ingredients of self regulation therapy are incorporated in hypnotherapy—self-responsibility, mastery, practice, positive imagery, information, and coaching. Summarizing their work, Gardner and Olness write:

> Treatment is conducted in the context of a safe, comfortable relationship in which the child capitalizes on imagery skills to enhance feelings of control and mastery and to recover a state of wellness to the greatest extent possible. Treatment should not require a passive submission but rather active and joyful participation. In the final analysis, we see ourselves as guides, coaches, teachers. It is the children who heal themselves.
>
> (Gardner and Olness, 1981, p. 6)

The treatment results of 505 children and adolescents who received hypnotherapy at the Minneapolis Children's Medical Center are extremely good (Kohen, Olness, Colwell, & Heimel, 1984), and are similar to results with biofeedback therapy. The 505 children were treated for a variety of complaints including asthma, chronic and acute pain, anxiety, hives, phobia, bed-wetting, side effects of chemotherapy, headache, and pain and trauma from medical procedures. Fifty-one percent of the patients eliminated the symptom, and half of these did so in one to two visits; 32 percent significantly improved, 10 percent improved initially and then the symptom recurred, and 7 percent had no change in symptom. The average length of training was four sessions.

Hypnotic techniques are particularly

BOX   16.2

ENURESIS

In hypnotherapeutic sessions with enuretic patients, we discuss in detail the best time for practice of suggested exercises. . . . We review the path from bed to bathroom and sometimes have the child draw us a map of this path. We encourage the child to decide on a specific reminder for practice (e.g., string around the toothbrush handle, ribbon around the neck of a favorite stuffed toy, sign on the door). We emphasize that the bladder is a muscle and that the patient has previously learned control of many muscles. We also use the analogy of the therapist being the coach asking the patient to practice muscle control, thereby further placing ultimate responsibility on the child.

We proceed to ask the child to explain likes and dislikes, such as hobbies, interests, favorite colors, and favorite dreams. We then choose an induction method which seems appropriate. Following the induction, we often ask the child to show us a "yes" finger and a "no" finger and then ask a series of questions, most irrelevant, . . . and without changing pace, insert the question "Would you like to have all dry beds?" or "Are you ready to work on solving the problem of wet beds today?" If the answer is no, as it is occasionally, this suggests that the child may be receiving significant secondary gain from the problem (e.g., being allowed to get into bed with parents when bed is wet) or simply that there is not sufficient motivation to work on the problem at this time. Following a yes response, we ask the child to imagine being in a favorite place and to signal a yes when ready to give instructions to his or her bladder. At this point, we might say, "Tell yourself that you will sleep well tonight. Tell your bladder to send a message to your brain to awaken you when it is full of urine (or pee). When you awaken, tell yourself to get out of your dry bed, walk across the room, through the door, down the hall to the bathroom, turn on the light, urinate in the toilet, turn the light off, return to your dry bed, and go back to sleep. Then think of yourself, awakening in a dry bed, knowing you will have a good day. Enjoy knowing your bed is dry because of your efforts, because you're the boss of your bladder muscle. Enjoy the good feeling of waking up in a dry bed as long as you like. Then, when you're ready, you can open your eyes and enjoy the rest of the day." The child is to practice this exercise daily.

From Gardner and Olness (1981), *Hypnosis and Hypnotherapy with Children*, pp. 132–133. Reprinted by permission of the authors and W. B. Saunders Company.

---

valuable for children who must undergo painful and traumatic medical procedures; we discuss this application in Section Two.

Whatever the techniques used in therapy, the goal of training is always to help the child gain self regulation skills, whether for symptom reduction, enhanced learning in school, behavioral management, overcoming a handicap, or handling frightening and painful medical procedures.

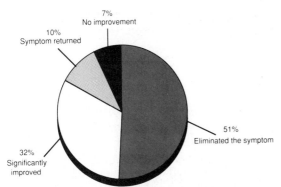

Figure 16.1.   Treatment Results for 505 Children and Adolescents Who Received Hypnotherapy at the Minneapolis Children's Medical Center. Adapted from Kohen, Olness, et al., (1984). "The use of relaxation-mental imagery (self-hypnosis) in the management of 505 pediatric behavioral encounters." *Journal of Developmental and Behavioral Pediatrics, Volume 5, 21–25.* **Reprinted with Permission of the Publisher and Author.**

In the remainder of the section, we describe in detail behavioral treatment of three disorders, hyperactivity, asthma, and migraine headache.

Hyperactivity

In 1971, the Office of Child Development defined hyperactivity as "an increase of purposeless physical activity and a significant impaired span of focused attention which may generate other conditions, such as disturbed mood and behavior within the home, at play with peers, and in the schoolroom" (Barkley, 1981). The following criteria are listed in the *Diagnostic Standard Manual* of the American Psychiatric Association (1980) for classifying children as hyperactive:

A. Inattention. At least three of the following:
   1. often fails to finish things he or she starts.
   2. often doesn't seem to listen.
   3. easily distracted.
   4. has difficulty concentrating on schoolwork or other tasks requiring sustained attention.
   5. has difficulty sticking to a play activity.
B. Impulsivity. At least three of the following:
   1. often acts before thinking.
   2. shifts excessively from one activity to another.
   3. has difficulty organizing work (this not being due to cognitive impairment).
   4. needs a lot of supervision.
   5. frequently calls out in class.
   6. has difficulty awaiting turn in games or group situations.
C. Hyperactivity. At least two of the following:
   1. runs about or climbs on things excessively.
   2. has difficulty sitting still or fidgets excessively.
   3. has difficulty staying seated.
   4. moves about excessively during sleep.
   5. is always "on the go" or acts as if "driven by a motor."
D. Onset before the age of seven.
E. Duration of at least six months.
F. Not due to schizophrenia, affective disorder, or severe or profound mental retardation.

Notice that the diagnosis or label, hyperactive, is based on behavior—behavior that is disruptive to the flow of school and family activities and may prevent the child from succeeding in school. Overworked classroom teachers have neither the time nor patience to help the hyperactive child, and parents of these children rarely have the skills, or learn the skills, that are needed to help the child gain self-control.

When teachers or parents are not able to tolerate the child's behavior or the behavior prevents learning, the child may be given Ritalin or a similar drug. Ritalin is a stimulant that paradoxically has a calming effect on children. In 1978, approximately 500,000 children in the United States were taking Ritalin, and by 1986 the number had risen to 1,500,000. Between 1975 and 1983 the rate of medication treatment for hyperactivity increased in Baltimore County, Maryland, by 74 percent for children ages 5 to 11 and 158 percent for students 12 to 15 (Safer & Krager, 1985). A recent survey of school and clinical child psychologists found that over 90 percent recommended the use of medication as the sole intervention or in combination with behavior and cognitive therapies for treatment of hyperactivity (Rosenberg & Beck, 1986). As with many drugs, the effectiveness of Ritalin decreases over time, and the dosage must be increased. The side effects of Ritalin include impaired physical growth, insomnia, loss of appetite, headache, and stomach-ache.

Drug intervention is popular because it is simple and costs less than behavioral treatments. Although Ritalin does not help the child gain self-control by virtue of the drug itself, its calming effect may reduce the child's negative experience in school and family and may help the child begin to succeed. These reinforcing experiences may help the child gain self-esteem and self-control.

It is rare that the cause or causes of hyperactive behavior in a child are known. Lead poisoning (David, Clark, & Voeller, 1972) and smoking or drug use by the mother during the child's gestation are fairly clear causes in some cases (Nichols & Chen, 1981). Some children are sensitive to a high-sugar diet (Swanson & Kinbourne, 1980), and others are sensitive to radiation from fluorescent lights and television (Mayron, Mayron, Ott, & Nations, 1976). Genetic abnormality is found in some hyperactive children (Shekim, Dekirmenjian, &

Chapel, 1977). The term "minimal brain dysfunction" is often used instead of "hyperactivity," suggesting that the behavioral problems are the result of neurological problems (Weiner, 1982). Although there is no direct neurological evidence for this, it does follow the biomedical model of disease and illness and lends support to the use of medication to control the child's behavior.

A dysfunctional family and poverty are also clearly implicated in hyperactivity (Barkley, 1981; Paternite & Loney, 1980; Schwarz, 1985). Twenty years ago a colleague of ours earning a graduate degree in learning disabilities was taught that hyperactivity is usually the result of neurological dysfunction. Today she works in the public school system as a special education teacher and tells us that 90 percent of the children with whom she works come from dysfunctional families in which physical or sexual abuse is common. In this case, the biopsychosocial model of the disorder seems particularly appropriate.

One cause of frustration and "burnout" in special education teachers is the simple fact that many families in which a child is labeled hyperactive need family therapy, and yet most of these families have neither the money nor the desire for help (Schwarz, 1985). There are few public resources for these families.

The fact that so many hyperactive children come from dysfunctional families suggests that the "neurological deficit" hypothesis is limited. It is also interesting that boys are more likely than girls to be hyperactive (Weiner, 1982). Is this because boys, more than girls, are neurologically deficient, or is it because boys, more than girls, are reinforced for being active and aggressive and have active and aggressive models in our society? When the classroom is overcrowded and the teacher is overworked, any boy who is unduly active might be classified as hyperactive. If the boy goes home to a family in which the parents are frustrated, intolerant, and angry, conflict ensues. Eventually the parents and teacher agree that the child is hyperactive, and the pediatrician recommends Ritalin or a similar drug.

Case Report: Carl

I was shocked when Carl's mother told me that she was mad at him because he was so good in my office. Indeed, he had been good in my office—he paid attention, sat still, understood what I was teaching, and raised his hand temperature higher than his mother's. His mother's statement told me a great deal about the family dynamics.

Carl was delighted to have his own hand temperature feedback unit to use at home, and within two weeks he had mastered hand-warming through relaxation and graduated to EMG training, with electrodes on his forehead. In the beginning Carl's biggest thrill with EMG training was preparing the electrodes and setting up the equipment, for which he took total responsibility. EMG training however, brought out the hyperactivity, and in the beginning we called it "wiggle feedback." Carl wiggled when the electrodes were on his forehead and when he was requested to hold still. In addition, he had an uncontrollable facial grimace, a side effect of Ritalin. The grimace faded away in about three weeks, with the aid of feedback from a mirror. The wiggling was another matter.

Carl's task in EMG training was to relax and lower EMG scores for one minute at a time. To complete the session he had to train for 10 minutes, but the beginning sessions were sometimes 40 minutes long because between every minute that was scored, Carl moved around and talked and fiddled with the electrodes and equipment. To compound the problem, Carl could not keep his eyes closed. After a few seconds with eyes closed, Carl's eyes popped open with a frightened look, as though something bad might happen to him if he were not constantly vigilant. Perhaps the greatest handicap to success, however, was Carl's fear of success. A good minute

of training was often followed by an out-of-control minute. This is why the standard deviations shown in Figure 16.2 are so large.

To help Carl with his task, during scored minutes I repeated autogenic phrases or told a story and gave continual reinforcement. I asked Carl to make up his own autogenic phrase, and he created "My hair is smooth." Between scored minutes I asked Carl to wiggle and grimace as much as possible to see how high the EMG would go; this helped to enhance his awareness of tension and relaxation.

The mean and standard deviation of Carl's EMG scores for each session are shown in Figure 16.2. The numbers are not microvolts but are equivalent. If you were to record your average score for 10 minutes of EMG training, it might be around 20. Figure 16.2 does not show the change in late November when Carl began training for two-minute intervals and total training minutes began increasing while total session time decreased. Nor can you see the bright purple line at the 20 level. Every day we plotted Carl's minute scores on a large graph on the wall of the children's training room. A purple "surprise line" was drawn across the chart at the 20 level. I told Carl that when he kept his scores under the surprise line for 10 minutes in a row he would get a fabulous surprise.

Sessions 9, 14, and 16 are noteworthy. Carl came to Session 9 with a stomach-ache and wanted to be covered with a blanket. You can see that the mean of EMG scores for that session was remarkably low, and the standard deviation was small. As the minutes went by with so little activity, Carl began to brighten, and after Minute 10 we were both smiling. I said, "Look how well you did! What is happening? Your stomach doesn't control your muscles, so how do you explain that?" Carl replied, "I guess I'm not retarded after all." I felt as though the sun had come up in the children's training room. Instead of saying, "I have a stomach-ache," Carl essentially said, "I did it, and if I can do that, then I can't be retarded."

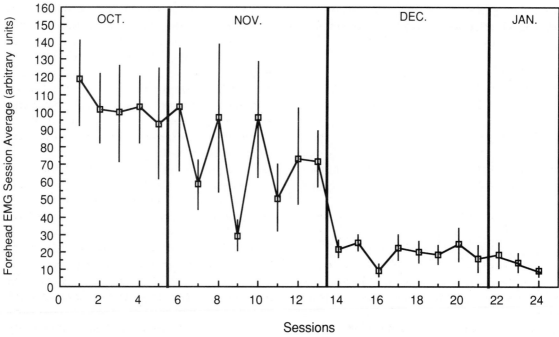

Figure 16.2. Carl's EMG Readings (Session Averages) and Standard Deviations.

To understand the importance of Session 14, you must know what happened in Session 12. In Session 12 Carl said to me, "You go to your office and type. I will do this myself." It was a self regulation therapist's dream, and at this point in Carl's training I had not thought of it myself! We placed a board across the arms of the recliner in which Carl worked, and placed the EMG unit, the start switch, and the score sheet in front of Carl, and then he told me to leave. Instead of going to my office I tiptoed into the next room and watched him through the one-way mirror. Carl kept his eyes glued to the numbers on the integrator that keep a running score of EMG activity, and he had the pencil ready to write the score when the minute was over. This was clearly an exciting task, and after six minutes Carl pulled off the electrodes and slipped under the board. I dashed to my office, and in a few seconds Carl ran in with his sheet saying, "I did it. Look what I did!"

After praise and a hug from me, he went down the hall showing everyone what he had done. This was the beginning of the metamorphosis from an "I can't" child to an "I can" child. In Session 13 Carl again went solo. He lasted 11 minutes, and again he openly sought and accepted praise.

Now look again at Session 14. Carl and I agreed that I should come back into the training room to help out with the start button and score-keeping because these activities created some tension, but this does not account for the dramatic change. Excessive activity during training was over. What do you think happened?

You might think that in Session 16 the child fell asleep. Carl held so still and relaxed so deeply that he looked as though he were asleep. This is what happened. In Session 15 I told Carl that if he could keep his scores under the surprise line in the next session he would get a wonderful surprise on that day. Carl's response was "I can't," but his first words in

Session 16 were "I think I can," and indeed he did. The surprise was a trip to the Nutcracker Suite ballet, in town only on that day.

After that success, the surprise line was lowered to 10, and in Session 25 Carl achieved the goal, graduated from EMG training, and won a trip to a nearby natural history museum.

Several important aspects of Carl's case make him more than a typical private practice client. During the biofeedback training and for three months after training, Carl had a nurturing male tutor who was earning college credits by interning with me. I worked with Carl twice a week, and Steve worked with him immediately after biofeedback training. Carl was in the supportive environment of the clinic about four hours a week. In addition, Carl and I became especially good friends because I drove him home after every session. Carl's mother was willing to drive him to the session, but she would not pick him up. Fortunately, Carl's house was near mine and I worked with him at the end of the day, so I drove him home. Several times Carl phoned home to ask his mother if I could stay for dinner. This gave me a chance to observe the family's poor diet, in which Kool-Aid was the dinner drink, and to note that the house with two children appeared to be childless—no drawings taped to the refrigerator, no children's magazines or books. The father was uninterested in Carl's progress, but after several hours of telephone conversation, Carl's mother began to understand the "logical and natural consequences" approach to child-rearing. She gained an appreciation of the benefits of reward, and occasionally she tried to apply these ideas, although they were not natural to her.

Carl was not retarded. In fact, his performance IQ was 114 and his verbal IQ was 92. He was given an IQ test in the children's training room by a tester who allowed him to stand up and move about; the test was given during Thanksgiving vacation when he was not taking Ritalin. The family myth had to be abandoned.

When we began discussing a reduction of medication after three months of training, Carl was against it. He could not remember being in school without his medication, and he was afraid. Nonetheless, by April, Carl began experimenting with medication reduction. His teacher reported that every time Carl reduced Ritalin by 5 mg she could tell because we was more "hyper" for a few days before returning to his usual behavior. By the end of the school year Carl was taking 15 mg Ritalin (he had started the year with 30 mg). Carl's parents did not give him Ritalin on weekends or holidays because they did not want to pay for the drug when he was not in school. Carl stopped taking Ritalin on the last day of school and did not take it again. Within two years Carl was in an appropriate classroom for his age and doing well.

What do you think about this case? Was this an example of minimal brain dysfunction? Did Ritalin hinder Carl's academic development? Was this a case of learned hyperactivity stemming from a dysfunctional family? Was hyperactive behavior Carl's attempt to get attention? Was the biofeedback training useful primarily because it facilitated self-image change? Should the school system or Carl's pediatrician have recommended family therapy instead of Ritalin? Is Carl typical of most hyperactive children who would benefit from behavioral treatment and a nurturing environment that says "You can" and enables the child to prove it?

Behavioral techniques with hyperactive children have a relatively long history. Texas psychologist Lendell Braud and co-workers developed nonpharmacologic techniques for working with hyperactive children. One of the earliest studies with children used EMG biofeedback training with an extremely hyperactive $6\frac{1}{2}$-year-old boy (Braud, Lupin, & Braud, 1975). Dramatic improvement occurred in his behavior, psychological tests, achievement tests, self-concept, and self-esteem, and he also had fewer headaches and allergies. Seven months later, however, the child's behavior became erratic again because his parents and teachers failed to reinforce the new behaviors. Consequently a program was developed for parents and children (Lupin, Braud, Braud, & Duer, 1976). The new program included progressive relaxation and guided imagery tapes. The tapes guide the listener to a peaceful setting and give suggestions for mind and body quieting and self-image change. Parents and children practiced the exercises at home. The results were positive. Children significantly reduced hyperactive behavior and improved on attention tasks, psychological tests, and the Wechsler Intelligent Scale for Children.

Based on this pioneering work, Denkowski and colleagues at the University of Houston have conducted several controlled studies that replicate the results (Denkowski, Denkowski, & Omizo, 1983; Omizo, 1980a, 1980b; Rivera & Omizo, 1980). Denkowski and colleagues found that children who received relaxation training had improved self-esteem, increased internal locus of control, and enhanced academic performance on reading and language tests, compared to a no-treatment attention control group (Denkowski et al., 1983).

The work of these psychologists demonstrates the efficacy of relaxation and guided imagery for the treatment of hyperactivity. Many children can gain self regulation without a drug and experience the added benefit of improved self-esteem and success in school.

Learning Disabilities

Doing poorly in school is frustrating and may be overwhelmingly discouraging. Fortunately, when I (RS) was in the first grade I was a good reader and speller. I had two classmates who were poor at reading and spelling. Almost every day of their first year in school they felt shame and humiliation. The first-grade teacher ridiculed them and hit them on the shoulder with a ruler, telling them to try harder.

My two classmates never became good readers and spellers even though they flunked first and third grade. Instead, they developed a poor self-image and felt looked-down upon by their peers because they had flunked. Their bodies got bigger but they did not get smarter, so they became very aggressive and were always picking fights.

The criteria for classifying a child as "learning disabled" were specified by the National Advisory Committee on Handicapped Children in 1968. These are:

1. Children with learning disabilities manifest a disorder of listening, thinking, talking, reading, writing, spelling, or arithmetic. These disorders are referred to as perceptual handicaps, brain injury, minimal brain dysfunction, dyslexia, developmental aphasia, and so forth.

2. They do not include learning problems that stem from visual, hearing, or motor handicaps; from mental retardation; from emotional disturbance; or from environmental disadvantage.

3. Children with learning disabilities have normal or above normal scores on intelligence tests.

There are many causes of learning disabilities. Some children suffer brain damage from lack of oxygen during the prenatal period or delivery. Children born to mothers who had German measles during pregnancy often have some form of brain dysfunction. Other children become disabled as a result of epileptic seizures. An entirely new group of brain-injured children is emerging as a result of medical technology that keeps the fetus and newborn child alive in spite of irreversible brain damage.

The need for effective methods to help the learning-disabled child improve academic performance and classroom behavior is greater than ever. Fortunately, new techniques and methods are evolving that may help these children.

Research with Learning-Disabled Children

While testing learning-disabled (LD) children at the University of Houston Diagnostic Center

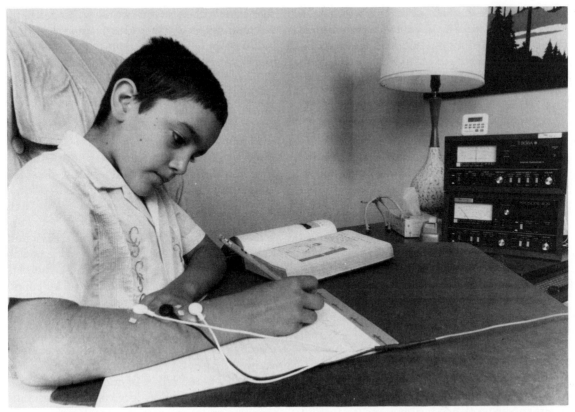

EMG Feedback from Forearm Helps this Child Relax While Writing. A Timer Creates Added Stress, Similar to Classroom Tests.
Source: Robert Waltman, Aims Community College, Greeley, CO.

in Clear Lake City, Texas, John Carter, director of the center, noticed that many of these children "tie themselves into knots" during the tests. The children squirmed, broke the pencil points from pressing too hard, became very tense, and had illegible writing. Carter wondered whether these children could learn to relax and improve their handwriting through biofeedback training. He recruited clinical psychologist Harold Russell, who used EMG feedback in his clinical work, and they trained four LD boys to deeply relax with EMG feedback from the forearm. As expected, handwriting significantly improved. Unexpectedly, the boys made a seven-month leap in reading and spelling skills. Parents and teachers reported that they were less impulsive and distractible,

made fewer careless errors, had more self-control, and were more interested in school.

Encouraged by these positive results, Carter and Russell (1984a) conducted a six-week controlled study with 16 LD children in the treatment group and 14 LD children in a no-treatment control group. The treatment-group subjects received six EMG feedback training sessions and listened to relaxation tapes three times a week at home for three weeks. The subjects in the control group received no training. In comparison to the no-treatment control group, the children in the treatment group made significant gains in handwriting, reading, and spelling skills, were less impulsive, and significantly improved their IQ scores.

News of Carter and Russell's success with LD children spread. Teachers and parents began referring LD children to Carter and Russell for biofeedback-assisted relaxation training. Over a period of three years they worked with 250 learning-disabled children. On the basis of this work, the Bureau of Education for the Handicapped awarded Carter and Russell a grant for a three-year controlled study with LD children. Their task was to create an effective biofeedback and relaxation training program that could be used in the public schools.

Carter and Russell designed an elaborate study with three phases. This is the largest study with children to date.

Phase One. During the first phase of the study, Russell and Carter (1984a; 1984b) used 11 experimental groups to determine the most effective procedures for LD children. One hundred thirty-two children were randomly assigned to one of the 11 groups: (1) biofeedback (EMG) and handwriting; (2) biofeedback and relaxation tapes; (3) biofeedback and homework (relaxation tapes and handwriting practice two times a week); (4) handwriting and relaxation tapes; (5) handwriting practice in school and at home; (6) relaxation tapes and homework; (7) biofeedback, handwriting, and tapes; (8) biofeedback, handwriting, and homework; (9) biofeedback, tapes, and homework; (10) handwriting, tapes, and homework; and (11) biofeedback, handwriting, tapes, and homework.

Subjects were trained in small groups by graduate students for 12 weeks. Measures on 11 dependent variables were derived from reading, spelling, arithmetic, and handwriting tests, and from scores on intelligence and psychological tests.

The analysis showed that children who gained self regulation through biofeedback training in combination with relaxation tapes (Group Two) had the greatest improvement on 10 of the 11 dependent variables. The improvements were both statistically and clinically significant. Handwriting practice was the most

significant factor in increased writing ability, although biofeedback and relaxation tapes did help children improve penmanship. At a 10-month follow-up, the LD children who received the relaxation tapes and biofeedback training maintained gains or continued to improve on 10 of the dependent measures. Only the information scale on the Peabody Achievement Test showed no improvement.

The results of the first phase of the study clearly showed that when learning-disabled children learn relaxation through biofeedback training and relaxation tapes, they improve in reading, spelling, handwriting, arithmetic, IQ, auditory memory, and self-concept. Carter and Russell concluded that "as children learned to control their internal level of arousal, their attention and memory improved and they coped more effectively with school learning tasks."

Phase Two The second phase of the research was with teachers. It was important to know whether or not teachers could use the biofeedback-assisted relaxation program with children. Nine teachers received 20 hours of instruction on the use of biofeedback training and relaxation tapes with LD children. Following the teachers' training, 90 LD children were randomly assigned to the following procedures: (1) EMG biofeedback training conducted by teachers, (2) EMG biofeedback training conducted by graduate students, (3) relaxation tapes administered by teachers, (4) educational games control condition (Phonics Bingo), and (5) no-treatment control condition. Biofeedback training was conducted individually, and children assigned to the tape or play conditions met in small groups. The dependent variables in phase two were the same as in phase one.

The greatest gains were made by the children who received biofeedback training from graduate students, and the least gains were made by children who received biofeedback training from the teachers. Children who listened to the relaxation tapes made intermediate gains. The teachers were not comfortable using the EMG instruments and training procedures, which may account for this result.

Phase Three Based on the results from phase two, Carter and Russell designed an instructional package for teachers that contained relaxation tapes and a handwriting workbook for LD children. In the third phase of the research, they distributed the kit to 82 teachers in 24 schools. Six hundred fifty LD children were assigned to either a treatment group, a no-treatment control, or an educational games control group. In comparison with the children in the control groups, the children who used the relaxation tapes and the workbook showed significant improvement on spelling, reading, and handwriting skills and enhanced self-image, auditory memory, attention, and IQ.

On the basis of this research, Carter and Russell recommended to the school system that teachers teach relaxation skills through the use of relaxation tapes and that school psychologists and counselors learn the principles and techniques of biofeedback training to use with LD children who need additional help.

Carter and Russell's extensive research demonstrates the benefit of EMG biofeedback and relaxation training for enhancing the IQ and academic skills of learning-disabled children. The intervention is simple and inexpensive and has only positive side effects. Children learn skills that can be used in a variety of stressful situations, and they gain a positive self-image and feeling of competency.

This three-phrase study exemplifies the complexity of research in behavioral medicine. Behavioral interventions involve skills that must be taught by the trainer and learned by the trainee. These two conditions involve several factors and complicate behavioral research, unlike drug research, for example. Administering a drug takes little skill, of giver or receiver. Administering a training procedure such as biofeedback training requires knowledge of the procedure and adequate teaching skills, and the learner must learn.

Furthermore, demonstrating the efficacy of self regulation methods may involve many subject groups and dependent variables. The process of weeding out the important variables and procedures may take time and long-term funding, which is often not available.

You may be wondering about the use of relaxation training with LD children today. Harold Russell tells us that few school systems include relaxation-training programs for helping hyperactive and LD children.

Asthma

Please read the brief description of asthma in Chapter 4.

An asthma attack is extremely frightening to have or to watch, and it is frightening to anticipate. It is easy to understand how asthma can become part of a family system in which the asthmatic child is overprotected and develops a self-protective stance toward the world. Asthma is complicated by the extreme sensitivity of the bronchial airways to allergens and stress, and by the conditionability of bronchiospasm. The extent to which factors like expectation of an attack contribute to the attack is never clear. It is clear that some children can "turn on" an asthmatic attack at will, and the fact that some people have attacks after simply being told that they are being exposed to the allergen is well known (Cluss & Fireman, 1985). It may be precisely the responsivity of the airways to mental and emotional processes that enable many children to counteract asthma, and, in some cases, to overcome it completely.

Case Report: Jessica

Jessica began biofeedback therapy at the suggestion of her pediatrician. To control nearly constant wheezing and the threat of severe asthma attacks, her medication use was increasing, and she hated medications. She also hated to stop playing when she was wheezing, and she often ran the risk of initiating a full-blown attack.

Jessica came to the first session with her father, a psychiatrist. She immediately understood the overall treatment plan for training mind and body, and she explained that her treatment goal was to take less medication, to be able to play longer, and to "stop asthma."

The first exercise for controlling asthma is abdominal breathing. Jessica naturally breathed correctly, so we moved to two-stage breathing and imagery. We studied a diagram of the lungs that shows the tubes leading to the air sacs and the circular muscles that cause bronchial spasm. The diagram is used to help the child visualize all the tubes open, relaxed, and comfortable.

The instruction is to fill the lungs slowly with two-stage breathing, and at the same time visualize the tubes open, the air sacs expanding with inhalation and relaxing with exhalation, while the little tubes remain perfectly round and open. This visualization is part of daily home training. Jessica understood that we use visualization to direct the body, and that even the inside of the body responds to images. This imagery and breathing exercise reduced her wheezing.

The rationale for hand-temperature training and EMG training for asthma is that relaxation opens constricted and clogged tubes and prepares the body to listen to the mind during desensitization training. Jessica became an expert at relaxation and imagery and was able to turn off wheezing even when it was quite severe, if she stopped her activities and concentrated on opening her lungs.

Relaxation and visualization skills also help counter the panic of the attack. The value of "having something to do" to prevent an attack when wheezing begins cannot be under-estimated.

When Jessica had mastered relaxation and felt confident in her ability to turn off wheezing, we began desensitization training. The first experiment was with molds. Using guided imagery, Jessica created a meadow surrounded by a dark forest; she followed a little brook into the forest. The forest floor was covered with moldy leaves and moldy dead trees, and Jessica discovered a grove of large molds and green spores. While exploring the forest Jessica got mold on her hands, but she visualized herself breathing perfectly. To enhance visualization, we grew molds on cheese and bread, and studied them under a microscope, discovering that molds are quite beautiful. Experiencing no reaction to the molds, Jessica graduated to feathers.

While Jessica was completely relaxed and breathing perfectly, I guided her through this scene:

> You are sitting in my office in the big brown chair. Notice how perfectly you are breathing. Now I come into the office with a baby quail in my hands [quail were available from an ethology research project nearby]. I hand you the baby bird. You notice how perfectly you are breathing and you say to yourself, "A feather is just a feather." Now you cuddle the bird against your cheek, and you say to your body, "A feather is just a feather." You notice how easily you are breathing while you talk to the little bird and cuddle it. Now you hand the bird to me and I take it back to the nursery. You continue to breathe perfectly.

After two rehearsals Jessica felt that she was ready to hold a baby bird, and so we acted out the imagery. To my dismay, the only bird available had recently hatched and was shedding tiny yellow feathers, yet Jessica cuddled the bird with no reaction. After this victory we moved on to feather pillows. When Jessica went to slumber parties she always had to take her own foam pillow.

The feather pillow desensitization went smoothly. A few weeks after we had used my feather pillow to act out the visualization we were surprised to find a feather sticking out of the pillow that Jessica used during relaxation and imagery training—then we realized that she had been using a feather pillow from the beginning of training, with no reaction. This turned out to be a valuable experience, because Jessica immediately knew that the allergic reaction was not inevitable and that the continual relaxation while she was exposed to the pillow must have prevented the reaction.

Jessica readily understood the concept of the unconscious mind. She created three phrases for directing her unconscious while she slept: "I will sleep peacefully and comfortably through the night," "Mind and body will heal the asthma while I sleep," and "My immune system is working perfectly." Nighttime awakening to take medications is a continual disturbance for asthmatic children and their parents. Jessica was on a medication that had to be taken every six hours, and she wanted to be able to skip the 2:00 A.M. medication without having difficulty breathing in the early morning.

Jessica's training sessions included a variety of relaxation techniques combined with hand-temperature and EMG feedback training and visualization for desensitization and body healing. We also talked about mind and body integration and the power of beliefs to help or hinder the body. Jessica was bright and verbal, and she conceptualized the work very well. When we had worked together for five months, we decided to write a summary of all the ideas and skills that Jessica had learned. I pretended to be a newspaper reporter interviewing Jessica about biofeedback therapy.

Jessica's home training included self-talk and hand-warming for relaxation and visualization. Midway through the training, I acquired a Mini-Wright peak flow meter for Jessica to use at home, and she kept records of her scores.

Over the year of intermittent treatment, Jessica had setbacks and gains, with gradual improvement in her ability to exercise harder and to tolerate exposure to allergens. During a respiratory infection, an X ray revealed spots on Jessica's lungs, and we created a healing visualization for the lungs. A severe reaction during a trip to the mountains put Jessica on a short course of prednisone, but before this she had a much reduced reaction while horseback riding. A significant change occurred when Jessica's mother gave her total responsibility for her medications. Jessica recorded medication use, but whether she took her medications or not was up to her. With this freedom, she developed a sensible plan for reducing medications, based on frequency of wheezing. Toward the end of training, Jessica broke her jaw in a car accident. The wiring of the jaws prevented Jessica from taking her regular medications, but she had no reaction to this reduction and gradually withdrew from all medications.

At one year after treatment, Jessica called me. She was symptom-free and wanted to know whether she could have a baby quail of her own. I felt that she met the ultimate challenge when she came to pick out a bird. The quail room was hot and stuffy, and there were hundreds of baby quails, all identical. Jessica stayed in the quail room for many minutes, handling the birds in the search of the right one. I know that I breathed a sign of relief when Jessica had no reaction to this unusual exposure.

Other Treatment Techniques and Research

Our friend and colleague, Erik Peper, a teacher at San Francisco State University and a biofeedback therapist, combines biofeedback training and family therapy in the treatment of asthmatic children. Peper was aware that family dynamics may play a role in a child's illness, and he notes that asthma symptoms can be reduced by 40 percent when the child undergoes a "parentectomy," that is, goes to summer camp (Stern, 1981). In Peper's program, parents participate in the first session and they learn correct breathing. They become a resource for the child by learning to be a good coach and to avoid escalating the anxiety of an attack. The first session with the family focuses primarily on breathing. Peper teaches correct breathing by coaching and demonstration, always emphasizing the importance of ease rather than effort. If the family quickly learns diaphragmatic breathing, Peper introduces an incentive inspirometer. The inspirometer measures inhalation volume and is a wonderfully simple device for inhalation feedback and reinforcement.

Parents are instructed to practice diaphragmatic breathing with the asthmatic child every day. This brings "health" attention to the child, rather than "sickness" attention, a dynamic that Peper believes is important in recovering from asthma when asthma has become an attention-getter for the child.

Once the child has mastered diaphragmatic breathing, the next step is upper-body relaxation. EMG feedback from scalene and trapezius muscles reflects breathing and is used to train relaxation of the chest and shoulders while breathing. The greater the effort and the higher the breath is in the chest, the higher the EMG reading. The importance of upper-body relaxation to breathing is dramatically demonstrated with the inspirometer. The person breathes into the inspirometer, as a

baseline. Then EMG electrodes are attached to trapezius and scalene muscles, and breathing with relaxation of these muscles is practiced. The next inhalation on the inspirometer is often surprisingly greater than the first. The combination of EMG feedback and incentive inspiration feedback is powerful. To lower EMG readings, the child must relax and breathe diaphragmatically, and the inspirometer shows the results.

When diaphragmatic breathing is mastered and the child can turn off exercise-induced wheezing, he is instructed to practice wheezing, a technique called "symptom prescription." This helps the child develop greater voluntary control over wheezing by turning it on and turning if off and reduces the child's and parents' fear associated with wheezing.

Other ingredients of therapy with asthmatic children include diet counseling, hand-temperature feedback, EDR feedback for relaxation training, and desensitization and flooding.

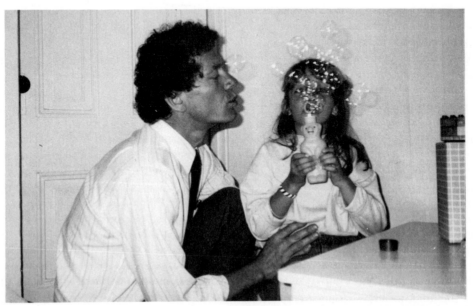

Erik Peper Teaches a Child to Breathe Correctly with the Aid of a Bubble Blower.

Peper reports reduced wheezing, attacks, hospitalization, and medication use with children and adults who gain control of breathing through this multicomponent approach to asthma (Peper, Smith, & Waddell, 1987).

Migraine Headache

Migraine headache is the most common chronic painful disorder of children. Pediatricians see about 50 migraine headache cases per 1,000 children. By age 15, about 5 percent of all children have migraine headache, and more than half of these children will continue to have migraine headaches into adulthood.

The causes of childhood migraine are similar to adult migraine (see Chapters 4 and 15). Potent medications such as ergotamine tartrate, prochlorpezine, and Elavil (amitryptaline) have side effects, and some medical researchers and physicians do not recommend medications as a long-term solution to childhood migraine. Behavioral techniques including biofeedback-assisted relaxation provide an effective alternative to pharmacologic treatment of childhood migraine.

Case Report: Teri

In our first biofeedback session, Teri was shy and unassertive. She spoke with a high, soft voice, in contrast to her mother, the verbal boss of the family. I had to ask the mother to let Teri speak for herself. Teri explained that she had a constant right-side headache that caused her to vomit, that she had missed many days of school in the past four months, that she had seen several doctors, and that her four medications did not really help. As the session progressed, Teri spoke more forcefully. She glowed when she found out that she would have her own biofeedback unit at home and that she was totally responsible for her training.

Unlike most children, Teri was unable to increase her hand temperature in the first session, perhaps because her initial finger temperature was low, 76.1°F. In two weeks of home training, Teri had not achieved a temperature of 96°, the training goal, but she received a prize for effort because she practiced hand-warming and relaxation many times a week. By the fourth week, Teri easily increased her hand temperature, and the number of hours of headache a week had decreased somewhat. Figure 16.3 has two keys, one for hours that Teri was free of headache, and the other for hours of headache per week. Teri had nearly continual headache at the beginning of training, and it was easiest for her to chart headache-free hours. By the sixth week, headaches had decreased so remarkably that she began charting headache hours per week.

Figure 16.3 does not show headache intensity, which decreased rapidly. By the third week Teri stopped taking medications, and by the fourth week she began going to school. During the training Teri did everything requested, and she even anticipated the importance of prevention before I explained it. In session four, Teri told me that she had been invited to a slumber party; before going she did extra hand-warming so that her headache would not get worse at the party. Her strategy worked.

Teri put colored dots around her bedroom and in school notebooks as reminders to practice the short relaxation exercises throughout the day, and I gave her a Biotic band for use at school and for continued training at home after she had returned the temperature feedback unit. The Biotic band is fastened around the finger, and the temperature sensitive crystals change color as the temperature of the skin changes.

By the eighth session, headache reduction had been so consistent that we ended therapy. As Figure 16.3 shows, at the one-month follow-up, Teri was almost free of headaches. Teri

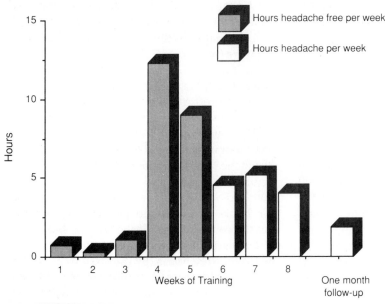

Figure 16.3. Teri's Headache Data.

reported that she continued to practice daily and could turn off headaches at will.

Teri is unusual in the duration and intensity of her headaches and initial vasoconstriction. To her advantage were a keen desire to eliminate headaches and an appreciation of the mind-body team. Midway through training, she asked whether it would be possible to get rid of a wart with the mind. A visualization was created, and by the follow-up the wart on her hand was gone.

Research

Behavioral treatment of childhood migraine has been consistently successful. Reports include clinical outcome studies in which patient results are analyzed as group data (Diamond & Franklin, 1975; Werder & Sargent, 1983), carefully designed single case studies using extensive baselines and follow-up (Labbe & Williamson, 1983), and studies with control groups (Fentress, Masek, Mehegan, & Benson,

1986; Larsson & Melin, 1986; Olness, MacDonald, & Uden, 1987).

Of all the stress-related disorders, migraine headache has the clearest genetic component. Family incidence is 61 percent when one parent has migraines and 83 percent when both have migraines (Deubner, 1977; Diamond & Franklin, 1975). People often think that if a disorder is genetic, then is it inevitable, and this misperception contributes to the belief that only traditional medical treatments, primarily medications, will help. The successful treatment results with both child and adult migraine sufferers clarifies this issue, showing that the genetic tendency to migraine headache can be overcome.

"Biofeedback: Treatment of Choice in Childhood Migraine" is the title of a presentation given in 1976 by the founder and director of one of the first headache clinics in the United States to use biofeedback training (Diamond, 1976). Biofeedback therapy is still the treatment of choice, taking advantage of the responsivity of the child's vascular system and the child's natural ability and desire to self regulate.

Summary

The three cases and supporting data that we have presented illustrate the use of biofeedback therapy and related techniques such as hypnotherapy. Treatment of migraine headache is short-term, and daily home training in peripheral vasodilation through relaxation and stress management is perhaps the essential ingredient in most cases. On the other hand, clinic sessions may have been the essential ingredient in the treatment of hyperactivity in Carl's case. Success in self regulation using EMG feedback, coupled with continual support and reinforcement, allows significant change in self-image. It is difficult for a child to fail at biofeedback training. Success can be engineered through progressive but easily achieved goals, reinforcement, and coaching. The fact is however, that few parents seek help for troubled children, and few special-education teachers have the time to work individually with difficult children. Braud and colleagues and Carter and Russell have demonstrated that programs for helping hyperactive and learning-disabled children through simple relaxation procedures can be used at school or at home, and are particularly effective when the parents participate.

Treatment of a long-term chronic problem such as asthma focuses on skills specific to the disorder, such as abdominal breathing, stress management, and desensitization. At the same time, the role of the family system in hindering or helping the child must be evaluated, and the family must be encouraged to help the child.

An underlying theme in self regulation therapy with children is: I can do something; I am not helpless. Skills, like tools, help us do something. Skills also give a psychological edge, the bonus of self-confidence and courage. These side effects of self regulation are the essential ingredients in helping children cope with hospitalization and traumatic and painful medical procedures, which are described next.

IIII➡

SECTION TWO: HELPING CHILDREN COPE WITH MEDICAL PROCEDURES AND CHRONIC DISEASE

Belle's mother called to find out whether I work with children who are very anxious about something that is going to happen to them. She explained that in one month her daughter was going to have surgery on her right leg; she needed surgery because she is a dwarf and her leg bones need straightening. This is her second surgery, and she is very afraid.

"Why is she afraid?" I asked.

Her mother explained: "Because her first experience was traumatic. She feels lied to and doesn't know what to expect. No one told her about the pain, and no one told her about the cast. She woke up in a lot of pain and in a huge cast and felt miserable, and she couldn't sleep. She is afraid that this will happen again. Her Dad thinks that Belle is being a baby, but I don't want her to go through that again." We set up four sessions.

Case Report: Belle

If a child on crutches can bounce, Belle bounces, and she radiates a cheerful, confident self. Very verbal and very bright, Belle's first question after the mandatory small talk was, "Did you hear about the boy who got rid of his brain tumor?" A little later, after hearing the idea, "We have a mind-body team, and we train the whole team," Belle wanted to know if I thought that this work would help her grow. "It is not impossible" is always a good answer when there is no way of knowing.

To help Belle with her crash course in self regulation for coping with hospitalization and pain, I printed an ideas list for the first session. These ideas made good sense to Belle and to her mother, who was with her, and we moved on to breathing, and then autogenic training with temperature feedback. Belle appeared to achieve deep relaxation very quickly, and her finger temperature rose from a high tempera-

ture at the outset, 92.3°F, to 93.0°. When she left the first session, Belle understood that learning the skill of relaxation was an important part of her training. At home after the first session, Belle achieved a finger temperature of 95.2°, and in 10 consecutive home training sessions finger temperature was never below 95° by the end of the session. In half of the home training sessions Belle's mother read the autogenic phrases to her. I encouraged this because Belle would need her mother's support

---

BOX 16.3

PAIN REDUCTION TECHNIQUES FOR BELLE

Relaxation

Body: To help the body listen to the mind.
To help the body decrease pain, and be comfortable.
To help the body heal faster.

Mind: Because the mind and body are a team, they work together. If the mind is upset, the body may get upset. If the mind is relaxed, the body will relax.

Positive mind: It is important to have a positive mind. Why? Because the body will try to do what the mind tells it to do. How do you tell the body? With words and with images.

Positive imagery: Seeing yourself in the hospital, and at home feeling comfortable, with bones and muscles healing perfectly.

Ways of making the pain less, and taking it away:

1. Breathing through the pain—feeling and seeing it float away.
2. See a long hallway. There are doors along the hallway. Each door is for a part of your body, and above each door is a light, which is on. You move down the hall, and when you turn the light off above a door, that part of your body becomes numb.
3. Get inside your knee and brain, and turn the pain hoses off.
4. Get inside your knee and any part that hurts, and with a big cotton ball, put on a special formula that takes away the pain.
5. Put your mind somewhere else:
   A meadow.
   Another part of your body.
   Into a fuzzy creature.
6. Pain-reduction tape and relaxation music.

and coaching in the hospital. In this case I also asked her mother or father to attend the sessions with Belle so that they would understand the techniques she had learned and how to help her.

A relaxation technique was a part of every session, as was visualization. A handout for Belle summarized the ideas and pain reduction techniques that we rehearsed several times (Box 16.3).

Belle thought it was neat that the hallway visualization was created by a boy her age who had cancer and used the hallway whenever he had a bone marrow sample taken (this technique was described by a child on *Donahue with Kids*, Project Peacock, 1981).

In our last guided imagery rehearsal, Belle imagined herself in bed the night before the surgery, relaxed and calm. Then she rehearsed getting up very early, dressing, eating breakfast, and riding to the hospital 50 miles away. Finally she rehearsed the procedures before surgery, falling asleep with the anesthesia, and waking up and feeling comfortable. In the last session, I gave Belle a delightful fuzzy creature with four floppy legs. I pinched Belle's leg, while she practiced putting her mind totally into her fingers, which were buried in the fluffy fur of the toy. This creature went with Belle to the hospital. Its floppy legs were a reminder to relax, and its fuzzy fur gave Belle a distracting sensory experience for putting her mind in another place, away from the pain. Belle also took a pain-reduction tape, a music tape, and the temperature feedback unit.

Belle woke up in a cast from her toes to her armpits. She was ready to cope with this cast because she had insisted on knowing in advance what the cast would be like. As soon as she felt uncomfortable, Belle began using her relaxation and pain-management skills, and when I called 24 hours after surgery she happily reported that she had raised her finger temperature to 96.3° and was doing well. This report was verified by Belle's mother, who said that compared to the previous surgery, Belle

was a different person. Unlike the first experience, she was cheerful, did not complain constantly, did not need her mother with her all the time, and slept well.

Belle's successful experience with the second surgery was the result of many factors. The medical team was more sensitive to her needs, her parents were more supportive and knew how to help, and Belle did not feel helpless; she had a variety of techniques to use and she went into the surgery with positive expectations and self-confidence. What an easy intervention for such an important payoff.

Belle and her parents worked with me in my private office. They came because Belle's mother had heard about biofeedback training and she thought that her daughter might benefit. Unfortunately, many parents and medical professionals are not familiar with this type of work and do not know how to help children, and children do not know how to help themselves. The trauma and pain that children experience is often underestimated by parents and medical staff, who themselves feel helpless and tend to discount or ignore the child's experience. Fortunately, this neglect is changing. One survey found that many hospitals have programs for helping children cope with hospitalization and stressful medical procedures (Peterson & Ridley-Johnson, 1980). Next we study a model program for helping children cope with hospitalization.

Helping Children Cope with Hospitalization

The University of Rochester Medical Center helps children cope with hospitalization through a two-stage program of information and coping-skills training (Zastowny, Kirschenbaum, & Meng, 1986).

In the first stage, the parents, the sick child, and siblings are invited to the hospital for an educational program about the hospitalization experience. The program begins with a

22-minute video, titled *Willie Welcomes You to the Hospital.* The star of the video is Willie, a frog puppet, who proudly describes his positive experience in the hospital. In an adventurous spirit, Willie describes beds with side rails and chest X rays, and he introduces the medical personnel, who are nice and helpful. Willie says that at first he was scared, but then he found out it is okay to be scared and to cry. He explains that he felt better after learning what was going to happen. After the video, the hospital staff answers questions and serves refreshments. Then the family is given a tour of the nursing unit, the patient's room, the playroom, the kitchen, and the admitting room.

The movie and the tour lessen the child's anxiety by providing accurate information, thus reducing negative fantasies about the hospital experience. Also, the hero of the movie, Willie the frog, models successful coping during hospitalization.

As with all types of self regulation training, information must be supplemented with coping-skills training.

In the second stage, parents are taught how to be "coping coaches" for their children. First, parents watch a 15-minute educational film that discusses the relationship between muscle tension and pain, feelings of hopelessness and pain, and expectations and pain. Parents are told that to function as good coaches, they must cope with their own stress and anxiety. Next parents watch another short film that describes the principles and procedures of stress inoculation developed by Meichenbaum (1977). The film teaches parents how to help the child use deep breathing, muscle relaxation, and coping thoughts to prepare for a stressor, handle a stressor, cope with feelings at critical moments, and reinforce oneself for successfully coping.

Finally, parents watch a film based on an illustrated booklet, *Good Thoughts—A Hospital Story.* The film and the booklet describe the use of coping skills by parent and child during

hospitalization. There are five major stressful events during hospitalization—admission, blood test, preoperative medication by injection, going to the operating room, and returning from the recovery room. In the illustrated booklet, cartoons show the nurse, the parent, and the child puppet preparing for each event. Parents use the booklet with the child to prepare for hospitalization. Parents are also encouraged to individualize the preparation by using coping skills that the child has used in the past.

Parents are also given a handout that summarizes methods and techniques for being effective coaches.

Psychologists Thomas Zastowny and Daniel Kirschenbaum and pediatric nurse Anne Meng (1986) conducted a controlled study comparing the effectiveness of the information and coping-skills training program to an information-only program and to an information-plus-relaxation program. Eleven children and their parents were assigned to the information-only program. They saw *Willie Welcomes You to the Hospital,* toured the hospital, and had refreshments. Eleven other children and their parents were assigned to a program that included the initial information, tour, and refreshments, and relaxation training. Parents were taught Benson's relaxation response to reduce their own stress and were encouraged to express their confidence about the forthcoming hospitalization to their children. Eleven other children and their parents were assigned to the initial information, tour and refreshments, and to the coping-skills training program described above.

In comparison to the other groups, the children in the information and coping-skills group showed fewer problems during the week before hospitalization, hospitalization, and the second week after hospitalization. Children in the relaxation group and the information/coping-skills group significantly reduced fearfulness and anxiety in comparison to the information-only group. Clearly, children can use information and skills effectively.

The information/coping-skills program of the University of Rochester Medical Center is a good model for helping children who must be hospitalized. Helping children cope with the pain of medical procedures is equally important. Special procedures are necessary for helping those children.

Helping Children Cope with Pain

For too long children's pain has been ignored or underestimated. In a review of 1,300 articles on pain, only 33 were concerned with children's pain (Eland & Anderson, 1977). Only three articles focused on helping children cope with pain. Fortunately, today the traumatic impact of pain is generally recognized, as is the importance of helping children cope with pain. Researchers and clinicians are studying the factors that contribute to a child's pain and methods for alleviating pain.

Pain is a complex phenomenon involving physical injury and psychosocial factors. To effectively help children cope with pain it is essential to understand these factors.

Physical and Psychosocial Factors in Pain

Painful and Traumatic Medical Procedures. Belle's dwarfism is rare: cancer, diabetes, hemophilia, kidney disease, sickle cell anemia, muscular dystrophy, and cystic fibrosis are more common in children. Medical procedures that accompany these diseases are painful and traumatic: bone marrow aspiration, bone marrow transplant, lumbar puncture, surgery, and chemotherapy. To aspirate bone marrow, a long needle is pushed into the bone, and tissue is drawn up the needle. An excruciating pain is felt as the marrow is suctioned into the needle and syringe. For many children, bone marrow aspirations are terrifying. The need to repeat painful procedures, sometimes for many months, is extremely difficult for children with chronic disease.

Undermedication. Several carefully conducted studies have found that children are often not given enough analgesic medication during medical procedures (Beyer, DeGood, Ashley, & Russell, 1983; Mather & Mackie, 1983; Perry & Heidrich, 1982). After surgery, children are often given lower doses of medication than recommended (Beyer, et al., 1983). Fearing the side effects and overdose, many professionals misjudge the amount of analgesic necessary for relief of pain in children. When my (RS) son was 10 years old, he broke two bones playing soccer. After a shot of an analgesic, the doctor proceeded to align Mike's bones without noting that the analgesia had no effect. My usually calm son turned white, flailed his arms, and screamed. He was suffering excruciating pain.

Mike has had several painful experiences, but in his estimation, having a bone set without analgesia was the worst. And, from his point of view, the doctor made a mistake. Adequate control of pain and suffering is deemed to be a fundamental responsibility by health professionals (Gross & Gardner, 1980).

Learned Pain and Fear from Previous Experiences. Painful experience with medical treatment can lead to anticipatory fear or terror. In Belle's case, the pain of bone surgery and the unexpected experience of waking up in a body case created extreme anxiety as she anticipated the second surgery.

Pain as Punishment. Often preschool children interpret medical personnel's actions as deliberately inflicting pain or as a form of punishment; this heightens the painfulness of the experience (Farley, 1981; Gross & Gardner, 1980; Melamed & Bush, 1985).

Separation. Separation from parents, fear of strangers, and encounters with other sick people who are in pain enhance the aversiveness of hospitalization (Bush & Holmbeck, 1987).

Emotional Contagion.   Anxiety and fear felt by parents, health-care professionals, and siblings are communicated to the child. Anxiety communicated through nonverbal behaviors increases the child's anxiety and negative coping (Melamed & Bush, 1985).

Emotional indifference and callousness of health professionals can also enhance the aversiveness of medical procedures. The following scene is described by the father of Alex, a young girl with cystic fibrosis (Defore, 1983, pp. 140–141).

A particularly officious young doctor brought a bunch of students over to examine Alex. He pointed to the tube in her chest, explaining that the incision of an inch or so had been made while she was under a local anesthetic, and then he declared, "This procedure is not very painful to the patient." Immediately, he proceeded with his lecture. All the years of hearing these cocky young experts talking at her as if she were a body on display, as if a child—a sick child—could not be a real person, welled up in Alex. "Wait!" she suddenly cried out.

But the doctor ignored her and kept right on with his spiel. "No, wait, you," she said again, louder still, and tugging at his sleeve this time, too.

He stopped. He had to. Alex had made him stop. And, only then, with a condescending look of annoyance, he turned down to her. "Yes, what is it, dear?"

"How do you know?" Alex asked.

"What, dear?"

"How do you know?"

"I'm sorry, but. . ."

"Have you ever had a big tube stuck in you and then taken out again?"

"Well, no, I, I. . ."

"Then don't you tell me—or them—it doesn't hurt. Because I don't like being lied to."

For Belle, as well, being lied to by health professionals who said "it won't hurt" had accentuated the trauma of hospitalization, because she felt betrayed and belittled.

Modeling.   Parents, siblings, friends, or relatives who perceive pain and cope with pain as an overwhelming experience perpetuate feelings of dread in the child.

Reinforcement of Pain Behaviors.   Reinforcement of the child's pain behaviors leads to greater attention to painful sensations and painful events, lowering the child's threshold for pain.

Family Dynamics.   Child psychiatrist Salvador Minuchin has identified family patterns that maintain the child's symptom and pain because the symptom fills a need in an unhealthy family system. For example, the child's symptom might diffuse marital conflict, provide a scapegoat for the frustrations of the family, or maintain the dependency of the child, thus fulfilling the need of a rescuing parent (Minuchin & Fishman, 1979).

Pain is complex. Probably every reader remembers a painful experience in childhood and might also remember that the amount of pain varied with the circumstances—when your parents were around, the pain was worse; when you were playing, pain was less. The fact that pain can be modified by attention, cognitions, and willpower can be used to advantage in working with children. A variety of factors influence a child's experience of pain. An effective program for helping children cope with pain must consider all of these factors.

Techniques

If you think of going to a hospital for medical diagnosis or treatment, your greatest concern may be pain. For children, a visit to the doctor or the hospital is synonymous with pain. Most children have felt the pain of inoculation, and children with chronic illnesses must undergo extremely painful and traumatic procedures. The child anticipating a bone marrow aspiration may become nauseated and vomit from fear, or may cry excessively or become exhausted from lack of sleep. During the procedure the child may fight vehemently, making repeated aspirations necessary and intensifying the child's terror. General anesthesia is not feasible because of the high risk and cost. Sedation with powerful tranquilizers is not always effective. One 7-year-old boy received Demerol, Thorazine, and Phenergan but thrashed violently during the aspiration (Jay, Katz, Elliott, & Siegel, 1987). These children need help.

A model program for helping children cope with bone marrow aspiration was developed by child psychologist Susan Jay and her colleagues at the University of Southern California School of Medicine (Jay, et al., 1987). The program, called the Cognitive Behavior Therapy Package, has five components: (1) breathing exercises, (2) positive reinforcement, (3) imagery, (4) behavioral rehearsal, and (5) modeling.

1. Breathing. Children are instructed: "Pretend that you are a big round tire. Take a deep breath and fill the tire with as much air as possible. Then slowly let the air out, making a hissing sound as the air slowly goes out of the tire. Let all the air out very slowly. Then pump it back up again and start over."

2. Reinforcement. The child is shown a trophy with her name on it. To get the trophy, she must lie quietly and use the breathing skill during the bone marrow aspiration.

3. Imagery. A drama is created, using the child's favorite hero: "Pretend that Wonder Woman has come to your house and told you that she wants you to be the newest member of her Superpower Team. Wonder Woman has given you special powers. These special powers make you very strong and tough, so that you can stand almost anything. She asks you to take some tests to try out these super powers. The tests are

called bone marrow aspirations and spinal taps. These tests hurt, but with your new super powers, you can take deep breaths and lie very still. Wonder Woman will be very proud when she finds out that your super powers work and you will be the newest member of the Superpower Team.

4. Behavioral rehearsal. Children role-play the bone marrow aspiration procedure with a doll and then with the nurse or psychologist. The child pretends to give a doll the bone marrow aspiration and then pretends to give the therapist the bone marrow aspiration. Finally, the therapist pretends to give the child the bone marrow aspiration. While pretending to give the bone marrow aspiration to the doll, the child is encouraged to tell the doll that the procedure is necessary to get well and that the nurses and physicians are her friends. While the therapist pretends to give the child the bone marrow aspiration, the child is encouraged to use the breathing and imagery skills.

5. Modeling. Children are shown a 12-minute film, *Joy Gets a Bone Marrow and Spinal Tap.* Joy says that she is scared, but she also expresses confidence because she has learned skills that will help her get through the bone marrow procedure. The film shows Joy practicing with the therapist, going into the treatment room, and successfully coping with the procedure.

In a three-year study with 56 children, ages 4–14, Jay and colleagues (Jay, Elliott, Ozolins, Olson, & Pruitt, 1985, and Jay, et al., 1987) compared responses to bone marrow aspiration in children who received the cognitive behavior therapy package (CBTP), or Valium, or nothing. In comparison to the others, the children in the CBTP program significantly reduce fear and anxiety and required no restraint during the aspiration procedure. They were very proud of having earned a trophy. The physicians and nurses were enthusiastic about CBTP and no longer felt a sense of dread when giving a bone marrow aspiration or lumbar puncture. Please read Box 16.4 now.

Visualization, relaxation, self-talk, and self-hypnosis help children cope with pain. They

---

take little time to learn and the child gains a sense of mastery and hardiness.

Helping Children Cope with Chronic, Crippling, and Terminal Disease

The development of crippling or terminal disease is a tragic and terrifying experience for children and parents. Traumatic medical procedures, loneliness, fear, pain, and neglect are a daily experience for many of these children. Many families break apart or parents abandon the sick child because they are unable to handle the strain of constant care of the child and because financial burden or bankruptcy and emotional exhaustion overwhelm them. Partly for this reason, the chronically ill account for one of five children in foster care (Hobbs, Perrin, & Ireys, 1985).

The plight of the parents is told in a moving account of the diagnosis, treatment, and death of their son with leukemia. Ross and Ross (1980) describe their frustration with the medical system as they attempted to get information and to provide support for their son who was in an isolation chamber as protection against infection while his immune system and leukemic cells were destroyed by chemotherapy. This is part of their story:

> It is so easy to say to someone who is devastated by the news of a terminal illness, "Don't cry," and offer them a tissue to wipe away the flood of tears. It makes a world of difference to say to that same distraught parent, "Go ahead and let it out," while comforting them with an arm around the shoulder. Someone must educate physicians to put away their handkerchiefs and offer their arms, a piece of themselves, the warmth of the body and the soul.
>
> For the patient's sake it is important that the health-care practitioners open the doors to the mystique and let us, the parents and family-at-large, in. Instead of acknowledging us as a viable part of the support system capable of contributing considerable love and sharing in the care of the child, we were cast aside. It was

very disturbing to be treated as if we already knew all possible was being done and thus were expected to observe in a nonparticipatory manner the mechanics of the health-care delivery system. It was even more irritating to be regarded as intellectual midgets incapable of comprehension, leaving us to make assumptions and presumptions about the techniques being utilized for our loved one. These irritations only added to our stress, anxiety and hurt and reduced our ability to cope with this unnatural situation.

> Our son, although under the sentence of death, was still a living being responsive to external stimuli and able to perceive our distress to such an extent that his anxiety increased. His ability to maintain confidence in the treatment and the hospital staff was reduced. He responded to our feelings, for we were his only link to the world of wellness.
>
> (Ross & Ross, 1980, p. 410)

The tragedy of the chronically ill child is compounded by the failure of medical professionals and society to meet the needs of these children and their families. Few families can afford the costs of medical, nursing, and mental health care. In 1978 average costs per year per family of the major childhood diseases were: kidney disease, $12,000; cystic fibrosis, $15,000; spina bifida, $13,000; hemophilia, $8,000 (Hobbs, Perrin, & Ireys, 1985). Today, care of a child who depends on a ventilator may exceed $35,000 *a month*. While home care is less expensive, costs for a child on a ventilator may surpass $15,000 a month for nursing services, therapies, equipment, drugs, and supplies (Ross & Thomas, 1987). Some insurance companies cover these costs but many do not, and some families do not have insurance. Some families have limited insurance through Medicaid, and some are dropped from Medicaid after the child develops the chronic disease.

Few schools have the programs and nursing staff necessary to handle the needs of the chronically ill child, and prolonged sickness and hospitalization may hinder the intellectual and social development of the ill child. Social services have minimal funds. The funds of many voluntary organizations such as the Muscular Dystrophy Association are primarily for research, and not enough governmental funds are appropriated for the care of chronically ill children.

You may be surprised to learn that 1 out of 100 children under the age of 18 has a major disability or sickness that interferes with normal functioning (Hobbs, Perrin, & Ireys, 1985). The most common disorders are leukemia, muscular dystrophy, hemophilia, sickle-cell anemia, spina bifida, cerebral palsy, diabetes, kidney disease, and cystic fibrosis.

This section briefly describes these disorders and the self regulation techniques that are used to help children cope with disease and with medical procedures. We can be brief because you are already familiar with the techniques that are used with children: relaxation, cognitive restructuring, hypnotherapy, breathing, and visualization and imagery techniques.

Spina Bifida (Myelomeningocele)

Spina (spine) bifida (cleft or fissure) is a congenital disorder in the vertebral processes during fetal development. Normally the vertebral column completely surrounds the spinal cord and its coverings, but in spina bifida a section of the bone fails to close, usually in the lumbosacral region. The fissure in the spinal canal allows the covering of the cord to protrude out of the vertebral column, forming a sac filled with cerebral spinal fluid. This process begins early in gestation and permanently damages the nerves that pass out of the cord in the area of the deformity. Depending upon the location and size of the sac, a variety of symptoms develop, such as poor coordination or paralysis of the legs and fecal and urinary incontinence. Children are often unable to walk or must use braces or crutches. Treatment involves repeated surgery and physical therapy. Many children

with spina bifida cannot attend school, because most schools lack the nursing services for their care. The cause of spina bifida is unknown, and there is no cure. Approximately 1 of 1,000 children is born with spina bifida.

As you know from Chapter 15, fecal incontinence can be treated with feedback from a balloon catheter or a perinometer. About 75 percent of the children with spina bifida who are trained with feedback and behavior modification techniques gain bowel control, and have maintained sphincter control at follow-up one to three years later (Wald, 1981, 1983; Whitehead, Parker, Masek, Cataldo, & Freeman, 1981; Whitehead, et al., 1986). Freedom from incontinence is a major victory for spina bifida children.

Cerebral Palsy

Cerebral palsy refers to a variety of motor disorders resulting from damage to the central nervous system during neonatal development or birth. The most common types of cerebral palsy are spastic (70 percent of cases), athetoid (20 percent of cases), and ataxic (10 percent of cases). Spasticity involves chronic muscle contractions causing a "scissors gait" or "toe-walking" and underdeveloped and weak arms and legs. Athetoid movement refers to slow, involuntary jerky movements that increase with tension and disappear during sleep. Ataxia refers to poor coordination in walking and in other motor movements. Most children with cerebral palsy are of normal or above-normal intelligence, although difficulty in speaking may give the impression of retardation.

A team of engineers, physicians, and physical therapists at the Ontario Crippled Children's Centre and Institute of Biomedical Engineering pioneered in the development of biofeedback instrumentation for motor-control training for children with cerebral palsy. These devices are shown in the photograph: head position trainer, joint position trainer, position/pressure sensor unit, drooling collection device, tongue position sensor, and a swallowing feedback device (Milner, 1983). These feedback instruments are linked with toys and computers to enhance motivation and learning. Since 1973, the center has helped many crippled children improve performance.

Behavioral skills cannot undo the brain damage of cerebral palsy, but the creative work of engineers and therapists has helped improve the quality of life of many children.

Kidney Disease

A variety of diseases of unknown origin cause kidney failure in children. Dialysis and kidney transplant are the only treatments. Hospitalization, surgery, catherization, and dialysis cause great stress for the child and the family. Uncertainty about the outcome of the kidney transplant and the possibility of early death compound the stress of chronic kidney diseases. Children with kidney failure need dialysis three times a week and must maintain a strict diet.

Pediatric nurses have pioneered in behavioral techniques to help these children adjust to the dialysis procedures and the strict diet. For hemodialysis, a large needle is inserted into an artery in the arm, and another is inserted into a vein; blood flows from the artery through the artificial kidney and returns to the body. Nurses on the pediatric hemodialysis unit at the University of Colorado Medical Center in Denver teach the children relaxation and breathing techniques and self-hypnosis, and distracting music is used during the insertion of the needles. An injection of lidocaine is used to deaden the skin where the large needles are inserted. Children are taught to inject the lidocaine themselves, a procedure that reduces anxiety and gives the children a sense of control.

To help children with kidney failure stick with a strict diet, the nurses record each child's diet on brightly colored charts that are posted on the walls of the unit. The nurses praise the children for maintaining the diet.

Cystic Fibrosis

Cystic fibrosis is a genetic disease characterized by the abnormal production of thick mucus in the pancreas, lungs, and small intestine. The mucus prevents normal function. Chronic coughing, wheezing, and respiratory infections are the most common symptoms of children with cystic fibrosis. Congestion from the excessive fluid in the lungs necessitates frequent hospitalization, and children often require respirators at home. There is no cure for cystic fibrosis. The average life span is 20 years and is increasing because of improved treatment of respiratory infections.

Psychologists Anthony Spirito, Dennis Russo, and Bruce Masek (1984) of the Children's Hospital Medical Center in Boston, Massachusetts, teach children with cystic fibrosis self regulation skills for coping with the anxiety and pain of the disease. Deep diaphragmatic breathing, autogenic training, progressive relaxation, and EMG biofeedback are the main ingredients of the program. Twenty-three children with cystic fibrosis learned self regulation techniques and experienced a decrease in anxiety, pain, insomnia, and episodes of hyperventilation. Nancy, a 19-year-old cystic fibrosis patient, used muscle relaxation to relieve the discomfort of tight back and neck muscles, and she used diaphragmatic breathing, which was particularly valuable during her last days of life. She practiced deep breathing to reduce anxiety and reported that her lungs felt better.

Sickle-Cell Anemia

Abnormal hemoglobin causes red blood cells to take a jagged, irregular "sickle" shape. Because of the shape, sickled cells cannot easily pass through small blood vessels. This may cause infarct in any organ of the body. Pain in bones and large joints may occur. Ulcers, pneumonia, swelling of hands and feet, and many other complications develop. Cold weather, stress, swimming in cold water, and even drinking cold water can precipitate a sickle-cell pain crisis because of the inability of the sickled cells to pass through constricted blood vessels.

Biofeedback-assisted relaxation for vasodilation has alleviated painful episodes of sickle-cell anemia (Thomas, Koshy, Patterson, Dorn, & Thomas, 1984). Zeltzer, Dash, and Holland (1979) used progressive relaxation, visualization, and temperature feedback to help adolescents with sickle-cell anemia learn to dilate peripheral arteries. At a 12-month follow-up, the adolescents had significantly reduced pain crises, use of analgesics, outpatient clinic visits, and number of days in the hospital.

Juvenile-Onset Diabetes

Insufficient secretion of insulin by the pancreas results in juvenile-onset diabetes. Control of juvenile diabetes requires a careful balance of diet, exercise, and insulin. Failure to maintain the balance can damage the kidneys, heart, and eyes. To maintain control, children must have daily shots of insulin and must monitor sugar in urine and blood with tests that they can do at home. Many children have difficulty with this daily procedure. To enhance compliance in children who are newly diagnosed, a variety of self-management techniques have been used, such as rewards, goal-setting, and contracts (Epstein, Figueroa, Farkas, & Beck, 1981). Biofeedback training, stress management, and family therapy help many diabetic children improve glucose tolerance and health (Rosenbaum, 1986). Gardner and Olness (1981) use hypnotherapy to help children turn off the "pain switches" during insulin injections.

Hemophilia

Hemophilia is excessive bleeding caused by abnormalities of blood-clotting factors. Without effective blood-clotting factors, excessive bleeding may occur from minor wounds, and internal bleeding may occur, particularly in joints. Bleeding in the joints causes arthritis and requires surgery to improve joint function. Pain is often severe and persistent, and addiction to narcotic analgesics is a hazard. Massive blood transfusions may be needed to replace lost blood. Hemophilia is genetically transmitted by the mother and affects only males. There is no cure for hemophilia, although new treatments can temporarily replace the blood-clotting material needed to prevent bleeding.

Some children with hemophilia spontaneously bleed during emotional stress (Chilcote & Baehner, 1980). For these children, stress management is vital. Hemophiliacs also use stress-management techniques to break the bleeding and pain cycle (Varni, 1981; Varni & Gilbert, 1982; Varni, Gilbert, & Dietrich, 1981). Jeff, age 9, was in a daily cycle of hemorrhage ⟶ pain ⟶ narcotic analgesics ⟶ joint immobilization ⟶ atrophy of muscles adjacent to the deteriorating joints ⟶ hemorrhage ⟶ pain ⟶ narcotic analgesics, and so forth. Jeff often used a wheelchair and missed many days of school each month. During pain episodes, his peripheral veins constricted, hindering injection of the coagulant. Larger doses of narcotics were needed to alleviate pain. As a last resort, Jeff was referred to the University of Southern California School of Medicine's behavioral pediatrics program, headed by James Varni (Varni, Gilbert, & Dietrich, 1981). Jeff learned progressive relaxation, diaphragmatic breathing, the relaxation response, and guided imagery, in which he visualized himself being healthy. He practiced these techniques daily. The results were remarkable. The cycle of daily bleeding, pain, and narcotic analgesics was broken; narcotic analgesics were no longer needed. During training, Jeff missed fewer days of school and was not hospitalized for bleeding and pain. At the one-year follow-up, Jeff's parents reported that he had not been hospitalized during the year and had missed only six days of school. In addition, Jeff's pain greatly diminished, he was less depressed, and he had a greater sense of self-control, self-esteem, and confidence in social relationships. Jeff also gained strength in muscles and joints and no longer needed a wheelchair. Again we note that simple, easy-to-teach and easy-to-learn techniques, consistently practiced, produce remarkable results.

Children also benefit from group training. In fact, Gardner and Olness found that many children prefer groups, saying, "It is our perception that younger children learn best from older children in the group setting. . . . They seem to learn by osmosis" (Gardner & Olness, 1981, p. 199). The group sessions for children and parents included 30 minutes of hypnosis exercises for relaxation, pain control, and reduction of bleeding. Children also had the opportunity to practice hand-warming with biofeedback training. The therapists found that the biofeedback instrumentation, with its visual display of control of skin temperature, encouraged the children to stick with the self-hypnosis training and practice.

Cancer

Cancer is the leading cause of death in children. Children rarely get the typical cancers of adulthood (breast, lung, and colon), which are solid tumors and often are more easily detected and treated than the childhood cancers. Treatment of cancer in children is often aggressive, traumatic, painful, and lengthy, and children suffer the typical side effects of chemotherapy and radiation (including nausea and vomiting), food aversion, baldness, and tissue damage from radiation. Today treatment of cancer has greatly reduced mortality, and about 60 percent of the children with cancer will live more than five years after diagnosis. This increase in survival makes cancer a chronic disease rather than an acute disease, and it brings additional complications and issues to the child and family. Marion Rose of the School of Nursing at the University of Washington, and Robin Thomas, project director of the Child and Family Support Project at the Children's Hospital and Medical Center in Seattle, describe the problems associated with the cure of children with cancer:

> To these definitions of cure must be added the consideration of quality of life for the survivor of childhood cancer, both as it relates to the demands of cancer treatment on daily living and to long-term sequelae or late effects of therapy. As more children survive the experience of cancer, it is becoming increasingly apparent that survival is not without its price. Growth delays, neuropsychological deficits, sterility, secondary malignancies, and organic dysfunction related to specific agents occur in a small but significant percentage of children who survive cancer treatment. The expression of short-term and long-term treatment effects account for the handicapping nature of the condition more so than does the disease itself.
>
> (Rose & Thomas, 1987, p. 188)

In a study of 117 children who survived cancer for at least five years, it was found that 47 percent had mild to severe adjustment problems, and many reported low self-esteem and low satisfaction with self compared with survivors who seemed to cope well with the diagnosis and treatment (Koocher & O'Malley, 1981). It is generally agreed, however, that children who are diagnosed with cancer are psychologically healthy and feel depression, withdrawal, hopelessness, and anger as a normal response to the trauma. Helping children prepare for and cope with survival of cancer is an important task for the health professional.

Of the childhood cancers, leukemia is the most common. Leukemia is characterized by the overproduction of white blood cells (leukocytes) from red bone marrow or from lymph nodes. The lymphocytes do not mature, and immunity is hindered. The leukocyte-producing cells may spread throughout the body, and eventually masses of leukocytes impede normal cell function. When red bone marrow is crowded out, the child becomes anemic, bleeds easily from lack of platelets, and feels pain.

In the past, leukemia was always fatal. Today, with chemotherapy and management of the secondary problems such an anemia, many children live. The treatment may last two or three years, and progress is monitored by repeated bone marrow aspirations.

Techniques that help children during bone marrow aspiration were described above. Although leukemia is no longer always life-threatening when it is treated, the disease and treatment are traumatic. Children with leukemia benefit greatly from behavioral training.

Hypnotherapy and self-hypnosis are the most commonly used behavioral techniques described in the literature on children with cancer. In addition, autogenic training, desensitization, breathing techniques, and play therapy are used. In the Children's Hospital Psychosocial Program at the Children's Hospital of Los Angeles, children and parents learn a variety of stress-management and coping skills for dealing with immediate crises and medical procedures, and parents may have individual or group counseling and receive orientation booklets and a hospital tour when the diagnosis of cancer is made (Kellerman, 1980).

The Psychosocial Program was created in 1976 as part of the Division of Hematology-Oncology at Children's Hospital; the psychology team includes psychologists, psychiatrists, social workers, social work assistants, counselors, paraprofessionals, and nurse coordinators with special training in psychiatry and oncology. All team members are staff of the hematology-oncology division. We comment on this because the integration of the psychosocial program with the medical division acknowledges the importance of psychosocial care for the child and the child's family, as an integral part of treatment of cancer. The medical staff routinely refers children to the program and understands the value of psychosocial therapy. The director of the program notes, however, that the oncology

center of Children's Hospital in Los Angeles is very large and that a comprehensive psychosocial program may not be possible in a smaller oncology department (Kellerman, 1980).

Regardless of the size of the institution, the needs of children with cancer are the same everywhere. All health professionals can learn to teach the basic procedures that help children gain mastery, confidence, and an enhanced quality of life.

Muscular Dystrophy

Muscular dystrophy (*dys* = bad, *trophy* = nourish) is a rare genetic disease that affects skeletal muscles. Gradual wasting of muscles, confinement to a wheelchair, and early death is the outlook for a child with muscular dystrophy, although some victims have lived for several years with the aid of a respirator, urinary catheter, and feeding tube. The cause of dystrophy is unknown. Muscular dystrophy usually is not diagnosed until the child is in school; consequently, other children may be born to the family before diagnosis. In some families, two or three children have the disease.

The Muscular Dystrophy Association administers more than 240 clinics across the country to help children and families cope with the agony and struggles of dystrophy. These centers provide professional medical support and organize parent-support groups. No home care is provided for the child. The association also operates summer camps for children in each state.

Eleven-year-old Peter has muscular dystrophy. He is in a hospital and on a respirator because he has a serious respiratory infection and his chest muscles are too weak to breathe; he cannot talk because the respirator's long tube blocks his throat. His mother comments:

> Peter begins to write. Because I must be standing to support his moving hand properly, I cannot see what he is writing. His hand blocks my view.

I stare at the top of his hand as it moves diagonally, from right to left in a downward stroke. Then he lifts his hand up ever so slightly off the paper and makes another downward stroke—this one from left to right. I know it's going to be a letter A before he draws the final horizontal line.

The next one is an M. He makes those strokes straight up and down, so I have to wait until the third stroke to make sure it's not an N.

I can't tell if the next one is going to be a T or an I or an L until he draws a horizontal line across the top and bottom, and then I know it's an I.

I'm pretty sure from the spherical way he starts out on the next letter that it's going to be an O, but I'm wrong. He stops in mid-circle and finishes it off as a G.

The next letter is an O. He is writing: "AM I GOING TO DIE?"

(Hobbes, Perrin, & Ireys, 1985)

The slow progressive dying of a muscular dystrophy child makes it difficult for health professionals and parents to respond appropriately to the psychological needs of the child. Health professionals need wisdom and knowledge in helping parents and children cope with death.

We find no literature on the use of behavior self regulation techniques for children with muscular dystrophy.

Death

Death is not a disease, but we include it here because, just as health professionals have much to give to a child who is overcoming disease, they have much to give to the child's family and to the child who is dying. We believe that the health professional who helps a child fight for life must also be able to support a dying child, appropriate to the needs of the child and family. We advise professionals to work with patients who have potentially life-threatening disease only when they themselves have come to terms with death and can talk freely about it within the patient's religious and cognitive framework.

Although the taboos about death have been lifted somewhat in this country, and death and dying are studied, shared, and understood as a natural part of life in adults, we find little mention of death and dying in childhood in the behavioral medicine literature. There have been several studies on children's beliefs about death and on the experiences of the family before and after a child's death (Spinetta, Elliott, Hennessey, Knapp, Sheposh, Sparta, & Sprigle, 1982). There is however, a growing hospice movement for aiding the dying child and the family. Increasingly, specialists are trained to provide home care for the child and family when it is planned that the child will die at home (Corr & Corr, 1985).

Health professionals who work with dying children are aware that the death of a child is often perceived by parents and caregivers as unnatural or as a failure. Above all, the death of a child is perceived as the greatest tragedy. Helping the dying child die as painlessly, peacefully, and consciously as possible takes courage, compassion, and skill. Some parents are able to provide the support that the child needs, but many cannot. There is a place for the sensitive health professional near the bedside of the dying child.

Summary

Children with chronic and life-threatening diseases feel isolation, helplessness, dread of repeated treatment procedures and relapse, and fear of death. The child's world of family, school, friends, and medical professionals can help the child, or it can hinder the child's psychological and physiological well-being. Like adults, children with chronic disease who must undergo traumatic medical procedures need social support, counseling, and behavioral skills to cope with treatment and to enhance healing in an atmosphere of hope.

The advent of behavioral treatment for children with chronic disease is a landmark in medicine and behavioral medicine. It may become a landslide as the benefit to child, parents, and caregivers is demonstrated and shared with the health professionals. Simple procedures that are easy to learn and easy to teach make up the basic treatment packages that provide profound relief: relaxation training, visualization and self-hypnosis, breathing techniques, distraction techniques, incentives, and information. Repeatedly, health professionals who use these procedures report the ease with which children learn and use self regulation techniques.

These techniques are of great value in helping the child cope with diagnosis, disease, treatment procedures, and death. As we reviewed the literature and talked with people who work with children with chronic and life-threatening diseases, however, we noted a missing element. Little is said about using these techniques to promote a cure or stabilize a progressive disease such as muscular dystrophy, cystic fibrosis, or cancer. Occasionally this possibility is alluded to, but it is not discussed nor researched directly. The apparent neglect of this area may stem from a lack of knowledge or belief in the possibility of cure, and it may also stem from the fact that the death of a child is particularly devastating to adults who most provide the help, including parents and health professionals.

Several years ago Stephanie Simonton, a pioneer working with cancer patients, told us that working with children was discouraging, not because working with a child with cancer is discouraging in itself, but because so often the family and caregivers either begin to withdraw or deny the seriousness of the disease. These psychological defense mechanisms may protect adults from grief, but they also prevent one of the essential factors in living—hope.

Many parents of children with cancer cannot allow themselves to be hopeful, and therefore they cannot help the child with a relaxation and visualization program or help the child fight for life. It was easier for these parents either to deny the severity of the disease and therefore minimize the importance of the training or to silently "let the child go" as a psychological protection against the seemingly greater grief of hoping that the child might live longer and then experiencing the child's death. Humans have an understandable weakness that can be overcome: fear of unbounded hope and dedication to a task that might fail. People believe that grief will be less when the worst is anticipated and happens than when the best is anticipated and does not happen.

We believe that this psychological protection must be overcome so that caregivers can go beyond helping children cope with disease and medical procedures, to helping children use their inner resources to overcome disease, regardless of the outcome.

IIII➡

SECTION THREE: THE CAREGIVERS

Parents, teachers, doctors, nurses, psychologists, counselors, friends, and even the hospital housekeeping staff are the caregivers to children. Unfortunately, having children to care for does not automatically confer wisdom in child care. Parents are the most glaring example of this and are the caregivers least likely to have training in child care.

The greatest challenge of parenting comes when the child is in psychological, behavioral, or physical trouble. Parents who themselves had good parents will naturally be more capable of helping the child over the hurdles. When you review the ingredients of health and wellness, it will be obvious that good parenting begins long before children are born. The challenge after people have become parents is to help the unhealthy adult become a healthy parent. Health professionals are challenged to work at this basic level by helping parents help their children.

The point here is that parents are care-givers and need many skills and personal qual-ities to provide care when a child needs help. When parents are able, they have a profound effect on the child's health and well-being. When parents are ignorant or abusive or when they otherwise abdicate responsibility, health professionals must repair the damage and make up the difference.

Classroom teachers play a role in the health and well-being of children. Overworked and underpaid teachers can teach the basics of re-laxation and stress management, but they can-not be expected to play a major role in therapy, even when the problem involves classroom be-havior. However, the classroom teacher can be a source of hope and positive expectations and can reinforce the use of self regulation skills. We think that we are correct in suggesting that every teacher could benefit, both personally and professionally, from courses on the dynam-ics of health and wellness.

Although school counselors are expected to help children avoid drug abuse, suicide, and behavioral problems and can teach the basics of relaxation and stress management, they can-not provide the support and counseling needed by children and adolescents who suffer from chronic emotional, physical, or psychophysio-logical disorders.

Behavioral therapies such as biofeedback training, hypnotherapy, and many other self regulation techniques enable psychologists to work effectively with children. A specialty within psychology, pediatric psychology (Tuma, 1982), uses behavioral therapies to help chil-dren cope with chronic disease. Pediatric psy-chologists work with children in hospitals and private clinics.

Unfortunately, few children have the op-portunity to work with health professionals who have the skills and knowledge to foster self regulation and healing. This is due to many factors: Parents and medical professionals are ignorant of behavioral medicine and of the potential that children have for self regulation and healing; physicians are reluctant to refer patients to other health professionals; the cost of private therapy is high; there is the belief that children will grow out of their problems; and there is the unspoken belief that because "terminally" ill children will die, self regula-tion therapy is not needed.

In the medical setting, anyone who inter-acts with the child and the family, from the housekeeping staff of the hospital to the physi-cian, is a potential caregiver. We mention housekeeping because in a unique program, pe-diatrician Karen Olness (1977) spent 18 months training the entire staff of the Minneapolis Children's Health Center in the use of hyp-notherapy and self-hypnosis. Olness realized that anyone who interacts with the child has the potential of enhancing the child's well-being and self-mastery. That person also can inadver-tently foster helplessness, fear, and a sense of failure in the child, the psychological factors that Olness and her colleagues were attempting to help the child overcome through hypnother-apy and self-hypnosis. When the entire staff understood the function and goals of hyp-notherapy and self-hypnosis, they were all able to give the children the encouragement that they needed, at every level of interaction and in every aspect of treatment. We applaud this work and can well imagine the benefit that it had for the children and their families.

In this chapter we have mentioned many programs for children, usually located in a chil-dren's hospital in such large cities as Boston, Los Angeles, Rochester, New York, and Min-neapolis. Several of these programs use a team approach in which the psychosocial practi-tioner—a term created by Kellerman (1980)—and other caregivers work with children and parents who ask for help, usually in coping with the diagnosis, home care, and medical pro-cedures. These programs are for children with serious and life-threatening disease who are in the medical system for long-term therapy.

Many children and their parents do not have access to such programs. In this case, help is given by the medical professional closest to the child during hospitalization and when home care is needed—the nurse.

Pediatric Nurses: The Unsung Heroes

Nurses are the largest group of health professionals who care for chronically sick children. Nurses obtain health histories, perform physical examinations, monitor vital signs, administer medications, and educate parents and children on self-care procedures such as catheterization and monitoring glucose. Nurses provide guidance and support for the child and parents during hospitalization and painful procedures. Nurses use play therapy, role-playing, and audiovisual aids to help children adjust to hospitalization, medical procedures, and daily self-care activities. Nurses function as advocates for the sick child and the families by helping parents and child use resources that can provide care and help.

Many pediatric nurse practitioners (PNP) specialize in working with chronically ill children and their families. The function of the pediatric nurse practitioner is to promote the "psychosocial, physical, and developmental well-being of children by functioning as a practitioner, as a collaborative member of the health team, and as an advocate of child health in the community (*The American Nurse*, 1974). The PNP visits the child at home and helps the family cope with the disease. The PNP is also available for telephone consultation. The PNPs at the Spina Bifida Center at New Haven Connecticut Hospital visit the home to help the parents care for the child, assess the psychosocial problems of parents and children, and provide encouragement and reassurance to the parents and children.

At the School of Nursing at the University of Washington and at the Child and Family Support Project in Seattle, nurses are trained to provide nursing and psychological help for families of chronically ill children. The job is described in this way:

> Knowledge of the pathophysiology, diagnosis, and treatment of the chronic condition is required, as well as information on the child's and parent's response to the impairment. Knowledge about family systems, crisis theory, development, vulnerability, and coping are therefore equally important. Nursing is central to helping the family deal with health and home management issues as well as mastery of the parenting role. Nursing plays a major part in the ongoing monitoring and management of the child; however, numerous other health care providers are likely to be involved as well. The nurse often serves in a case management role, helping to coordinate services and advocating on the child's and family's behalf. The nurse is often the only health professional who has the scope of expertise in the biological, behavioral, and sociological sciences to appreciate all the issues involved in these complex cases.
>
> (Barnard, 1987, p. x)

The complex role of the nurse specialist may also include organizing parent support groups and teaching basic stress-management skills to child and parents.

School nurses are essential to help chronically sick children function at school. The nationwide School Nurse Achievement Program (Igoe, 1980) prepares nurses to care for handicapped children. Workshops, workbooks, and learning packages give school nurses the knowledge and skills for working with chronically sick children.

Several nursing programs include stress-management and biofeedback training. The University of Washington School of Nursing provides an extensive program in stress-management and biofeedback training (Nagawaka-Kogan, et al., 1984). The University of Wisconsin at Madison has established a joint doctoral program in nursing and psychology in which students learn behavioral methods and nursing skills (Keller & Baumann, 1986).

We expect that as the benefits of self regulation skills are increasingly appreciated, teaching these skills to all patients will become an accepted element of care.

Chronically sick children and their families need support from health professionals and community agencies. Nurse specialists cannot carry the burden of helping so many people with so many needs. Existing programs are a small drop in a big bucket. Federal, state, and local programs must be created to help children and families at all levels of need, from financial to psychological, and through all phases of diagnosis, treatment, and recovery or death of the child.

This comprehensive caring task cannot be met by a single health professional, but it can be met by a team in a hospital or community.

Center for Attitudinal Healing

Consider for a moment what it would be like to an 8-year-old who has felt a little sick for a few days. You go to the doctor, who sends you to another doctor in a hospital, who sticks a huge needle in you and sucks out bone. You cannot go home; instead, you are put in isolation, and when people talk to you they have to wear a mask and gown. Lots of people poke needles in you, and your mom is crying and you hurt all over. You might live or you might die. Finally, after several weeks of this treatment, you are skinny and pale, but you can go home. Now chemotherapy continues in a clinic, and every few weeks you go to the hospital for a "bone marrow." What would be your greatest need at this time? Courage, hope, laughter, serious talk about dying, and getting on with life.

Like adults, children need psychological help and social support to cope in a healthy way with chronic and life-threatening disease. Child psychiatrist Jerry Jampolsky created an institution in Tiburon, California, where children with catastrophic disease and injury can share any fear, ask any question, and dream any dream, in an atmosphere of mutual love where people believe in possibility, not limits, and where every child has an incomparable support group—other children.

The first Center for Attitudinal Healing opened its doors in 1975 as a free service for children, functioning entirely on voluntary help and a great deal of love. Soon after, a group of parents was started, and next a group for the brothers and sisters of children with serious disease, then support groups for adults and young adults with life-threatening disease, and finally a group for children who have a parent with cancer. The center recently initiated a group for children with AIDS. Children who cannot come to the center can phone; the center has a hotline for children with cancer and a hotline for children with AIDS. A child anywhere in the United States can call the center, free, and talk to a child who understands.

Focus for a moment on the concept of attitudinal healing. The foundation of the work at the center manifests three beliefs or attitudes: (1) Love is the greatest healer; (2) healing is letting go of fear; and (3) health is inner peace. The feelings of love and inner peace come from giving and receiving love, living in the present, by forgiving rather than judging oneself and others, by looking at life as a whole and death as a process, and by feeling eternal love. These attitudes are the teaching of the center, and the children themselves are the teachers and the learners, with the guidance of the adult volunteers. At the center, children come to know these attitudes through the experience of "connectedness" with others, through giving and receiving love and comfort, through freedom from fear, and through a profound acceptance of the healer within. In *Teach Only Love* (1983), Jampolsky writes: "The attitudinal healer does not counsel adjustment to pain and death or compromise with misery because it is possible for anyone to quietly listen to his inner guide, who will teach him the way to freedom. Love knows no place it cannot go and no person it cannot bring rest" (p. 41).

To facilitate the process of attitudinal healing and to help children cope with chronic disease and medical procedures, children are taught relaxation skills and the use of positive mental imagery. Drawing is an important tool in helping the children express and explore feelings, and in 1978 the center produced a book of the children's drawings, *There Is a Rainbow Behind Every Dark Cloud* (Center for Attitudinal Healing, 1978). The drawings express children's perceptions of disease from diagnosis to death. The drawings in Figure 16.4 need no explanation.

The Center for Attitudinal Healing was founded with the idea that it would not be involved in physical treatment, and it is not, in the traditional sense. It is not surprising, however, that physical healing sometimes accompanies attitudinal healing. Perhaps the most important attitude, the underlying belief that promotes healing at all levels is described by Jampolsky in this statement:

> To have inner rest and contentment and an increasing experience of freedom and release, it is necessary for us to question our old sense of identity. Are we really only a body that lives a few moments and dies? Does the body set the limits to our strength, dictate how we must feel and define the tiny range of activities in which we can engage? Or is there a potential within us that knows no limit of any kind and is unending in its capacity to make happy and set free?
>
> *(Teach Only Love, p. 40)*

Jampolsky's repeated message: There are no limits to what can be done.

Against this backdrop of hope, children learn that attitudes determine how we feel and that we can choose to have positive attitudes. Children learn to look at the positive results of the struggle with disease, and they learn that they have a choice in the way that they respond to events. Children learn that they can work through pain and let go of fear. As a 10-year-old with cancer said:

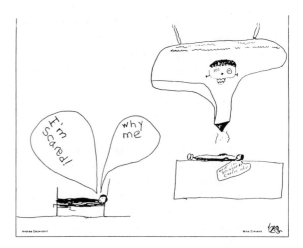

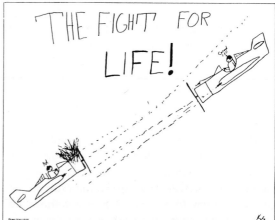

Figure 16.4. Children's Drawings Expressing Fear and Courage. From *There Is a Rainbow Behind Every Dark Cloud.* © **1978 by the Center for Attitudinal Healing. Published by Celestial Arts, Berkeley, CA. Reprinted with Permission.**

Why worry about something that may not ever happen? Why always put illness ahead of what you can do and what you can't do? Yes, you do have an illness. But we're not making that our number one priority. We're putting that on the back burner and just going on with our lives.

(Stacy, 1987)

Children who participate in the groups at the Center for Attitudinal Healing are learning to be healthy in ways that most adults have never learned.

Several years ago we attended a conference for health professionals who work with children. Jampolsky described the center, and then several children told their stories. Very few eyes remained dry, certainly not ours. These were not tears of despair or pity, but the tears that come when we witness courage, hope, and victory. The children were living proof that nothing is impossible.

We highlight the Center for Attitudinal Healing as an illustration of what can be done to help children help themselves, through attitudinal healing. Severely ill children need a place where they can let go of fear, where their natural tendency to be hopeful and to heal can be nurtured, and where they can feel love and give love regardless of handicaps and disease.

The idea is spreading. The center now conducts training seminars for health professionals and others who are dedicated to the idea of being of service and plan to start a center in their area. As of this writing there are 44 centers in the United States and Canada and 6 in other countries (*New Realities,* 1987). All of these centers operate without fee and rely extensively on volunteer help and private and corporate donations.

The advent of attitudinal healing centers is an important trend in children's advocacy—psychological support. Young children lack the skills and resources for starting their own self-help groups, a source of support for many adults. The groups for children give children an opportunity to relate to other children on many levels, in an environment that supports physical, emotional, and spiritual healing, where death is not a taboo subject, and where anything is possible.

With an emphasis on wellness, health professionals have much to offer and to learn from these centers. The focus on wellness is stated nicely in the phrases "Health is inner peace"

and "Healing is letting go of fear." Wellness in spite of sickness is an invaluable concept and an achievable goal for children and adults with life-threatening disease and severe handicaps.

Summary

Caregivers are paramount in the sick child's world, whether parent, teacher, health professional, nurse, social worker, psychosocial practitioner, pediatric psychologist, or physician. Children cannot form support groups on their own. They do not read self-help books; they do not research their disease; they do not demand explanations of treatment from medical staff; and they do not ask for a second opinion. The psychological and physiological well-being of children with problems, from nail-biting to life threatening, depends to a great extent upon the wisdom of the caregiver.

⦀➡ CONCLUSION

It would be wonderful if all children grew into healthy adults as inevitably as acorns grow into oak trees in good soil. Many children do, but many children do not. Many children suffer the consequences of a disrupted family or social environment, many suffer from the stresses of everyday life, many have accidents, many live with chronic disease and the possibility of death, and many undergo painful and traumatic medical procedures. These children can be empowered with self regulation skills and a sense of mastery for overcoming immediate problems and for smoothing the way through the tough times ahead.

With amazing ease, children learn self regulation skills—relaxation, visualization, cognitive restructuring, role-playing, self-hypnosis, and psychophysiological control through biofeedback training. Health professionals who work with children, whether in classrooms, clinics, or hospitals, observe that children are fast learners who enjoy self-responsibility and self-mastery. The self regulation techniques for children are easy to teach and easy to learn. The benefits are extraordinary, ranging from simple relaxation in the classroom to the elimination of cancer.

Most children are blessed with a belief system that says "I can if you say that I can." Because children are sensitive to the beliefs and expectations of adults, negative and positive, the caregiver must also be a believer. The caregiver must be a good coach and teacher, and above all must be able to get inside the world of a child and provide understanding and support.

If you want to feel hopeful, helpful, inspired, dedicated, selfless, compassionate, lighthearted, and childlike, work with children. And be prepared to be both sad and glad, frustrated and encouraged, alone and united, humble and triumphant, student and teacher.

PART SIX

Personality and Health

We ask our students, "Can your personality play a role in how healthy or how sick you are?" and the answer is an unequivocal "yes." When we ask, "How does your personality affect your health?" students immediately say, "By the way that you look at things, the way that you perceive the world, how much stress you feel." The biopsychosocial approach also suggests that this is true. The dynamic of mind ⟶ body is the mechanism.

Given a relationship between personality and health, obvious and intriguing questions arise: "What personality traits predispose a person to disease and illness, and what personality traits foster health?" "Do particular personality traits correspond to particular diseases?" Today another intriguing question is asked, and is beginning to be answered: "If a person changes or eliminates negative per-

sonality traits and adopts prohealth traits, will the risk of disease be reduced, or will the course of a disease already diagnosed be changed?" Part Six concerns these questions, focusing on personality characteristics associated with coronary heart disease and cancer, and on prohealth characteristics that may counteract these diseases.

Chapter 17, Coronary-Prone Personality, Type A, examines the history and research on the Type A personality pattern, a constellation of traits that is associated with heart disease. An evaluation of research is important in personality studies, and the Type A research raises several issues that are discussed. We also describe a program for helping chronic Type A people overcome the destructive behaviors that are associated with heart disease. The success of the program verifies the Type of the program verifies the Type A construct and demonstrates that seemingly hard-core personality characteristics are changeable.

Chapter 18, Personality and Cancer, reviews research on personality variables as precursors of cancer and as a factor in the progression of cancer. The data and clinical impressions of many therapists are suggestive but not conclusive. We also review research on the link between psychological factors, such as stress, and immune system suppression, a research area in psychoneuroimmunology that may eventually pinpoint the mechanisms through which psychological states affect the immune system.

The bulk of research on cancer and personality has focused on the characteristics of people who develop cancer and who succumb to it. Research on survivors and on people who outlive their prognosis is sparse, and yet knowledge of the characteristics of survivors provides invaluable information for helping all cancer patients increase their chances for survival. Several clinicians have written about their observations and programs for cancer patients, and survivors have written about and shared their experiences with others. We include the characteristics of survivors in Chapter 18 because survivors provide insight into the dynamics of health and wellness and point the way for prevention and treatment of cancer.

Chapter 19, The Development of the Personality Characteristics of Healthy People, pulls together and augments information from throughout this text. It is the culmination of the question raised at the outset, "Who stays well?" In this case, we address psychological wellness, reviewing the characteristics of psychologically healthy people and examining the role of the caregiver and the school in the development of personality characteristics and skills of healthy children who become healthy adults.

The characteristics of healthy people—hardiness, stress resistance, a sense of self-efficacy and high self-esteem, empathy, friendliness, purpose in life, and well-being—can be nurtured, taught, and encouraged in children. Children learn primarily from adult models and from experience, and although it may seem miraculous that anyone grows up healthy, the process is natural when the right conditions of nurture and support are met. When the right conditions are met, children grow into healthy adults, as inevitably as acorns in good soil grow into oak trees.

CHAPTER 17

Coronary-Prone Personality, Type A

IIII➡

June 11, 1972

Rrrrrrrrring: Rrrrrrrrring. Rrrrrrrrring.

That darn phone. Who could be calling this early? I look at the clock—it is only 7:00 A.M. Should I answer it? Maybe not; after all, this is the first Saturday morning of summer vacation. The phone continues to ring.

Then I hear Kim answer the phone. She is 4 and loves to answer the phone.

She hollers, "Dad, come to the phone! A lady wants you to wake up and talk to her!"

I roll out of bed and go to the phone.

"Hello, Robert, this is Mrs. Friesen. Your father died this morning, at about 1 o'clock. He had a heart attack. He died in his sleep."

A surge of feelings overwhelms me. I block them. I don't know what to say. How can this be? He has never been sick!

"How is my mother taking it?"

"Poorly. She was totally unprepared. She would like you to come home as soon as you can."

"Okay. I'll catch the first flight I can out of Chicago. Should I call her now?"

"Wait until you get your plane reservations, so she can know when to expect you."

"Okay."

Flying home on the plane, I wonder why my father died so early. He was only 66. That is young. He had no signs of heart trouble.

My father never smoked. He walked regularly for exercise. He ate moderately and was just a little overweight. He retired a year ago, so there was no unusual stress in his life. He had a good retirement pension, so everything seemed to be going fine. Maybe it was genetics. But his parents lived into their 80s. None of his brothers died early of heart disease. He did

not have high blood cholesterol. So why would he die at 66?

A week after the funeral, I am talking with my father's physician.

"Why do you think my father died? You knew him for at least 20 years."

"I don't know."

"Perhaps it's genetic?" I ask. "If it's genetic, is there anything I can do to prevent the same thing happening to me?"

"I doubt that it's genetic, given your father's family history. But there are some new tests out that measure the amount of fat in your blood. Deposits of fat in the arteries that supply the heart can cause heart trouble. You may want to take those tests."

When I return to Illinois, I have a blood test to see if I have unusually high levels of fatty lipids. The cardiologist says that the test results are normal. He tells me I do not have to worry.

RS

June 1975

Three years after my father's death, I am reading everything I can find on heart attack. One Saturday afternoon, I am browsing through the books in the medical and health section of my favorite bookstore. I spot a bright red paperback, *Type A Behavior and Your Heart*, written by two cardiologists, Meyer Friedman and Ray Rosenman. The book is new. I begin to read and I cannot put the book down.

"At least half the people who get heart attacks can be linked to none of the known and suspected causative factors—smoking, diet, exercise habits, other contributing diseases, and so forth. . . . Plainly, another factor is at work here, and this is the one we have discovered and dubbed Type A Behavior Pattern. It is a particular complex of personality traits, including excessive competitive drive, aggressiveness, impatience, and a harrying sense of time urgency." (pp. 14, 15) . . . "YOU POSSESS TYPE A BEHAVIOR PATTERN. . . . If you always move, walk, and eat rapidly. . . . If you become unduly irritated or even enraged when a car ahead of you in your lane runs at a pace you consider too slow. . . . If you frequently do two or more things simultaneously. . . . If you almost always feel vaguely guilty when you relax and do absolutely nothing for several hours to several days. . . . If you attempt to schedule more and more in less and less time, and in doing so make fewer and fewer allowances for unforeseen contingencies. . . . A concomitant of this is a chronic sense of time urgency, one of the core components of Type A Behavior Pattern."

(Friedman & Rosenman, 1974).

I am stunned as I read the book. The description of the Type A person describes my father, and it is a description of me! As a psychologist I can hardly believe what I am reading. Two cardiologists are telling me, a psychologist, that personality factors are one of the main reasons for heart attack before the age of 70. In addition, the personality characteristics they describe are true of my father and of me. Dad always drove faster than the speed limit, and so do I. He worked day and night trying to get more and more done in less and less time, and I do the same! (In fact, my daughter is already rebelling at my fast pace of life. Whenever I hold the door for her to get into the car she stops, pauses, and looks around as if saying, "You can't rush me.") My father was impatient with us if we were not on time, and I am the same way. And my father could not tolerate "sitting around," and I can't either. I feel guilty when I am not doing something productive all the time.

After reading, *Type A Behavior and Your Heart*, I begin to study the research on Type A behavior and heart disease to evaluate the

evidence. I do this because I am not particularly thrilled about changing my lifestyle, and I reason that I will not change unless the evidence is clear.

In this chapter we explore the link between Type A behavior and heart disease and describe a program that meets the challenge of changing Type A behavior. The discovery of a connection between personality and the cardiovascular system and the demonstration that people can change these destructive patterns are significant contributions to knowledge of the dynamics of health and wellness. In Section One, the history of the concept of Type A behavior and the main studies that established the link between Type A behavior and heart disease are discussed. Over the years research has found that the lethal components in Type A behavior are hostility and anger. In Section Two, the reliability and validity of the measures for determining Type A behavior are critically examined in the context of understanding conflicting data. Section Three answers an important question, "Can personality traits be changed?" In the Recurrent Coronary Prevention Project, chronic Type A individuals learned to eliminate destructive habits and adopt cognitive and behavioral habits that reduce the risk of coronary heart disease. The methods and results of the project are described.

||||➡

SECTION ONE: HEART DISEASE AND TYPE A BEHAVIOR

Heart disease is the number one cause of death in the United States. Over half of all deaths among middle-aged men are caused by heart disease. One fourth of the people who die from heart disease are younger than 65 (American Heart Association, 1985).

Coronary heart disease, also known as coronary artery disease, is the main cause of heart attack. Coronary heart disease refers to inadequate blood flow to the heart because the coronary arteries are blocked by atherosclerosis. Atherosclerosis is the thickening of the artery walls with deposits of fat and minerals. Angina pectoris (severe chest pain) and myocardial infarction (heart attack) result from lack of blood flow to the heart muscle.

My father's physician told me that my father died of a "massive coronary." This means that a major coronary artery was blocked in some way, either by a blood clot or a spasm that prevented the flow of blood to the heart muscle. The cells of the heart muscle died from lack of oxygen. What caused the blockage of the arteries?

High blood pressure, cigarette smoking, obesity, diabetes, lack of exercise, family history, and high blood cholesterol are known to increase the likelihood of coronary heart disease. When considered singly or in combination, these risk factors account for less than half of the coronary heart disease in middle-aged men (Jenkins, 1971), the population that has the highest risk for coronary heart disease in the United States. Obviously, more is involved in coronary heart disease than these known risk factors.

Cardiologists Meyer Friedman and Ray Rosenman were not satisfied with the usual explanations for heart disease, partly because their research on high-fat diets indicated that dietary fat is not the major cause and because they knew that the known risk factors could not account for all cases. When the wife of an executive in the diet study informed Friedman and Rosenman that she knew that stress caused heart attacks, they were willing to explore the possibility. The hypothesis that emotional stress affects the cardiovascular system was new, but it seemed reasonable. Like the evolution of most hunches into concrete concepts, the evolution of the concept of Type A behavior and its link to coronary heart disease took time and persistence.

The New Risk: Type A Behavior

As a first step in testing the hypothesis about stress, Friedman and Rosenman sent a questionnaire to several hundred businessmen. The businessmen were asked, "What do you believe was the cause of a heart attack in someone you know?" Over 70 percent believed that the cause was the stress associated with deadlines and excessive competition at work.

Friedman and Rosenman sent the same questionnaire to 100 cardiologists. Sixty physicians believed that the stress associated with deadlines and competition was the main cause of heart attack. Surprised by these responses, Friedman and Rosenman said, "We were startled to find so many physicians ascribing lethality to a factor that was neither mentioned nor described in medical textbooks or professional journals of the day" (Friedman & Ulmer, 1984, p. 5). Surprise is understandable; when Friedman and Rosenman began their research in 1955, the effect of stress on disease and illness was not common medical knowledge, as it is today.

The next step was to determine whether the stress from deadlines and competitive pressures does in fact affect physiological processes that might in turn affect the cardiovascular system. Friedman and Rosenman measured the blood cholesterol level of 40 accountants from January 1957 to June 1957. During that period, the accountants' eating habits, exercise habits, and life patterns did not change. What happened, of course, was an increase in stress as the April 15 tax deadline approached. In January, February, and March, blood cholesterol and the blood-clotting rate were normal. During the first two weeks of April, the average blood cholesterol level rose abruptly, and blood clotting rate increased. In May and June, with the tax deadline past, blood cholesterol and the blood-clotting rate returned to normal levels. Friedman and Rosenman were amazed. "For the first time in medical history, a clear-cut demonstration of the power of the mind alone to alter man's blood cholesterol and clotting time had been achieved" (Friedman & Ulmer, 1985, p. 5).

It is significant that two cardiologists, trained in traditional medicine, described this discovery as a clear link between the mind and physiological processes. This happened at a time when the treatment of cardiovascular disease focused primarily on the mechanical nature of the heart. As one heart surgeon said, "It is a matter of plumbing."

Friedman and Rosenman observed that in response to pressures from the environment, some people become worried and competitive. They work harder and faster; they do not take time off for recreation and relaxation; their toleration for frustration decreases; and they are frequently angry. Friedman and Rosenman realized that many of their patients with heart disease were hard-driving, competitive, and always on edge. They labeled this aggressive, time-pressure personality style "Type A." Individuals who are easygoing, relaxed, and noncompetitive were labeled "Type B."

Having determined that stress affects two physiological parameters that could affect the cardiovascular system, the next step was to find out whether people with Type A behavior have elevated blood cholesterol and blood-clotting time. If so, this would indicate that people who exhibit Type A behavior also have physiological signs of stress.

In 1958, Rosenman and Friedman studied 80 men who exhibited Type A personality characteristics, 80 men who were Type B, and 40 men who were chronically anxious. The diet and exercise patterns of all the men were the same. The Type A men had significantly higher blood cholesterol levels and blood-clotting rates than the men in the other groups. In addition, "the most surprising and terrifying finding was that the Type A group already possessed a seven times greater incidence of coronary heart disease than those in the other groups"

(Friedman & Ulmer, 1984, p. 8). Friedman and Rosenman were surprised to find that some of these Type A men with coronary heart disease were only in their 40s.

In 1960, Friedman and Rosenman presented their research on Type A Behavior and coronary heart disease at a medical conference. The presentation was greeted with silence. The idea that attitudes and behavior can affect the heart contradicted the biomedical model's premise that physical diseases have only physical causes.

Over the next 30 years, Friedman and Rosenman responded to the challenge of skepticism with several excellent studies. The major study was the Western Collaborative Group Study, in which the health and sickness patterns of 3,500 men were recorded over 8½ years. Subjects were classified as Type A or Type B. At the end of the first year of the group study, Rosenman and Friedman examined the health records of the subjects. It was found

WHY TYPE A?

Friedman and Rosenman submitted two research proposals on emotional stress to the National Institutes of Health for a research grant to study the relationship of heart disease and emotional stress. The proposals were rejected. The director of the review team informed Friedman and Rosenman that the proposals had been rejected by psychiatrists who said that cardiologists were not competent to investigate emotions. The director suggested using the term "Type A Behavior Pattern" instead of "emotional stress." With this change, the proposal was accepted, funding an elaborate study of Type A behavior and coronary heart disease.

that 113 men had coronary heart disease, and 80 of these had been classified as Type A. Over the 8 1/2-year study, a total of 257 heart attacks were recorded. One hundred seventy-eight of the heart attack victims had been classified Type A. The study revealed that Type A individuals are two times more prone to having a heart attack than Type Bs.

The tool used by Friedman and Rosenman for determining Type A behavior is called the Structured Interview, created by them. The 45-minute interview follows a format of 26 questions and follow-up questions. The interview is scored by content of replies and by mode of communication and other nonverbal behaviors. A skilled interviewer elicits Type A behavior by interrupting the subject, speaking very slowly and seeming confused at times, and detects the Type A responders' clipped speech, lack of humor, hidden hostility, fist clenching and jaw-tightening in response to frustrating questions. Type A responders interrupt the interviewer frequently and try to hasten the conversation with "yes, yes," or "right, right," or nodding the head. Type As display impatience by tapping their fingers and jiggling their feet. Questions about time, such as, "How do you feel about waiting in lines—bank lines, supermarket lines, post office lines?" elicit vehement responses from Type As such as "I HATE waiting in lines."

Shortly after Friedman and Rosenman published the results of the Western Collaborative Group Study, similar results were found in a study conducted by a professor of psychology and Trappist monk, Bernard Caffrey (1968, 1970). Caffrey knew that Trappist and Benedictine monks in the United States are three times more likely to suffer coronary heart disease than Trappist and Benedictine monks in Europe. Caffrey suspected that Type A behavior might explain the difference; he studied with Friedman and Rosenman and learned to conduct the structured interview. Caffrey interviewed monks throughout Canada and the United States. Medical records obtained after

the interviews disclosed that Type A monks were five times more likely to have coronary heart disease than Type B monks. This was the first replication study of Friedman and Rosenman's work, and it gave further credence to the link between Type A behavior and coronary heart disease.

By 1978, the work of Rosenman and Friedman and other research on Type A behavior had attracted the attention of lay people and professionals alike. The idea that personality influences health was accepted as a clear possibility. In that year, the prestigious National Heart, Lung, and Blood Institute sponsored a conference on Type A behavior. The conference concluded:

> The review panel accepts the available body of scientific evidence as demonstrating that Type A behavior is associated with an increased risk of clinically apparent coronary heart disease in employed, middle-aged U.S. citizens. This increased risk is greater than that imposed by age, elevated levels of systolic blood pressure, serum cholesterol, and smoking, and appears to be of the same order of magnitude as the relative risk associated with the latter three of these other factors.
>
> (Cited in Price, 1984 p. 9)

Refining the Concept of Type A: Anger and Hostility

To determine the personality factors that are the strongest predictors of coronary heart disease within the global Type A pattern, Karen Matthews, David Glass, Ray Rosenman, and Rayman Bortner (1977) reanalyzed the original Western Collaborative Group Study interviews. As part of such an analysis, factors that play a role in coronary heart disease but are not personality characteristics, such as smoking or obesity, are eliminated. One could hypothesize that more Type A people than Type B people smoke, and it is smoking that accounts for the increased coronary heart

IS THERE A TYPE A PERSONALITY?

What is personality? Most definitions are based on the observations that different people respond to the same event in distinctive ways and that people develop patterns that are consistent ways of coping with life. A common definition of personality is "the distinctive patterns of behavior (including thoughts and emotions) that characterize an individual's response to the environment" (Mischel, 1976, p. 2).

A major issue in current personality theory is whether "personality" should be defined as a constellation of stable characteristics, called traits, or defined as a constellation of behaviors determined by the situation. Some theorists argue that Type A behavior refers to a complex of traits and is thus a personality type. Traits are stable dispositions that shape behavior.

Walter Mischel (1968) argues that "trait theorists" have failed to show that traits are consistent across situations. For example, a person may be passive at work but aggressive at home. In this case, the situation would be the explanation of behavior, not the person's personality traits. Mischel argues that people alter their personality and behavior according to the situation.

Friedman and Rosenman take the position that Type A behavior is an interaction between stable personality traits and situations, and that only in certain types of situations will the aggressive Type A pattern emerge. In other words, a Type A trait is a predisposition to respond in a particular way in a particular situation, and it is a personality type.

How do these traits develop? Are they inborn or learned? Friedman and Rosenman believe that our society rewards Type A behaviors, such as aggression and competitiveness, and values people on the basis of their accumulation of material possessions. Friedman and Rosenman state, "We have rarely encountered this behavior pattern in any person whose religious beliefs take precedence over his preoccupation with the accumulation of 'numbers' or the acquisition of personal power."

(Friedman & Rosenman, 1976, p. 169)

---

disease. The contribution of smoking and other risks are eliminated statistically in the analysis of personality risk factors.

The research team analyzed the personality characteristics and behaviors that are seen during the structured interview to determine which ones were highly correlated with coronary heart disease. They discovered six characteristics:

1. Potential for hostility.
2. Angry more than once a week, and anger directed toward others.
3. Irritability at having to wait in lines.
4. Competitiveness in games with peers.
5. Explosive voice modulation (talking in loud, staccato bursts).
6. Vigorous responses to interview questions rather than calm, deliberate answers.

Of these characteristics, **anger** and **hostility** were the most predictive of coronary heart disease.

To explore the anger dimension of the constellation of Type A behavior, Charles

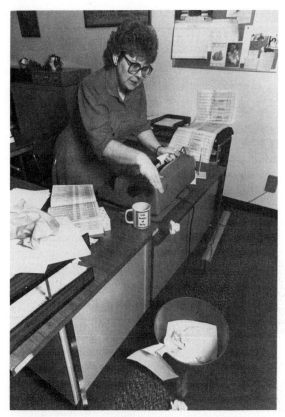

Frequent Anger and Hostility Are the Most Harmful Aspects of Type A Behavior.
Source: Robert Waltman, Aims Community College, Greeley, CO.

Spielberger, author of a widely used test for measuring anxiety, developed an anger scale to measure this core characteristic. The test includes items such as "I am quick-tempered," "I get angry when I'm slowed down by other's mistakes," "When I get mad, I say nasty things," and "I feel infuriated when I do a good job and get a poor evaluation." Spielberger found that people who score high on the anger scale are more likely to have coronary heart disease than those who do not (Spielberger, Jacobs, Russell, & Crane, 1983).

The current research on Type A behavior indicates that chronic anger is a risk factor for coronary heart disease. The more times a person feels rage and anger, the more destructive anger and rage are to the body.

The ancient Chinese had a proverb:
"The fire you kindle for your enemy
often burns you more than him."
(Spielberger & London, 1982, p. 56)

Other research on the relationship of anger and heart disease found that people who hold in anger, a characteristic referred to as **anger-in**, are also at high risk for heart disease. Anger-in is the inability or unwillingness to express anger, irritation, or annoyance, particularly if expressing the feeling would cause interpersonal conflict. In the structured interview, the question "When you get angry, do people around you know about it?" is answered, "No, I hold it in" or "I never let people know when I'm angry." The question "Would you say anything about being kept waiting for an appointment?" is answered, "No, it wouldn't help anyway." Haynes, Feinleib, and Kannel (1980) analyzed data from the 1,674 subjects who participated in the prospective heart study in Framingham, Massachusetts, and found that of all the Type A characteristics, hostility and anger-in were the highest predictors of coronary heart disease. MacDougall, Dembroski, Dimsdale, and Hackett (1985), who studied 126 male patients at Massachusetts General Hospital in Boston who received the Type A structured interview and an angiogram, also found that hostility and anger-in were the best predictors of coronary heart disease.

To verify the importance of hostility and anger in coronary heart disease, Michael Hecker and colleagues (Hecker, Chesney, Black, & Frautschi, 1988) reanalyzed the data of the Western Collaborative Group Study and replicated the 1977 results. In the meantime, researchers at Duke University (Williams, Haney, Lee, Kong, Blumenthal, & Whalen, 1980) also found that hostility and anger behaviors are the toxic elements in Type A personality. These researchers studied 1,000 patients who had coronary angiograms to determine the cause of angina pectoris (chest pain). Subjects were given the hostility scale from a popular personality test, the Minnesota Multiphasic Personality Inventory (MMPI). Subjects who scored high had 50 percent more coronary blockage than low scorers; this was true of women and men. The Duke.team also studied 255 male physicians who had taken the MMPI 25 years earlier in medical school. Men who scored high on the hostility scale had five times the number of coronary events (angina pectoris and heart attack) than low scorers (Barefoot, Dahlstrom, & Williams, 1983). Several other studies have found a highly significant correlation between hostility and coronary heart disease (Dembroski, MacDougall, Williams, Haney, & Blumenthal, 1985; Shekelle, Gayle, Ostfeld, & Paul, 1983; Weinstein, Davison, DeQuattro, & Allen, 1987; Williams & Anderson, 1987).

To clarify the concept of hostility, John Barefoot and his colleagues at Duke University Medical Center (Barefoot, Dodge, Peterson, Dahlstrom, & Williams, 1989), examined the items on the hostility scale of the MMPI and found that they actually measure several characteristics that are part of the global concept of hostility: cynicism, hostile beliefs, hostile feelings, aggressive behavior, and social avoidance. Examples of these characteristics and items on the hostility scale of the MMPI are:

Cynicism—"I think most people would lie to get ahead." "Most people are honest chiefly through fear of being caught." "It is safer to trust nobody."

Hostile beliefs—"I commonly wonder what hidden reason another person may have for doing something nice for me." "My way of doing things is apt to be misunderstood by others."

Hostile feelings—"People often disappoint me." "There are certain people whom I dislike so much that I am inwardly pleased when they are catching it for something they have done."

Aggressive behavior—"When someone does me a wrong I feel I should pay him back if I can, just for the principle of the thing." "I have at times had to be rough with people who were rude or annoying."

Social avoidance—"I am likely not to speak to people until they speak to me." "I prefer to pass by school friends, or people I know but have not seen for a long time, unless they speak to me first."

Barefoot and colleagues (1989) examined the specific responses on the hostility scale of 118 lawyers who had taken the MMPI 22 years earlier, and found that cynicism, hostile feelings, and aggressive behavior were the best predictors of early mortality.

You might now ask, "What is the difference between anger, anger-in, hostility, aggression, and cynicism, and how can they all be related to coronary heart disease?" One answer is that these are uniquely different personality characteristics that predispose a person to heart disease. As Barefoot and colleagues suggest, however, another answer is that these characteristis are different ways of describing aspects of a common pattern and appear to be different only because they are determined by different measures and because they reflect different aspects of a person—beliefs, feelings, and behaviors. When the aspects of the Type A personality that predispose a person to heart disease are finally clarified and understood, we will probably find that the most lethal combination of traits centers on a broad meaning of hostility and involves beliefs, feelings, and behaviors.

Summary

Friedman and Rosenman identified a behavior pattern, Type A, that predicts coronary heart disease. This pattern is identified most clearly through the structured interview in which facial and vocal behaviors, gestures, posture, and communication patterns can be measured to determine the person's level of impatience, hostility, time-pressure, frustration, and anger. Over time, the most important Type A characteristics for predicting coronary heart disease are being separated from the less important. As measured today, the traits most predictive of coronary heart disease are hostility (which includes aggression and cynicism) and anger-in. In August 1989 a new scale was added to the MMPI, the Type A Scale, which incorporates many of the items from the original hostility scale. This new scale will stimulate research and encourage continued exploration of the fascinating link between personality traits and heart disease.

▐▐▐▐▶

SECTION TWO: RELIABILITY, VALIDITY, AND TYPE A BEHAVIOR

Many studies in the 1960s indicated that Type A behavior is a risk for coronary heart disease. In the 1970s and 1980s, however, conflicting results were reported. Some studies showed a connection between Type A behavior and coronary heart disease and some did not. When results conflict, the research evaluation check list discussed in Chapter 5 is useful for comparing studies. In this section we examine the contradictory results of Type A research, focusing on issues of reliability and validity of Type A measures.

Validity of Pencil-Paper Assessments

In the 1970s, research on the link between Type A behavior and coronary heart disease took a turn toward simpler methods of assessing behavior than the structured interview, and a variety of pencil-paper tests of Type A behavior were developed. The most common test is the Jenkins Activity Survey. There are 54 questions, centered on characteristics of hard-driving, speed, impatience, and job involvement. Typical questions are:

1. Do you ever set deadlines or quotas for yourself at work or at home?
   a. Yes, once per week or more often.
   b. Yes, but only occasionally.
   c. No.
2. Has your spouse or some friend ever told you that you eat too fast?
   a. Yes, often.
   b. Yes, once or twice.
   c. No, no one has told me this.
3. How would your wife (or closest friend) rate you?
   a. Definitely hard-driving and competitive.
   b. Probably hard-driving and competitive.
   c. Probably relaxed and easygoing.
   d. Definitely relaxed and easygoing.

Pencil-paper tests, like the Jenkins Survey, are much easier to administer and score than the 45-minute structured interview used by Friedman and Rosenman, making large studies of Type A behavior and coronary heart disease possible. For example, using pencil-paper assessments of Type A behavior, 2,411 subjects in France and Belgium (French-Belgian Collaborative Group, 1982), 2,200 men of Japanese descent in Honolulu (Cohen, Syme, Jenkins, Kagan, & Zyzanski, 1979), 1,672 subjects in Framingham, Massachusetts (Haynes, Feinleib, & Kannel, 1980), and 2,000 subjects in Belgium (DeBacker, Dramaix, Kittel, & Kornitzer, 1983) were studied. The results of these studies were contradictory. The French-Belgian study showed that Type A behavior predicts coronary heart disease, but the second Belgian study showed that Type A behavior does not predict heart disease. The Honolulu study showed that Type A behavior does not predict heart disease, but the Framingham study showed that it does (Haynes & Matthews, 1988).

One explanation for the contradictory results of these studies is that pencil-paper tests lack construct validity. The Type A personality pattern is a "construct." *Construct* is another word for concept or hypothesis (Hogan & Nicholson, 1988). For a Type A pencil-paper test to have validity, it must accurately measure the trait or behavior patterns that reflect the Type A construct. Friedman and Rosenman argue that pencil-paper tests do not accurately measure Type A behavior, and therefore lack construct validity, because they cannot measure nonverbal behaviors such as tone of voice, posture, interrupting the interviewers, and facial expressions. Also, most Type A individuals are not aware of their Type A behaviors and may not respond true to form on a pencil-paper test, while hostile behavior patterns reflected in the tone of voice and the manner in which questions are answered are seen during the structured interview. Several studies comparing pencil-paper tests with a structured interview have found low correlations between the two assessment methods (Chesney, Black, Chadwick, & Rosenman, 1981; Dembroski, et al., 1985). These studies support Friedman and Rosenman's position that pencil-paper tests do not capture the important characteristics of Type A individuals. Tests that lack construct validity will have invalid results.

Reliability and Validity of the Structured Interview

The best evidence for the link between Type A behavior and coronary heart disease is based on studies that used the structured interview, notably the Western Collaborative Group Study conducted by Friedman and Rosenman. However, in 1980 a significant study using the structured interview and the Jenkins Survey failed to show a connection between Type A behavior and coronary heart disease. Type A behavior did not predict heart disease, and the researchers concluded that Type A behavior is not a risk

(MRFIT Study Group, 1982). This study was the Multiple Risk Factor Intervention Trial (MRFIT, known as "Mister Fit"). MRFIT, conducted by the National Heart, Lung, and Blood Institute, recorded the health history of 3,110 men from 1973 to 1980. MRFIT was an intervention study in which subjects were encouraged to change lifestyle habits, and the research also included measurement of Type A behavior. The men were classified as Type A or Type B.

To understand the contradictory results of the MRFIT study and the Western Collaborative Group Study, it is important to assess the reliability and validity of the measures used in the two studies.

Reliability

As discussed in Chapter 5, one of the best ways to determine reliability is to conduct a test/re-test study. The test is given twice to the same group of subjects. If the scores are very similar on both tests, the test is reliable. The WCGS study included reliability assessments of the Type A structured interview method. Re-tests were given at 12 and 20 months (Jenkins, Rosenman, & Friedman, 1968). Reliability scores averaged .82. This means that the structured interview used in the WCGS study was highly reliable.

When human judgment is used to determine a variable such as a subject's voice quality, another source of error, human error, is introduced. Human error is compounded when several raters are used to score the interview. To determine the amount of error caused by errors in judgment, **inter-rater** reliability measures are obtained. In the WCGS, inter-rater reliability measures were obtained by having three interviewers assess the same subjects. The inter-rater reliability correlations ranged from .75 to .90 (Caffrey, 1978; Dembroski, 1978).

In the structured interview assessment procedure, the interviewers must be skilled and the inter-rater reliability must be high. The inter-rater reliability of the structured interview procedure of the MRFIT study was assessed by videotapes of the interviewed subjects scored by different interviewers (MRFIT Group, 1979; Scherwitz, Graham II, Grandits, Billings, 1987). The inter-rater reliability results varied from .16 to .69, with an average of .42 (MRFIT, 1979). Rosenman trained the interviewers for the MRFIT study and reviewed their tapes, but he comments, "The interviewing in MRFIT was sadly deficient. I didn't select the interviewers, and I refused to train some of them, because they were so incompetent" (Fischman, 1987). Larry Scherwitz, a psychologist at the University of California, San Francisco, listened to the taped interviews from the Multiple Risk Intervention Trial and from the Western Collaborative Group Study. He believes that the MRFIT interviews were flawed enough to invalidate the results (Scherwitz, Graham II, Grandits, & Billings, 1987). Scherwitz states that many of the interviewers engaged in verbal tennis with the subjects so that questions and answers were volleyed back and forth with little chance for the subject to express real feelings. Thus, the interviews in the MRFIT study were not reliable. Consequently, the structured interview assessments in the MRFIT study were not valid because the interviewers hurried the subjects and interrupted their answers excessively. According to Scherwitz, the interviewers made the Type A people suspicious and they hid their real feelings, appearing less Type A than they were (Fischman, 1987).

Concurrent Validity

Type A assessments have concurrent validity when they indicate the presence of a criterion or variable of interest, in this case coronary heart disease. If measures from Type A assessments indicate that a person has coronary heart disease at the time the assessment is given, the assessment has concurrent validity. Friedman and Rosenman's 1958 study found that the group of Type A men had a seven times greater incidence of coronary heart disease than the

other groups. In their Western Collaborative Group Study, the Type A assessment accurately predicted 80 of 113 men who already had coronary heart disease. The MRFIT study found no relationship between measures of Type A behavior and measures of coronary heart disease. This would be expected, given the low reliability of the assessment measures.

Predictive Validity

As described in Chapter 5, predictive validity refers to the ability of measures to predict a condition. Do Type A assessments accurately predict coronary heart disease? As demonstrated in the prospective WCGS study and replicated in the prospective study of Trappist monks (Caffrey, 1968, 1970), highly reliable structured interview assessments predict coronary heart disease. It is plausible that the MRFIT study did not predict coronary heart disease because the interview assessments were unreliable and lacked validity.

Summary

Many of the early studies of Type A behavior were carefully conducted with trained interviewers with assessments of the inter-rater reliability of the interviewers and assessment of the stability of Type A behaviors over time. A pencil-paper questionnaire cannot capture the nonverbal behaviors that are most revealing of Type A, such as the speech intonations that reflect hostility. Contradictions regarding Type A behavior arise from failure to rigorously replicate the original Structured Interview Assessments that were used in early studies such as the WCGS study, the Recurrent Coronary Prevention Project (Friedman, Thoresen, Gill, Ulmer, Powell, Price, Brown, Thompson, Rabin, Breall, Bourg, Levy, & Dixon, 1986), and the Trappist and Benedictine study done by Caffrey.

Failure to replicate original studies exactly

is a continuing problem for research. In attempting to expand a data base or verify an original observation on a large scale, shortcuts are taken that may compromise the results, a pencil-paper questionnaire may be substituted for a lengthy interview, or, as in the MRFIT study, unskilled and inexperienced interviewers are used. In comparing research results and evaluating conflicting data, it is important to compare the reliability and validity of the measures that are used. When highly reliable and valid methods have been used for assessment of Type A behavior, Type A behavior is predictive of coronary heart disease for white North American men. Sufficient studies have not been conducted on other segments of the population to demonstrate the universality of Type A behavior as a predictor of coronary heart disease.

||||▶

SECTION THREE:
MODIFYING TYPE A BEHAVIOR:
AN EXPERIMENT IN CHANGING
PERSONALITY

Can Personality Be Changed?

"In most of us, by the age of 30, the character has set like plaster and will never soften again."

William James

Can Type A behavior be changed? If you had asked Friedman and Rosenman this question 25 years ago, they might have said "no." In *Type A Behavior and Your Heart*, Friedman and Rosenman were skeptical that Type A behavior could be modified. They believed that the Type A behavior pattern is deeply entrenched in early childhood and persists through adulthood as a result of the social reinforcement and underlying insecurity that has been found in Type A people.

Today, after working with more than a thousand Type A individuals, Friedman

concludes, "In our view, Type A behavior—however induced and however deep-seated—is neither purely genetic nor inaccessible. It can be changed by the individual himself or herself, and we have proved it" (Friedman & Ulmer, 1984, p. 111). Friedman and Ulmer refer to the Recurrent Coronary Prevention Project, a $4 \frac{1}{2}$-year study of Type A individuals who had already suffered one myocardial infarction and who were treated with either cardiac counseling or with a combination of cardiac and behavioral counseling. Several hundred people learned to modify Type A behavior and reduce the risk of myocardial infarction.

The significance of the Recurrent Coronary Prevention Project has been recognized by many as an intervention program for reducing the risk of heart attack, but its significance as a demonstration of personality change is also significant.

The fact that people can reduce negative personality traits and acquire positive traits is of particular interest in a textbook on the dynamics of health and wellness. The Recurrent Coronary Prevention Project is the largest controlled study on an intervention program for personality change. But a critic might say, "The Type A pattern refers to a behavior and not to a personality type. The Recurrent Coronary Prevention Project modified behaviors, not personality." As discussed earlier in this chapter, a common definition of personality is "consistent behavior patterns." Using this definition, Type A behaviors are personality traits because they are stable over time and are pervasive, influencing all aspects of a person's life. In this section we discuss the evidence that Type A is a stable personality type that can be significantly modified.

Stability of the Type A Behavior Pattern

University of Pittsburgh School of Medicine researchers Karen Matthews and Karen Woodall

(1988) contend that the Type A behavior pattern is stable, beginning in childhood and continuing throughout life. In a comprehensive review of the research literature, Matthews and Woodall point to longitudinal studies, twin studies, and family studies as evidence for the stability of the Type A behavior pattern. A Swedish study of 170 13-year-olds, showed that Type A behavior, as rated by school teachers, was highly correlated with self-reported Type A behaviors at age 27 (Bergman & Magnusson, 1986). In another study, 183 children were rated for five years by their classroom teacher. Type A scores were significantly stable throughout the study. Longitudinal studies indicate that Type A behaviors in children are similar to Type A behaviors in adults—Type A children are aggressive, competitive, impatient, and experience more anger than other children.

Studies of Type A behavior in identical and fraternal twins conclude that loudness of speech, competition, and hostility are heritable (Carmelli, Rosenman, & Chesney, 1987; Matthews & Krantz, 1976; Rahe, Hervig, & Rosenman, 1978). On the other hand, family studies reveal that parents of Type A children are more critical, more demanding, and more anxious, and that they model Type A behavior in comparison to parents of Type B children (Matthews, Rosenman, Dembroski, McDougall, & Harris, 1984). In summary, a number of studies point to the stability of the Type A behavior pattern throughout life.

Pervasiveness of the Type A Behavior Pattern

Friedman and Rosenman found that the core aspect of a Type A behavior pattern is a hostile "struggle with life" that pervades a person's entire personality and experience: interpersonal relationships, work, and play. The pattern is manifested in temperament, values, sense of self, and physiology.

Temperament

Type A people become hostile and impatient in many situations. They get angry at drivers and are impatient with co-workers and family members.

Values

Type A people focus on the quantitative dimensions of life and evaluate success in numbers, such as number of achievements and how much money they accumulate. Friedman and Ulmer call this value system a "numbers consciousness" (Friedman & Ulmer, 1984). For example, a famous track star is described in the following way, "What you've got to understand is that she judges her worth as a person solely by what she accomplishes on the track. It is scary to contemplate, but the competitive nature that we so admire in this woman is actually a huge personality flaw" (Powell & Thoresen, 1987, p. 189).

Interpersonal Relationships

Relationships with people are competitive, with an attempt to dominate. Interactions with people are competitive because the Type A's self-esteem is at stake; this person cannot lose an argument or game without feeling worthless. Nonsupportive interactions characterize a Type A's interpersonal relationships (Watkins & Eisler, 1988).

Self-Concept

Type A individuals have low self-esteem (Houston & Kelly, 1987). Most of them have felt a chronic insecurity since early childhood (Fontana, Rosenberg, Kerns, & Marcus, 1986; Friedman & Ulmer, 1984). They worry that a situation might arise in which they will appear inadequate and incompetent.

Physiology

As a result of feeling on guard and in a struggle with life, Type As have a chronically over-aroused physiology (Fontana, Rosenberg, Kerns, & Marcus, 1986). Type A people, in comparison to Type Bs, respond to stressful events that involve challenge or frustration with higher blood norepinephrine levels (Matthews, 1982; Schmieder, Friedrich, Neus, Rudel, & von Eiff, 1984). As discussed in Chapter 4, the effects of norepinephrine include elevated blood pressure, increased blood-clotting rate, increased insulin, and elevated blood cholesterol. David Elliot, a cardiologist and pioneer of the "hot reactor" personality, suggests that "hot reactors" who respond to stress with high elevations of noradrenaline and adrenaline make the heart increasingly more vulnerable (Elliot & Breo, 1984).

Characteristics of Type A people are summarized in Table 17.1.

The Type A behavior pattern pervades many dimensions of a person's life. To significantly modify such a pattern, a comprehensive, multicomponent approach was developed by Friedman and the team at the Recurrent Coronary Prevention Project.

The Recurrent Coronary Prevention Project

In 1978, Friedman and associates began a $4\frac{1}{2}$-year study of men and women who had already suffered one myocardial infarction. The goal was to determine whether or not Type A behavior can be modified and what effect this would have on cardiac disease and mortality (Friedman, Thoresen, et al., 1986). Eight hundred sixty-two participants were randomly assigned to either a cardiac counseling group or a group offering cardiac counseling plus behavioral counseling. One hundred fifty-one subjects served as a no-treatment control group. The average age of the participants was 53.

The 1,013 subjects received physical exams, blood tests, and ECGs, and they completed an extensive questionnaire. To assess Type A behaviors, the interview was conducted by an expert who had been using the structured interview for more than 20 years. In addition to the structured interview, the 592 subjects who received behavioral counseling were required to have a spouse, a close friend, or a business associate meet with a member of the team to complete questionnaires about the participant's Type A behavior. Information from the "confidant" was obtained throughout the project.

The 270 subjects in the cardiac counseling group met for an average of 25 group sessions in which anxieties about heart disease and other matters were discussed. Information was presented about diet, exercise, and the physiology of the cardiovascular system. Subjects in the cardiac and behavioral counseling group met an average of 38 sessions in small groups. These people practiced Type B behaviors (stopping at yellow lights, driving more slowly) and learned relaxation, cognitive restructuring, and social skills. Methods for enhancing self-esteem were used. Social support from the group leader and other group members was inherent in the program. Over a three-year period, subjects who received Type A behavioral counseling and cardiac counseling had 45 percent fewer second myocardial infarctions than subjects who received cardiac counseling alone. At $4\frac{1}{2}$ years the results were the same (Friedman, Thoresen, et al., 1986).

Table 17.1   Type A Characteristics

Values	Number consciousness
Self-esteem	Low, chronic insecurity
Temperament	Hostile, impatient
Interpersonal	Dominating, alienating
Physiology	Hyperarousal

The success of the behavioral and cardiac counseling program in significantly reducing Type A personality patterns and in preventing the recurrence of myocardial infarction warrants a detailed examination of the methods and procedures of the program.

The training goals of the combined cardiac counseling and behavior counseling program were to help chronic Type A individuals modify Type A behavior and develop healthy behaviors. The treatment goal was reduction of the risk of a second myocardial infarction. Participants met in groups of 10 led by a facilitator who helped them become aware of the Type A behavior pattern and taught skills for developing healthy behaviors. A variety of methods were used.

Awareness of Type A Behavior through Group Discussions and Educational Materials

A variety of audiotapes and videotapes were used in which Type A behavior was clearly described. For example, widows described the lifestyles of their deceased Type A husbands, and Type A men described destructive habits in a hurried and irritated tone of voice. Participants read and discussed biographies of Type A people such as General Douglas MacArthur

---

BOX 17.1

OCTOBER

Monday: Set aside 30 minutes for yourself.

Tuesday: Practice smiling.

Wednesday: Practice removing your grimaces.

Thursday: Eat more slowly.

Friday: Recall memories for 10 minutes.

Saturday: Verbalize affection to spouse/children.

Sunday: Linger at table.

1. "The only future we can conceive is built upon the forward shadow of our past"—Proust
2. "If you make the organization your life, you are defenseless against the inevitable disappointments"—Peter Drucker
3. "The moment numeration ceases to be your servant, it becomes your tyrant."
4. "Habit is the hardiest of all the plants in human growth."

Powell and Thoresen (1987)

and Lyndon Johnson. Discussions and lectures were used to help participants become aware of the cognitive shifts that must occur to overcome Type A behavior, from "I don't believe in Type A" or "It might be true of other people, but not me" to "I do have Type A characteristics, and I can change how I behave and how I think."

After developing an awareness of Type A behavior, participants became aware of their unique pattern and how it might be a problem for them. Awareness of their unique Type A behaviors was achieved through self-monitoring and feedback from the leader and group members.

Drills

The technique of "drills" is exactly as the word suggests, practicing new behaviors over and over again. Each participant in the treatment group received a *Drill Book* of 12 pages, one page for each month. On each page were seven drills—one drill for each day of the week. Also on each page were aphorisms that participants were asked to think about. Box 17.1 is an example from one page in the *Drill Book*.

A quotation by William James was presented as the rationale for using the drills.

> If we wish to conquer undesirable emotional tendencies in ourselves, we must assiduously, and in the first instance cold-bloodedly, go through the outward movements of those contrary dispositions which we prefer to cultivate.
>
> William James, from the
> *Principles of Psychology*

Drills were developed for all facets of an individual's life (Friedman & Ulmer, 1984; Powell & Thoresen, 1987).

Temperament Drills.

"Drive in the slow lane of the highway to reduce your urge to drive faster than anyone on the road."

"Leave your watch off."

"Do absolutely nothing but listen to music for 15 minutes."

"Find a long line in a supermarket and get at the end of it. As you wait and find yourself becoming restless, ask yourself why you find it so boring to be alone with yourself."

"Look at yourself in the mirror at midday and again when you first arrive home in the evening to see if your face exhibits irritation, aggravation, or anger."

Value Drills.

"Visit an art museum, a park, a zoo, or an aquarium."

"Eliminate 'how much' and 'how many' from your everyday vocabulary."

"Note carefully the various components making up a tree, a flower, a bird, a sunset, or a dawn."

"Seek beauty wherever and in whatever form you may find it."

"Become aware of the transcendental. Man cannot flourish if his entire world consists only of objects that he can see, hear, touch, taste, or smell."

"Daydream, meditate, read the classics."

Interpersonal Drills.

"Deliberately say to someone 'Maybe I'm wrong' at least twice today, even when you are not at all certain that you are in error."

"Say 'Good morning' in a pleasant, cheerful manner to each member of your family, and later to those you meet at your place of work."

"Surprise your spouse by taking her or him to the theater, a concert, the ballet, the movies, or a nice restaurant. As you go, keep in mind that you once thought of this person as your sweetheart."

"Invite someone to lunch and keep your friend talking about his/her interests—not yours."

Self-esteem Drills.

"Remind yourself every morning of the fact that life is by its very nature unfinished. . . ."

"What did I do right today and what happened that is worth remembering?"

"Recall positive memories for 10 minutes."

"Employ understanding, compassion, and forgiveness when dealing with others and self."

Physiological Drills.

"Interrupt long sessions of working with periods of relaxation. . . . Take a 5- or 10-minute break every hour during work sessions. Stretch out, or daydream, or talk with an associate."

"During an entire workday, practice moving your entire arm, not just your fingers, when writing. This maneuver tends to lead to muscular relaxation."

In the group meetings, participants reported how often that they had used the drills, and they shared their experience of practicing the drills. The daily practice of drills was viewed by many participants and group leaders as a major factor in helping participants change Type A behaviors.

Skills

Skills training was the core of the program, including relaxation, cognitive, behavioral, and social skills. Participants learned and practiced many relaxation skills. The weekly group sessions began with the practice of relaxation—progressive relaxation, autogenic training, guided imagery, the quieting response, or temperature biofeedback using a temperature-sensitive "dot" that sticks to the skin, a device that many patients found very helpful (Powell & Thoresen, 1987). Participants were taught to identify irrational thought patterns, confront rationalizations, and develop rational thinking.

Participants also learned to recognize situations that elicit Type A behaviors, called "hooks."

Suddenly, a hook drops before us with attractive bait and we make the decision to bite (get angry, irritated, annoyed) or to let the hook float by. Whatever is done with any particular hook is relatively unimportant because inevitably another one will follow and we must again make the choice about taking the bait. Perhaps as many as 30 hooks drop in front of us each day. Sometimes they come close together; other times they are spaced widely apart. What is important is to consider the actual number of hooks we swallow as we go through each and every day, how many we have remaining in our mouths when we go to sleep, and how many we have ignored or taken but then successfully spit out.

(Powell & Thoresen, 1987, pp. 183–184)

Many Type A people are poor listeners and poor communicators. In group sessions, participants learned to listen, and through assertiveness training participants learned to communicate rationally without becoming hostile or angry. Role-playing was used to ensure acquisition and transfer of skills from the counseling sessions to everyday life.

Dreams

Participants were urged to keep a record of their dreams and to share them in the group sessions. The purpose was to teach participants to use dreams as feedback about stressors and coping with stressors. Participants soon learned to understand dream symbols as messages about daily life. A busy lawyer had several nightmares of being back in law school cramming for exams only to discover that the classrooms had vanished; this was followed by chasing a train and carrying a briefcase with a broken handle. The lawyer became aware that the frustration dreams represented the frustrations in his life, of not being able to accomplish all of his goals. Frustration dreams were common for many participants. The use of dreams as a source of information was undoubtedly a novel experience for Type A people, who are focused outwardly rather than inwardly. This element in the program may have facilitated the shift to greater self-awareness.

Modeling, Caring, and Social Support

Careful attention was paid to selecting group counselors who could model the skills and behaviors that the participants were learning. The most important characteristic of a leader was ability to care. "Perhaps more than any other thing a leader can do for these patients is to provide them with what many did not adequately secure in childhood—unconditional love and affection from a respected parent figure. . . . This caring and competent leader must at times be tough on certain patients. But if the tough approach is blended with respect and genuine caring, growth can emerge" (Powell & Thoresen, 1987, p. 202). The entire Recurrent Coronary Prevention Project staff were caring, supportive people who created a sense of community. The quality of this caring community was vividly seen in the field director, Diane Ulmer. Friedman writes:

> Diane Ulmer became a sort of surrogate mother to hundreds of our male participants. Possibly the fact that she was the first person to interview and examine them for the study had something to do with it; in any case, they quickly sensed both her professional competence and her feminine gentleness—stiffened as it was with just a hint of maternal discipline—and adopted her as their own. She of course did just the same in reverse—she still knows both the surname and the given name of each and every one of our participants.
>
> While we had been aware of the importance of inadequate maternal love and affection in the formation of Type A behavior in men, we did not realize until we were well along in the study that such deprivation could be to some degree compensated for in adult life. Diane Ulmer was able to do this. Presumably someone else as warm and dedicated could do the same. We must note in passing, however, that the wives of our male participants were rarely able to fill the role, one reason being that many of them were themselves Type A, and thus busy searching for (and not finding) the unconditional parental love missing in their own childhoods.
>
> (Friedman & Ulmer, 1984, pp. 128–129)

"There is no learning to live without learning to love."
John Powell S.J., cited in
Friedman and Ulmer (1984, p. 293)

The Recurrent Coronary Prevention Project's multicomponent program integrated the major dynamics of health and wellness into a format that helped Type A individuals replace Type A behaviors with Type B behaviors. Many of the resources and tools for stress resistance discussed in Chapters 6 through 10 were incorporated: relaxation, social support, love, biofeedback training, self-monitoring, cognitive restructuring, and the use of imagery in dreams.

The effectiveness of the program was assessed with results of a second structured interview, reports from friends and group leaders, and self-reports. The majority of the participants were able to significantly modify Type A behavior in comparison to the no-treatment control and cardiac counseling groups (p < .001). The project demonstrated that a persistent and pervasive personality pattern can be significantly altered and that a new healthy behavior pattern developed. In addition, the project demonstrated that coronary heart disease is reduced when Type A behavior is reduced. Figure 17.1 shows the difference between the cardiac counseling group and the behavioral counseling group in recurrence rate of heart attack. At the end of 4.5 years, participants in the behavioral counseling groups had a 45 percent lower recurrence of myocardial infarction than the cardiac counseling group.

In comparisons to studies using aspirin, medications, or surgery to reduce recurrence of myocardial infarction, the behavioral

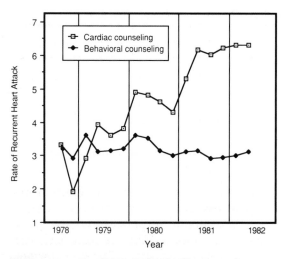

Figure 17.1. Participants in the Recurrent Coronary Prevention Project Who Received Behavioral Counseling Had a Lower Rate of Second Attack than Patients Who Received Cardiac Counseling Only. Rate Was Calculated Every Three Months. From Friedman et al., (1986). Alteration of Type A Behavior and Its Effect on Cardiac Recurrences in Post Myocardial Infarction Patients: Summary Result of the Recurrent Coronary Prevention Project. *American Heart Journal, 112,* **653–675. Reprinted by Permission of C.V. Mosby Company.**

counseling treatment subjects had a 40 percent lower recurrence (Friedman, Thoresen, et al., 1986). On a smaller scale, more than 15 other studies have replicated the findings of the Recurrent Coronary Prevention Project; these studies are summarized by Levenkron and Moore (1988).

The "hidden" results of the Recurrent Coronary Prevention Project are perhaps the most impressive, from the standpoint of personality change, and are the basis for overt behavior change and reduced risk of second myocardial infarction, namely the "enhancement of the quality of the person's familial and vocational relationships" (Friedman, Thoresen, et al., 1986, p. 664). This enhancement in the quality of life of the Type A participant resulted from a significant modification of the Type A pattern,

in the five areas in which Type A characteristics are manifested.

1. Value: Participants become less preoccupied with acquisition of possessions and money and developed interests in art, music, theater, religion, and relationships.
2. Self-esteem: One of the most significant changes for participants was the development of a greater sense of self-worth. The unconditional love received by the participants from the group leaders, the project director, and eventually from other group members, boosted the feelings of self-worth and feelings of security (Powell & Thoresen, 1987).
3. Temperament: Participants learned to slow their pace of life and became more patient, less hassled, more cooperative, and more agreeable.
4. Interpersonal relationships: Participants learned to listen to and become more focused on other people; they learned how to express feelings and thoughts in rational, assertive ways, which resulted in improved relationships with family and colleagues (Friedman, Thoresen, et al., 1986).
5. Physiology: Through daily relaxation and slowing the pace of life, participants lowered physiological arousal levels, with a significant reduction in the severity of coronary disease and the risk of a second myocardial infarction. Table 17.2 outlines the positive shifts from Type A behavior to healthy behaviors.

IIII➡

CONCLUSION

To health professionals, the history of research on Type A behavior is an adventure. Two physicians ventured into an area unexplored

Table 17.2   Modification of Type A Behaviors to Healthy Behaviors

	Type A Characteristics	Modification of Type A
Values	Number consciousness	Transcendental (beauty, love, spiritual)
Self-esteem	Low, chronic insecurity	Self-acceptance, secure
Temperament	Hostile, impatient	Agreeable, patient
Interpersonal	Dominating, alienating	Empathic, assertive
Physiology	Hyperarousal	Relaxed

by medical science. They were open to new ideas even when the ideas came from "unlikely" sources—a furniture upholsterer and the president of the Junior League of San Francisco. They risked the disapproval and silence of their colleagues to develop and test a new hypothesis about the cause of coronary heart disease. For more than 30 years, Friedman and Rosenman have persisted in their research effort to understand the causes, mechanisms, and patterns of Type A behavior and coronary heart disease. They established a reliable and valid procedure for assessing Type A behavior, the structured interview. They conducted prospective studies to demonstrate the association of Type A behavior and coronary heart disease. In addition, Friedman and colleagues created a model program for reducing Type A behavior and the risk of recurrent myocardial infarction.

The relationship between Type A personality and coronary heart disease is a clear example of mind $\longrightarrow$ body because it demonstrates that thoughts, attitudes, feelings, and behaviors can alter the cardiovascular system. We have come a long way from the germ theory of disease and the belief that the role of the mind is irrelevant to a scientific study of health and sickness. Today, physicians, epidemiologists, psychologists, and the general public are aware of the Type A personality pattern and its link to coronary heart disease. Prevention programs in industry and business include Type A inventories, and clinicians in private practice assess the Type A

characteristics of their clients. Books and articles on stress and stress management usually include a section on Type A behavior, a questionnaire for assessing Type A characteristics, and suggestions for changing Type A behavior. Clearly, Type A behavior has taken a place with other factors as a demonstrable and treatable risk for heart disease.

Over the years, the work of Friedman and Rosenman and their colleagues supported the broadest implication of Type A research: that stress, in this case stress sustained by pervasive personality characteristics, plays a significant role in the development of disease and illness. At the same time, research on Type B behavior provides significant insights into the healthy personality. The recent work of Friedman and colleagues on modifying Type A behavior answers the question, "Can personality be changed?" To theorists who argue that personality cannot be changed, we refer to the hundreds of people in the Recurrent Coronary Prevention Project who changed a long-standing personality pattern, Type A behavior.

Clinicians and researchers already studying the relationship of personality and illness, particularly in cancer, were encouraged by the Type A research. In Chapter 18 we describe the research on personality and cancer, which, with Type A research, forms a solid basis for understanding the importance of personality in disease etiology, and consequently, in the dynamics of health and wellness.

CHAPTER *18*

Personality and Cancer

IIII➡

The day he received his diagnosis, Jerry resigned from life, he quit his job and, after taking care of his financial affairs, he settled in front of the television set, staring blankly hour after hour. Within twenty-four hours he was experiencing severe pain and lack of energy.

No one was able to get him interested in much of anything. He did remember that he had always wanted to make some bar stools for the house, so for a week or two he worked in his shop, with some signs of increased energy and reduced pain. But as soon as the bar stools were completed, he returned to the TV. His wife reported that he did not really watch it as much as he watched the clock, for fear that he would miss the time for taking his pain medication. Jerry showed no signs of response to radiation therapy, and within three months he was dead.

Bill was also diagnosed with cancer of the lung, which had spread to his brain. The prognosis for his survival and the treatment were nearly identical to Jerry's. But Bill's response to the diagnosis was very different. For one thing, he took the illness as a time to review the priorities of his life. As a traveling sales manager he had been constantly on the go and, he said, had "never taken time to see the trees." Although he continued working, he rearranged his schedule so that he could take more time to do things that were enjoyable to him.

At our clinic, he participated actively in the therapy group and regularly used a mental imagery process he had learned there. He responded favorably to radiation therapy and became virtually symptom-free. All the while he remained active. Approximately a year and a half after Bill left our program, he experienced several major emotional blows and, within a short time, he suffered a recurrence and died shortly thereafter.

(Simonton, Matthews-Simonton & Creighton, 1978, pp. 15–16)

Probably every physician and healer has wondered why some people succumb to disease rapidly while others with the same diagnosis and prognosis do not. In the fields of cancer research and treatment, the focus on personality variables as a factor in this puzzle has been certainly interesting, although not conclusive. Some patients give up psychologically, while others do not. Does this account for the difference in outcomes? And who gets cancer in the first place; do certain personality characteristics predispose a person to cancer? And why do people such as Bill recover, only to regress during a crisis? If personality characteristics do play a role in the development and progression or regression of cancer, can these characteristics be changed? If so, will the risk of cancer or the progression of cancer decrease? These issues are the subject of this chapter.

In Chapter 1 we described the case of Mr. Wright, the cancer patient whose beliefs and expectations strongly affected the regression and progression of his tumors. In Chapter 2, we described several examples of mind ⟶ body. In Chapter 4, the effects of stress on the immune system were described, and in Chapter 6, we discussed social support as a buffer against these effects. In the previous chapter, on Type A behavior, the relationship between personality characteristics and coronary heart disease was described. In this chapter we explore the link between personality and immune system functioning, focusing on cancer. Although the case of Mr. Wright is definitely unusual, there is increasing evidence that personality characteristics affect diseases of immune system dysfunction such as cancer.

You might say, "Mr. Wright's case seems so unusual. It is hard to believe that it happened. Even though nurses and doctors witnessed the progression and regression of Mr. Wright's tumors, it is still hard to believe. How could the mind have that much influence on cancer?" This question is not yet answered, but there are several approaches through which the answer is being pursued.

In Section One we describe research on personality and cancer. We begin with the **early retrospective studies**. These studies were conducted primarily by clinicians who were intrigued by the observation that cancer patients seem to have certain personality traits in common. We then look at the **prospective longitudinal studies** in which subjects take a set of personality tests, and their responses are correlated with health status many years later. In Section Two we examine studies that correlate personality characteristics and the progression of cancer, and we present data on the immune system mechanisms that may be the links between mind and disease.

While the data supporting the concept of the cancer-prone personality are suggestive and have led to the hypothesis, or "construct," of the Type C personality (Temoshok & Heller, 1981), they are by no means conclusive; as with Type A research, difficulties abound.

The characteristics of cancer survivors and the work and observations of health professionals who help patients become cancer survivors are the topics of Section Three. The growing use of nonmedical interventions with cancer patients, such as psychotherapeutic techniques, visualization, relaxation training, diet, and support groups, provides increasing evidence of the ability of patients to change the course of cancer, perhaps by overcoming personality traits that suppress immune functioning and by adopting behaviors and attitudes that enhance the immune system.

Intervention studies are not common, but the increasing use of interventions in clinical

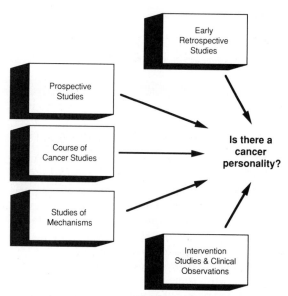

Figure 18.1. Sources of Information for Investigating the Link Between Personality and Disease.

practice provides information on the relationship of personality variables and outcome of cancer. The study of cancer survivors yields invaluable insight into the dynamics of health and wellness and provides a roadmap for helping all cancer patients.

Like heart disease, cancer is undoubtedly multicausal, meaning that many factors contribute to the development of cancer. The biopsychosocial approach to the study of cancer and to the treatment of cancer is appropriate. In this chapter, we look primarily at psychological factors, but we emphasize the fact that if psychological factors do play a role in cancer, these factors interact with other variables. Figure 18.1 summarizes our sources of information.

The material in this chapter underscores the importance of the biopsychosocial model of cancer and of multicomponent treatment, which brings together conventional medical treatment with lifestyle change, stress management, personality change, and change in a person's social environment.

||||➡

SECTION ONE: PSYCHOSOCIAL PRECURSORS OF CANCER

In this section, we examine research on psychological factors that may predispose a person to cancer, with this question in mind "Do cancer patients have particular personality traits that distinguish them from other patients?" Knowledge of the psychological factors in the development of cancer is a step toward prevention and successful treatment.

Early Retrospective Studies on Personality and Cancer

For centuries physicians have noted a relationship between emotions and cancer. In 1759, an English physician described women who were prone to cancer as "sedentary, melancholic disposition of mind, who meet with such disasters in life as occasion much trouble and grief" (cited in Stolbach & Brandt, 1988). Melancholia and depression were the first characteristics that seemed to distinguish cancer patients from other patients.

Depression and Hopelessness

In the late 1800s, Herbert Snow, a London physician, noticed that cancer patients differed from other patients and healthy people. Snow studied 250 women with mammary and uterine cancers at the London Cancer Hospital. He found that before the development of the cancer, 156 patients experienced the death of a parent or relative and responded with depression.

> "The number of instances in which malignant disease of the breast and uterus follows immediately antecedent emotion of a depressing character is too large to be set down to chance, or to the general liability to the buffets of ill fortune which the cancer patients, in their passage through life, share with most other people not so afflicted."

(Snow, 1883, cited in Simonton, Matthews-Simonton, & Creighton, 1978)

The pattern of significant loss, followed by hopelessness and depression, was observed by other clinicians. In 1926, Dr. Elida Evans interviewed 100 cancer patients and found that many of the patients had lost an important relationship before the onset of the disease. The typical response to the loss was a "giving up" on life, a hopelessness. (Evans, 1926, cited in Simonton, et al., 1978). Please read Box 18.1 now.

Several other studies investigated depression as a precursor of cancer (Renneker, Cutler, Hora, Bacon, Bradley, Kearney, & Cutler, 1963; Giovacchini & Muslin, 1956: LeShan, 1966, Bahnson, 1969a). Schmale and Iker (1966) found that women with cancer of the cervix differed little from non-cancer control subjects in the incidence of recent stressful experiences, but the cancer patients were significantly more likely to report feelings of hopelessness as a reaction to their stressors. Miller and Jones (1948) studied six patients with chronic myelocytic leukemia who showed "marked emotional stress" before leukemia was diagnosed. The authors speculated that the frequent occurrence of emotional difficulties in patients with leukemia may be more than coincidental. Over a period of 15 years, Greene and Miller (1958) observed that cancer was frequently preceded by personal losses to which the patient responded with hopelessness and despair.

Suppression of Emotions

In the late 1950's, Lawrence LeShan, a clinical psychologist, and Richard Worthington, a research psychologist, gave the Worthington Personal History Test to 540 hospitalized cancer patients (LeShan, 1977). A control group of 12,000 healthy subjects also took the test. LeShan and Worthington were surprised to

---

LEARNED HELPLESSNESS

Martin Seligman, a pioneer in the study of depression and learned helplessness, is currently studying the relationship between learned helplessness and disease (Peterson & Seligman, 1987). In his early research, Seligman showed that depression results from an experience in which a person learns that effort to change a situation has little effect on the outcome of the situation (Seligman, 1975). Faced with stressful situations, a person with this history may not try to surmount the difficulties, and may become helpless, passive, and depressed. When this reaction to stressors becomes habitual, learned helplessness can be thought of as a personality trait.

After 104 experiments involving nearly 15,000 subjects, Seligman is convinced that the core of the helplessness pattern is a "pessimistic explanatory style." Events that are ambiguous are always interpreted negatively, such as "This problem will last forever," "It's going to ruin everything," "It's all my fault," and "There is nothing I can do about it."

Working with the data of George Vaillant (1977), a psychiatrist who is following the health status of members of the Harvard classes of 1939–1944, Seligman is examining the relationship between explanatory style and physical health. Although the results are preliminary, the data indicate that a person's explanatory style is a reliable predictor of physical health 25 to 30 years later. At the University of Michigan, Seligman's colleague, Christopher Peterson, recorded the explanatory style of 172 undergraduates. One year later, he found a strong positive correlation between helpless explanatory style and the number of visits to the student health center (Peterson & Seligman, 1987).

---

find that the cancer patients had a distinctive profile. Cancer patients had a history of loneliness and failure to establish satisfying relationships. Intrigued by these results, LeShan studied 250 cancer patients in greater depth, with a control group of 125 healthy subjects. Subjects in both groups took a variety of personality tests and were given a thorough interview lasting two to eight hours. The clinical interview included these questions:

1. When sad or depressed, do you always put on a brave front and keep your feelings to yourself?

2. Are you doing what you want to do with your life?

3. Are your relationships with others deeply satisfying?

4. If you were told that you had six months to live, would you continue the same work and activities that you have now?

5. If you should lose your job, your child or your spouse, would you feel you had no reason to go on living?

6. Do you frequently feel worthless and unlovable?

7. Are you plagued by secret dreams and ambitions that you never expect to realize?

8. If you learned you had a fatal disease, might you feel a surprising sense of relief as well as fear?

The results were striking. Seventy-two percent of the cancer patients had a particular personality and life history pattern that occurred in only 10 percent of the control subjects. This pattern was:

1. Feeling rejected and unloved from an early age, the individual continually tried to please others as a way of ensuring love.

2. Fearful of losing friends, the individual almost never expressed feelings of anger, loneliness, hopelessness, and negative beliefs about themselves.

3. Although feeling hurt, frustrated, and angry, the individual was considerate, sweet, gentle, and uncomplaining.

4. The cancer appeared only after stressful life events, to which these individuals responded with rage, grief, and hopelessness but did not express these feelings openly.

According to LeShan, the core of the cancer personality pattern is reflected in the following statement by a cancer patient. "Last time I hoped, and look what happened. As soon as my defenses were down, of course I was left alone again. I'll never hope again. It's too much. It's better to stay in a shell" (LeShan, 1977).

Suppression of feelings as the primary characteristic of cancer patients was also found by psychologist Claus Bahnson of Jefferson Medical College in Philadelphia. After interviewing 400 cancer patients, he concluded that cancer patients tend to be "emotion suppressors." "They seemed to be out of touch with their own wants and needs, choosing to affect a permanent pleasant attitude and personality regardless of the bleakness of their inner lives" (Bahnson, 1969).

The most exemplary early studies were conducted by a psychologist and a chest physician, who combined resources to study the causes of lung cancer. D. M. Kissen, a lung specialist, was intrigued by the relationship between smoking and lung cancer. He observed that there is no direct relationship between the number of cigarettes a person smokes and lung cancer. Light smokers may develop lung cancer and heavy smokers may not. Furthermore, nonsmokers develop lung cancer. Kissen wondered whether nonsmokers and light smokers who develop cancer have certain common personality characteristics that make them susceptible to lung cancer, while heavy smokers who do not develop lung cancer are in some way protected by their personality.

To answer these questions, Kissen enlisted the help of Hans Eysenck, the British psychologist who developed the Eysenck Personality Inventory, which measures introversion and extroversion. Kissen and Eysenck conducted a series of controlled studies in which they examined the personality characteristics of cancer patients who were light smokers, heavy smokers, and nonsmokers, and compared the cancer patients to a control group of 123 healthy smokers and nonsmokers. Kissen and Eysenck used a variety of standardized personality tests and personal interviews. They ranked the lung cancer patients on the basis of lung tissue exposure to smoke. (The medium smoker/inhaler has greater exposure than heavy smoker/non-inhaler, and nonsmokers have the least exposure).

The results were clear. Lung cancer was associated with poor "emotional discharge," that is, the inability to appropriately express emotions, especially emotions that would create conflict. This was true regardless of smoking habit. Furthermore, the researchers found that the poorer the ability to express emotions, the less smoke was needed to produce lung cancer. Kissen was so intrigued by these results that over the next eight years he and his co-workers replicated this study several times (1963, 1964, 1967, 1969).

Critique of the Early Studies

This section began with the question "Do cancer patients have personality traits that are different from other people?" The investigations of Bahnson, Kissen, and LeShan indicate that cancer patients have a profile that distinguishes them from healthy people and from patients with other types of disease. These studies however, were retrospective; the subjects had cancer at the time of the study, and the attempt was to determine personality factors that predated the cancer. Retrospective cancer research is problematical because having cancer could cause a person to feel depressed; the depressive traits might not have predated the cancer diagnosis and might not have played a role in the development of cancer. Hospitalization, fear, chemotherapy with its side effects (nausea and hair loss) and the threat of death could lead to depression. Depression could bias the person's self-report of current feelings and bias memories of early life. Having cancer could cause the person to appear to have a depressive personality, while in fact, the depressive responses were merely the result of having cancer. Although LeShan attempted to overcome these difficulties, the relationship between personality and cancer is more accurately determined through prospective studies.

Prospective Studies

The best way to determine the relationship of personality and disease is to determine the personality characteristics of people before they become sick. This approach is prospective, as noted in the description of Type A research. A prospective study surveys the personality characteristics of a large group of healthy people; after many years, the health status of the subjects is determined and correlated with the personality characteristics measured years earlier.

Johns Hopkins Study—Loners and the Inability to Express Emotions

The longest prospective study to date is being conducted by Carolyn Thomas and her colleagues at Johns Hopkins Medical School (Thomas, Dusynski, & Shaffer, 1979; Shaffer, Graves, Swank, & Pearson, 1987). In 1948, Thomas gave a battery of psychological questionnaires, including the Rorschach, to 1,337 male students entering medical school and has followed their health status for over 30 years. By 1978, 200 subjects had cancer, benign tumors, coronary heart disease, high blood pressure, or mental illness. The 1948 psychological tests revealed that the students who developed cancer had a distinctive personality profile and were different from other groups on three measures: a lack of closeness to parents, a lack of emotional expression, and a lack of intimacy. They were "loners." An analysis of the data by Shaffer and colleagues found that the loners were 16 times as likely to develop cancer as people who acted out and expressed their emotions (Shaffer, et al., 1987).

The Alameda Study—Social Isolation

Similar results were found in the Alameda study. As you may remember from Chapter 6, in 1965, 6,928 residents of Alameda County responded to an extensive questionnaire on personal health practices, psychosocial variables (focusing on social support), and demographic characteristics. Mortality data for this sample population were collected in 1974. In a re-analysis of the data, Reynolds and Kaplan (1986) found that cancer deaths were most frequent among women who felt socially isolated. Please read Box 18.2 now.

BOX 18.2

LONELINESS AND HEALTH

Loneliness is one of the most stressful experiences in life, and yet a national survey in 1985 revealed that almost one-fourth of the population, 50 million people, feels extremely lonely at some time during any month (Meer, 1985).

Loneliness can be a risk to health. Lonely people are more susceptible to colds, sore throats, flu, and mononucleosis. A two-year study of people over age 65 observed that lonely people were four times more likely to die early than the least lonely people (Russell & Cutrona, 1985).

Who are the loneliest people in our society? Senior citizens? Surprisingly, older people are the least lonely of all age groups. In a survey of 25,000 people on the East Coast, conducted by a New York University team, the most lonely group is between ages 18–25, while the least lonely are age 70. In a University of California, Los Angeles, study (Cutrona, 1982), more than 75 percent of all undergraduates thought loneliness was a major problem. However, more senior citizens live alone and see their friends less often than young adults. What accounts for the age difference in loneliness?

The loneliness of young adults is explained partly by their many transitions: moving away from home, going to college, leaving good friends behind, venturing into new social worlds. Philip Shaver and his colleagues at the University of Denver (1985) studied 400 college students. The majority reported that going to college was the most difficult transition that they had ever experienced, due primarily to the loss of friendships and love affairs. When the freshman year was completed, half of the precollege romances had ended. Students reported that when a precollege romance did survive the first year of college, the relationship was less satisfying.

Personality factors are a second cause of loneliness among young people. Warren Jones (1982) and his colleagues at the University of Tulsa videotaped lonely college students meeting a new person. Students high in loneliness were matched with "not lonely" students. Compared to the "not lonely" students, lonely students asked fewer questions of their partner, talked more about themselves, arbitrarily changed the topic of conversation more often, made more negative evaluations of their partner, were less accurate in describing the partner's personality, and liked their partner less. In another study of college students, Solano, Batten, and Parish (1982) found that lonely students disclose less intimate information about themselves to others and are perceived by others as "difficult to get to know." These studies portray lonely people as insensitive in new social situations, self-focused, unresponsive, and lacking in social skills, all of which may be the result of, and contribute to, loneliness.

A third cause of loneliness is the widely held belief among young people that "love solves all social problems." People who believe this neglect friendships at work or school and put all their energy into "falling in love." Cutrona's study (1982) of college freshmen at UCLA found that students who overcame loneliness made many friends. Those who remained lonely said that they were still seeking a boyfriend of girlfriend as the solution to their problem.

Another cause of loneliness is low self-esteem (Peplau & Goldston, 1984). Chronically lonely people feel uninteresting, unattractive, and unlovable. Psychiatrist David Burns (1985) describes his first 26 years of life: "From the time I was a child, I felt ugly and awkward. . . . I was rarely invited to parties. . . . In high school, people respected me for my seriousness and intelligence—but I was lonely and didn't feel close to very many people" (pp. 17–18). Low self-esteem can lead to a vicious cycle of loneliness. The lonely person needs to reach out and make contact with people but, feeling inadequate, does not; this leads to greater feelings of loneliness and inadequacy.

Researchers at New York University are pessimistic about the ability of people to overcome loneliness. They believe that many social forces cause loneliness and that these forces are difficult to change. In the NYU study, recently divorced people and young singles were the most lonely. Researchers and students on the "sunny" West Coast are much more optimistic; they believe that loneliness can be overcome if a person tries hard enough.

Are researchers on the East Coast right or are researchers on the West Coast right? If loneliness is a result of external situations, can people overcome loneliness? If personal expectations and attitudes cause loneliness, can people overcome it? Perhaps the best answer is the pragmatic one—the optimistic answer. Loneliness can be overcome or reduced by developing social skills and satisfying friendships. Even when loneliness is due to factors such as the loss of a lover or a parent, or not finding someone special, people can overcome loneliness. Warren Jones (1982) at the University of Tulsa teaches students the interpersonal skills that are necessary for developing friendships by counteracting the habits of lonely people noted above. Many counseling centers in colleges and universities offer programs to help students develop social skills.

Western Electric Company Study—Depression

Shekelle and his colleagues at the University of Chicago studied the health of 2,000 male industrial employees at Western Electric Company over a 17-year period (Persky, Kempthorne-Rawson, & Shekelle, 1987; Shekelle, Raynor, Ostfeld, Garron, Bieliauskas, Liu, Maliza, & Ogelsby, 1981). The employees who died of cancer were twice as likely to have had depressive character traits, measured 17 years earlier with the Minnesota Multiphasic Personality Inventory. The increased cancer risk could not be explained by smoking or drinking habits of the depressed men (Shekelle, et al., 1981).

Interestingly, the Alameda study did not find a relationship between depression and cancer (Kaplan & Reynolds, 1987). How can these conflicting results be explained? One

answer is that the studies used different measures of depression and perhaps different definitions of depression. The Alameda study used 18 items to determine depression, and the Chicago study used the 60 items on the depression scale of the MMPI. Perhaps the MMPI measures factors other than depression that may predict cancer, such as a lack of social support or an inability to express emotions. The Alameda study found a significant correlation between unhappiness and certain types of cancers. Women who were unhappy were more likely to develop cancer and die of it than women who were happy (Reynolds & Kaplan, 1987). Are unhappiness and depression different? Perhaps the results of these studies are not conflicting; perhaps they just reflect a difference in use of terms and measurements.

The Crvenka Study—Rationality and Anti-Emotionality

In 1965, Grossarth-Matticek, Bastiaans, and Kanazir (1985) began a prospective study with residents of Crvenka, a small industrial town of 74,000 residents in Yugoslavia. A total of 1,353 townspeople completed a psychosocial questionnaire and assessment of smoking habits. Smoking was a variable in this study because the project was funded by the Reynolds Tobacco Company, which was interested in smoking habits and disease. Ten years later, Grossarth-Matticek returned to Crvenka to examine the health histories of the study participants. Responses on a single scale of the questionnaire predicted the incidence of cancer over the 10-year period with 93 percent accuracy. Because the results of the study were highly significant, and therefore controversial, we examine it in detail.

Subjects. The subjects, 965 men and 388 women, were selected for the study either because they were elderly or because preliminary questioning indicated that the person was at risk for disease, indicated by chronic helplessness or anger. In other words, subjects were selected who might be expected to develop disease or die within the period of the study. As morbid as this sounds, this sampling technique was used because in order to study the relationship between a variable and disease, disease must be likely. Subjects were physically healthy at the time of selection. Health status at the 10-year follow-up was determined by subject reports, reports from friends and relatives, and medical records.

Method. A 109-item psychosocial questionnaire was used that measured eight psychosocial risk factors from which risk scores were calculated, based on the number of responses in each factor category. The eight categories were: (1) adverse life events or situation leading to long-lasting helplessness; (2) anger;

(3) rationality/anti-emotionality; (4) need for harmonious interpersonal relationships; (5) ignoring signs of illness; (6) lack of positive emotional relevance; (7) absence of self-reported psychopathological symptoms, especially anxiety; and (8) acquiescence, that is, the tendency to give a positive answer regardless of the content of the question. Information on smoking included total number of years up to 1965, average number of cigarettes smoked daily for five years before 1965, whether or not the subject inhaled the smoke, and whether or not the cigarette had a filter.

In 1976, Grossarth-Matticek returned to Crvenka to determine the health status of the participants. One hundred sixty-six people had died of cancer. Upon analyzing the data from the psychosocial questionnaire, Grossarth-Matticek found that the rationality/anti-emotionality scale with a total of 11 items had the highest predictive value. Amazingly, 158 of the 166 cancer deaths, and all 38 of the lung cancer deaths, occurred in people who scored 10 or 11 out of the total 11 points on the rationality/anti-emotionality scale (Box 18.3). The cancer incidence was 40 times higher for people who answered positively on 10 or 11 of the questions than for people who answered positively on only three or fewer questions.

The authors of the Crvenka study claim that they have identified a risk factor for cancer death that is independent of other risk factors. Because it is extraordinary that an 11-item personality scale could predict 158 of 166 deaths, these data are being re-analyzed by an independent team.

Rationality and anti-emotionality seem like odd traits to be so predictive of cancer, but if we look deeper, we see a reflection of Kissen's findings and the Johns Hopkins study, the suppression of feelings. People who score high on the rationality/anti-emotionality scale seem to have adopted a purely rational stance in life, at the expense of feelings.

To explore further the relationship between

BOX 18.3

RATIONALITY/
ANTI-EMOTIONALITY SCALE

1. Do you always try to do what is reasonable and logical?
2. Do you always try to understand people and their behavior, so that you seldom respond emotionally?
3. Do you try to act rationally in all interpersonal situations?
4. Do you try to overcome all interpersonal conflicts by intelligence and reason, trying hard not to show any emotional response?
5. If someone deeply hurts your feelings, do you nevertheless try to treat him rationally and to understand his way of behaving (so that you hardly ever attack and deprecate him or treat him purely emotionally)?
6. Do you succeed in avoiding most interpersonal conflicts by relying on your reason and logic (often contrary to your feelings)?

7. If someone acts against your needs and desires, do you nevertheless try to understand him?
8. Do you behave in almost all life situations so rationally that only rarely is your behavior influenced by emotions only?
9. Is your behavior frequently influenced by emotions to such a degree that from a purely rational point of view it would have to be regarded as nonsensical or detrimental?
10. Do you try to understand others even if you do not like them?
11. Does your rationality prevent you from attacking others, even if there are sufficient reasons for doing so?

Reprinted with permission from *Journal of Psychosomatic Research, 29* Grossarth-Matticek, Bastiaans, and Kanazir, "Psychosocial factors as strong predictors of mortality from cancer, ischaemic heart disease and stroke: The Yugoslav prospective study." Copyright 1985, Pergamon Press PLC.

personality and cancer, Grossarth-Matticek and colleagues conducted at 10-year prospective study with 100 subjects who were at high risk for cancer, based on the rationality/anti-emotionality scale (Grossarth-Matticek, Eysenck, Vetter, & Frentzel-Beyme, 1986, cited in Eysenck, 1987, 1988). It was hypothesized that modification of the rationality/anti-emotionality trait would reduce the risk of cancer. In an intervention study of this type, when changes in one variable, such as rationality/anti-emotionality, affect a second variable, such as incidence of cancer, then the causal link between the two variables is more firmly

established. If the hypothesis were correct, this study would further substantiate the relationship between cancer and rationality and anti-emotionality. Subjects were assigned to either a no-treatment control group (N = 50) or a treatment group (N = 50). The treatment group subjects were taught a variety of behavioral techniques for expressing emotions, thus overcoming the tendency to respond to events with rationality, while suppressing emotions. The results were highly significant—no subjects in the treatment group contracted cancer in 10 years, while 16 subjects in the control group died of cancer.

Grossarth-Matticek and colleagues also conducted an intervention study to determine the effect of cognitive-behavioral therapy on survival (Grossarth-Maticek, Kanazir, Vetter, & Jankovic, 1983, cited in Eysenck, 1987, 1988). Seventy-five women with breast cancer were assigned to one of the three groups: chemotherapy, cognitive-behavior therapy, or cognitive-behavior therapy and chemotherapy; the survival time of 25 women who received no treatment was used for comparison. Women who received no treatment survived an average of 11.28 months, women in the chemotherapy group survived an average of 14 months, women in the cognitive-behavior group survived an average of 15 months, and women in the chemotherapy and cognitive-behavioral combined group survived an average of 22.5 months. The combination of chemotherapy and cognitive-behavioral therapy was twice as effective as no treatment at all, and 1.5 times as effective as chemotherapy or cognitive-behavioral therapy alone. The Grossarth-Matticek studies have identified lack of emotional expression as a precursor of cancer. This variable is also implicated in the progression of cancer. The retrospective

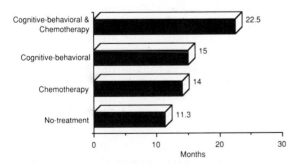

Figure 18.2. Comparison of Three Treatments and No-Treatment on the Survival Time of Cancer Patients. Adapted with Permission from Eysenck, H.J. (1987). Anxiety, Learned Helplessness, and Cancer: A Causal Theory. *Journal of Anxiety Disorders, 1*, **p. 95. Adapted with Permission from the Author and Publisher, Pergamon Press.**

and prospective studies attempted to identify personality characteristics that predispose a person to cancer. In the next section we describe studies that attempt to identify personality characteristics that affect the course of cancer.

SECTION TWO: PERSONALITY FACTORS THAT INFLUENCE THE COURSE OF CANCER

In 1959, the president of the American Cancer Society, Eugene P. Pendergrass, concluded his presidential address in this way:

> Anyone who has had an extensive experience in the treatment of cancer is aware that there are great differences among patients. . . . I personally have observed cancer patients who have undergone unsuccessful treatment and were living and well for years. Then an emotional stress such as the death of a son in World War II, the infidelity of a daughter-in-law, or the burden of long unemployment seem to have been precipitating factors in the reactivation of their disease which resulted in death. . . . There is solid evidence that the course of disease in general is affected by emotional distress. . . . Thus, we as doctors may begin to emphasize treatment of the patient as a whole as well as the disease from which the patient is suffering. We may learn how to influence general body systems and through them modify the neoplasm which resides within the body. As we go forward . . . searching for new means of controlling growth both within the cell and through systemic influences, it is my sincere hope that we can widen the quest to include the distinct possibility that within one's mind is a power capable of exerting forces which can enhance or inhibit the progress of this disease.
>
> (Cited in *Getting Well Again*,
> Simonton, et al., 1978, pp. 26, 27).

Like Pendergrass, other clinicians have noted that patients with similar diagnosis and prognosis may have very dissimilar outcome of cancer, some succumbing immediately, some recovering completely. It was this observation that prompted Carl and Stephanie Simonton to pay closer attention to the beliefs and visualizations of their cancer patients (Box 18.5). And like Pendergrass, many health professionals, physicians and psychotherapists alike, are "widening the quest."

Bruno Klopfer, the psychologist who studied Mr. Wright's Rorschach (ink blot) test, widened the quest by correlating the progression of the disease and treatment outcome with the patient's personality characteristics as indicated on the Rorschach test.

Bruno Klopfer

Klopfer began his research by examining the Rorschach tests of six patients, three with fast-growing tumors and three with slow-growing tumors. Two physicians conducted the medical examinations to assess the growth rate of the tumors. Based on the patients' answers to the Rorschach test, Klopfer determined personality patterns that differentiated the patients with fast-growing tumors from the patients with slow-growing tumors. Following this initial success, Klopfer examined the Rorschach tests of 24 recently diagnosed tumor patients; he knew only their age and sex. Nine out of 11 individuals who developed fast-growing tumors, and 10 out of 12 individuals who developed slow-growing tumors, were accurately predicted. Klopfer was undecided about one patient, who turned out to be Mr. Wright. Please read Box 18.4 now.

Klopfer found that patients with fast-growing tumors were "loyal to reality" and invested energy in being good and loyal people. The patients with slow-growing tumors were not particularly invested in being good and loyal.

Blumberg and colleagues (1954) found similar results. In a study of 75 patients, they accurately identified the cancer growth rate of 75

BOX 18.4

THE PERSONALITY OF MR. WRIGHT

Did Mr. Wright's personality foster his mercurial cure and rapid death? Dr. Klopfer, who studied Mr. Wright's Rorschach test, described Mr. Wright as having a "floating ego" personality structure. Klopfer meant that Mr. Wright lacked an internal locus of control. Mr. Wright depended on external input and was susceptible to external influence; he lacked an internal base. His ego was "simply floating along." Mr. Wright uncritically accepted suggestions from his doctor and suggestions from the press about Krebiozen. Thus, when the AMA reported that Krebiozen was a "worthless" drug, Mr. Wright uncritically accepted this pronouncement, even though his own internal experience contradicted the AMA statement. Dr. Klopfer wrote, "To use a symbolic analogy, while he was floating along on the surface of the water under the influence of his optimistic auto-suggestions or suggestion, he was transformed into a heavy stone and sank to the bottom without any resistance at the moment when the powers of this suggestion expired."

Klopfer, 1957, p. 339

---

percent of the subjects based on Rorschach and MMPI results. Blumberg described the patients with fast-growing tumors as having a need to create a good impression of themselves, defensive, and denying a need for affection.

Greer, Morris, and Pettingale

Greer, Morris, and Pettingale (1979) have conducted rigorous research on personality and cancer for many years. The major study followed 69 women with breast cancer for five years after diagnosis. The patients' psychological reactions to the diagnosis were classified as stoic acceptance, denial, fighting spirit, and helpless/hopeless. The women with a fighting spirit or denial of the disease lived for at least five years following diagnosis. The women who responded with feelings of helplessness or stoic acceptance had recurrences and a shorter survival time.

A similar response pattern was observed by Simonton and Simonton (1976). In their study of 250 patients, the Simontons used a battery of personality tests including the MMPI. The patients who died within one year of diagnosis tended to be docile and obsequious. Please read Box 18.5 now.

Goodkin (1986) at Stanford University and Linda Temoshok (1985) at the University of California at San Francisco have results similar to those of Greer, Morris, and Pettingale, and

---

BOX 18.5

CARL SIMONTON AND STEPHANIE MATTHEWS-SIMONTON

In 1968 Carl Simonton, M.D., was a resident in oncology at the University of Oregon Medical School. He was puzzled by the fact that a few cancer patients behaved as if they did not want to live. These patients missed their appointments for treatment. They did not change habits closely linked to cancer; liver cancer patients continued to drink alcohol and lung cancer patients continued to smoke. Simonton observed that some cancer patients were more apathetic, depressed, and hopeless than other patients with terminal disease. Simonton searched the medical and psychological literature for explanations of these patterns. He was amazed to find considerable research and discussion of the relationship between personality and cancer. The research explained the patterns he observed in his patients and the patterns in his own life. Simonton had had cancer at the age of 17. From his own experience with the disease, he came to believe that cancer and personality might be related.

After his residency, Simonton and his wife, Stephanie, developed a cancer treatment package that includes conventional medical treatment and many visualization and relaxation techniques that help the patient develop the personality characteristics that seem to promote cancer regression and health. Their observations and program are described in their book, *Getting Well Again*.

The Simontons observed that people who respond to stress with chronic hopelessness and helplessness seem to be vulnerable to cancer. They also found that some patients appear to retard the progress of cancer by adopting positive attitudes and coping skills.

The creative, pioneering work of the Simontons stimulated cancer programs and research around the country. Today Carl Simonton continues the program at the Simonton Cancer Counseling Center in Pacific Palisades, California.

the Simontons. Goodkin and colleagues found that precancerous cells of the cervix were more likely to change from benign to malignant in women with pessimistic attitudes toward life than in optimistic women. In a series of studies of patients with malignant melanoma, a form of skin cancer, Temoshok and her colleagues attempted to relate psychosocial factors and aspects of cancer, such as severity at diagnosis, delay before seeking medical diagnosis, and measures of the body's resistance to the tumor. One study compared psychosocial variables of patients who died or had accelerated disease with patients who had no cancer development following surgery. Another study compared cancer patients with coronary heart disease patients on a task that compared self-reported reaction to anxiety-provoking statements. The studies showed fairly consistent psychosocial factors, a tendency to be emotionally unexpressive and to repress feelings. The expression of emotions, such as sadness and anger, appeared to be beneficial.

Lack of emotional expression is a primary trait that seems to negatively influence the course of cancer. In fact, based on research evidence and theory, Temoshok and Heller created a construct, the Type C personality, that depicts the cancer-prone person as cooperative, unassertive, and patient, a person who suppresses negative emotions and accepts external authorities (1985). Temoshok and Heller suggest that the Type C person is the opposite of the Type A person.

In a study of the survival time of 34 breast cancer patients begun in 1979, Sandra Levy and her colleagues found that patients with shorter survival time reported significantly less joy and greater depression at the time of the diagnosis than long survivors (Levy & Wise, 1988). A study by Reynolds and Kaplan (1986) at the University of California, Berkeley, found that women with breast cancer who expressed less well-being and happiness at diagnosis had shorter survival times than women who expressed greater well-being and happiness.

In 1981 Levy and her colleagues (Levy, Herberman, Maluish, Schlien, & Lippman, 1985) initiated a study of 75 women with a diagnosis of Stage I (lymph nodes free of cancer cells) or Stage II (lymph nodes containing cancer cells) breast cancer. Immediately following surgery but before the diagnosis was made, subjects were given a structured interview and several measures of psychological status, and blood was drawn for assessment of natural killer cell activity against "foreign" cells. As predicted, patients with greater natural killer cell activity tended to have fewer nodes involved. When natural killer cell activity was compared with psychosocial variables, three variables were found to be related to decreased activity: The patient was rated as "well adjusted" to the disease, felt that she did not have satisfactory interpersonal support, and described symptoms of fatigue, such as lack of vigor and apathy.

Levy and Wise (1988) also report a joint study with Seligman of eight women with recurrent breast cancer and eight matched patients without recurrence from the original 1981 study. The interviews were analyzed according to Seligman's multidimensional helplessness construct, looking for a tendency to attribute negative events to oneself and a belief of helplessness in changing oneself as the cause of negative events. Data indicate that helplessness concerning personal cause of negative events was linked to disease recurrence. In this ongoing study, the concept of social support has been broadened to include the patients' sense of support from the medical team and friends, and urinary epinephrine and norepinephrine level is measured as an indicator of stress level at the time of the initial interview. In summarizing this research and the results of other studies, Levy and Wise (1988) describe three psychosocial factors associated with biological risk factors as indicated by reduced natural killer cell activity: inadequate social support, cognitively generated helplessness, and inadequate expression of negative emotion.

Hypothesizing that a person's consistent

coping style and personality characteristics will be manifested in response to a severe stress, Wirsching and colleagues (Wirsching, Stierlin, Hoffman, Weber, & Wirsching, 1982) interviewed 62 women the day before biopsy of a lymph node that might indicate breast cancer; subjects also completed two questionnaires related to the Grossarth-Matticek's concept of rationalization. Nineteen subjects had malignant cancer. Five years later six women were healthy, seven had worsened, five had died from cancer, and one had died from another cause. Responses on the interview proved to be the most valuable indicators of future health. In comparison to the other patients, the women who worsened or died expressed helplessness and said that they received little family support. They described themselves as "rationalizing," and they reported extreme psychological stress in the years before the diagnosis.

These studies indicate that some of the factors that may predispose a person to cancer may also influence the course of the disease. Altogether, 20 different variables are reported to be correlated with the development or progression of cancer. Several of these variables, like depression and repression of emotions were found to be significant in more than one study. Twenty variables would seem to be too many to delineate a cancer-prone personality, however. Table 18.1 lists many of these variables, grouped into five categories. Grouped in this way, the variables indicate a constellation of characteristics

that are found fairly consistently: rational, accepts reality; does not "make waves"; does not express negative emotions; feels helpless or depressed or both; and lacks social support. The Simontons observed that some of their patients tended to consider others' needs before their own and failed to follow their own goals. One can imagine that a person with these characteristics might respond to the diagnosis of cancer with a loss of will to live, albeit unexpressed, stoically accepting fate rather than fighting it because fighting, "making waves," and expressing feelings and needs is not a natural response to events in life. The data from the studies described here, and the observations of health professionals who work with cancer patients, indicate that this pattern is associated with a shorter survival time than that of people who take a fighting stance against cancer and may become cancer survivors. This passive or depressive response, and the opposite, are discussed in detail in *Getting Well Again*, (Simonton, Simonton-Matthews & Creighton, 1978) and in *Love, Medicine and Miracles* (Siegel, 1986). The work of surgeon and cancer counselor, Bernie Siegel, a "student" of the Simontons, is described in Section Three.

If there is a dynamic of health and wellness referred to as "will to live," as many have argued, (Cousins, 1979; Hutschnecker, 1951), and as seems intuitively correct, and if the will to live promotes life, whereas the loss of the will to live hastens death, then it is

Table 18.1 Possible Personality Characteristics of the Cancer-Prone Personality

Interpersonal Style	Temperament	Emotional Style	Cognitive Style	Social Factors
Effort to look good and be good	Depressed Helpless/hopeless	Pleasant Suppresses negative emotions	Stoic acceptance Rational, loyal to reality	Loner Lack of social support
Accepts authority	Fatigue (apathy)		Pessimistic	Lack of intimacy
Docile and loyal				

understandable that patients who accept the diagnosis of cancer fatalistically could shorten their lives.

That these personality characteristics might be associated with the development of cancer, however, implies that they jeopardize the health of the healthy person. This could happen only if these characteristics suppress the immune system or are factors in a lifestyle that predisposes a person to cancer. Next we describe data on the mechanisms that may link psychological states and of immune suppression; knowledge is incomplete, but provocative.

Mechanisms of Cancer

There is no longer doubt that the nervous system and the endocrine system communicate with components of the immune system; every year knowledge of these interactions increases, ultimately enhancing our knowledge of how the mind affects immunity, and therefore disease. In Chapter 4, The Stress Response, we described some of these findings. We also described several studies on the effect of stress on components of the immune system. In a series of studies with medical students during the stress of academic exams, Kiecolt-Glaser and Glaser and colleagues at the Ohio State University College of Medicine found a decrease in natural killer cell activity, a decrease in percent of helper T cells in blood, a decrease in interferon production, and an increase in the antibody to latent herpes virus, compared to a control period before exams (Kiecolt-Glaser & Glaser, 1987). Not surprisingly, these researchers found that when the medical students practiced a relaxation technique during the exam period, the percent of helper T cells increased with frequency of relaxation practices. In another study on the effects of relaxation (Kiecolt-Glaser, Glaser, et al., 1985), nursing home residents who learned and practiced relaxation skills over 12 sessions had increased natural killer cell activity and

decreased antibodies to herpes simplex. They also reported fewer stress-related symptoms in comparison to a social contact control group and a no-treatment control group.

In Chapter 6, Psychosocial Dynamics of Stress Resistance, the effects of positive experiences such as love, social support, and happiness in marriage were described; the effects on immune system functioning were an increase in helper T cells, a decrease in antibodies to virus, and an increase in S-IgA. In Chapter 7, Relaxation, effects of relaxation training on immune system activity were described. In Chapter 9, Imagery for Health and Wellness, studies of the effect of visualization and relaxation on immunocompetence were described.

These data indicate that stress, relaxation, positive emotions, and visualization affect elements of the immune system. Direct evidence of a relationship between immune functioning and the personality characteristics of people who develop cancer is sparse. One study of psychiatric inpatients with severe depression indicated immunosuppression, but the data are difficult to interpret because other variables such as medications may also affect immune function (Krueger, Levy, Cathcart, Fox, & Black, 1984). In a study of medication-free patients with major depressive disorder, Schleifer and colleagues found a decreased mitogen-induced lymphocyte response and a decreased number of T and B cells compared to matched controls (Schleifer, et al., 1984). As noted above, Levy and colleagues found that breast cancer patients who felt that they lacked adequate social support, experienced symptoms of fatigue such as apathy, and were well-adjusted to the disease (meaning that they did not take a fighting stance against it), tended to have decreased natural killer cell activity. Using pathologist reports and light microscope examination of the melanomas of patients in her study, Temoshok and colleagues found that patients who tended to be unexpressive had fewer lymphocytes and macrophages and other indicators of a reduced response against the cancer than patients who expressed emotions, particularly sadness and anger (Temoshok, 1985).

Although comparison of laboratory animal research and human functioning may be questioned, it has been demonstrated that in comparison to rats that can control an electric shock, rats that cannot control the delivery of the shock have a reduced immune response to challenge. Perhaps the lack of control over a stressor is analogous to helplessness in humans.

Cancer-causing agents damage the DNA in cells, producing a mutant cell. The body defends against this by destroying chemical carcinogens, by repairing DNA, and by destroying the mutant cell. To study the effect of depression on DNA repair, Kiecolt-Glaser, Stephens, Lipetz, Speicher, and Glaser (1985) took blood samples from 28 nonmedicated psychiatric inpatients. The subjects' white blood cells were exposed to X rays that damage cellular DNA, and DNA repair was measured. Subjects who were more depressed, as measured by the MMPI, had significantly poorer repair of DNA than less depressed subjects in the sample.

Like the search for psychosocial variables that may predispose a person to cancer, the search for the biological mechanisms is complex and fraught with problems of measurement. Nonetheless, certain measures, such as natural killer cell activity, may be accurate indicators of overall immune system competence.

Is There a Cancer-Prone Personality?

Do certain personality characteristics predispose a person to cancer and shorten life when cancer is diagnosed? There is another way to ask this: "Is Type C a valid construct?" "Construct" is another word for "concept" or "hypothesis" (Landy, 1986). Based on hunches and evidence, Rosenman and Friedman developed the Type A construct, and over many years of research they established its validity. If the Type C construct is valid, then it is empirically true; that is, Type C characteristics, such as

suppression of emotions, do increase the risk of cancer in people who have these characteristics. The answer to the question is "Perhaps." We have no definitive answer yet. To evaluate the evidence for the components of the Type C construct, review the results of the studies in Table 18.2.

After examining Table 18.2, ask yourself, "What is sufficient evidence?" Can we assume that a personality characteristic is associated with cancer because several studies support it? Obviously not all studies are equal in quality and significance. The criteria developed in Chapter 5 would be helpful. For example, prospective studies would have more significance than retrospective studies. However, the Chicago and Alameda studies conflict, illustrating a common problem in the research, the use of different assessment instruments for measuring an attribute, such as depression.

The Chicago prospective study found a significant association between depression and cancer, using the depression scale of the MMPI. The Alameda study did not find this association but used a different scale. To thoroughly evaluate the disparity in results, the depression scales must be examined. The MMPI depression scale of 60 items is complex and measures many dimensions of health. For example, there are four items that involve social dimensions of a person's life: "I am a good mixer," "I prefer to pass by school friends, or people I know but have not seen for a long time, unless they speak to me first," "I go to church almost every week," and "I enjoy many different kinds of play and recreation." The MMPI depression scale also includes many items concerning physical symptoms: nausea, convulsions, vomiting, constipation, coughing up blood, weight loss, hay fever, and asthma. Questions about general health are also included: "I am in just as good physical health as most of my friends," "During the past few years I have been well most of the time," and "I feel weak all over much of the time." At least 15 items on the MMPI depression scale are related to physical health. In contrast, the

Table 18.2   Studies of Personality Characteristics and Cancer

Studies	Lack of emotional expression	Loners and/or lack of social support	Helpless and/or depression	Cooperative
Retrospective				
LeShan	X	X	X	
Bahnson	X		X	
Kissen-Eysenck	X			
Prospective				
John Hopkins	X	X		
Alameda		X	No	
Chicago			X	
Crvenka	X			
Course of Disease				
Klopfer	X			X
Blumberg	X			X
Greer	X		X	
Temoshok	X	X		X
Mechanism				
Kiecolt-Glaser		X		
Levy	X	X	X	
Temoshok				
Intervention				
Kiecolt-Glaser		X		
Simonton	X	X	X	
Grossarth/Matticek	X			

Alameda scale has no items on physical health as seen in Table 18.3.

The items used in the Alameda are strikingly different from the MMPI. Which scale most accurately measures depression? What is depression in the first place? These questions must be raised when evaluating any construct or content of a construct: How are the variables defined, and how are they measured? The differences in the Chicago and Alameda studies may be due to the difference in measures. Based on the results of the Alameda and Chicago studies, we cannot say that depression is or is not a component of the Type C personality and associated with cancer. On the other hand, the Alameda study found that "unhappiness" is associated with cancer; are depression and unhappiness the same phenomenon?

The same question can be asked of other factors. Are unassertiveness, loyalty, acceptance of authority, docility, and failure to express emotions, particularly negative emotions, all manifestations of the same basic characteristic? Until standardized assessment tools are developed that reliably measure these characteristics, and are used consistently, this question will be unanswered.

Two personality factors, lack of emotional expression and social isolation, have the clearest association with the development and progression of cancer. Yet here, too, studies used different measures to assess these factors, and the

Table 18.3   Items in the Alameda Depression Index

Felt depressed or very unhappy
Appetite poor
Trouble getting to sleep or staying asleep
Felt lonely or remote from other people
Felt on top of the world
Felt too tired even to do things I enjoy
Little enjoyment from leisure time
Less energy than other people
Felt pleased about accomplishing something
Felt bored
Felt so restless, could not sit still long
Felt left out, even in a group
Felt excited or interested in something
Hard to feel close to others
Never satisfied with performance
Cannot relax easily
Bothered by getting tired in a short time
Felt vaguely uneasy without knowing why

Source: Kaplan & Reynolds, 1987

concepts were interpreted somewhat differently. For example, Grossarth-Maticek emphasized the intellectual rationalizing aspect of the lack of emotional expression, while the Johns Hopkins study emphasized interpersonal isolation that emerges from failure to share feelings, and Temoshok emphasized a lack of assertiveness. These studies demonstrate an important factor in relationships that may predispose a person to cancer, but the variety of measures complicates the interpretation.

The variety of instruments and procedures used to identify personality traits that might predict cancer is a major problem in cancer and personality research. A single, reliable procedure has not been developed, and the reliability of the tests used is rarely reported.

Type A research has clearly shown that pencil-paper tests do not accurately measure Type A behavior because they cannot measure nonverbal behaviors such as tone of voice, posture, interruption of the interviewer, and facial expressions. Also, most Type A individuals are not aware of their Type A behaviors and may not respond "true to form" on a pencil-paper test, while hostile behavior patterns reflected in the tone of voice and the manner in which questions are answered are seen during the structured interview. Reliance on pencil and paper assessments is a weakness of many personality and cancer studies. Although several researchers have used interviews, a standardized interview is needed.

A primary problem, then, is a lack of standard measures that measure the content of the cancer-prone construct, that is, a repression of emotions or inadequate social support. Another problem, stemming from the first, is a lack of replication studies. Because so many different measures have been used, there are no replication studies of personality characteristics and cancer to date. Even though significant links have been established between personality and cancer in individual studies, without reliable and valid assessment measures and without replication, concise identification of the cancer-prone personality will not be achieved. Nonetheless, as noted above, the data are provocative and point a way to understanding the link between personality and cancer.

Summary

Several retrospective studies demonstrate a correlation between the development and progression of cancer and personality characteristics such as depression, hopelessness, and a lack of emotional expression. Correlation, however, does not mean causality; clearly the diagnosis and treatment of cancer could foster depression, hopelessness, and lack of emotional expression, and therefore these characteristics would be the result of the situation and not of stable personality traits. In an attempt to reduce the effect of having cancer on results of personality assessment, Sandra Levy and other researchers interview cancer patients before the cancer is diagnosed or the severity of the disease is explained to the patient. At the same time, the person's response to the situation may reflect a consistent pattern of coping with life events and influence the course of the disease over many years.

To rule out the possibility of measuring only situationally determined psychological states instead of underlying personality traits, prospective studies are undertaken. The Chicago and Alameda studies produced inconsistent results regarding depression as a precursor of cancer. Consistent results, however, were found in the Johns Hopkins, Grossarth-Matticek, and Alameda studies, indicating that a lack of emotional expression predisposes a person to cancer. In fact, the Grossarth-Matticek study found that a lack of emotional expression (rationality/anti-emotionality) is a stronger predictor of lung cancer than smoking.

The results of a prospective study are based on correlation. Although a lack of emotional expression, for example, is correlated with incidence of cancer, it may not be a causal factor; a third variable might be involved. A causal relationship between two variables is more clearly demonstrated when the removal of one variable affects the second variable. For example, if it can be shown that when people learn to be emotionally expressive they are less likely to develop cancer, or if it can be shown that cancer patients have a longer survival time when they learn to be emotionally expressive, then it is more likely that a lack of expressiveness is related to cancer. The Grossarth-Matticek controlled study, with 91 subjects at high risk of cancer on the rationality/anti-emotionality scale, demonstrated that teaching people to be emotionally expressive significantly reduces the incidence of cancer in comparison to a control group with no training. This substantiates the relationship between a lack of emotional expressiveness and cancer.

The studies listed in Table 18.2 focused on two or three variables. Others measured many psychosocial variables, and only two or three were associated with cancer.

In spite of the diversity of these studies, certain personality characteristics distinguish cancer patients from non-cancer patients and from patients who recover or exceed the expected survival time. These characteristics center on a lack of emotional expression and a cluster of factors related to helplessness, depression, passivity, and a lack of social support. It must be remembered that the results of the studies reported here, such as the Type A behavior studies, are based on group data. Many people who lack social support, who do not express emotions, and who respond to life events with helplessness do not develop cancer, and many cancer patients do not have these characteristics. The study of personality and cancer is important, however, because if personality characteristics can be established as a risk factor, then, like all other risk factors, personality characteristics can be taken into account in the prevention and treatment of cancer.

In the next section, we look at the characteristics of cancer survivors. In Chapter 1 we said that health includes recovery from disease and illness; by studying survivors we learn about the dynamics of health and wellness and how better to help people stay healthy and recover when not.

|||►

SECTION THREE: THE CANCER SURVIVORS

As a teenager Louise developed cancer of the ovary with metastases to the lungs and abdomen. Her oncologist "gave" her six to twelve months to live with chemotherapy. She told him only God could decide when her number was up, and began to take her life into her own hands. She left home because of stressful living conditions there, got her own apartment, and spent her last ten dollars to place a newspaper ad, looking for other cancer patients who needed her help. At one point her oncologist had refused her any further treatment because she was "too far gone," but six months after she had taken the path of her own choosing, all her tumor had disappeared. Her doctor couldn't even tell her this out loud. Instead, with tears in his eyes, he handed her a prescription form on which he'd written, "Your cancer has disappeared." On the day she was supposed to be dead, Louise sent him a joking note asking, "Where should I send the casket?"

Love, Medicine and Miracles,
Bernie Siegel, M.D., 1986, pp. 40–41

Take a minute: Ask yourself, "Why did Louise live?" Based on information in this chapter and in the rest of this book, make a mental list of the characteristics of people who survive life-threatening disease. Or, to make this exercise more meaningful, imagine that you have a life-threatening disease. What characteristics do you need to be a survivor?

Do It Now.

How common are people such as Louise, and why do they survive? It is true that many cancer patients are cured with modern medical treatments, such as surgery, chemotherapy, and radiation. Yet some cancer patients, who are not expected to live regardless of treatment, live beyond the predicted prognosis. Some are cancer survivors who live many years beyond the prognosis, and when death occurs, it is not related to cancer.

Do cancer survivors have particular personality traits that we might refer to as the "survival-prone personality"? The answer appears to be a fairly certain "yes," as evidenced by the patients' descriptions of themselves, by their physicians' and therapists' descriptions, and by research, albeit scarce, on the healthy cancer patient—the patient who fights for life and who survives against the odds.

Journalist Judith Glassman interviewed more than 100 cancer survivors for her book, *The Cancer Survivors and How They Did It* (1983). These patients described themselves as fighters; stubborn; often angry at the physician who gave them a "death sentence"; tenacious in sticking with their treatment, whether medical or "nonmedical"; and dedicated to living. Bernie Siegel writes:

Exceptional patients refuse to be victims. They educate themselves and become specialists in their own care. They question the doctor because they want to understand their treatment and participate in it. They demand dignity, personhood, and control, no matter what the course of the disease. . . . It takes courage to be exceptional. . . . Physicians must realize that the patients they consider difficult or uncooperative are those who are most likely to get well.

(Siegel, 1986, pp. 24, 25)

The "uncooperative" patient is one who questions every procedure, requests information, insists on having medical records, and may decide upon "alternative" adjunctive therapy such as a diet or other health program in addition to traditional therapy or as a substitute for it. The Simontons found that cancer patients who are recovering gain a new perspective on life and decide to change. One of the most beneficial attitudes is expressed as "What can I learn from this experience?" Several children who survived cancer were interviewed on the *Phil Donahue Show* in 1981. A common idea was shared by one child: "I added up all the bad things since I got cancer, and I added up all the good things, and there were more good things than bad things." This child, who had had a leg amputated, said, "I learned to do the things that I could do, and work on the things that I couldn't do." Another child said, "Even though I had cancer, that was the best year of my life." We note that these children were from strong families, whose parents were fighters themselves.

Patricia Norris, a psychologist and biofeedback therapist who has worked with many cancer patients, children and adults, writes "Another group of patients is willing to do anything to get well. No effort seems too great. This is a characteristic shared by survivors of catastrophic and life-threatening disease (Norris & Porter, 1987, p. 133). This characteristic is translated into action. Norman Cousins, no stranger to life-threatening disease, describes his decision to take action after learning that he had a 1–in–500 chance of surviving a collagen disease: "All this gave me a great deal to think about. Up to that time, I had been more or less disposed to let the doctors worry about my condition. But now I felt a compulsion to get into the act. It seemed clear to me that if I was to be that one in five hundred I had better be something more than a passive observer" (Cousins, 1979, p. 31). Becoming an active participant in treatment earns some of these people the reputation of being a bad patient. They become knowledgeable about medical treatment, question the physician's approach, and dedicate themselves to alternative therapies.

The majority of cancer survivors interviewed by Judith Glassman followed very strict and difficult alternative programs, particularly nutrition programs. Survivors pursue a therapy, stick with it, and do not give up. The Simontons' first cancer patient with whom visualization and relaxation techniques were used in conjunction with conventional medical treatment practiced three times a day, every day, until the cancer was gone. People who follow dietary programs must make a considerable lifestyle change and maintain that change.

These people are responding to a need that is so powerful in humans as to seem innate—the need for control. We noted in Chapter 3, Stress, that stressors are less troublesome when a person has a sense of control. We have noted repeatedly that a sense of self-efficacy is a dynamic in health and wellness, and in this chapter we briefly mentioned research on immune responses to lack of control in laboratory animals. There are few events in life that can destroy a person's sense of control as rapidly as the diagnosis and aggressive treatment of cancer. Survivors fight the loss of control in a healthy way, refusing to feel helpless; they strive for control, cognitively and in many other ways. One of the children on the *Phil Donahue Show* said, "You own the disease; it doesn't own you." Hand in hand with the belief in control over the disease, survivors act as a way of gaining control and consider themselves to be in a partnership with the medical team. If the physician does not support the patient's independence or use of adjunctive cancer treatment, the patient may find a physician who does.

People who survive far beyond their prognosis, who persist with difficult therapies, and who take control in action and in thought have another characteristic in common, an extraordinary will to live. Bernie Siegel writes, "Exceptional patients manifest the will to live in its most potent form. They take charge of their lives even if they were never able to before, and they work hard to achieve health and peace of mind (Siegel, 1986, p. 3). Garrett Porter, who used visualization to eliminate a brain tumor when he was 9, said, "You have to decide if you are going to live or die. I decided that I was going to live." A survivor interviewed by Judith Glassman said, "My whole thing as far as survival was concerned was total will. I became healthy because I wanted to live" (Glassman, 1983, p. 334). Some survivors have an immediate response to the diagnosis and prognosis: "I knew I would live, I never doubted it, even when they said I would die." One of Glassman's interviewees said, "I resolved that in my case the disease was not going to be fatal." Glassman comments, "A strong will to live did not guarantee survival, but it played a major role for those patients who did get better and was notably absent in nearly all who did not" (p. 335).

The anger that some survivors express is often will-to-live expressed emotionally. In a study of Stage V (most severe) patients with breast cancer, Achterberg, Matthews, Simonton, and Simonton (1977) found that women who lived beyond the expected survival time were argumentative, in fact, ornery. These women also expressed feelings of personal adequacy and vitality, and had "ego strength" as measured on a variety of psychological tests. A positive correlation between expression of anger and survival has been found in other studies as well.

Characteristics of Survivors

Based on her extensive interviews with cancer survivors, Glassman identifies eight outstanding characteristics.

Hope and a Positive Attitude

Regardless of their prognosis or physical condition, these people maintained an unbeatable optimism.

Anger and Fight

Survivors take a fighting stance against cancer and for life. The survivor mobilizes energy for this fight rather than languishing in depression. The anger of the survivor is expressed; more importantly, it is turned into action.

Responsibility and Involvement

Survivors accept responsibility, not necessarily for the cancer (although some patients do see a link between previous lifestyle habits or psychological state and the development of cancer), but for fighting the cancer and for choosing life.

Belief

Survivors believe completely in their therapy, whether it is traditional medical treatment such as chemotherapy or adjunctive procedures such as diet or visualization.

Tenacity and Determination

These characteristics are another manifestation of a strong will to live. Survivors are able to hang on even when in pain, when suffering severe side effects of treatment, and when the disease is progressing. They stick tenaciously to their treatment programs. The poem "I Will Prevail" written by Garrett Porter when he was 12 years old reflects his tenacity and determination.

I WILL PREVAIL

I won't settle for just surviving
I will settle for prevailing,
Overcoming all obstacles.
I have fought a war, and won,
I have seen death, and cried,
I have seen life, and felt joy.
I will prevail.

Garrett, 1981, in *I Choose Life*, Norris and Porter, 1986. Copyright by Stillpoint International Press. Reprinted by permission.

Goals

In Chapter 6 we said "Goals pull a person toward life" in the description of survivors of extreme conditions, such as the Nazi war camps, and we noted then that goal-setting is one of the first steps in the Simontons' cancer treatment program. Short-term goals and long-term life goals reinforce a person's will to live, because goals give meaning to life. Some cancer survivors report that the reality of death was the impetus for reevaluating goals, and some make the important discovery that they are living by someone else's expectations and have failed to pursue the goals that were once precious.

Love and Support

Survivors are likely to have the unconditional support of another person. Glassman writes, "Repeatedly patients told me that their will and strength and fight was bolstered by the presence of a powerful, caring mate, who said in essence, 'I will not let you die. You must be strong, live, and share your life with me'" (Glassman, 1983, p. 347). The supporting persons often made great sacrifices themselves, helping the patient through treatment and maintaining hope and love. The children who appeared on the *Phil Donahue Show* were unanimous in their appreciation of a strong family in which feelings and love were openly shared.

The importance of social support to health has been mentioned many times in this text. In recovery of any type, whether of addiction or disease, support of other people "in the same boat" is a dynamic of inestimable value. Judith Glassman interviewed a woman with this story:

> I ended up driving a couple of folks back down from Boulder with me. They were also patients and we got to know each other. One lady was eighty-one, a metastatic breast patient who was getting radiation, a little maiden lady. And another was a Chicana lady who had just had a breast removed, and couldn't speak English very well. We were so different, and we *really* needed each other. Those car trips were something, with everyone feeling really crummy and throwing up, and laughing and crying, and we loved it. I just will never forget that. You never would imagine, looking at a car with these three women driving, what was going on. It was such a help to me. We just all really loved each other.
>
> (Glassman, 1983, pp. 25–26)

Survivors sometimes begin support groups themselves, recognizing the need for support from other patients and recognizing that this need is common to all patients. The Cancer Connection, Make Today Count, and We Can Do!, which have chapters in several states, were founded by cancer survivors.

The connection of love and health is not new to you. We described this relationship in Chapter 6, and we can say unequivocally that giving and receiving love is a dynamic in health and wellness. Jerry Jampolsky, child psychiatrist and founder of the Center for Attitudinal Healing, described in Chapter 16 on children, believes that love is the greatest healing force.

Jampolsky created an environment in which children experience unconditional love. In *Love, Medicine, and Miracles,* Bernie Siegel writes, "If I told patients to raise their blood levels of immune globulins or killer T cells, no one would know how. But if I can teach them to love themselves and others fully, the same changes happen automatically. The truth is: Love heals" (Siegel, 1986, p. 181). Survivors receive and give love. Survivors also have a quality that can be called "self-love," as Siegel mentions, which is manifested as high self-esteem and as the force behind the survivors' ability to get needs met and pursue personal goals.

The Doctor

Glassman found that all survivors she interviewed felt the support and caring of the physician. Early in their work, the Simontons described three belief systems that are important in recovery—the patient's, the patient's family's, and the patient's physician's. If the physician believes that the cancer is incurable or does not support the patient's effort to live, then the person must fight both the disease and the beliefs of the medical authority. The negativity or disapproval of the physician can be extremely difficult to counteract, even for the most determined patient. Survivors seek out physicians and other health professionals who will join them in the fight for life. Norman Cousins wrote of his physician, "Dr. Hitzig said it was clear to him that there was nothing undersized about my will to live. He said that what was most important was that I continue to believe in everything I had said. He shared my excitement about the possibilities of recovery and liked the idea of a partnership" (Cousins, 1979, p. 39). Dr. Hitzig did not object when Cousins moved out of the hospital and into a hotel, and began taking large doses of vitamin C and laughter.

Many people survive cancer. The survivors Glassman interviewed and survivors described by physicians and therapists, such as Garrett and Louise, survive against sometimes great odds. In addition to surviving long beyond the prognosis, these people have common traits. The remarkable finding is that these traits are the opposite of those found in people who succumb to cancer as predicted. Perhaps the survivors are among the people in the prospective studies who develop cancer but do not fit the pattern of depression, or emotional inexpressiveness, or helplessness and pessimism.

Some people seem to be natural survivors, and their fight against cancer reflects who they are. Garrett began biofeedback and visualization therapy having already made a decision to live. We study these people to help those for whom survival skills do not come naturally. The Simontons began their treatment program based on observations of the differences between survivors and people who succumb quickly. The hope was that both quality and length of life could be increased by helping cancer patients develop the traits of survivors.

Can it be done? Can people who are not fighters, who do not have a strong will to live, and who respond to crises with feelings of helplessness or with acceptance, learn to have hope and a fighting spirit and dedicate themselves to recovery with a perseverance and optimism? For health professionals who work with cancer patients the answer is: It is worth a try. It is our experience, however, and the experience of many therapists, that this is not an easy task. People who have the characteristics that are associated with the development of cancer, and with short survival time, have these characteristics for profound reasons, often stemming from childhood experiences. As noted above, in her prospective study of medical students, Caroline Thomas found that people who developed cancer were likely to have felt that their parents were "distant." About his own experience of unconditional love and support as a child, Siegel writes, "The hardest lesson for me to learn was that most of my patients are not the products of such love. In fact, I would estimate that 80 percent of my patients were unwanted or treated indifferently as children" (Siegel, 1986, p. 85). The Simontons found that many patients for whom a recent loss seemed to be a precipitating factor in cancer, or in the recurrence of cancer, had also experienced a significant loss in childhood.

The challenge for the patient is to overcome the cognitive and behavioral patterns that have become habitual personality traits. Some patients must overcome a deep sense of lack of self-worth that they have harbored for years and have attempted to overcome, perhaps unconsciously, by seeking approval of others at the expense of personal feelings, needs, and goals. Lawrence LeShan writes:

> Once the patient realizes how much he has condemned and rejected his inner self, it is sometimes useful to discuss this process in terms of a metaphorical trial. In his childhood, the patient in effect held a trial in which he was judge, jury and defendant. At this trial, on the basis of half-understood evidence and a child's limited understanding, he condemned himself as guilty. Having long forgotten that this trial ever took place, the patient has been responding to himself on a basis of that false verdict.
>
> (LeShan, 1977, p. 140)

LeShan describes two essential tasks for the patient in the "retrial": accepting the rejected child within and discovering what she or he *really* wants in life.

The process of self-discovery and self-healing is an important aspect of recovery that is experienced by some patients as a personal awakening and by others as a spiritual awakening. The author of *Mind as Healer, Mind as Slayer*, Kenneth Pelletier (1977), found that some survivors have profound intrapsychic and interpersonal changes.

As the Simonton treatment evolved, two approaches developed. One was a self-help program that focused on diet, exercise, relaxation, visualization, and play. The other program included those self-help procedures plus group or individual psychotherapy for self-discovery and growth. Two programs developed because many patients declined therapy and felt that exploration of psychological issues was not necessary, but they were interested in lifestyle change.

After meeting the Simontons in 1978, Siegel initiated a similar program called Exceptional Cancer Patients (ECaP). Patients meet for two-hour sessions each week in which every aspect of the fight for recovery is shared. Siegel describes the group as "instant family." Before joining ECaP, a person is required to draw a picture of himself, the disease, the treatment, and the white blood cells destroying the cancer. The drawing is a tool for helping the person begin the journey of self-discovery and recovery. Participants must also answer four questions, for the same purpose: Do you want to live to be a hundred? What happened to you in the year or two before your illness? What does the illness mean to you? Why did you need the illness? Undoubtedly the last two questions evoke much thought and may provide a direction for personal growth.

Like others, Siegel has found that people who recover from serious disease have a strong faith in themselves, in the physician, and in the treatment. Spiritual faith or spirituality is another crucial ingredient, described by Siegel as acceptance, forgiveness, peace, and love. "These characteristics *always* appear in those who achieve unexpected healing of serious illness" (Siegel, 1986, p. 178).

Programs such as ECaP help people make lifestyle and intrapersonal changes; they help people replace helplessness with hope and action, isolation with social support, and ambivalence with will to live. The characteristics of survivors can be cultivated, learned, nourished, and unveiled. Potential survivors can become survivors. That is the experience of therapists, physicians, and other health professionals who are involved in programs that foster these characteristics.

Is every person a potential survivor? Perhaps, and yet it is also the experience of health professionals that many people do not choose to try. Some people do not follow recommended lifestyle changes. They have many reasons for not using relaxation and visualization techniques, and although they speak of a desire to live, it is without conviction. LeShan (1977) describes a patient who explained that if she continued in therapy she would discover that she would have to give up her marriage, and she would rather lose her life than her marriage. Because no one can choose life for another person, people have the choice to fight for life as best they can, or not.

We return to the question, "Can a person who is not a survivor learn to be a survivor, and if so, do survival skills prolong life?" We believe, as do our colleagues, that the answer is "Yes, it is possible." This is based primarily on clinical observation, but the little research that has been done on the survival of patients who learn to be survivors supports this observation (Siegel, 1986).

Summary

This section is about survivors, the people who have lived far beyond their prognosis and recovered from a life-threatening disease against great odds. The characteristics of these people—hope, action, persistence, self-confidence, emotional expressiveness including anger, an ability to create meaning in life, and a strong will to live—teach us about life and point the way for helping all people with life-threatening disease. Teaching, facilitating, and nurturing these characteristics is an essential part of a multicomponent treatment program.

There are many interacting domains of human experience—physical, emotional, mental, and spiritual—and healing can occur in all domains. Survivors teach us about this healing.

||||➡

CONCLUSION

The evidence for a link between personality and cancer is like the evidence for cigarette smoking and lung cancer: The research evidence accumulated over many years and many studies contributed to the data. The evidence from several sources—retrospective, prospective, and intervention studies; clinical observation; and survivors—does point to a personality pattern of emotional unexpressiveness (particularly of negative feelings), depression, and helplessness that is correlated with the development and progression of cancer. This personality pattern may develop early in life as a result of insufficient parenting or as the result of loss when a parent or other family member dies or leaves the family. A person with this personality pattern may be physically healthy for years until another significant loss occurs, threatening the person's meaning and purpose in life. This second loss triggers the pattern, and the person responds with depression and suppressions of feelings. Studies of immunocompetence, stress, and disease and health may eventually establish the mechanisms through which personality variables affect the immune system.

The data are suggestive, but not conclusive. This is partly because research methods vary, and replication studies have not been done. This is also undoubtedly because cancer, like heart disease, has a hierarchy of interacting causes. Cancer can be described from the biopsychosocial perspective (Figure 18.3). There are several well known biological risks for cancer, such as smoking and exposure to carcinogens (the Environmental Protection Agency classifies 1,500 chemicals as carcinogenic). Some "biological" risks, particularly smoking, obesity, and diet are lifestyle risks that are supported by cultural values and habits. The presence of carcinogenic pollutants in air, water, and land is a societal problem. Social forces, such as social support and the medical system, are also variables in sickness and recovery. As we have seen, evidence for the effect of psychological factors in cancer is increasing. The biopsychosocial approach to cancer suggests that the personality characteristics that may predispose a person to cancer are not independent

causes of cancer; these factors are each only one element in a complex picture. Many people with these characteristics do not develop cancer, and many people without these characteristics do. Nonetheless, the evidence points to an important cognitive component of treatment.

Carolyn Thomas, the physician who initiated the Johns Hopkins longitudinal study in 1946, writes: "In the end, the likelihood that traits of character may join with genetic and environmental factors to play a causal role in cancer is a challenging possibility, the truth of which can only be determined by further study" (Thomas, 1988, p. 57).

What does this mean for you personally? Can you apply the results of these studies of personality and cancer to your life? If you are chronically lonely and depressed, will you get cancer? If you respond to life events with a fighting spirit, if you are optimistic and emotionally expressive, are you immune to cancer? The probability that your health will be affected by a risk factor or a "survivor factor" is derived from studies of groups. A risk factor based on

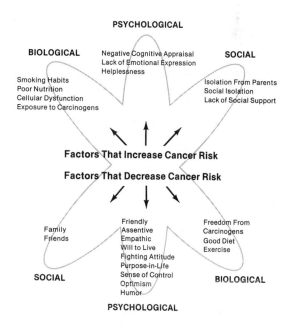

Figure 18.3.   Many Biological, Psychological, and Social Factors May Play a Role in Cancer.

group data does not necessarily apply to a particular person.

Nonetheless, knowledge of risks enables you to make wise decisions about your lifestyle. You already know that certain risks, such as smoking, should be avoided. If you don't smoke, the chances of getting lung cancer are decreased by 600 percent and your chances of dying from coronary heart disease are decreased by 200 percent (American Cancer Society, 1984).

Personality risk factors for disease are more complex. Nevertheless, practical insights for prevention of disease are derived from the clinical and experimental studies of cancer and other immune disorders. These are:

1. If you always respond to stressors with chronic feelings of hopelessness, you may be at increased risk for illnesses such as a cold, sore throat, mononucleosis, and upper respiratory infections. Later in life you may be more susceptible to cancer.

2. To decrease your susceptibility to immune disorders, learn skills and techniques that will help you respond to life with positive attitudes and positive actions instead of "learned helplessness." Develop a meaningful purpose in life.

3. If you have difficulty coping with negative emotions and keep angry feelings bottled up, learn problem-solving and communication skills. Many of these skills and techniques are discussed in Chapters 6 through 13.

4. Do not permit unhappy, conflict-laden relationships to go on indefinitely without resolution. Take action! Join classes and groups that will help you resolve these conflicts. Consult specialists who are skilled in helping people cope better in marriages, families, and other interpersonal relationships.

5. Develop the characteristics of survivors.

Researchers in medicine, immunology, medical sociology, public health, and psychology are asking: Can personality affect immunity, and if so, what personality characteristics are involved? Can stress affect immunity? If negative emotions contribute to disease, can positive emotions such as hope and love enhance health? What are the biochemical mechanisms through which emotions affect the body? By daring to ask these questions, investigators have contributed significantly to understanding mind $\longrightarrow$ body. They have widened the search for the causes of disease, for the dynamics of health and wellness, and for the best tools for prevention and treatment.

The fact that personality characteristics influence health presents a clear challenge to the study of the dynamics of health and wellness: (1) identify the characteristics with reliable and valid measures, (2) create methods for determining these characteristics in people before illness develops, and (3) devise strategies for teaching the skills needed to change disease-prone personality patterns into pro-health patterns.

A few years from now the studies described in this chapter may seem like a science in its infancy. Today, they provide clues to treatment and to the prevention of a major cause of death. The door is open for the development and application of therapeutic procedures for cancer treatment that promote biological, psychological, social, and spiritual healing.

CHAPTER *19*

Development of the Personality Characteristics of Healthy People

IIII➡

I believe that we form our own lives, that we create our own reality, and that everything works out for the best. I know I drive some people crazy with what seems to be a ridiculous optimism, but it's always worked for me. I believe in taking a positive attitude toward the world, toward people, toward my work. I spend a few minutes in meditation and prayer each morning, trying to determine, or stay in tune with, the purpose of my life. . . . I find it's important for me to stop every now and then and get re-charged, re-inspired. Nature and the beauty of nature has been one of the great inspirations in my life. Growing up as an artist I've always been in awe of the incredible beauty of every last bit of design in nature.

Jim Henson, creator of the Muppets,
in Berman (1986)

My personal vision started with my parents who were Italian immigrants. They left their homeland, loved ones, and security to actualize a dream. They were not unusually adventuresome, tireless, or fearless; they were immensely human. They settled in Los Angeles with little more than a willingness to work hard, a spirit of adventure (or was it naiveté), and an unending sense of humor. They raised a family, acquired a small home and struggled to maintain an Italian-American culture in dignity, despite poverty and contending with strong anti-Italian prejudice. I remember our home as continually filled with the sounds of life, and too small for the myriad people moving through it. We seemed always to be living on the cusp between triumph and disaster, despair and celebration, tears and laughter, birth and death. Still, I never recall, even for a moment, fearing life or experiencing any sense of helplessness or hopelessness. Never did I question where I belonged. It was in this environment that I learned much of what I still believe. Without ever defining the terms, I was

taught love, responsibility, commitment, the dignity of work and the importance of laughter, song, dance, good food, and God.

Leo Buscaglia, author and lecturer,
in Berman (1986)

You already know a great deal about healthy people, people for whom the dynamics of health and wellness are no mystery. Hardiness, stress resistance, self-efficacy, high self-esteem, learned resourcefulness, Type B characteristics, optimism, and a fighting spirit are personality characteristics of healthy people, using a broad meaning of health. The term *healthy person* has two meanings—a person who is physically healthy, and a person who is psychologically healthy. In this chapter on personality characteristics, we use "healthy person" to refer to someone who is psychologically healthy, who has the characteristics of hardiness, stress resistance, and so forth, remembering that psychologically healthy people tend to be physiologically healthy as well. The concept of *healthy personality* refers to the psychological characteristics of healthy people: their attitudes, perceptions of self and others, cognitive coping skills, values, communication style, and a host of other attributes that make up one's personality. By definition, healthy people have healthy personality characteristics: not anger and aggression but tolerance and empathy, not depression but cheerfulness, not helplessness but courage, not pessimism but optimism.

We begin this chapter with a characteristic of healthy people that we mentioned briefly in Chapter 17—transcendental values and goals that move a person beyond materialistic, personal needs. Transcendental values and goals are a characteristic of people who are self-actualizing, a term coined by Abraham Maslow to describe people who have achieved the highest levels on the hierarchy of needs, presented in Chapter 3, Stress. Transcendental values and goals are also characteristic of people of high well-being. Section One concludes with a snapshot view of four other characteristics of healthy people, as a review.

Section Two addresses the intriguing question that must be asked in a textbook on health and wellness: "How do psychologically healthy people get that way?" This is perhaps the most fascinating question in the field, and yet the development of hardy, healthy personality traits in childhood has not been extensively researched. The obvious answer—the caregiver—is the focus of this section. We discuss two essential tasks, nurturing and teaching.

The caregiver and the home environment are the primary sources for the development of the healthy personality. Sometimes, however, healthy people survive unhealthy homes because another person or the environment has provided the necessary ingredients. In Section Three the role of public education is described. The school environment can be very influential in the development of a healthy child. We end this chapter with a discussion of an effective outdoor education program, Outward Bound.

IIII➡

SECTION ONE: THE PERSONALITY CHARACTERISTICS OF HEALTHY PEOPLE

Sometimes I think of a priest who, many years ago, predicted that if I did not change my ways I would spend my life in prison. He was my religion teacher, and up to this day I do not know whether or not he was right. He taught me in the first few grades of grammar school and kept track of my development. He was aware of my hypersensitivity to truth, my desire to have it revealed no matter what the price

may be. If I believed that something was one way and not another, I'd always do all that I could to have the truth surface, no matter who was hiding it or trying to obscure it. . . . I think that my character was and still is a little bit warped whenever truth is at stake; it's something I just won't compromise, no matter what.

Lech Walesa, winner of the
Nobel Prize for peace and a
leader in the Solidarity movement
in Poland, in Berman (1986)

As I write these words I am of an age older than most of those who have taught me, and of almost all of those who will read me. But although considered, and sometimes referred to, as an old man, I feel no different from the days when I set out on my career, from the earlier days when I resolved to add to the store of truth and beauty that inspired me when young.

Sidney Hook, philosopher and recipient
of the 1985 Presidential Medal of
Freedom, in Berman (1986)

Commitment to Transcendental Values and Goals: A Key to Well-Being

Commitment, particularly commitment to self, is a characteristic of hardy people. This means "an ability to recognize one's distinctive values, goals, and priorities, and an appreciation of one's capacity to have purpose" (Kobasa, 1979, p. 4). Of all the personality variables studied in the hardiness research, commitment to values and goals is most predictive of health and well-being.

But are all goals, values, and priorities equal in facilitating psychological health? We have noted that goals "pull a person toward life" and are an important element in healing. But is the goal of having two Mercedes-Benzes in the garage, for example, as salubrious as the goal of building a park for inner-city children, or visiting the great museums of Europe, or growing spiritually? In recovering from disease, it may be that any goal or value that enhances the will to live is good. But life goals that a person

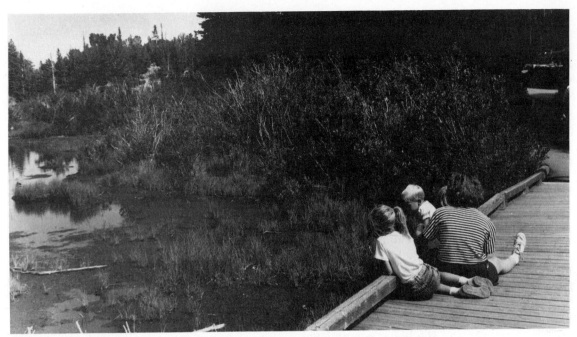

Children Can Develop Transcendental Values Such as Appreciation of Nature.
Source: Judith Green.

pursues for many years—goals that determine the quality of a person's life—are not equal. Friedman and Rosenman found that Type B people characteristically have goals and values that transcend materialistic needs. Type B people value and seek spirituality, beauty in nature and art, and meaningful relationships. In contrast, Type A people focus on possessions and have a "number consciousness"; they spend their days pursuing things that they believe are worth having, rather than pursuing characteristics worth being. The pursuit of materialistic goals and numbers consciousness are driving forces behind the competitiveness and aggression of the Type A person. Helping Type A people shift from number consciousness to transcendental consciousness was an important component of Friedman and Rosenman's treatment program for Type A people who had already suffered one heart attack.

Abraham Maslow's description of the self-actualizing person, who has reached the highest level on the hierarchy of needs (Figure 19.1) discussed in Chapter 3, is similar to the Type B personality. The person pursues transcendental goals—spirituality, beauty, truth, or justice. Based on his study of the lives of exceptional people, Maslow (1968) believed that once a person moves beyond the first four needs in the hierarchy—physical, safety, belonging, and esteem—the way is prepared for self-actualization. We use the phrase "move beyond" to emphasize the fact that a person may never achieve the basic needs for shelter and safety, for example, or may give up these needs, and yet may "rise above" these needs and pursue transcendental goals. We have no doubt that all over the world there are exceptional people whose basic needs were never met and yet who have dedicated themselves to a transcendental goal, such as helping others.

The human being needs a framework of values, a philosophy of life . . . to live by and understand

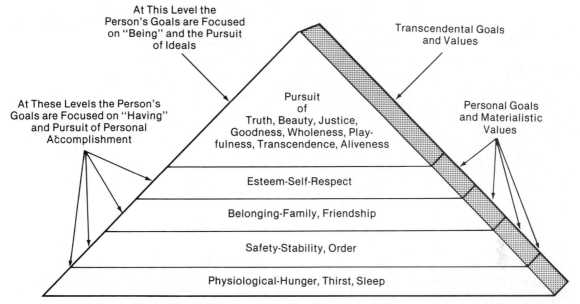

At This Level the Person's Goals are Focused on "Being" and the Pursuit of Ideals

Transcendental Goals and Values

At These Levels the Person's Goals are Focused on "Having" and Pursuit of Personal Accomplishment

Personal Goals and Materialistic Values

Pursuit of Truth, Beauty, Justice, Goodness, Wholeness, Play-fulness, Transcendence, Aliveness

Esteem-Self-Respect

Belonging-Family, Friendship

Safety-Stability, Order

Physiological-Hunger, Thirst, Sleep

Figure 19.1.   Maslow's Hierarchy of Needs and the Development of Transcendental Goals and Values.

by, in about the same sense that he needs sunlight, calcium, or love.

Maslow (1968, p. 206)

Transcendental goals and values are the centerpiece of life for people who surmount life crises and exhibit well-being. Author Gail Sheehy describes major changes and life crises as "passages." Sheehy wondered why some people successfully navigate these passages, becoming more mature and more creative, and radiating well-being, while other people slip backward, blame others for their troubles, and become less mature. In collaboration with sociologist Phillip Shaver and psychologist Carin Rubenstein, Sheehy conducted an elaborate study to identify the characteristics of healthy people.

Shaver and Rubenstein developed a 100-item life history questionnaire that included a subset of items designed to measure well-being such as: "How often do you feel bored? How have you been feeling about your friends and social life? How have you been feeling about

your religion and spiritual life?" (Sheehy, 1985). The questionnaire was given to sixty thousand people from all segments of American society: congressmen and their wives, congresswomen and their husbands, corporate chiefs and their spouses, entrepreneurs, lawyers, brokers, bankers, athletes, homemakers, union representatives, semi-skilled and technical workers, and college students. "Well-being" was defined as having high scores on satisfaction in the areas of work, love, children, success, finances, and health, and having high scores on meaningfulness of life, inner control, and self-responsibility. Shaver and Rubenstein identified people with well-being, and a group was selected for extensive interviews. Sheehy interviewed these people. "It would be enlightening, I thought, to compare the experiences of people who feel exceptionally good about themselves and to explore the qualities of mind and heart they call upon at important crossroads. This was the task that excited me" (Sheehy, 1985, p. 13).

Sheehy found that people with exceptional well-being radiated enthusiasm for life, were attractive, and made people around them feel good. "Like the dance of brilliant reflections on a clear pond, well-being is a shimmer that accumulates from many important life choices made over the years by a mind that is not often muddied by pretense or ignorance and a heart that is open enough to sense people in their depths and to intuit the meaning of most situations" (Sheehy, 1985, p. 12).

The single item that was most highly correlated with high well-being was "My life has meaning and direction." Sheehy found that invariably the object of "meaning and direction" in people of high well-being was involvement with something beyond themselves, transcendental goals such as work, an idea, other people, a social objective, or spiritual growth. Many had discarded dogmas accepted in youth and adopted spiritual values more in harmony with their goals.

> Lay up your treasures in heaven
> Where neither moth nor dust doth
>   corrupt
> For where your treasures are,
> there will your heart be also.
> —The Bible

Having a meaningful purpose in life and being committed to the higher values of love, spirituality, and beauty are characteristic of people with well-being. From the interview and questionnaire responses, Sheehy found 10 characteristics that were highly correlated with well-being; she calls these the "Ten Hallmarks of Well-Being." These characteristics are:

1. Life has meaning and direction.
2. Important transitions in the adult years have been handled in an unusual, personal, or creative way.
3. Life has not been disappointing.
4. Long-terms goals have already been attained.
5. There is satisfaction with personal growth and development.
6. In love with partner.
7. Many friends.
8. Cheerful person.
9. Not thin-skinned or sensitive to criticism.
10. No major fears.

In addition to transcendental goals and values, four characteristics of healthy people emerge from the studies of hardiness and of people high in well-being: high self-esteem, cheerful temperament, positive interpersonal relationships, and the ability to accept change as a challenge.

Self-Esteem

Healthy people feel good about themselves (high self-esteem), they feel confident in their ability to cope (self-efficacy), and they have a sense of control. Sheehy found that people with optimum well-being were not free of difficulties and had experienced failures, the death of a spouse or child, divorce, a severe accident, the loss of a job, or transitions such as going back to school or starting a new career. These people took the necessary steps to complete the transition and gained new confidence in the process. "I'm forty-five and next year I'll graduate from college. . . . I started this new life after staying home for ten years so my husband wouldn't feel inferior. If I die tomorrow I've had a ball. The confidence I have now is in myself" (Sheehy, 1985, p. 103).

In describing learned resourcefulness, Israeli psychologist David Rosenbaum pointed out that healthy people know how to self regulate and how to use resources to cope effectively with life. In Sheehy's study, the item scored second-most often by people high in well-being was "I have experienced one or more important transitions in my adult years and I have handled these transitions in an unusual, personal, or creative way" (Sheehy, 1985). In contrast to people who are low in well-being and who blame others for their difficulties, people high in well-being are more resourceful in coping with difficulties and accept responsibility for change.

Kobasa found that hardy people respond to stress with a sense of control rather than with helplessness. They gain control through problem-solving and by incorporating the stressor into a philosophical framework. For example, religious beliefs help people cope with the death of a loved one; the belief that events do not occur by chance, but are "lessons," helps many people grow through stressful events. Muppet creator Jim Henson expressed an unquenchable optimism, believing that whatever happened was "for the best"; this philosophy helped him through life changes. Antonovsky found that people who survived concentration camps with some measure of psychological health were able to incorporate the stressful event into a meaningful framework that he called "sense of coherence."

Self-esteem and its companions—self-efficacy, self regulation and a sense of control—are common themes that run through the studies of healthy, stress-resistant people.

Cheerful Temperament

In his study of telephone workers, Hinkle found that cheerful, pleasant workers maintained mental and physical health in spite of many life changes. Type B personalities are easygoing and cheerful and have few incidents of coronary heart disease. In a replication of Kobasa's hardiness studies, Charles Holahan at the University of Texas and Rudolf Moos at Stanford University studied 493 people. In addition to hardiness, Holahan and Moos measured temperament with questionnaire items such as "Describe the way you see yourself" and "How do other people see you." People highest in hardiness qualities were easygoing and happy (Holahan & Moos, 1986). In Sheehy's study, people with high well-being described themselves as cheerful.

Interpersonal Relationships

The healthiest telephone workers studied by Hinkle were friendly people who had many friends. Sheehy found that people high in well-being reported having many friends and described themselves as tolerant of criticism and tough-skinned. People high in well-being are able to accept criticism without sinking into anger or depression (Sheehy, 1985). In their middle years, many people high in well-being felt greater love and intimacy with their partner than in previous years. Sheehy found that honoring loving relationships was an important value for people of high well-being. People with high well-being were unwilling to jeopardize their families' needs for personal needs and professional achievement. The people lowest in well-being were willing to sacrifice friends, spouse, or children in pursuit of a career. Economic status was not tied to well-being, but the capacity to love and be loved was.

Longitudinal studies of personality and cancer indicate that the healthiest patients expressed feelings and have close, meaningful relationships.

Change as Challenge

Kobasa found that hardy people perceive the stressors of life as challenges to overcome rather than as overwhelming events. In Sheehy's study, a subgroup of people survived extreme stress and life change and yet radiated a sense of confidence. She called these people "pathfinders." The pathfinders confronted a crossroad, chose a path, and emerged with new strength and expanded potential. They looked upon life changes as interesting challenges. They were optimistic about the present and the future, and they were not "stuck" in the past. Sheehy was struck by the fact that pathfinders were willing to take risks to develop their own potential and the potential of others.

CHARACTERISTICS OF THE HEALTHY PERSONALITY

Commitment to transcendental values
Perceiving change as a challenge
Easygoing temperament
Positive relationships
High self-esteem

Summary

Commitment to transcendental goals and values, high self-esteem, positive interpersonal relationships, an easygoing temperament, and perceiving change as a challenge are characteristics of healthy people. This summary is no surprise. Whenever we describe personality characteristics associated with health and stress resistance, these stand out.

SECTION TWO: THE ROOTS OF THE HEALTHY PERSON

I am deeply impressed by the potentialities of human beings—to love generously, to dedicate themselves to causes, to be loyal and honest, to forgive, to create beauty in all the arts and to appreciate them, to make experiments and discoveries. What wonderful creatures! Yet of course, humans can also be cruel, vengeful, ungrateful, deceitful, and greedy. Child psychiatry tells us that our good and evil traits come mainly from the way we were treated as children and from the examples we had in our parents. . . . My mother was totally devoted to her children. She particularly loved and enjoyed babies. . . . Every year at the Easter ceremony at Sunday school, when the small children carrying lighted candles led the march, my mother's face would turn red as a tomato, and tears would stream down her cheeks. We Spock children

hardly dared look at her because all of us would then weep, too, sensing that this symbolized the positive bond between us. Of her six children, five went into child psychology or school teaching.

Benjamin Spock, author and
pediatrician, in Berman (1986)

We introduced this book as an examination of the dynamics of health and wellness; the study of psychologically and physically healthy people is vital to this task. By studying healthy and well people we learn about health and wellness. Having determined the characteristics of healthy people, the next question arises: "How do healthy people get that way?"

Take a minute: So you just had a baby. You want this child to grow up to be a hardy, stress-resistant, Type B person with high well-being and the characteristics of a survivor. Answer this question: How will you foster these characteristics in your child?

Do It Now.

In this section we focus on the characteristics of parents who raise psychologically healthy children. From extensive interviews of both hardy and nonhardy people, Salvatore Maddi and Suzanne Kobasa concluded that certain parenting styles facilitate hardiness. George Vaillant (1977) found that parents of healthy men were quite different from parents of unhealthy men. The research on Type A and Type B children indicates that parents of Type B children are quite different from parents of Type A children. The principle characteristics of the parents of children who become healthy adults can be classified as "nurturing caregiver" and "teacher."

Nurturing Caregiver

Maddi and Kobasa (1984) found that parents of hardy children provide a nurturing, supportive environment that fulfills the child's basic needs. These parents give love, encourage independence, and support the child's goals in school, sports, and hobbies. Maddi and Kobasa (1984) emphasize that a nurturing environment fosters the three components of hardiness—commitment, control, and challenge—because the child experiences the world as meaningful, interesting, and challenging. Maddi and Kobasa found that nonhardy executives had rigid or punitive parents who used the child to fulfill their own needs. Parents with rigid expectations impose on the child their own ideas of who the child should be, even if it contradicts the child's natural capabilities. Executives with rigid parents felt alienated, and their worlds seemed empty and worthless. Many of the nonhardy executives were successful in their jobs, but inwardly they felt that something important in life was missing (Maddi & Kobasa, 1984).

Type A people feel an underlying insecurity because of a lack of unconditional love in childhood. "One of the most important influences fostering status insecurity is the failure of the Type A person in infancy and very early childhood to receive unconditional love, affection, and encouragement from one or both of his parents" (Friedman & Ulmer, 1984, p. 46). As discussed in Chapter 17, the success of the treatment program for Type A men was due in part to the unconditional love that they received from the staff and from other members.

Many studies have demonstrated the importance of a supportive and nurturing caregiver for the development of a healthy person. Vaillant's prospective study of 185 Harvard men found that the healthiest men experienced a warm, intimate family life in childhood (Vaillant, 1977). The healthiest people in the 30-year prospective Johns Hopkins study characterized their early family experiences as warm and intimate (Thomas, et al., 1979).

Warm, nurturing parents help fulfill the child's needs for intimacy and warmth. Nurturing parents also foster independence in the child. After an extensive examination of the research on locus of control, Kansas State University psychologist Jerry Phares, in his book on internal locus of control, states:

> Parental child-rearing practices that can be characterized as warm, protective, positive, and nurturant with only minor exceptions are linked to children who develop an internal locus of control. On the other side of the coin, many pathological populations (schizophrenics and others) are described as having sprung from cold, rejecting, negative parents.
>
> (Phares, 1976, p. 147)

Nurturing parents who provide warmth and support, and encourage the independence of the child, foster creative children. In 1968, Jeanne and Jack Block, researchers at the University of California, Berkeley, initiated a longitudinal study of 53 boys and 53 girls who were enrolled in the nursery schools at the University of California, Berkeley (Harrington, Block, & Block, 1987). Most children enrolled at age 3. During the child's first year in nursery school, the parents were asked to describe their child-rearing attitudes and practices. When the children were 4½ years old, parent-child interactions were observed between father and child and mother and child in situations in which the father or mother helped the child solve a battery of thinking tasks. These sessions were videotaped, and the teaching strategies of the parents were evaluated twice. Based on the self-reported child-rearing practices and the observations of parent-child interaction on the thinking tasks, a global score was created that reflected the parents' child-rearing and teaching styles. At ages 3½, 4½, and 5½, the children were assessed for intelligence, creativity, and psychological maturity. During the sixth and ninth grades, the children's creativity was assessed and rated by classroom teachers, a clinical psychologist, and examiners who administered a variety of tests. A composite score based on these creativity ratings was positively correlated with the global child-rearing and teaching style score of the parents. Children who were high on creativity had parents who provided psychological safety and freedom. Psychological safety is created when the child is given a sense of unconditional worthiness, when external evaluation is absent, and when the child is understood empathically. Psychological freedom is created when the child is allowed to engage in fantasy freely and experiment with ideas and symbols. The characteristics of the parents who were positively correlated with creative children are presented in Table 19.1

Harrington, Block, and Block (1987) concluded that the data from their longitudinal studies of children support the idea that creativity is fostered when parents provide psychological safety and psychological freedom.

Children have a natural tendency to explore their environment and to do things for themselves. When parents encourage a child to explore the environment, the child develops a

Table 19.1

Teaching Patterns of Parents that Fostered Creativity in Children	Characteristics of Creative Children, Sixth and Ninth Grades
Parent was warm and supportive. Parent reacted to the child in an ego-enhancing manner. Child appeared to enjoy the situation. Adult derived pleasure from being with the child. Parent praised the child. Parent established a good working relationship with the child. Parent encouraged child to proceed independently. Parent encouraged the child.	Appears to have a high degree of intellectual capacity. Is productive; gets things done. Unconventional thought processes. Genuinely values intellectual and cognitive matters. Is an interesting person. Enjoys esthetic impressions and is esthetically reactive. Behaves in ethically consistent manner; consistent with own standards. Has high aspiration for self. Concerned with own adequacy as a person. Is concerned with philosophical problems, e.g. values, the meaning of life, religions, etc. Values own independence and autonomy.
Teaching Patterns that Did Not Foster Creativity in Children	**Characteristics of Uncreative Children, Sixth and Ninth Grades**
Parent tended to overstructure the tasks. Parent tended to control the tasks. Parent tended to provide specific solutions. Parent was critical of child; rejected child's ideas and suggestions. Parent appeared ashamed of child, lacked pride in child. Parent was hostile in the situation. Parent gave up and retreated from difficulties. Parent pressured child to work at the tasks. Parent was impatient with the child.	Is uncomfortable with uncertainty and complexities. Feels a lack of personal meaning in life. Gives up and withdraws where possible in the face of adversity. Reluctant to commit self to any definite course of action; tends to delay or avoid action. Is self-defeating. Is emotionally bland; has flattened affect. Feels cheated and victimized by life; self-pitying.

Source: From Harrington, Block, and Block (1987). Testing aspects of Carl Roger's theory of creative environments: Child-rearing antecedents of creative potential in young adolescents. *Journal of Personality and Social Psychology,* pp. 52, 851–856. Copyright 1987 by the American Psychological Association. Reprinted by permission.

strong sense of competency and a sense of control. Parents can discourage the sense of competency by not allowing children to do things for themselves. The world-renowned child psychologist Rudolf Dreikurs said, "Every time you do something for a child that he can do for himself, you are discouraging the child" (Dreikurs & Stoltz, 1964). If you dress children when they can dress themselves, or clean up for them when they can clean up for themselves, you are sending messages of incompetence. Dreikurs states, "Spilled milk is less important than loss of confidence" (Dreikurs & Stoltz, 1964).

In summary, nurturing caregivers provide intimacy and support, foster a sense of purpose in life, model positive attitudes toward change, and encourage independence in their children. The longitudinal research of Harrington, Block, and Block confirmed Maddi and Kobasa's observations that nurturing parents foster healthy, hardy children. Loving, caring parents provide the basic conditions for the development of the healthy, hardy person. But love is not enough; parents must also be teachers for their children.

Parents as Teachers

I was raised until age thirteen by my grandmother, Omi. An anti-fascist both prior to and during the time of Hitler, she has always been a very courageous woman who, as a war widow, learned to live without men supporting her. She

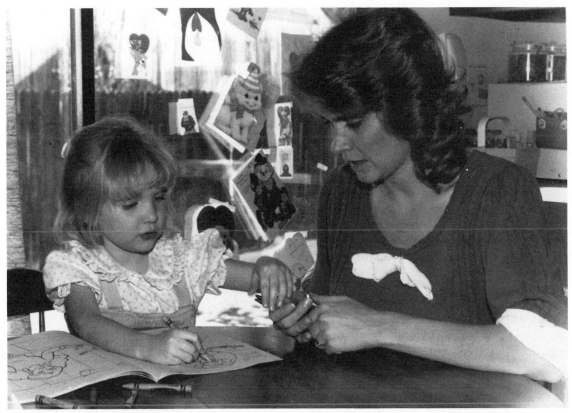

Nurturing Caregivers Provide Encouragement and Support While Allowing the Child Freedom to Be Creative and Self-Sufficient.
Source: Gordon Steward, Denver, CO.

took care of both my mother and me during the hardest times. When I was six years old, she began reading newspapers and news magazines to me, going through them page by page.

Petra Kelly, founder of the
West German Green political
party, cited in Berman (1986)

My grandmother has been the most influential person in my life. Articulate and dynamic, she became a leader in both church and community. I am convinced that had opportunities for furthering her education been available, she would have been a powerful force in our society. Fortunately for me, she was not only my mentor but my best friend. She constantly told me that I was somebody and could be or do anything on this earth if I would only study hard and keep faith in God.

M. Deborah Hyde-Rowan, M.D., one of
two black female neurosurgeons in the
United States, cited in Berman (1986)

As parents, we are in a sense, our children's first hypnotists and can give them positive post-hypnotic suggestions.

Bernie Siegel, M.D. (1986) from
Love, Medicine, and Miracles (p. 87)

Teaching "Change as a Challenge."

Children learn through the examples of parents, teachers, peers, television heroes, and even fairy-tale characters, but parents play a primary role. Through what they say and what they do, parents teach children how to adapt to the world. Please read Box 19.1 now.

It is no surprise to find that hardy people have hardy parents and that nonhardy people have nonhardy parents. Maddi and Kobasa's research showed that the parents of hardy people view life changes as natural and challenging. For example, Chuck was brought up in a poor family. When Chuck's father lost his job, his mother, who had never worked before, became a seamstress. She was proud of her skills and modeled an attitude of challenge in confronting stressful events. Chuck was one of the hardy executives. In contrast, the parents

of nonhardy people were overwhelmed by life changes, as in the case of Jim, a nonhardy executive. When Jim's father died, his mother withdrew into helplessness and depression. For Jim, helplessness was modeled as a response to life change. When the Illinois Bell telephone company reorganized as a result of divestiture, Jim was frightened by the change and responded with regressive coping patterns—he drank excessively and avoided major problems (Maddi & Kobasa, 1984).

Describing a cancer survivor, Bernie Siegel writes:

> I have a patient, a frail woman named Edith, who weighs all of eighty-five pounds. She told me, "I don't need you and your group. My mother always told me when I was a youngster, 'You're scrawny, but whatever happens, you'll always get over it. You'll live to be ninety-three, and then they'll have to run you over with a steamroller.'"
>
> (Siegel, 1986, p. 87)

Parents of hardy people also teach their children to view change as challenge by teaching them skills for confronting new challenges. Many parents of the hardy executives taught their children how to read a map and get around in a city. Others emphasized learning new activities, such as music, sports, or crafts. Chuck described his father as a good teacher who taught him how to fix things around the house. Bill, another hardy executive, described his early family life as very active. Everyone had a hobby or sport. Bill specialized in building model airplanes and drawing comic strips. Years later, when his wife died, Bill overcame depression through the challenge of new hobbies.

Teaching Social Skills

There is no substitute for good social skills. Three characteristics—friendliness, empathy, and nonaggressiveness—are particularly important. How do children learn to be friendly, empathic, and nonaggressive?

BOX 19.1

FAIRY TALES

Fairy tales were once an important medium through which children learned about the characteristics of hardiness and stress resistance, honor and courage. The classic *The Little Engine that Could* is a case in point. As an illustration, we include a story taken from a six-volume set of beautifully illustrated fairy tales that provided continual entertainment, and instruction, when we were young.

SHINGEBISS
A Chippewa Indian Tale

In his lodge on the shores of the great Lake Huron lived little brown duck, Shingebiss. When the fierce North Wind swept down from the white and glittering Land of Snow, four great logs for firewood had little brown duck, Shingebiss, one for each month of winter.

Brave and cheery was Shingebiss, and no matter how the North Wind raged, he waddled out across the ice and found what food he needed. With his strong bill he pulled frozen rushes up from the pond, and dived down through the holes they left, to get his fish for supper. Then away to his lodge he went, dragging a string of fish behind him. By his blazing fire he cooked his supper and made himself warm and comfortable.

So at last the North Wind shrieked angrily:

"Woooo-oo-oo! Woo-oo-oo! Who dares to brave Big Chief North Wind? All other creatures fear him. But little brown duck, Shingebiss, heeds Big Chief North Wind no more than Minnewawa, little, gently blowing squaw-breeze."

So the North Wind sent out cold, icy blasts, and made high drifts of snow, till not a bird or beast dared venture forth—save Shingebiss. Shingebiss went out the same as before and paid no heed to the weather. He got his fish every day and cooked his supper every night and warmed himself by his glowing fire.

"Ah!" raged the North Wind. "Little brown duck, Shingebiss, cares not for snow or ice or wind! Big Chief North Wind will freeze his holes, so he gets no food and then Big Chief will conquer him."

But when Shingebiss came and found his holes all closed so he could not reach the water, he did not even murmur. He went cheerily on till he found a pond that was free of snow and had more rushes. Then he pulled up the rushes and made new holes through which he could do his fishing.

North Wind grew angrier still.

"Brown duck shall know who is Big Chief!" he howled, and for days he followed close on the little duck's footsteps, froze up his holes in the ice almost as soon as he made them and covered his ponds with snow. But Shingebiss walked fearlessly forth as before, and always managed to get a few fish before each hole was frozen, or found some other pond that was free and made new holes. So he still went cheerily home every night dragging his fish behind him.

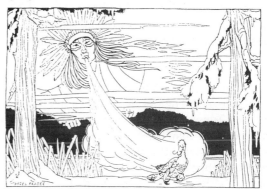

At last the North Wind roared in a fury!

"Woo-oo-oo! Woo-oo-oo! Big Chief go to brown duck's lodge, blow in at his door, sit down beside him, and breathe icy breath till he freezes."

Now Shingebiss had just eaten his supper, his log was burning bright, and he sat cozily warming his little webbed feet by the blaze.

Carefully North Wind crept up to his door, holding his breath, so Shingebiss should not know he was coming. Quietly, quietly, he crept along over the snow. But Shingebiss felt the icy cold come in through the cracks of the door. He thought "I know who is there" and he began to sing sturdily:

"Ka neej, ka neej,
Bee in, bee in,
Bon in, bon in,
Ok ee, ok ee,
Ka weya, ka weya"

Now the North Wind know this was his way of saying:

"North Wind, North Wind,
    fierce in feature,
You are still my fellow creature;
Blow your worst,
    you cannot freeze me,
I fear you not, and so I'm FREE."

Then North Wind was angrier than ever:

"Little brown duck to sing so boldly! Big Chief can bite him, sting him, freeze him!"

So North Wind crept in under the door, slipped up behind Shingebiss and sat down by the fire. Now Shingebiss knew he was there, but he paid no heed. He kept on singing louder than ever:

"Ka neej! Ka neej! Bee in, bee in."

"Big Chief stay here till he freezes," whistled North Wind, and he tried to breathe more fiercely than ever. But at that moment Shingebiss stirred his fire till the sparks leaped up the smoke-flue and the log glowed ruddy gold. Then all at once North Wind's frosty hair began to drip, his icy beard began to drip, the tears ran down his cheeks, and his breath came puffing more and more faintly. Still Shingebiss warmed his little webbed feet by the blaze and sang:

"North Wind, North Wind,
    fierce in feature,
You are still my fellow creature."

At length North Wind gave a shriek.

"Big Chief is melting!" And he rushed headlong through the doorway, fled out into the darkness, and fell upon a snowbank.

"Strange little brown duck, Shingebiss," he murmured weakly. "Big Chief North Wind can't starve him, can't freeze him, can't make him afraid! Ugh! Ugh! North Wind will let him alone. The Great Spirit is with him."

Miller (1925)

Children of empathic parents spontaneously express empathic behavior at an early age. A 12-month-old girl saw her mother crying. She ran over to her mother and patted her mother's face and then put her head in her mother's lap (Zahn-Waxler & Radke-Yarrow, 1979). A 13-month-old girl overheard her mother's friend share feelings of sadness; the little girl walked over and offered her beloved doll to the sad friend (Hoffman, 1977). Anthropologist Margaret Bacon and associates (1963) examined data on 48 nonliterate societies in Africa, North and South America, Asia, and the South Pacific. Social conflict and violent crime were absent in societies with nurturing and empathic parents. Parents who model helpfulness, empathy, and friendliness raise children with these qualities (London, 1970; McClelland, Constantian, Regalado, & Stone, 1982; Rosenhan, 1970; Yarrow, MacTurk, Vietze, McCarthy, Klein, & McQuiston, 1984).

Parents teach empathy by modeling empathy, and by using "affective explanations." Affective explanations such as "She doesn't want to play now" or "You might hurt him" encourage awareness of the feelings of others, and encourage the child to behave in ways that show sensitivity and concern for the needs of others. Children who are exposed to affective explanations demonstrate high levels of social maturity, helpfulness, and empathy, and they are rated by peers as generous and helpful (Brody & Shafer, 1982; Hoffman, 1982; Radke-Yarrow & Zahn-Waxler, 1984). Parents who use force and threats teach fear of punishment as a motivation for behavior, not empathy, and raise children who are not sensitive to the needs of others and who lack the ability to self regulate (Baumrind, 1973; Kuczynski, 1983; Lepper, 1983).

Adolescents with strong ties to friends and parents are not likely to be depressed, commit suicide, or become addicted to drugs (Harlow, Newcomb, & Bentler, 1986). How do strong social ties develop? The answer is clear. Parents who are friendly and empathic with their children teach their children to be friendly and empathic with others, which enhances social ties. Adolescent girls who are treated democratically and affectionately by their mothers tend to form more intimate ties to best friends than do girls whose mothers are distant and autocratic (Gold & Yanof, 1985). In a study of 18,000 adolescents, grades 7 through 12, those who perceived their parents as warm, interested, understanding, sharing, and helpful felt closer to their friends than those who perceived their parents as cold, strict, and harsh (Curtis, 1975).

Nonaggressiveness in children is a significant predictor of social success, health, and educational and occupational success. Aggressive behavior in children is a significant predictor of social failure, psychopathology, aggression, and low educational and occupational success (Eron, 1987). The characteristic of nonaggressiveness is also taught through modeling. Parents teach their children to be aggressive or nonaggressive primarily through the type of discipline they use when conflicts arise.

Parents of nonaggressive children teach problem solving as a way of dealing with conflict and do not use physical punishment (Cummings, Iannotti, & Zahn-Waxler, 1985; Eron, 1987). In a prospective 22-year study, University of Chicago psychologist Leonard Eron and colleagues studied 600 children and interviewed their parents. The most significant predictor of aggressive behavior in children was the use of physical punishment by the parents. In contrast, nonaggressive children had parents who used reason and logical consequences to resolve conflict and enforce rules (Eron, 1987; Eron & Huseman, 1984), as described in Chapter 12.

Parents of nonaggressive children are generally rational and consistent in the development and application of rules. Parents of aggressive children are generally arbitrary and inconsistent in the development and application of rules (Baumrind, 1971, 1973). Children from families with consistent rules are more competent and less aggressive (Patterson & Stouthamer-Loeber, 1984).

Teaching Values

One of my earliest memories is of a night during a visit to my grandmother at her cottage on the dunes above a great, sandy beach. It must have been an unusually beautiful night for someone to have said, "Let's wake the baby and show her the stars." The mosquito netting was untucked, I was picked up and carried out onto the beach, and there above me was the night sky, luminous with stars and the great flowing river of the Milky Way. I was too young to understand in any conscious way that this sight of the glory of creation was to set my way of looking at the universe, and at my small place in it.

Madeleine L'Engle, author,
cited in Berman (1986)

"Values" refer to a person's beliefs about what is important and what is unimportant. Education is a value for most people, because they believe that education is important. Values are the principles that govern decisions. The decision to go to college is based on the value of education, the belief that education is important.

Parents model values by what they say and do. Children of parents who listen to classical music appreciate classical music; children of parents who value the equality of all people have this value; children whose parents are adventurers and love nature become adventurers and love nature. This is the general rule unless parents are abusive, demeaning, or "pushy" and insist that the children adopt their values, in which case the effort may backfire (Cooper, Grotevant, & Condon, 1982). Parents are not the only source of values for children, but for most children, they play a central role.

Friedman and Rosenman observed that parents of Type B people taught the importance of values such as beauty, religion, and unconditional love (Friedman & Rosenman, 1975; Friedman & Ulmer, 1984). However, systematic study of the transmission of transcendental values from parents to children has been neglected.

Summary

Good parenting is so important to the development of the child that it must be considered a dynamic in health and wellness. Nurturing caregivers have unconditional positive regard for their children, they model openness to change, and give their children the freedom to develop a sense of independence and control.

The parents of hardy children avoid the pitfalls of parenting, such as rigidly requiring the accomplishment of unrealistic tasks or believing that doing things for the child that the child can do herself is a sign of love.

Through modeling, parents teach important social skills. They teach children how to be friendly and empathic, and how to solve problems through reason, logic, and the application of fair rules.

It is true that resilient children, described in Chapter 6, are healthy in spite of bad parenting, but they are the exceptions and they usually have another adult who provides the needed nurture and modeling. The foundations of a healthy person are in the child's parenting. It must be obvious to you that a caregiver who teaches the child to be hardy and stress-resistant must be a hardy, stress-resistant person; a caregiver who teaches empathy must be an empathic person. If you are raising children or plan to, evaluate yourself. Learn to transmit to your children the characteristics of hardiness, stress resistance, creativity, and well-being, which will prepare them for a lifetime of health and wellness.

||||➡

SECTION THREE: EDUCATION AND THE DEVELOPMENT OF HEALTHY CHILDREN

Nine seems to have been a magical year in my life, for it was also at that age that I moved into the class in my elementary school where my teacher for the next four years was George Bidgood. It was from Mr. Bidgood that I learned the most important of all the lessons from my life: the nature and necessity of love. It was not that Mr. Bidgood, so far as I recollect, ever uttered the word, nor do I think that any of us were ever aware of the fact that something remarkable was happening in his class. It was only years later that I understood what had occurred. Mr. Bidgood not only loved children, but considered it a privilege to be with them. He kept a notebook on each child, evaluating each one's aptitudes, personality, intellect, and other traits, each child being treated as a person and respected as such. He would call on parents to discuss their children with them, always with encouraging words, often suggesting that it would be a good thing if they could send their children to a better school in which their talents could bloom more fully.

Ashley Montagu, anthropologist
and author, cited in Berman (1986)

The importance of a healthy adult model cannot be underestimated, but children who do not have healthy parents are not lost; other adults can fulfill the parental role—ministers, relatives, friends of the family, coaches, and teachers (Foster & Seltzer, 1986). The school is an important setting for the development of a healthy personality. In this section we examine educational programs that foster the personality characteristics of healthy people.

Preschools

In 1986, 9 million preschoolers spent their days in the care of someone other than their mother or father. Fifty percent of working women return to work before their child's first birthday; most mothers say that they must return to work to pay the bills. High-quality day-care centers can foster social skills and may compensate for inadequate parenting. After learning to share and interact with peers, children in these day-care centers continue to demonstrate social skills in kindergarten and elementary school (Clarke-Stewart & Fein, 1983; McCartney, 1985; Rutter, 1983; Scarr, 1984). An experimental group of 4-year-old Head Start children learned social skills through games, dialogues, and videos in 20-minute lessons over a 10-week period. At the end of the program, these children had made significant gains in empathy, friendliness, and assertiveness compared with children without training. The gains were maintained at follow-up a year later (Spivack &

Shure, 1974). Long-term follow-up studies have shown that for many children, being in Head Start improved IQ, social skills, and cognitive skills, in comparison with children who did not participate in Head Start (Consortium for Longitudinal Studies, 1983; Lazar & Darlington, 1982; Miller & Bizzel, 1984).

The quality of the preschool program is the key to its effectiveness. Programs that have a low teacher-student ratio and nurturing teachers provide the best care. For very young children, the ideal ratio is not more than five children to one adult. Harvard psychologists Jerome Kagan, Richard Kearsley, and Philip Zelazo (1978) established a day-care center in Boston for children ages 4 to 29 months. The ratio was one day-care worker to three children. The day-care children were equal in intellectual, emotional, and social areas to children kept at home.

Elementary and Secondary Schools

"Schools Make a Difference" is the title of a comprehensive critique of public schools written by University of Missouri researcher Thomas Good and University of California, Berkeley, researcher Rhona Weinstein. Good and Weinstein (1986) concluded that there are good schools and bad schools. In contrast to students in mediocre or poor schools, students in good schools have higher levels of achievement, less delinquency, and higher self-esteem and competency. In contrast to teachers in ineffective schools, Good and Weinstein found that teachers in effective schools believe that all children can learn and that the school has a primary responsibility in helping children learn. This is an interesting finding at a time when many school teachers and administrators feel, perhaps rightly, that parents are abdicating responsibility and expect the school to "do everything." In any case, the enhancement of self-efficacy and self-esteem in children is a major contribution of good schools.

Self-Efficacy

Jane, age 5, is in kindergarten. She loves school. She is the first to raise her hand when the teacher asks a question, and she tackles assignments with enthusiasm. Jane likes to do things for herself. She is proud that she can wake herself up, dress herself, and make breakfast for herself. Jane believes that she is one of the brightest children in the class. In fact, her natural ability is no greater than most of the other kindergartners.

Mary, age 6, is in the first grade. Her progress is slow. She never raises her hand when the teacher asks a question. Mary does her assignments without enthusiasm. At home, her mother wakes her up, helps her get dressed, and fixes breakfast for her. Mary thinks that she is one of the least intelligent children in the class. In fact, her natural ability is greater than most of the children in her class.

It is clear that Jane has a sense of self-efficacy and is confident in her ability to accomplish what she sets out to do. Mary is the opposite and lacks a sense of self-efficacy. Because Jane has a sense of self-efficacy, she uses available resources to effectively cope with her school environment, while a lack of self-efficacy prevents Mary from using her resources. As we have noted many times, people who have a sense of self-efficacy cope more effectively with stressful events than people who do not. In Chapter 6, you learned that self-efficacy is an element of learned resourcefulness: people with a sense of self-efficacy initiate coping skills, expend more effort, and persist longer in the face of stressful experiences than people who lack a sense of self-efficacy. Self-efficacy is crucial for becoming a hardy, stress-resistant person. Stanford psychologist Albert Bandura found that self-efficacy is developed by observing people successfully confront difficult situations. In a study of people who are frightened by snakes, Bandura and Adams found these people can overcome fear by watching other people behave in a nonfearful manner in the presence of snakes (Bandura & Adams, 1977). Children develop self-efficacy by watching their parents, teachers, siblings, friends, and even television characters confront difficult situations. Again we note that fairy tales have this function.

It is clear that teachers can enhance the self-efficacy of children. To foster self-efficacy, the teacher must first expect the student to be capable of significant learning. Second, the teacher must establish challenging goals that the student can accomplish. Third, the teacher must provide procedures and feedback for helping the child accomplish the goal. Fourth, the teacher must help the student develop a cognitive framework for understanding failure as a lack of effort or appropriate strategy, rather than as a lack of ability. Fifth, a pleasant emotional climate must characterize the learning environment.

An overworked teacher with a crowded classroom might wonder how all this can be accomplished for every child with low self-efficacy. We do not know. As schools lose teachers and as class size increases, the task of helping each child becomes more difficult unless the child is placed in a special-education classroom. In any case, these are the ingredients to fostering improved sense of self-efficacy in children.

Research indicates that challenging tasks are more motivating for children than frequent praise for easy tasks (Brown, Palincsar, & Purcell, 1984). Robert Rosenthal (1971) misled a group of teachers by telling them that certain students had high IQ scores but were "late bloomers" and that these students might show unusual intellectual development during the school year. Later in the year the "bloomers" were rated by the teachers as more curious, interested, and happier than other students. At the end of the year, the "bloomers" had increased their IQ scores by more than 15 points compared to the "non-bloomers." Rosenthal showed that teachers' expectations enhanced the performance of the children because the

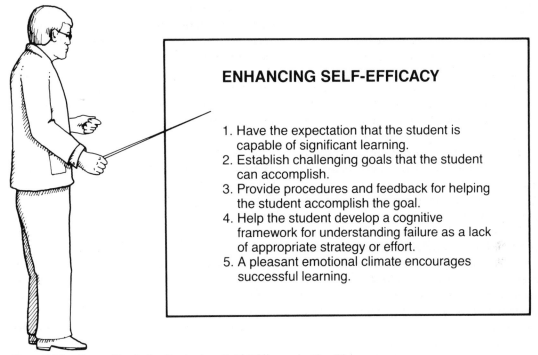

ENHANCING SELF-EFFICACY

1. Have the expectation that the student is capable of significant learning.
2. Establish challenging goals that the student can accomplish.
3. Provide procedures and feedback for helping the student accomplish the goal.
4. Help the student develop a cognitive framework for understanding failure as a lack of appropriate strategy or effort.
5. A pleasant emotional climate encourages successful learning.

Figure 19.2. Ingredients for Fostering Self-Efficacy in the Classroom.

teachers had given challenging goals to the children who thought they were of high intelligence. The teachers also gave unchallenging goals, with too little and too easy work, to children who thought they were of low intelligence (Dweck, 1986).

When children learn skills, when they do things for themselves and feel good about accomplishing goals through effort and appropriate strategies, they develop a sense of competency and self-efficacy. This in turn encourages further effort, harder goals, and greater competency and self-efficacy.

Social Skills

Children can learn important social skills at school through instruction. To learn problem-solving skills, third-, fourth-, and fifth-graders watched videotapes of children struggling with problems such as conflicts with friends,

and then saw the children using problem-solving skills to resolve the problems. Later, when confronting similar problems in real life, the children applied the skills for resolving the interpersonal conflicts (Stone, Hindz, & Schmidt, 1975).

Norma Feshbach, a professor in the Department of Education at the University of California, Los Angeles, is a pioneer in teaching empathy skills to children. Feshbach (1984) assessed empathy skills and gave empathy exercises to third-, fourth-, and fifth-grade students who were identified as aggressive by their teachers. Twenty-four children, the control group, were tested but did not participate in the empathy exercises. In 30 hours of training, children in the experimental group learned empathy skills for identifying emotions felt by others, understanding situations from another person's perspective, and personally experiencing another person's emotions. The children learned to identify emotions of others conveyed in photographs, in tape recordings of emotion-laden conversations, in videotaped pantomimes, and in psychodramas. Children also role-played both parts of an emotional scene involving two children, first one part and then the other. The dramas were videotaped, and the children reviewed the tapes and discussed the emotions of the characters. The results were impressive. There was a 50 percent gain in prosocial behaviors such as cooperation, and a reduction in aggression. The behavior of the children in the control group did not change.

Empathy is a key ingredient in healthy social relationships. It is clearly possible to enhance empathy skills of young children, even children who are aggressive. Feshbach points out, however, that the gains made in a school program can be overwhelmed by family and social forces that perpetuate aggression. We note also that few schools provide empathy training. Educators and researchers have demonstrated the value of empathy training, but enhancing empathy in children is not part of many school curriculums.

Social psychologists Irwin and Barbara Sarason, a husband-and-wife team at the University of Washington, pioneered in programs for adolescents at risk of delinquency and dropping out of school (Sarason & Sarason, 1981). One out of three poor children drop out of school (U.S. Department of Education, 1986), and programs that stem this tide are important. Sarason and Sarason pioneered in research on programs for prevention of delinquency and dropout. As part of a health class curriculum, 127 ninth-grade students with dropout and delinquency records were randomly assigned to a control group or to one of two experimental groups. The control group received the regular health class curriculum. The curriculum for the experimental groups included observing models role-playing cognitive and social skills in the following situations: job interview, peer pressure, asking for help in school, asking questions in class, getting along with the boss, dealing with frustration on the job, cutting class, asking for help at work, and getting along with parents. One experimental group observed "live" models, and the other experimental group watched the same situations on video. The following script is an example of a "role-play module" that students witnessed.

Scene: Cutting class.

Tom: Hey, Jim, you want to go down to Green Lake fourth period?

Jim: What are you gonna do down at Green Lake?

Tom: A bunch of us are gonna take the afternoon off and party it up.

Jim: I don't think I can go. Sixth period Mr. Smith is reviewing for the algebra exam.

Tom: What about coming over and staying until sixth?

Jim: Well, I kind of like Mr. Jones's class. Besides, it's too hard to get to Green Lake and back in an hour and 40 minutes. I could come after school.

Tom: You know, Lydia is going to be there.

Jim (noticeable interest): She is?

Tom: Yeah. And by the time school is over, who knows if the party will still be there. We might go over to someone's house.

Jim's cognitions: *Gee, I really want to go to that party. Maybe I can get up the nerve to ask Lydia out. But I should stay for that algebra review, at least. The test will be hard enough without missing the review.*

Tom: You know, it is Friday afternoon and a beautiful day.

Jim's cognitions: *I wish Tom would let me make my own decision. This isn't easy. Maybe I could study hard during the weekend. Then I won't need to go the the review. But will I really study on a Saturday?*

Tom: Well, are you going to come?

Jim: I don't know, Tom. I'll have to think about it some more. Maybe I'll see you there fourth. If not, I'll probably come later.

Tom: Okay, I hope you come.

After observing a role-play module, the students and teacher discuss the consequences of Jim's decision from the perspective of students, teachers, and parents. The key principles involved in Jim's decision are discussed; students form small groups to role-play a similar situation.

At the one-year follow-up, students in the two experimental groups had significantly better school attendance, had fewer behavioral problems, and had demonstrated improvement in social and cognitive skills, in comparison with the students in the control group. There were no significant differences between the two experimental groups.

Social skills are essential for positive interpersonal relationships. Because children may not learn these skills at home, training programs must be implemented in the school systems. Empathy, friendliness, and problem-solving skills can be taught in school. The work of Sarason and Sarason demonstrates effectiveness of these programs. If you went to an average high school, you know that problems abound. Theft and violence are common, and a high percentage of students drop out. Teaching an adolescent basic skills such as problem-solving, assertiveness, and empathy could conceivably change the course of that person's life. Unfortunately, such programs are rare. Longitudinal studies on the effectiveness of these programs are even rarer, because of a lack of funding.

Values and Moral Reasoning

The development of transcendental values through educational programs has not been studied. However, a related area, moral development, has been studied, and programs for helping children develop moral reasoning have led to another area, values clarification.

Lawrence Kohlberg, for many years a professor in the Department of Education at Harvard University, was the leading theorist and researcher on moral development in this country. Kohlberg studied the moral reasoning of thousands of adults and children in several countries. A person's level of moral reasoning was determined by responses to a series of moral dilemmas. A typical dilemma is presented in this story:

> In Europe a woman was near death from a special kind of cancer. There was one drug that the doctors thought might save her. It was a form of radium that a druggist in the same town had recently discovered. The drug was expensive to make, but the druggist was charging ten times what the drug cost him to make. He paid $200 for the radium and charged $2,000 for a small dose of the drug. The sick woman's husband, Heinz, went to everyone he knew to borrow the money, but he could only get together $1,000, which is half of what it cost. He told the druggist that his wife was dying and asked him to sell it cheaper or let him pay later. But the druggist said, "No, I discovered the drug, and I am going to make money from it." So Heinz got desperate and broke into the man's store to steal the drug for his wife.
>
> (Kohlberg, 1969, p. 379)

Take a minute: Answer this question: "Was Heinz right to steal the drug for his wife?" In answering this question you are tackling a moral dilemma. When you have answered this question, imagine that you are being interviewed; the interviewer asks you to explain your answer. A good interviewer would lead you to the reasoning behind your answer, so think through your reasoning until you come to the core of your immediate response.

Do It Now.

Kohlberg found that responses to moral dilemmas can be categorized into six levels of moral reasoning, and he found that to some extent, moral reasoning changes with age and is therefore developmental (see Figure 19.3)

Now compare your response to the question "Was Heinz right to steal the drug for his wife?" to typical responses at each stage of moral development: (1) No, God would punish him if he did that; he would get punished; he might fall out of a tree or something. (2) Well,

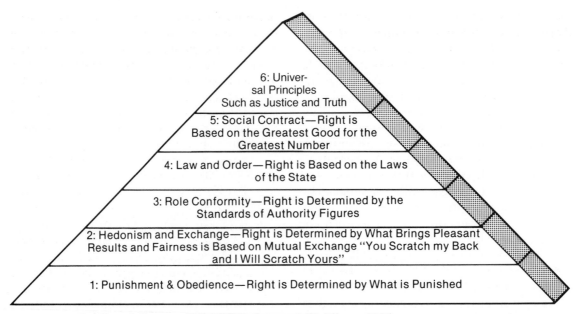

Figure 19.3. Kohlberg's Stages of Moral Development (Kohlberg, 1969).

Heinz should steal the drug. He is a good husband, and he loves his wife very much, and she loves him, and it would make her very happy. He should apologize to the druggist, but the druggist was not being very nice; he should have given Heinz the drug. (4) No, Heinz should not steal the drug. That would be against the law. He should try to change the druggist's mind or get more money, but he should not break the law. (5) In this case, Heinz should steal the drug for his wife, because, whether he loves her or not, this is a moral obligation, and people must be responsible for one another. Actually, the druggist was being immoral, and society should prevent this sort of thing. (6) Yes, Heinz should steal the drug to save his wife because the value of life comes before everything else. Even though the druggist may have had a right to sell the drug, and even though Heinz was breaking the law, these conderations are not as important as the value of life itself. This is the highest principle.

Kohlberg found that many adults do not move beyond stages 3 or 4, and that moral reasoning based on universal principles was uncommon unless the person was educated in a religious or academic setting in which universal principles were taught and valued.

Kohlberg's research sparked intense interest in the development of values and moral reasoning in children. Several educators, including Kohlberg and his colleagues, took up the challenge of designing programs for enhancing the moral values of children and adolescents. Typically, children were presented dilemmas such as the Heinz story. After presenting the dilemma, the teacher led the students in a discussion of what the moral action would be: steal the drug or let his wife die. Several researchers found that these discussions involving moral reasoning led to an upward shift of at least a half-stage in most children (Schaefli, Rest, & Thoma, 1985).

The small shift in moral reasoning, however, does not improve behavior, as measured in the classroom. In an interesting study with delinquents, William Niles (1986) at Fordham University attempted to facilitate moral reasoning by having a group of adolescents discuss moral dilemmas and reach a consensus on how the dilemma should be solved. Niles thought that the consensus requirement would force the participants to seriously consider the beliefs of others, including the facilitator. Compared with a control group and a group that only discussed the dilemmas, a few students in the consensus group did increase moral reasoning by one stage. While this is encouraging, the move was from stage 1 to stage 2 moral reasoning. Stage 2 is characteristic of delinquency: "I have the right to whatever I want"; therefore, the shift in moral reasoning had no effect on behavior. Participants who were at stage 2 stayed at that level. Even after 32 sessions, no one had moved to stage 3 reasoning.

To improve moral behavior as well as moral reasoning, values-clarification programs became popular in the 1970s. The purpose of most values-clarification programs is to encourage students to express their values in concrete actions. Education professors Simon, Howe, and Kirschenbaum (1972) developed a values-clarification handbook for teachers with activities that help students clarify, critically analyze, and follow through on their values. In one exercise children publicly affirm their values in response to forced-choice questions such as "Which do you identify with more, a Volkswagen or a Cadillac?" Adolescents face tougher questions: "If you were a 16-year-old girl who had been raped, and were pregnant from the rape, would you have an abortion?" Students discuss their choice with a classmate who made the opposite choice. Another values-clarification activity is the "public interview." In this strategy, students volunteer to be interviewed by the rest of the class and publicly affirm their stand on various issues.

After students have clarified and critically analyzed their values, they act on their values. In an action exercise, students list five changes that would improve the nation, and then each student sends a telegram to an important

person who could influence national policy. In another exercise, students propose five changes that would improve their community or state. Then a list of action steps is handed out, and each student decides on a particular course of action. The student makes a contract on the steps that she or he will take to improve the community or state. A month later students report on their action projects.

Critics of values clarification argue that classroom discussions of values, and even action projects, will not carry over into real life. Critics also argue that simply clarifying values does not mean that the students will adopt values that enhance their well-being. In an evaluation of the literature, Lovin (1988) states that values-clarification programs have yet to demonstrate the effectiveness of actually enhancing the values of students. Most students maintain the values of their parents and their culture. Values-clarification programs simply clarify values that children have already accepted.

The most effective program for enhancing moral values and eliciting behavior change was the "just environment" program designed by Kohlberg and colleagues (Higgins, Power, & Kohlberg, 1984). The program involved two schools in the Boston area. A separate "community" of 60 students was formed in each school—a "school within a school." All rules, and methods of enforcing rules, were established in meetings in which each student and teacher received one vote. The program was referred to as a "just" environment because it was based on a system of justice that was created by all. Students were responsible for establishing and enforcing the rules. The results were highly significant. Stealing and petty crime virtually disappeared among the 60 students, and students jumped two stages in moral development. Cooperation and caring became group norms.

If stealing or not stealing and caring and cooperation are moral issues, then certainly morality changed when students were given the opportunity to create their own system of justice and a community. Most importantly, moral reasoning was enhanced.

Kohlberg (1981) hypothesized that moral reasoning is a necessary condition, but not a sufficient condition, for moral behavior. To improve moral behavior, the school experience must represent a real life experience. The success of the "just environment" program demonstrates this.

A 20-year longitudinal study by sociologist Melvin Kohn and colleagues (1959, 1983) has shown that socialization forces embedded in the family, school, and workplace are the most powerful in shaping values. Similar results were found in a longitudinal study by Cornwall (1987). In 1933, John Dewey, America's leading educator and theorist, said that schools provide moral education by virtue of a "hidden curriculum" that teaches both obedience to and defiance of authority, rather than democratic principles and moral reasoning. Today it is recognized that the school is a moral system and teaches values explicitly or implicitly (Santrock, 1987). Whether they mean to or not, teachers and administrators serve as models of ethical behaviors and values. Classroom rules and peer relations also manifest values and ethical attitudes.

Values-clarification programs and moral-discussion classes will not significantly enhance values unless the hidden authoritarian curriculum is replaced with a democratic and just curriculum (Haan, 1985; Higgins, Power, & Kohlberg, 1984). The "just community" has been the most effective program for enhancing moral reasoning and moral behavior. The success of the program may be due in part to the fact that the "hidden curriculum" was altered so that students participated in a school structure that required students to use moral reasoning in order to establish a fair system.

Dewey emphasized that "experience-based learning is the best teacher." This is borne out in the history of values-clarification and moral-discussion programs for enhancing moral behavior. The most significant learning occurred in programs that combined thought and action, such as the "just environment" program. An excellent example of the power of experience-based education is described at the end of this chapter. Now we proceed to another type of experience-based education, also very important to the development of the healthy person.

Stress-Management Programs

You are well aware of the importance of stress management for health and wellness. Because children are not immune to stress, and because the school is a stressful environment for many children, the school is an excellent setting in which to teach and practice stress-management skills.

Several stress-management and relaxation programs have been developed for children. One of the first programs was conducted by Loretta Englehardt in Spearfish, North Dakota (Englehardt, 1976). Englehardt is an innovative educator with training in nursing, counseling, and biofeedback therapy. From 1976 to 1978, 194 students in grades 1 through 12 and 54 administrators, teachers, and parents participated in a biofeedback training and relaxation program created by Englehardt. The project began with a six-week program for adults, staff members, and parents. Parents and staff had 18 sessions of relaxation training at the school. EMG and temperature feedback were used to enhance learning. All participants completed the six-week course and were enthusiastic about biofeedback and relaxation training. The enthusiasm of the staff and parents spread to the students. Students eagerly began 18 biofeedback and relaxation sessions. The students liked the program and reported many positive benefits.

> "I can relax when I am having tests and remember."
> "I used to be tense when skiing, now I am relaxed."

"It is easier to figure out answers to questions just by relaxing totally."

"I relax every night before I go to bed, it helps me sleep and makes me feel good about me."

"Relaxation helps my headaches, my work in school and helps me when I'm in trouble."

Pre- and post-training measures showed that the children had significantly reduced their levels of anxiety and enhanced their self-image. Students' self-reports were positive and enthusiastic. Soon, six other South Dakota schools began a relaxation program for children in high school, junior high, and elementary schools.

Elizabeth Stroebel, director of the Behavioral Education and Self Regulation Institute in Hartford, Connecticut, developed a set of short relaxation exercises for children called the Kiddie QR (quieting response) (Stroebel & Stroebel, 1980). The Kiddie QR (described in Chapter 16) guides the child through 16 lesson plans. The lessons help children identify stressful situations, Type A behaviors, and unproductive worries and helps them learn relaxation and cognitive skills. Metaphors such as "Rigid Robot," "Fighty Fists," and "Grouchy Head" help children discriminate negative body states. Other metaphors, such as "Breathing Pores," "Magic Jaw String," "Finger Balloons," and "Octopus," are called "body friends" that help the child relax and overcome negative states. "Breathing Pores" are described as magic breathing holes that bring heaviness and warmth into the body (Stroebel & Stroebel, 1984). Over 850 school districts have adopted the Kiddie QR as part of the regular curriculum. No studies have been reported on the effectiveness of the Kiddie QR for helping children relax. Two controlled studies found that the Kiddie QR training helped improve attention (Petosa & Oldfield, 1985) and short-term memory (Disorbio, 1985).

Elizabeth Stroebel has translated many concepts of health and wellness into language and techniques that are understandable and interesting to children. The Kiddie QR is fun for children and provides a curriculum for teaching children to be stress resistant. Research is needed to assess its long-term effectiveness.

One of the largest relaxation programs was conducted by Doris Matthews, a professor of education at South Carolina State College, with rural students in South Carolina. Matthews conducted her first study with 571 seventh-grade students. The students were randomly assigned to either an experimental or a no-training control group. Students in the experimental group practiced relaxation training skills aided by EDR and temperature feedback, 15 minutes every morning for nine months. Autogenic training, progressive relaxation, guided imagery, and diaphragmatic breathing exercises were practiced throughout the year. Paper-pencil pre- and post-training measures of self-concept were made, as were observer ratings of classroom behavior.

In comparison to the control group, girls in the experimental group had better self-concept, and both boys and girls had fewer discipline infractions. No improvement in self-concept was found for the boys, and no improvement in academic performance was found for either boys or girls.

Most children learn relaxation skills and gain psychophysiological self regulation with ease. The studies noted here were beneficial, as indicated by a number of measures. The mastery of relaxation and stress-management skills was not tested in these studies, however, and training to mastery would undoubtedly have improved results (Shellenberger & Green, 1986).

In a program for five children with stress-related symptoms, we combined relaxation training and mastery tasks. The relaxation task was to increase finger temperature to 95°F in five minutes and lower forehead EMG to 2.5 µV peak-to-peak or less in 15 minutes. In the mastery tasks, the children had to demonstrate self regulation skills in stressful situations. The first task was to put one hand into a bucket of ice water for 30 seconds and after the hand was removed, warm the other hand to 95° in five minutes. In the second task, the child was provoked by our 200-pound colleague for five minutes and then challenged to warm both hands to 95° in five minutes. For the third task, a parent, sibling, or friend was enlisted to provoke the child for five minutes, and then the child was challenged to warm the hands up to 95° in five minutes. Large graphs in the shape of a thermometer recorded each child's progress and were placed on a wall in the training room. The children were motivated by the challenging tasks and practiced relaxation exercises diligently at home. All five children mastered all of the tasks and significantly reduced their symptoms. For accomplishing these mastery tasks, each child received a beautiful liquid crystal ring that monitored skin temperature.

Mastery tasks also help college students. In a biofeedback and stress-management class at the University of North Carolina at Asheville, Professors Buckalew and McDonagh (1987) give a performance examination as well as an academic examination. Twenty percent of the student's grade depends on the performance examination. The student must demonstrate mastery of warming and cooling the hands by warming for 10 minutes and then cooling for 5 minutes. In a class of 44 students, 41 elevated their hand temperature, but only 32 decreased their hand temperature. Student reports indicated that the majority felt that the mastery tasks helped them perform under pressure.

In general, goals of relaxation and stress-management programs for children have not been challenging enough. In a comprehensive relaxation program conducted by Matthews (1984), students became bored with passive activities such as guided imagery and relaxation every school day for five months. Such activities need to be supplemented with challenging goals such as demonstrating relaxation and stress-management skills in mastery situations. The research on effective education demonstrates the importance of establishing challenging goals for children that enhance motivation and self-efficacy.

Now we introduce a model educational program that excels in establishing mastery tasks for helping children and adults develop the personality characteristics of healthy people.

Outward Bound—Training in Hardiness

Take a minute: Everyone has had an adventure of some sort, no matter how seemingly simple. Almost any challenging experience can be an adventure. Go back into childhood or adolescence, and recall a challenging adventure. Try to recapture your feelings during the adventure and when it was over.
Do It Now.

Michael is scared. He is over 15 feet off the ground tied to a rope held by a belayer above him. The rock which offered so many footholds at the beginning of the climb is becoming smoother and smoother and steeper. Michael has been ascending the rock by jamming his feet into cracks and footholds. Only one foot is wedged in now. It hurts. The foot supports all his weight; the weighted leg twitches spasmodically. His other foot skitters aimlessly and frantically over the rock face in search of a purchase. His fingers, which tightly grip the chalky sandstone, begin to sweat, turning the chalk into a thick, slippery film of mud. Michael looks up. The top of the climb is guarded by an intimidating bulge of rock. If he wants to make it to the top, he has a choice. He can either muscle over the ledge or circumvent it entirely by climbing out and onto the face. Some choice. He imagines himself falling. Michael, a 15-year-old who is in trouble with the law and at school, begins to cry. His peers, who have either climbed the rock or are about to, cheer him on. His instructors, who have trekked with Michael in the wilds for a week, exhort him to succeed. Michael inches up, tears streaking his dusty face. Occasionally relying on a taut rope from his belayer, Michael manages the bulge. Over the lip, untying the rope, he whoops triumphantly, and slaps his seated belayer on the shoulder in appreciation. He turns around to gaze out at the vista below him. Blood trickles down a small gash on his knee; he wonders when he cut it. He did not feel it. His knuckles are chaffed white by the rock; his palms are pitted and coarse like sandpaper. He feels good. He feels complete. He feels heroic.

(Adapted from Gerald Golins, 1980. *Outward Bound and Troubled Youth.* Reprinted by permission of Outward Bound USA.)

Michael is participating in an Outward Bound course for juvenile offenders. Outward Bound is a worldwide adventure-based educational program with 48 schools on five continents. The purpose is to "enhance in its participants self-confidence and self-esteem, leadership, teamwork and empathy for others, service to the community and sensitivity to the environment" (Outward Bound, 1988, p. 4). The method is "learning by doing" through outdoor adventures that are mentally and physically strenuous.

Outward Bound began in Great Britain in 1941 as a training program for British seamen, hence the name. After the war, it evolved into an outdoor education program, and soon similar programs were started in the United States and elsewhere. Outward Bound is the most extensive of all outdoor education programs, with courses for college and high school students, for disadvantaged and handicapped adolescents, and for adolescents and young people who are in trouble with the law or who are overcoming alcohol and drug addiction. Recently, Outward Bound expanded its programs to include adults and senior citizens. In 1988, the U.S. Congress and president approved a presidential proclamation acknowledging Outward Bound's many years of educational service to youth.

Mountain-climbing, backpacking, canoeing, white-water rafting, kayaking, rock-climbing, mountaineering, cross-country skiing, sailing, and bicycling are the activities of Outward Bound. Through these activities, students encounter challenging situations in which they must overcome obstacles through teamwork, skill, and persistence. Focus for a moment on the significance of these elements—*challenge, teamwork, skill, and persistence.* Participants are challenged, but not without the skills to succeed. They are part of a team that provides social support and friendship, while requiring empathy, cooperation, and communication skills. Participants learn to persist in spite of discouragement and fatigue. These elements explain the success of the Outward Bound experience in fostering the key personality characteristics of the healthy personality.

Outward Bound courses involve five phases:

1. The first phase is training and preparation. Students get in condition for the upcoming adventure by running, swimming, and hiking. They learn first-aid techniques, search-and-rescue procedures, food planning and preparation, map and compass use, and how to plan an expedition. In this phase, students receive technical training in the activity of the expedition (rock-climbing, kayaking, sailing, and so on). During this training period students encounter the "wall." The wall is a 70-ft. vertical structure with handholds and footholds to a ledge halfway up. After reaching the ledge, students have to shinny up ropes to the top.
2. The second phase is the expedition, in which 8 to 12 students, accompanied by an instructor, carry out the expedition that they have planned.
3. The third phase is the solo, in which the student spends three days and three nights in the wilderness alone, with a minimum of equipment.
4. The fourth phase is discussion and reflection, in which students share their fears and discoveries during the program.

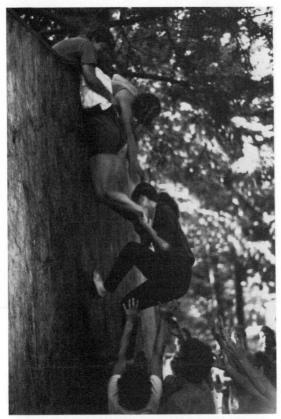

Outward Bound Participants Prepare for the "Wall" Through Teamwork and Courage.
Source: Outward Bound.

5. The final phase is a student-led expedition, in which the students receive little help from the instructor.

You know from your own adventure that the feelings of confidence, courage, and self-esteem stayed with you for some time. They may have been so powerful that your self-image changed, and you are who you are today because of your adventure. The intention of Outward Bound is to create an experience in which a positive self-image change can occur rapidly. An adventure can induce that quintessential experience of self such as Michael had when he made it over the top of the rock wall—good, complete, and heroic. Intense personal experience of success and personal

confrontation during the solo become referential experiences, the kind of experience that one refers back to as a reminder of personal accomplishment. Abraham Maslow coined the term "peak experience" to describe moments of intense happiness, relief, joy, and satisfaction. Peak experiences have powerful effects on a person's life, and life events are interpreted in the light of the experience. A peak experience becomes a ruler by which other events are measured. Students in Outward Bound programs have powerful peak experiences of mastery by overcoming difficult situations. At the same time, Outward Bound programs foster leadership, cooperation, and empathy, and teach two important transcendental values (the beauty of nature, and the importance of preserving it).

Outward Bound's success lies partly with its instructors. The instructors are empathic and encourage independence. They provide knowledge and feedback on survival skills, teach social skills, challenge the student with difficult tasks that develop competence and self-mastery, establish a structure that requires the student to be self-responsible and to cooperate with others, and model the characteristics of a healthy person.

Although the Outward Bound experience justifies itself, the researcher will ask "Is Outward Bound effective—does the experience have lasting effects?" More than 50 studies have been conducted on the effectiveness of Outward Bound programs (Burton, 1981; Swan, Stark, Hammerman, & Lewis, 1983). The results are consistent. For example, controlled studies on the effectiveness of Outward Bound programs with juvenile offenders and emotionally disturbed adolescents show improvement in self-esteem, locus of control, interpersonal competence, social acceptance, academic achievement, academic self-concept, physical fitness, and a decrease in recidivism (Bacon, 1987; Burton, 1981; Outward Bound, 1988; Wetmore, 1972). In a five-year follow-up of Outward Bound graduates, 98.6 percent of 2,400 students

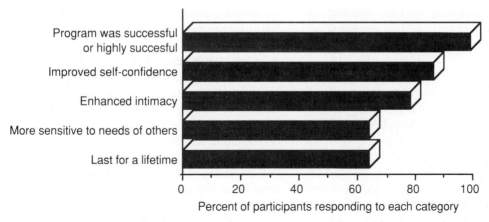

Figure 19.4.   A Five-Year Follow-Up of 2,400 Graduates of Outward Bound Indicates Lasting Benefits of Being in the Program. Adapted from S. Bacon (1987), *The Evolution of the Outward Bound Process.* **Adapted with Permission of the Publisher.**

said that the Outward Bound experience was either "successful" or "highly successful." Eighty-six percent reported that their self-confidence had improved, 78 percent felt that they had increased in general maturity, 64 percent believed that they had become more sensitive to the needs of others, and 64 percent believed that the positive changes would last for a lifetime (Fletcher, 1970).

We include Outward Bound in this chapter because we found that it facilitates the characteristics of health in a special way—adventure-based education. The setting in nature, the teamwork, the teachers, and the adventure generate a peak experience for young people that may last for a lifetime.

||||➡

CONCLUSION

In this chapter we enlarged the picture of the healthy person, shifting the focus from people who handle life stressors with hardiness and stress resistance to a more complete picture that includes transcendental values and goals. Self-actualization describes the process of evolving beyond the pursuit of personal, materialistic

goals to the pursuit of transcendental goals and the acceptance of transcendental values.

The concepts of transcendental goals and values and self-actualization describe the effort of the healthy person to reach "beyond the personal self," to have values and to strive for goals that encompass the larger spheres of humanity, nature, beauty, justice, and spirituality. People who survive the "slings and arrows of outrageous fortune," as Hamlet described life's events, who navigate the passages of life intact, and who have every advantage and choose to dedicate their lives to a cause—whether art, peace, justice, or knowledge—seem to be the psychologically healthiest among us.

This correlation between the healthy person and transcendental values and goals is not mere chance. It is related to the importance of purpose in life, to the healthful effects of high self-esteem, and to the development of characteristics that promote both psychological and physical health. These characteristics— hardiness and stress resistance, cheerfulness, optimism, and a sense of self-efficacy—facilitate and are facilitated by transcendental goals and values. Nor is the development of a healthy personality a matter of chance. We described the importance of a nurturing caregiver who provides an environment of love and unconditional support and teaches empathy, social skills, and values through modeling and coaching.

Nurture and healthy modeling from parents are the foundations of psychological health in the child; when absent, the child is at risk. Fortunately, another adult can provide the support. The school is a natural setting for the development of healthy personality characteristics because many of the child's challenges and triumphs are experienced at school. The classroom teacher provides nurture and instruction, and by promoting programs that help children develop social skills, stress-management skills, and values, the school system can be a force for health and wellness. However, as we write today, we are discouraged by the lack of school programs for helping children develop the personality characteristics and skills of healthy people. The busy classroom teacher cannot be expected to conduct special social-skills or moral-development programs, and most school systems have neither the funds nor curricula for doing so. Society has a long way to go to provide the opportunity for all children to develop the

personality characteristics of healthy people, but although the path is not well trodden, it is at least known.

Outward Bound, an adventure-based educational program, challenges students to new heights of self-mastery and cooperation, and to leadership and self-discovery, while instilling a love of natue and appreciation of beauty. Yet not all children who could rise to the challenge of an adventure have access to Outward Bound and similar programs. Parents and educators must bring the adventuring spirit to the child's everyday experiences.

We are encouraged by the fact that the characteristics of the healthy person are not a mystery and that the essentials of healthy development are known. In the introduction to Part Six we said, "When the right conditions are met, children grow into healthy adults, as inevitably as acorns grow into oak trees in good soil." This chapter is about the right conditions and the possibility of providing the right conditions and experiences for children and adolescents when they do not occur in the family.

PART *Seven*

Society and Health

This textbook is about the dynamics of health and wellness. We have examined many variables that promote psychological and physiological health, and we have examined personality characteristics and lifestyle habits that contribute to disease and illness. We have emphasized self regulation skills and personal self-responsibility as key elements in health. Self regulation and self-responsibility are characteristics of the individual.

But individuals are not isolated islands. We live in a societal and cultural milieu that influences every aspect of health and wellness, from the way that we are born to the way that we die. A textbook on the dynamics of health would not be complete without examining the larger picture, the social forces that influence the health and wellness of the individual.

The trend in medicine, and particularly in

behavioral medicine, is "holistic." That means that symptoms, illness, and disease are not separate from the person; the whole person is involved in illness and in health, and the whole person must be considered in treatment and prevention. The study of the dynamics of health and wellness would be incomplete if it focused only on the whole person and failed to take interest in the societal and cultural forces that influence the health of the individual. Ultimately the health and well-being of individuals depends on society, and therefore societal issues must concern everyone.

A variety of disciplines contribute to the subject of society and health: health psychology, health education, medical sociology and medical anthropology, behavioral medicine, community nursing, political science, community health, environmental health, and public health. As we were gathering material for Part Seven, a friend said "Society and Health? That is like writing on 'God and humanity.'" She was right. Society and Health is an extensive topic that could easily fill a volume. We have selected a few central topics that will extend your knowledge of the dynamics of health and wellness to the level of society; other topics could have been chosen.

Like many of the factors in life that affect health and wellness, society has both positive and negative effects and plays a role in promoting sickness and in facilitating health. We begin with the negative.

Chapter 20, Societal and Cultural Factors against Health and Wellness, introduces two dynamics that underlie worseness, the quick-fix mentality and forces in a free-market economy, or in any economy in which the profit motive is strong. Next, we examine several markets that promote worseness directly (such as the tobacco and alcohol industries), and that promote worseness indirectly, by involvement in treatment without promoting health and the prevention of illness and disease (the pharmaceutical and medical industries).

We include two social conditions that nearly guarantee a lack of psychological and physical health—violence and poverty. Finally we discuss specific ways in which government fails to safeguard the health and well-being of all people. Chapter 20 highlights both blatant and subtle forces in society that undermine health and work against self regulation and self-responsibility.

As the cost of treating disease and illness increases, so does concern for promoting health and preventing disease. In Chapter 21, Societal Forces for Health and Wellness, we focus on model programs that promote health and wellness, both in the "private sector" of business, and in the "public sector" of government, schools, the community, and prisons. The success of these programs is supported by a growing health consciousness in this country. Another important force that safeguards and promotes the health of all—private citizens groups—is described. We conclude Chapter 21 by broadening the focus to the international level.

As we move from the dynamics of health and wellness at the level of the person to the dynamics of health and wellness at the societal level, we also move from the emphasis on self regulation and self-responsibility to an emphasis on social responsibility through public action. It is our thesis that social responsibility is required of all people who live in a society that influences human and environmental health.

We believe that it is the responsibility of all to understand and change societal and cultural forces that promote illness and disease and to understand and promote societal and cultural forces that enhance the health and well-being of all. These chapters present a challenge and a direction for everyone who is interested in the dynamics of health and wellness.

CHAPTER 20

Societal and Cultural Forces against Health and Wellness

Take a minute: Imagine this. Tomorrow, with no warning whatsoever, all physicians, hospitals, clinics, drug companies, drugstores, health insurance companies, dentists, and all associated personnel will vanish from the face of the earth.

Think of that for a moment; nothing medical or pharmaceutical is left on earth. Medicine and medical research gone, no surgery, no checkups, no doctor to see.

Now answer these questions: Would you live your life differently beginning tomorrow? What would you do that you are not doing today? How would society help or hinder your goal of staying healthy?

Do It Now.

If you smoke, would you quit? If you drink, would you stop? If you live in a polluted, violent city, would you move? If you have been living on junk food, would you change your diet? If you have been sedentary, would you start getting in shape? If you have been stressed, would you take a class in stress management? Would you lose weight, start a support group, develop hardiness, and establish positive goals? Would you change your work environment? Would you learn to be assertive and play more? Would you become politically involved in promoting health?

If you grasp the implications of the "no medicine" scenario, you might be surprised to discover that you, like many other people, have two profound beliefs that work against your wellness lifestyle—that you are immune to the diseases of lifestyle that other people get, and that if something does happen, medicine will fix it.

There is much in society that supports these beliefs. In this chapter we examine the obvious and not-so-obvious forces in society that promote worseness and a lack of self-responsibility. This is not because the people behind these forces say "Let's create some worseness and lack of self-responsibility today," but because, as you will see, worseness and a lack of self-responsibility are by-products of these forces. Section One describes two foundations of worseness, different but interestingly complementary—the quick-fix mentality and the free-market economy that makes profit, not health, the guiding principle in industries that affect the health of the individual and the environment. In Section Two we discuss facts and figures related to four industries that we hope will be food for thought—the food, tobacco, alcohol, and pharmaceutical industries. These industries represent specific ways in which worseness is promoted or wellness is not, or both. In Section Three the medical industry is described, not because it promotes worseness per se, but because traditionally it has not promoted health and wellness and yet has authority in determining "health care" in this country. Section Four focuses on two societal problems that epitomize worseness and that are directly related to the health and well-being of hundreds of thousands of people, and therefore to us all, poverty and violence. In Section Five we discuss the role of the federal government, which has the financial power and structure to promote health and wellness for all. We discuss the role of government in worseness, a role that is characterized by passivity in regulating worseness industries and reluctance to make personal health and the health of the environment national priorities.

The food, pharmaceutical, and medical industries and the government are clear forces for health and wellness; in this chapter, however, our interest is on the ways in which these institutions threaten health and wellness. These are the forces that would be of no help if you had to rely solely upon yourself for health, and would not have prepared you to do so.

We include this chapter in a textbook on the dynamics of health because the study of health cannot ignore societal conditions that jeopardize health. The biopsychosocial approach recognizes societal factors that influence the individual's health, for better or worse. The biopsychosocial approach is also a systems approach, which is another way of talking about interconnectedness. Figure 20.1 highlights the elements in the system relevant to this chapter, elements that affect everyone, directly or indirectly.

We have repeatedly, and we hope persuasively, emphasized the necessity of self regulation and self-responsibility for personal health and wellness. In this chapter we emphasize social responsibility as part of the total picture. This means that individuals must do more than attend to personal health and wellness. Because everyone is part of the system and the system influences health and wellness, each individual must also promote health and wellness by a personal effort to change the social institutions that promote worseness.

Social responsibility requires knowledge. This chapter is not meant to provide all the knowledge needed to be an informed consumer or voter, a political activist, or a leader of a citizens' group. This chapter is meant to bring to your attention certain issues that are of immediate concern to you, as well as issues that may seem removed from your daily life.

As health professionals, we can hope that individuals will be self-responsible and will always make wise lifestyle choices, that everyone will become an informed consumer and wise voter, and that people become socially responsible. Health professionals know, however, that for many people, perhaps the majority, this is expecting a great deal. Furthermore, being an informed consumer does not guarantee a healthy lifestyle when environmental conditions—polluted water, air, and food, for example—are beyond personal control and choice. Social responsibility, therefore, does not lie solely with the individual; social responsibility extends to all elements of the system. No element in a system can be exempted from taking responsibility for the health and wellness of the individuals that it affects.

Individuals must be sensitive to societal forces that work against health and wellness. Some of these forces are obvious, such as the effects of tobacco on health and its enormous cost to society; other issues may seem quite unrelated to our topic, such as the manner in which campaign funds are acquired. Yet, you will find that the topics we have chosen are interrelated, and all exemplify basic issues that are related to health. We hope that you will be challenged by the immediacy of these issues, by the difficulty of changing the larger picture, and by the importance of doing so.

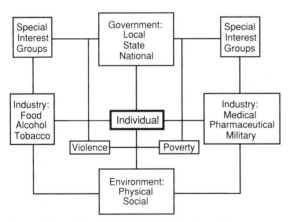

Figure 20.1.   These Interacting Societal Forces that Affect the Individual Are the Topics of This Chapter.

IIII➡

SECTION ONE: UNDERPINNINGS OF WORSENESS

If our scenario of "no more medical services" came true, you would become aware of subtle and not-so-subtle forces in society working against you. You could easily list several societal factors that promote worseness, illness, and disease in our society. Now review a hierarchy-of-causes diagram (Figure 20.2) that describes Roger's death.

Everything on the hierarchy of causes of Roger's death are either directly or indirectly influenced by "society," meaning, in its broadest sense, everything outside of us that has to do with human habits and institutions. Because we live in society, we are subjected to societal influences. To a greater or lesser extent, we are a product of society, including the way that we are born, the way that we live, and the way that we die. Even our genetic structure is not immune from environmental and maternal factors that are influenced by society.

We live in a society that encourages worseness of all sorts: Type A behavior; obesity; malnutrition; alcoholism; violence; smoking; drug use; overuse of medical services; abuse of children and spouse; sexual promiscuity; depression; loneliness; bigotry and racism; "sickness mentality"; poverty; stress of all types; traffic accidents; a lack of responsibility for self, for others, and for the planet; and the endless search for the "quick fix." Many commentators have described the American propensity for seeking instant gratification and instant solutions as a foundation of American worseness.

The Quick-Fix Mentality

This phrase *quick fix* may have started with the drug culture, where it means instant gratification and good feeling, but the search for the quick fix is becoming a cultural norm: instant solution to every problem, instant anti-depression, instant anti-anxiety, instant entertainment, instant transportation, instant sex, instant high, instant cure, instant food. Literally, the term applies perfectly to worseness trends in cooking—fix-it-quick TV dinners.

Quick fix also means instant results with little effort. From the patient's point of view this means "Doctor, you fix me up (and please don't ask *me* to take responsibility)." From the physician's point of view this means treating the symptom but not the complex psychosocial causes of disease and illness. In finances this translates as the "strike it rich" mentality, the eternal hope for the quick deal, the fast buck. In education quick fix translates into a dislike for tough teachers, a "you mean I have to work to get a grade" mentality. In child-rearing this means "the school is responsible" mentality, television as baby-sitter, and violence as problem-solver. And in nutrition this manifests itself as eating out at fast-food places, and the use of processed foods at home. In feeling good the quick fix translates into drug use. In going to the next floor this means taking the elevator. In psychotherapy it means "Give me a drug. Don't make me work." In conflict resolution quick fix means violence or withdrawal. And in government it means patchwork solutions to fundamental, long-term societal problems.

Probably every generation has said to its children, "You have it too easy," and in many ways this seems true. Young people have more cars, more computers, more telephones, and more entertainment than ever before. A lot of kids work for these privileges, often at the expense of study time, community service, or stress management. The availability of goods and services that "instantize" life promotes the quick-fix mentality and lifestyle. When there is no quick fix, what happens? Boredom, anger, frustration, helplessness, the search for another drug, another doctor, a faster food.

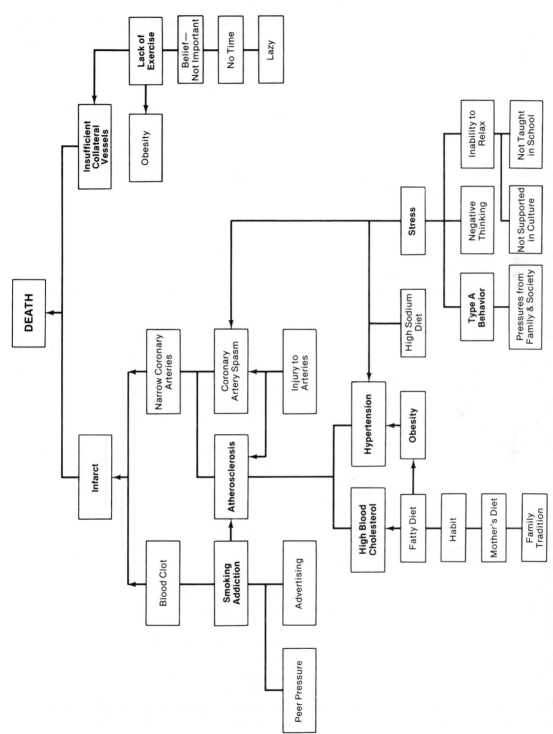

Figure 20.2. The Hierarchy of Causes of Roger's Death Can Be Examined from the Perspective of Societal Forces Against Health and Wellness.

595

The quick-fix mentality is antithetical to self regulation. Self regulation takes time, patience, effort and a sense of self-responsibility. This is true in all endeavors, whether they be education, attaining financial security, parenting, physical and psychological well-being, protecting the environment, or world peace. The quick fix mentality runs not far beneath the surface of many worseness habits and hazardous conditions in this country.

In 1976, the Commission of Critical Choices for Americans, chaired by Nelson Rockefeller, invited John H. Knowles, M.D., president of the Rockefeller Foundation, to organize a group of experts to study problems of health care in America. The group prepared a collection of essays, *Doing Better and Feeling Worse* (Knowles, 1977). Knowles wrote a landmark article, "The Responsibility of the Individual," in which he said, "I believe the idea of a 'right' to health should be replaced by the idea of an individual moral obligation to preserve one's own health—a public duty if you will." Knowles noted, however, that much conspires against self-responsibility:

> . . . A credit-minded culture which does it now and pays for it later, whether in drinking and eating or in buying cars and houses; an economy which depends on profligate production and consumption regardless of the results to individual health, or to the public health in terms of a wide variety of environmental pollutants; ignorance (and therefore a lack of conviction and commitment) on the part of both producers and consumers as to exact costs and benefits of many preventive and health-education measures, a reflection of the sparse national commitment to research in these areas; the failure, conceptually, to view health holistically, i.e., its interdependence with educational attainment, poverty, the availability of work, housing and the density of populations, degree of environmental pollution (air, water, noise, mass-media offerings), and levels of stress in work, play and love; and finally, the values and habits of the health establishment itself. One cannot hope to develop a rational health system if the parts of the whole

that bear on health are moving in irrational ways.

> From "The Responsibility of the Individual" in *Doing Better and Feeling Worse* (1977)

Knowles summarizes the key elements in worseness, and points to the individual's "public duty" to assume responsibility for health. Knowles also observes that the selling of worseness, and worseness as a by-product of selling, is part of the problem.

Selling Worseness

The economic foundation of any society impinges on the health of its citizens. For all of its achievements, our economy promotes personal and planetary worseness, when worseness sells or when the by-products of production threaten health. The bottom line of the marketplace is buying and selling; someone sells, we buy, and the seller makes a profit. When everyone is buying, America is strong—the markets, banks, and economy do well; people have jobs, earn money, and buy more. The free-market economy works extremely well, but to do so it promotes rapacious consumerism and throwaway products. As the demand for goods and energy increases, the burden on the environment increases, as witnessed by acid rain, garbage barges that cannot be unloaded, landfills that overflow and seep toxins into groundwater, debris on the beaches, and toxic-waste dumps that threaten whole communities. The by-product type of environmental worseness that affects humans and destroys plant and animal ecosystems is becoming an issue for producers and consumers. This is one front on which social responsibility must proceed. The direct selling of worseness is a front on which both self-responsibility and social responsibility must proceed.

What is for sale? Any kind of worseness that people want, and a lot that they do not want, such as pesticides and preservatives in

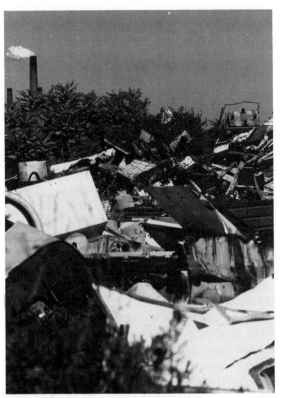

Trash and Toxins Accumulate in Our Energy-Wasting, Throw-Away Society.
Source: S. Kittner, Greenpeace, 1988.

food. People can buy all the salt and sugar and fat-loaded foods that they want, all the alcohol, tobacco, and over-the-counter drugs they want, and all the street drugs they want. People can buy violence and the tools to be violent. People can pay to be sedentary and never walk or ride a bike. In other words, it is possible to buy a lifestyle that kills, by choice or by ignorance.

Of the several ways to keep people buying, one is of particular interest to us. It is the **externalization of value**—personal worth based on things external to the person, such as clothes, cars, and the other things that money can buy. Externalization of value promotes worseness because it is hard to be self regulating and self-responsible when "self" is determined by external forces and values that are not prohealth. In

the language used in Chapter 6, Psychosocial Dynamics of Stress Resistance, we are talking about "external locus of control."

To let health be determined by external societal forces works only if one is lucky enough to be in an environment that is prohealth. Peers or role models who drink and smoke or steal to buy street drugs, or who are sedentary or rely on prescription drugs to solve every problem, teach these behaviors to people who cannot or do not choose to make better choices. Individuals with an external locus of control are likely to be victims of habits, susceptible to advertising, and satisfied with a medical system that alleviates symptoms without promoting health. They may believe that external forces cause sickness and cure sickness. The result is a lack of self regulatory behaviors.

When worseness is for sale, it is valuable to have a population that is externally oriented, that lacks knowledge and a sense of personal responsibility for health, and lacks willpower and skills for wellness. In subtle ways these deficits result from, and encourage, worseness industries.

The selling of worseness habits is often not subtle at all. Cigarettes, liquor, fast foods, and sugar-coated cereals are worseness products that get the "big sell" treatment. More money is spent advertising these products in one year than is spent on cancer research in a decade.

We raise these questions for your consideration: Who is responsible for all this worseness? Is it the individual; is it business; is it the government, with its power to regulate worseness and promote wellness; or is it the media? Or is responsibility an issue for all elements in the system? A traditional response is "the individual; if people want to kill themselves, that is their privilege." Another response is "the individual; people must be educated to make better choices." On the face of it, these answers are logically correct; practically, however, they do not solve the problem of 400,000 deaths a year from smoking and alcohol abuse. People are not becoming educated fast enough.

Another response is also logically correct: "Stop manufacturing the products that enable or promote worseness." Business rarely regulates itself, however, unless forced to do so by consumers or by the federal government. Social responsibility is not the guiding principle in business; profit is. Profit and social responsibility can go hand in hand, and they may do so when the public demands that industry and "corporate America" become socially responsible. Here we focus on the fact that social responsibility is not an integral part of doing business. It is unlikely that the tobacco industry, for example, will disassemble itself for the sake of national health.

If people will not assume self-responsibility and social responsibility, and if business will not regulate itself on behalf of wellness, what about the government? Through its agencies, the government can regulate business and people. This is often ineffective, however, and traditionally government does not interfere with business and the lives of private citizens, although this philosophy and practice depend somewhat upon the administration in power. Arguments against governmental regulation of both business and the lifestyle of citizens usually include Prohibition as an example of a failed attempt. Prohibition failed because it was impossible to stop bootlegging and the demand for alcohol, even though it may have benefitted thousands of people who had no access to alcohol. Today it is unlikely that mandating wellness will be attempted again. So we return to our original question, who is responsible?

If the answer to this question is "the individual," then is anyone responsible for helping the ignorant or the unwise make better choices and become socially responsible? Local, state, and federal governments can play a key role through schools, public information, and programs of various sorts. The school programs that we described for preventing and changing problem behaviors in Chapter 13 are not part of a national school curriculum because funding is not available for these extensive programs.

There is no easy answer to the question of who is responsible for promoting wellness. We return to the perspective of the systems approach, in which all elements of the system affect the health and wellness of the individual, and all elements share responsibility for promoting health and wellness.

An Issue of Rights

For the sake of the discussion, imagine that you are the head of the cigarette division of a large tobacco company. A reporter with a lot of disease data is interviewing you, and she wants to know specifically how you justify your business. How would you respond?

Here are some responses made by people in the worseness business: *It's a free country. We just make cigarettes, we don't make people smoke them. If you don't like smoking, don't smoke. It is not our fault that people become addicted. People have the right to choose. There is no evidence that smoking is bad for health. I just work here. My family and I have been smoking for years and we are healthy. If people would stop smoking immediately when signs of disease develop, there would be no problem. We recommend moderation, not addiction. We are only giving the public what it wants. We are not responsible for misuse of our product. We do not advertise to children.* In your opinion, which of these arguments for selling a worseness product is the most persuasive?

"It's a free country," and "people have the right to choose" are usually the most persuasive. "Rights" in this country are sacrosanct. Of course, the right to engage in certain worseness habits is reserved for adults, who are expected to be mature enough to have the wisdom to choose wisely. Children and adolescents have fewer rights to worseness than do adults, but this does not prevent many from launching a worseness career very early.

Two kinds of rights are intermingled in this issue: the right of people to choose lifestyle habits without governmental regulation, and the right to make a profit, also unhindered by governmental regulation. Of course, "rights" are often determined by society (sometimes only after great struggle, as the right of women and blacks to vote was), but once a right is established or is accepted *de facto,* it is protected. Cigarette companies have the right to sell cigarettes because they have always done so (and also because they are "big business" with a powerful lobby in Washington). The point is that these important rights of free choice and free enterprise support worseness, disease, and illness, but it is unlikely that the battle against worseness will be won by negating these rights. It is for this reason that responsibility must accompany rights. People have a right to choose lifestyle habits, but without responsible choices, the right becomes a threat. The sellers of worseness have the right to sell, but without social responsibility, this right becomes a threat to the buyer.

The laissez faire approach to business would work well if businesses of all types were dedicated to protecting and promoting health and well-being and had complete knowledge of the long-term impact of their activities on human and environmental health. Government becomes involved because neither of these are true. In this country people also have a right to protection.

Government plays a role in protecting the public against dangerous and worthless goods, hazardous industrial processes and worksite conditions, and against price-fixing, monopolies, and fraudulent practices. But the road to protection is long and arduous. We discuss the failure of government to safeguard public health later, in Section Five.

Through this economic landscape three deep-running rivers work against wellness: the failure of the consumer to be informed and to accept social responsibility for changing worseness institutions and conditions; governmental reluctance to regulate business; and the failure of business to regulate itself on behalf of human and environmental health.

REGULATION IN THE U.S. BUT . . .

Flammable pajamas for children can no longer be sold; nonnutritional milk formula for babies cannot be sold; certain carcinogenic or environmentally dangerous pesticides cannot be sold; certain weapons cannot be sold, and certain drugs cannot be sold in the United States. If you have followed these products, however, you know that when banned in the United States, the sellers moved to foreign markets, particularly Third World countries, where regulations are looser. The profit motive is stronger than social responsibility.

The underpinnings of worseness are so much a part of the fabric of our economic system and culture that they are difficult to perceive and change. You will appreciate the problems of changing societal institutions and cultural values and habits as you proceed through this chapter.

SECTION TWO: THE MARKET

Think now of the vast marketplace of goods that is at your fingertips. Visitors from less developed nations are stunned by the American cornucopia. If you are not poor, you have choices undreamed of even 20 years age. For this section we have chosen four "corners" of the marketplace that directly and indirectly affect the health and well-being of everyone in this nation, perhaps in ways that are only suspected: the food industry, the tobacco industry, the alcohol industry, and the pharmaceutical industry.

The Food Industry

If tomorrow our scenario of "no more medical services ever" came true, what food choices would you make today? How would the food industry hinder your quest for lasting health? Perhaps in more ways than you know.

In her classic book on the food industry, *Consumer Beware!*, Beatrice Hunter began:

> 'Let the buyer beware!' has always been sensible advice in the free marketplace. Today this admonition is especially meaningful for food consumers—in other words, for everyone. The 1960s was a decade marked by growing awareness of a rapid deterioration of environmental quality. Although air and water received ample publicity, soil and food were neglected. Our basic foodstuffs, how they are grown, modified, and processed, relate to the overall quality of life.
>
> (Hunter, 1971, p. xi)

Today, many scientists, nutritionists, and informed citizens believe that Hunter's advice continues to be good advice. From planting to the plate, from factory to fat cells, the food industry controls our food. The story of the processing of real food and the creation of "fake food" is the story of "chemicalization," "artificialization," and preservation—all, the food industry claims, for the sake of the consumer, who wants brighter food, tastier food, packaged food that never decays, food shipped from distant places, instant food, apples that stay red for months, flour that always flows, potato chips that never get soggy, and on and on. The quick-fix approach to eating is keeping pace with the need to fix quickly. Nutritionists and others who have worked inside the industry (Stitt, 1981) claim that as high-technology processing increases, the nutrient value of food decreases; to compensate for lost flavor and texture, many dangerous additives are used.

Today more than 2,800 substances are added to food or can be used to make fabricated foods. Thousands of compounds are used in food or in processing, packaging, and storage (Harrington, 1987). Many of these substances are common additives used to color, soften, harden, stabilize, emulsify, bleach, flavor, leaven, thicken, sweeten, or preserve food. A few additives, particularly coal-tar dyes, have been banned by the Food and Drug Administration because they are carcinogenic in laboratory animals. Many others are known to be carcinogenic in laboratory animals but are used by the food industry because the government does not enforce the law as stated in the Delaney Clause of 1958 prohibiting the use of any food additive known to be carcinogenic in animals.

In *Unsafe at Any Meal*, nutritionist Earl Mindell describes many additives that may affect health, including the sulfites that have killed several people, although they keep vegetables looking fresh. The sulfites are now banned from use on produce, but may be used in other foods (Mindell, 1987).

When the Delaney Clause became law in 1958, the federal government created a list of additives, called the GRAS list, an acronym for "generally recognized as safe." Additives on this list were in use when the law was created and were exempt from testing for safety. Many of these additives have since been removed, notably the dyes and the sulfites, but many have escaped testing and could be hazardous to health. Harrington writes:

> Additives that keep food from going stale . . . or rancid, make it moister or fluffier or crunchier than it would be naturally, are no boon to the consumer. Anything that keeps something "fresh" when it is really too old to be good food any longer—the 'Shangri-La' vegetables that have not been allowed to wither and die—anything that is totally artificial but propped up by modern technology is something that you don't really want to eat. And there is always the possibility that more advanced technology may—in the future as in the past—disclose that these substances are harmful.
>
> (Harrington, 1987, p. 279)

The repeated question that is raised by the food industry in fighting regulation of the chemicalization of foods, particularly those known to be carcinogenic to animals at a given dose is: How much of a known carcinogen is "safe" for humans; at what level does the substance become harmful? This question is a major stumbling block to the elimination of unsafe chemicals in food. This question applies to pesticides and all other chemicals that are consumed in food. Many "foods" are not real foods but are fabricated from proteins, carbohydrates, and fats, buoyed up by additives. When food is actually grown, the food industry faces problems that seem insurmountable without chemicals, an idea that is voiced by Monsanto, a major chemical manufacturer: "Without chemicals, life itself would be impossible" (Regenstein, 1986).

The growers of plants and animals for food rely on an armamentarium of chemicals to enhance productivity by killing insects, rodents, fungi, and weeds, and by enhancing growth. The Environmental Protection Agency has registered more than 35,000 pesticides, made from 600 basic chemical compounds. Over 2 billion pounds of pesticides are used on crops annually (*Congressional Quarterly*, 1982). Many of these chemicals end up in food.

Even before seeds are planted, the soil is prepared with herbicides highly toxic to humans. Before harvesting, plants may be sprayed several times with pesticides. They may be treated with a variety of chemicals that change or enhance growth to ensure a uniform crop that ripens simultaneously. After harvest, chemicals retard spoilage of stored grains and preserve fruits and vegetables during transport. Then processing begins.

The production of poultry, beef, and pork has undergone chemicalization of frightening dimensions. Chemicals keep animals alive in the poor conditions of feedlots and chicken houses, fatten animals artificially, change the reproductive cycle, destress the animals, and clean the flesh after slaughter. This is done with antibiotics, hormones, and tranquilizers in animal feed, and a chlorine bath for the fresh meat. And these chemicals are consumed by meat-eaters. So pervasive and potentially threatening to health is the problem that in 1985, the National Residue Program was established for monitoring chemicals in meat.

Approximately half of the antibiotics manufactured in the United States are used in animal feed. The use of antibiotics, primarily penicillin and tetracycline, is creating a phenomenon that concerns medical professionals in particular, but it will eventually concern everyone if the trend continues—an increasing bacterial resistance to antibiotics. That resistance is passed on to humans, rendering these antibiotics

---

THE CHEMICAL INDUSTRY: THE POISONING OF AMERICA

A few facts:

Pesticide manufacturers make over $2 billion a year.

There are more than 35,000 pesticide products on the market.

Dioxin, the most toxic substance known, is banned for some uses and not for others; in 1981 Dow Chemical, the primary producer of products that contain dioxin, sued the Environmental Protection Agency over the ban.

Pesticides that are banned in the United States are sold to Third World countries, where they are used by the ton, threatening the health of thousands; they return to the United States in bananas, coffee, tea, tomatoes, sugar, and other foods.

Russell Mokhiber (1988)

ineffective. Experts agree that the use of antibiotics poses a greater health threat than the use of hormones (Schell, 1985); but in both cases, long-term risks are difficult to assess.

You might think that nothing more can happen to food, but that is not so. Chemicals in the environment can end up in food, including mother's milk. The toxic by-products and substances used in industry enter the food chain through water, air, and soil and through other circuitous routes. Every year thousands of chemicals are synthesized by the petrochemical industry, and hundreds of these are used in industry; many appear to be nontoxic, but the toxicity of some is discovered only after disaster. Some of these chemicals get into foods. The poisoning of fish of the Great Lakes is well known.

As an example of the problem, D. Peter Drotman of the Centers for Disease Control (Drotman, 1985) describes food contamination by polychlorinated byphenyl (PCB). PCBs are semi-synthetic oils that are heavy, nonflammable, and stable; they have a high boiling point and are good electrical insulators, which is why they are used in transformers. Drotman writes:

> An illustration of how ubiquitous and insidious PCB contamination is involves an incident in 1979. An unused transformer at a hog slaughterhouse in Montana was punctured accidentally. The PCBs leaked out and entered the plant's recycling system for grease, waste meats, and the like. The waste was sold to a large chicken farm in Idaho in the form of meatmeal protein supplement for chicken feed. Over the next several months the chickens laid eggs laced with PCBs. The eggs were sold to groceries all over the western United States and to commercial food processors such as bakeries and mayonnaise makers. The contamination was discovered, and literally millions of dollars worth of food had to be recalled from across the United States to be destroyed. Human absorption of PCBs was documented by correlating egg consumption with breast milk PCB levels in the small town where the chicken farm was located. The incident pointed out the need for continued vigilance and chemical surveillance of the food supply. There is no doubt that similar incidents go undetected.
>
> (Drotman, 1985, p. 61)

Clearly the food that we eat contains more than we know, and for some consumers, more than they want to know. Moreover, the long-term accumulative effects on humans of the hundreds of chemicals that enter our bodies, either in food or as food, are unknown. Yet, the common advice is always "be a cautious consumer; err on the side of safety." It is not possible to be cautious and err on the side of safety if one does not know about food and processing, about pesticides and the chemical contamination of food. Unless you have time to do your own research, the best way to be an informed consumer is to read the literature from the citizen "watchdog" groups that do the research. We describe this force for health in the next chapter.

We have described certain hazards in the production, processing, fabrication, and delivery of foods, depicted in Figure 20.3. What about the seller? Does the seller manipulate our food choices?

Food is a good example of quick fix, and the food industry is well aware of this. Not only is food advertised as the instant solution to every problem, it is also the reward for every achievement and the appropriate medium of all celebration. Agribusiness, food processing, and marketing combined make up the largest industry in America. As with all business, the bottom line of the food industry is profit, not the health of the consumer, unless "health" sells. You are at the mercy of food growers, processors, and sellers, unless you become an informed consumer, take self-responsibility, and stop buying products that undermine health. No one is going to get the salt out of ketchup and the sugar out of peanut butter until consumers demand it and stop buying.

In the meantime you can read labels, although labels can be deceiving and make use of

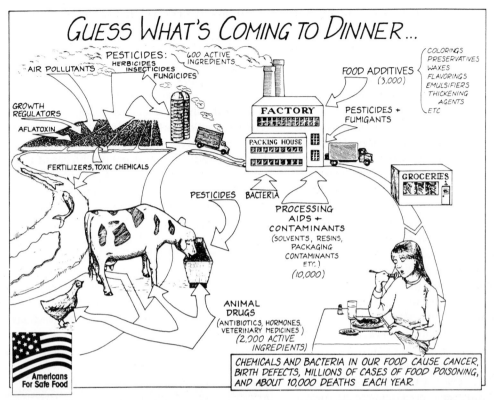

Figure 20.3.   The Contamination of Food, from Farm to Plate. Reprinted from *Guess What's Coming to Dinner: Contaminants in Our Food* (1987). Available from the Center for Science in the Public Interest, 1501 16th Street, N.W., Washington, D.C. 20036 for $3.50, Copyright 1987.

loopholes. Produce growers are not required to use a pesticide label, and meat growers are not required to use an antibiotic/hormone label. There are also loopholes in advertising. The words "lite" and "lean" and "natural," for example, can mean almost anything.

Worseness in food is big business, and the food industry is a slow-to-change, multinational, multibillion-dollar business. In the end, we come back to the basics described in Chapter 12—know what you are eating, and keep it simple and unprocessed. Now we add that washing might help. As Americans seek a better diet with more fresh fruits and vegetables, new hazards arise. The hopeful note is that the hazardous contamination of food can be stopped—when consumers are knowledgeable and take

action, and when they stop "demanding" bright red apples.

The Tobacco Industry

The tobacco industry is immense. In 1982, the American public spent over $14 billion on tobacco products, and American farmers harvested 2.1 billion pounds of tobacco (Higgins & Whitley, 1982). The industry spends more than $2.1 billion in advertising each year (*Consumer Reports*, 1987)—$33 million on ads in *TV Guide* alone—reaching 6.1 million children. Magazines that accept cigarette advertising seldom print articles on the negative effects of smoking. *Redbook* magazine and

U.S. News & World Report had no articles on smoking from 1982–1985, although *U.S. News & World Report* had 18 articles on cancer. Recently the fourth-largest tobacco company, Loews Corporation, acquired major control of CBS news. Will news of tobacco harm be omitted?

The federal and state governments receive $6 billion in taxes from tobacco sales. The medical system and drug companies get $22 billion repairing the damage of tobacco use, and mortuaries do well accommodating the 350,000 deaths connected to smoking each year.

Tobacco is the leading cause of death in the United States. Death by tobacco involves primarily the cardiovascular system, causing strokes, heart attack, and lung cancer, which is the most common cancer in men and is increasing in women. Tobacco causes chronic lung disease and infant mortality, and it contributes to peptic ulcer and vascular disease. It is a complicating factor in many other conditions.

By 1960, it was known that cigarette smoking is the major cause of lung cancer. Yet the federal government continues to subsidize the tobacco industry. In a seemingly cynical but perhaps correct analysis, Cairns (1985) says that the federal government is reluctant to promote the elimination of tobacco use because the more people who die around retirement age, the more money the government saves. Each smoker who dies prematurely saves the government $35,000 in Social Security payments; through premature deaths caused by tobacco use, the government will save more than $10 billion dollars in the next five years.

In 1988 the surgeon general of the United States, Dr. Everett Koop, announced that nicotine is addictive. Many people already knew this. The official government statement, however, eliminated one of the tobacco industry's primary arguments against regulation of the industry. But even though nicotine is classified as an addictive drug, Koop said it would not be banned; instead, more money will be invested in helping people quit. When Koop announced that nicotine is addictive and gave statistics on deaths attributed to tobacco use, he stated his hope for a smoke-free society by the year 2000. Will people, notably teenagers, take responsibility for health and quit smoking or not start? Will the tobacco industry stop manufacturing cigarettes and other tobacco products? Will state and federal governments increase regulations or ban cigarettes altogether? Will businesses and schools pass their own "laws" against smoking? In your opinion, what is the best approach for achieving a smoke-free society by the year 2000? Based on trends from 1974 through 1985, by the year 2000, 22 percent of the adult population will be smokers (Pierce, Fiore, Novotny, Hatziandreu, & Davis, 1989), which is not very encouraging.

In the meantime, the tobacco industry serves as an example of the strength of a worseness industry, particularly one that has a long

---

COUNTERATTACK, AFTER THE FACT

Three months from now, Oregon physicians signing death certificates will be asked, "Did tobacco use contribute to the death?" The question will be answered by checking one of four boxes: "yes," "no," "probably," or "unknown."

State health officials say data from the revised 1989 death certificate—believed to be the first in the nation to pose this question—will be used in studies of links between tobacco use and mortality rates.

Gunby, 1988a

history, a powerful lobby, a multimillion-dollar advertising and legal defense budget, and one that is condoned by millions of Americans who indulge in the worseness habit. The reluctance of government to regulate business, to allow a major industry to fail, and to cut off a source of revenue is a key problem.

It is likely that in time the United States will be a smoke-free society. This will happen because government will take action, because non-smoker's rights will become law (a trend that is rapidly growing), and because the government, private insurers, and citizens will no longer tolerate the spiraling medical bill for tobacco-related disease. Third World countries are not so fortunate.

Between 1971 and 1981, the number of cigarettes smoked increased by 41.5 percent in Africa, by 31.4 percent in Latin America, and by 28.5 percent in Asia (*World Health Organization*, 1987). This increase was promoted primarily by Western tobacco companies. The executive director of the Hong Kong Council on Smoking and Health writes:

> The tobacco industry is looking east for expansion and creation of new markets. The industry's designs are even in print. The September 1986 issue of the tobacco industry journal *World Tobacco* ran a major article entitled "Bright Future Predicted for Asia Pacific," which stated that the prospects for the year 2000 were "promising" and contained headlines such as "Growth Potential" and "More Smokers." The article particularly emphasized the market in China and concluded with the comment that the most conservative estimation is that sales in Asia will increase by 18 percent by the year 2000.
>
> (Mackay, 1989, p. 28)

In the United States, we have a case of the right hand either not knowing or not caring what the left hand is doing. While some agencies of the federal government encourage a smokeless society in the United States, others pressure foreign countries to import more U.S. tobacco products. In 1987, when the Hong Kong government decided to ban the import of smokeless tobacco from the United States, the tobacco industry mobilized several federal agencies and senators to fight the ban. Senators Bob Dole, Christopher Dodd, Robert Kasten, and Lowell Weicker warned the Hong Kong government that the ban would "constitute an unfair and discriminatory restriction on foreign trade." When Japan attempted to maintain its tariff on U.S. cigarettes, Senator Jesse Helms of North Carolina cautioned the Japanese government, "Your friends in Congress will have a better chance to stem the tide of anti-Japanese sentiment if and when they can cite tangible examples of your doors being opened to American products. I urge that you make a commitment to establish a timetable for allowing U.S. cigarettes a specific share of your market. May I suggest a goal of 20 percent within the next 18 months" (Mackay, 1989, p. 29). To pressure the Japanese further, the Office of the U.S. Trade Representative prepared retaliatory tariffs on Japanese exports. The Japanese suspended the tariffs on U.S. cigarettes. On a hopeful note, Mackay said, "If tiny Hong Kong of 404 square miles can stand up to the mighty tobacco giants, then maybe other countries can as well" (Mackay, 1989, p. 29). It is amazing to us that Third World countries must fight both the tobacco giants and the U.S. government.

We were also dismayed to learn that cigarettes have been included in the "food for peace" program to Third World countries, and that cigarettes are advertised extensively abroad, even when this is against the laws of the country, as it is in China. The United States' food for peace program has helped increase the incidence of smoking-related diseases in the Third World. Lung cancer, chronic bronchitis, emphysema, and ischemic heart disease have all increased in these countries. The inside story on how cigarettes got into the food for peace packages would be interesting indeed.

The Alcohol Industry

Alcohol abuse kills more dramatically and more disastrously than nicotine abuse, and it often kills more than the user. Following tobacco, alcohol is the second-leading cause of death in the United States. Here are facts:

5 percent of the population is alcoholic.

10 percent of the population is problem drinkers, including 4 million to 6 million adolescents ages 14–17.

20 percent–50 percent of all general hospital admissions are alcohol-related.

24,000 traffic deaths were caused by alcohol in 1980; 45 percent of all auto deaths that year.

19,751 deaths from medical problems in 1980 were related to alcohol.

31,914 other deaths were related to alcohol (homicide, fires, falls, and so on) in 1980.

300,000 disabilities were related to alcohol in 1980.

$116.7 billion was the total cost of alcoholism; 61 percent of that was the indirect cost of decreased productivity, lost employment, and so forth.

$7.6 billion is the direct cost for treatment of alcohol abuse.

$42 billion was made by the alcohol industry on the sale of beverages in 1982.

$1.1 billion was spent on advertising in 1982; $535 million was spent on television alone. The industry receives a 35 percent tax deduction on advertising.

$6 billion is paid to the federal government annually in excise taxes.

The immediate effect of alcohol is depression of the central nervous system, causing impaired coordination and judgment. Long-term physical effects of alcohol abuse include mental disorders, cardiovascular disease, liver damage, certain cancers including an increase in breast cancer among women who drink only moderately, fetal alcohol syndrome, and impaired fetal development. The social effects

---

COUNTERATTACK

"The three major television networks and 13 studios in the Los Angeles area that are responsible for more than 70 percent of prime-time programming will participate in a coordinated attack against drinking and driving.

"The campaign will encourage the use of designated drivers. These are persons who agree beforehand, when a group is to be in a situation where potentially intoxicating beverages will be served, to refrain from drinking and to take responsibility for transporting the others to their homes.

"Announcement of the initiative comes from Jay A. Winsten, PhD, assistant dean, Harvard School of Public Health, Boston, and director of the university's Center for Health Communication, which initiated this 'Harvard Alcohol Project.' Starting around Thanksgiving, the networks will include mention of designated drivers in dialogue of popular entertainment show characters supposedly talking at parties or in bars and—probably beginning in December—they also will schedule public-service advertising to familiarize viewers with the idea."

Gunby, 1988b

---

of alcohol abuse are equally devastating. Alcohol abuse begets violence of all types—in the home, in public, on the highways, at the worksite. Alcohol abuse is a primary cause of absenteeism, worksite injury, and loss of employment. Alcoholism is a major cause of broken homes and abandonment.

When we consider the cost/benefit ratio of alcohol use, not from the perspective of the industry but from the perspective of society, it is clear that the costs far outweigh the benefits of this industry.

The Pharmaceutical Industry: The Drugging of America

No one would deny the miracles of pharmacology that prolong life and enhance its quality for many people. This section is about a different use of medication—the use of medication as a substitute for learned self regulation, as a solution to the stress of everyday hassles, as a way of coping with the depression of a bad marriage, and as a form of treatment that replaces psychotherapy or behavioral medicine. These uses, which undermine self regulation and self-responsibility and are not without the danger of overdose, addiction and side effects, are the focus of this section. We begin with vignettes to capture several aspects of the problem, including drug ads. Drug advertisements in medical journals for physicians tell the story very succinctly.

Visualize this scene: A high-powered stock broker nicknamed Tiger Lady, who is about to be made vice president of her New York firm, is sitting on the floor of her apartment with a baby girl that she just inherited across her lap, bare bottom up. This brilliant, competent woman has a baby book in one hand and a thermometer in the other, and she looks thoroughly distressed. In the middle of this ordeal, she puts the book down and says, something like "Oh, I can't do this without a Valium." She reaches for a large bottle of pills and takes one.

This is a scene from the 1987 movie Baby Boom. In that moment millions of women got the message that a tranquilizer is a good way to handle stress. Our heroine did not use a short relaxation technique or a cognitive coping strategy. She took a pill, the quick fix. In another popular movie, the heroine mentions Xanax as the drug that everyone takes.

Visualize this scene: The client comes into the office for her weekly biofeedback therapy session; she is learning to lower blood pressure. She says, "Tonight I am going to take two Valium" and explains that she is going to take an extra Valium because that afternoon she must have the old and sick family dog put to sleep and she does not want to cry all night. Here we see a common occurrence—buffering or eliminating normal human emotions with a drug.

Another client was given a prescription for an antidepressant on the day that her husband was diagnosed with cancer; the physician told her that she would need it.

Visualize this drug ad in a medical journal: A cutaway of a pleasant, upper-income family home. The attic looks cozy, with old toys, a tricycle, trunks, clothes, and old pictures. Below the attic are two bedrooms, one decorated in blue, with a baseball and bat and sports letters on the wall, the other decorated in pink, with dolls and a canopy bed. On the first floor are a dining room and a comfortable living room. The house is empty, almost. There is Mom, an attractive woman in a blue dress. Mom is sitting on the couch, staring blankly out of the picture. Below the photo is the caption, "Empty nest syndrome." The next page says "Triavil for mild depression with anxiety."

This advertisement is seen only by physicians; it tells the physician that the normal feeling of loss that comes when the children have moved away from home should be treated with a drug. The ad does not say "The best medical advice for this patient is career counseling," or any other advice for action that would lead to self-responsibility, self regulation, and joy in life. The pharmaceutical company hopes that the physician will believe that the best solution to empty nest syndrome is a drug.

Visualize this advertisement in a medical journal: In a series of photos of an elderly woman, each photo portrays her with a different emotion and is labeled "confused," "untidy," "forgetful," and "depressed." The drug is a tranquilizer, and the caption says, "Give enough, soon enough, long enough." In other words, give an elderly woman a high dose, right now, for the rest of her life; eliminate the signs of aging with a drug.

As a group, the elderly are the victims of overuse of medications, prescribed by physicians. One drug company advertises a tranquilizer as having "a side-effect profile suitable for the elderly." One third of the 1.5 billion drug prescriptions written yearly in the United States are for people over age 65; at 20 doses per prescription, this equals 10 billion tablets (Watterson, 1988).

Consider these captions: "Depression: The hidden diagnosis. The ulcer shows, the depression may not. Think of depression as the underlying cause." "When you can find no cause for headache think of depression, the hidden diagnosis." Currently the pharmaceutical companies are emphasizing depression as the underlying cause of psychosomatic disorders; with this "hidden diagnosis" the physician can give a drug for the symptom and a drug for the depression. This ad also highlights an important trend. Any physician, in any speciality or in general practice, can prescribe drugs for emotional problems. Cardiologists, neurologists, gynecologists, and gastroenterologists all prescribe antidepressants and tranquilizers, thus treating the emotional symptom without providing therapy.

These represent the 15 to 20 advertisements that appear weekly in the leading medical journals at a cost of millions of dollars annually, paid to the journals and paid for by the consumers.

Every year 20 to 30 new prescription drugs are marketed. Physicians have neither the time nor staff to investigate the safety, side effects, and efficacy of the drugs that they prescribe; they rely primarily on the pharmaceutical companies for drug information.

Visualize this paperweight: A plastic model of the limbic system, the part of the brain that is involved in the experience of emotion. One side of the oval pedestal holding the model says Librium, the other side says LaRoche. Researchers working for pharmaceutical companies are experts in creating chemicals that affect the limbic system and therefore affect emotions. The paperweight is like scores of other gimmicks—coffee cups, pens, note pads, calendars—that display drug names and are liberally distributed by sales representatives, along with free patient samples of the medications. One drug company gives Easter baskets with drug names on chocolate eggs.

The pharmaceutical industry is an international multibillion-dollar business with subsidiaries in many fields, including the media. In 1986, sales exceeded $34 billion for prescription drugs. A total of 1.56 billion prescriptions were dispensed from retail pharmacies in 1986, an average of 6.5 prescriptions for every person in the United States. This average breaks down into 13 prescriptions for every person over 65 years of age and 3.8 for every person under 65 years of age. Total prescriptions include contraceptives, vitamins, and medications used during pregnancy; total prescriptions for treating disease and illness is somewhat less than 1.56 billion. Drug facts are shown in Table 20.1. In 1986, 20 new drugs were approved for marketing. In the period 1980–1986, about 160 new drugs were marketed.

Drugs are often prescribed to counteract the side effects of other drugs. Deaths caused by overdose, by an adverse reaction to medication, or by interactions of medications is about 2 percent of the total deaths annually.

When drugs are marketed in countries with less stringent laws, pharmaceutical companies sometimes exclude the side-effect profile material and may recommend standard doses that are double those in the United States (Jayasuriya, 1981).

The quick-fix mentality of Americans and the quick-profit mentality of business fit well with the needs of the pharmaceutical industry

Table 20.1   Drug Facts: Number of Prescriptions

Disorder	Under 65 years of age	Over 65 years of age
Cardiovascular disease	65,409,000	95,279,000
Viral and bacterial infections	157,705,000	34,252,000
Pain	68,889,000	25,090,000
Cough/colds*	54,892,000	
Arthritis	16,746,000	33,237,000
GI disorders	11,242,000	19,388,000
Lung disease/asthma	21,358,000	12,328,000
Anxiety	23,284,000	17,159,000
Depression*	20,562,000	
(*Data combined)		
Top Sellers		
Hypertension—Atenolol (Tenormin, Tenoretic)	15,319,000	
Anxiety—Alprazolam (Xanax)	14,728,000	
Ulcers—Ranitidine (Zantac)	11,403,000	
Male/Female Differences	**Female**	**Male**
Anti-infectives	104,476,000	79,923,000
Cardiovascular agents	81,901,000	71,677,000
Analgesics	53,694,000	36,740,000
Minor tranquilizers	19,705,000	10,244,000
Antidepressants	16,123,000	8,739,000
Total of all classes of drugs	689,686,000	449,849,000
Average Prescription Cost		
1987	\$15.52, an overall increase of 8.1 percent from 1986	

Source: Drug Utilization in the U.S. —1986, Office of Epidemiology and Biostatistics, FDA

to create and sell drugs for every human condition. We have become a drug culture. We anticipate that this trend will increase as medical costs soar and the medical industry tries to reduce costs by limiting patient access to non-medical treatments such as psychotherapy and behavioral therapy, family therapy, acupuncture, massage, and physical therapy. The quickest, simplest treatment for most complaints, including stress-related disorders, will continue to be medications. The increasing ability of pharmaceutical companies to create drugs for every symptom, with fewer side effects and the

reduced possibility of addiction, will promote this trend.

The pharmaceutical industry has two fronts, over-the-counter drugs and prescription drugs, which are available only when a physician prescribes them. The prescription drug market is unusual. The buyer cannot buy these drugs directly, but depends on the physician, and the seller advertises not to the buyer, but only to the physician. The physician is not the purchaser of the drugs, but he or she controls distribution and functions as a partner of the pharmaceutical industry. Over-the-counter

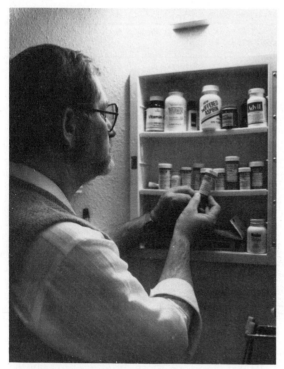

Medications Are Becoming the Solution to Every Problem and Are Used to Treat the Side Effects of Other Medications.
Source: Gordon Steward, Denver, CO.

drugs are advertised directly to the public. The message is clear: Drugs are the solution to every problem, even overeating. The hidden message is: You are helpless; you need an external agent to help you. And the very hidden message is: Mind and body are not related—if you have a mental problem, such as stress, take a pill; if you have a body problem, such as low-back pain, take a pill.

Anyone who believes in "skills, not pills" must be dismayed by the proliferation of legal drugs, by the fervor with which pharmaceutical companies produce and market mind- and brain-altering drugs (as indicated in "Big Money in Anxiolytics," Box 20.1), and by the difficulty of changing the pharmaceutical approach to treatment. The medical industry supports this approach, the pharmaceutical industry strenuously promotes it, the government hesitates to

---

BOX 20.1

BIG MONEY IN ANXIOLYTICS

"The antianxiety market also holds a great deal of promise for the future. . . .

"Upjohn's Xanax, on the other hand, was the sleeper that took off, producing $250 million in 1987 sales, up 20 percent from 1986. An impressive 17.2 million Xanax prescriptions were dispensed in 1987, up 14 percent from 15.0 million in 1986. Commenting on the drug's success, Smith said, 'Upjohn was a superb marketer.'

"'This market is going to explode over the next 10 or 15 years.'" Sammon said. 'It's a hydra-headed situation. Whereas the cardiovascular area is a little more specific in its effects, anti-anxiety agents can have many different uses.'

"'The down side,' he continued, 'is that because of the chemistry of the brain, we may be doing undesirable things without realizing it. But there's a lot of opportunity here. I get excited when I hear about a company that's making a major research commitment into these drugs.'"

Drug Topics (1988, April 4). "Big Money in Anxiolytics."

---

regulate it, and many patients prefer medications to a behavioral program that involves changing lifestyle and learning skills.

We have included the pharmaceutical industry in this chapter because the extensive use of medications, particularly for the treatment of stress-related illness, behavioral problems, and emotional problems, are often quick-fix solutions that are convenient for the physician and patient, but that may jeopardize rather than enhance health. Relying on drugs to counteract the emotional and physical effects of stress can only reinforce an external locus of control and sense of helplessness. Medications are effective, and sometimes essential, but as a substitute for learning self regulation skills and developing stress resistance, they do not enhance health and wellness.

Summary

These four industries provide the clearest example of the extraordinary impact of commercial enterprise on our lives. The tobacco industry promotes and sells an addictive substance that is a major cause of death and disease, and yet it receives government support, an example of conflicting priorities. The alcohol industry promotes and sells the second-most abused substance in this country, which, like tobacco, causes death, disease, and disability and has other profound social effects, including child abuse and other types of violence, divorce, absenteeism, and loss of production. The cultural norm, depicted vigorously in advertising, is drinking for pleasure and entertainment, far removed from the destruction by alcohol abuse that is the destiny of 10 percent of our population. These industries are the starkest examples of the legalization and commercialization of addictive drugs that are passively condoned by the government, actively promoted by the industries, and staunchly protected by users and sellers as a "right."

In comparison, the "chemicalization" of food seems tame. If death is associated with food chemicalization, including the use of pesticides, it lacks public drama and is difficult to prove unless a tragic accident happens. Undetectable, too, are the effects of hundreds of chemicals that can be added to food. The buyer does not know what he is buying; pesticides,

antibiotics, steroids, and many other additives never appear on a label. Restaurants and fast-food outlets do not use labels. Increasingly the dictum "Let the buyer beware" applies to food choices, but the buyer must be knowledgeable in order to beware and must be motivated to make prohealth choices.

We include the pharmaceutical industry in this chapter because it has the potential for harm, because it does not promote self regulation or self-responsibility, and because the drugging of America is philosophically an important issue for health professionals. We end with this question: If a safe drug were available for every human discomfort—if people could take a nonaddicting drug to control the slightest twinge of anger, anxiety, fatigue, boredom, grief, or pain—would this be a benefit to humanity?

||||➡

SECTION THREE: THE MEDICAL INDUSTRY

If our scenario came true, and all things medical vanished from the earth, the medical industry would have neither helped nor hindered you directly in your effort to maintain health. As with the pharmaceutical industry, no one would deny the miracles of medical science and treatment that prolong life and enhance the quality of life. We include the medical industry in this chapter, however, because in particular ways, the medical industry inadvertently promotes worseness, does not promote wellness, and would have contributed little to your ability to stay well, although it has assumed the guardianship of health care in this country.

In this discussion we use "medicine" and "medical industry" to refer to the entire spectrum including physicians, hospitals and staff, medical insurance systems, diagnostic procedures and treatments, delivery of care, pharmaceutical companies, and medical equipment manufacturers. Combined, these make up the third-largest industry in America, with sales of over $404 billion in 1986. For their numbers, physicians are the highest-paid professionals in the United States.

The term "industry" also refers to the fact that medicine is a for-profit business and is called a growth industry. As a business, medicine has gained extraordinary power to control health care in the United States, akin to other monopolies. This power arises from the legal, social, and scientific authority that physicians have gained in society, and it is manifested in physician control of medical services, medical payments, insurance-reimbursement policies, and health-care delivery through laws that prohibit professionals from delivering health care without a medical license.

Today the United States has the largest medical bill of all nations. As the costs of diagnosis and treatment have soared in the past 15 years, medicine has come under scrutiny, and occasionally under attack, for failure to promote health, failure to provide service for all at a fair price, and failure to contain costs. The analysis runs the gamut from the thesis of Ivan Illich, described in *Medical Nemesis* (1975), that the medical industry ultimately destroys health to the promotion of a national health-care system and regulation by government. In general, medical and nonmedical commentators make four observations: (1) Medicine plays a minor role in the health of people; (2) there is little equality in the distribution of health services, a situation that should be remedied; (3) medical costs are soaring partly because the medical industry is a for-profit enterprise and cost containment is opposed to profit-taking; and (4) the solution to rising cost is primary prevention, not the development of more costly diagnostic and treatment procedures.

The World Health Organization defines health as "a state of complete physical, mental, and social well-being, and not merely the absence of disease and infirmity." The practice of medicine has been, and perhaps will always be,

the art and science of diagnosis and treatment of disease and illness. Treating people after they have become sick does not substantially improve the health of the nation. In addition, a healthy lifestyle is an essential ingredient in health. From this perspective, modern medicine has had little to do with health promotion until the 1980s.

Promoting health and wellness has not been an integral part of the practice of medicine, and even today medical students are given little information on the elements of healthy lifestyle and the dynamics of health and wellness. This is changing, but whether or not it will fundamentally change the practice of medicine is unclear. Whether or not the practice of medicine should change is also unclear. If the practice of medicine included the tasks of providing behavioral treatments and of helping patients become self-responsible and self regulating, the physician would need to understand these ingredients of health, would need to be a good teacher, and would need to take the time to teach.

While these conditions are met by some physicians, and can be met in a team approach to patient care, it is unlikely that physicians will assume these tasks. The threat to health then is that prevention and the use of therapies that promote self regulation and self-responsibility will not become an integral part of medical treatment. Today physicians are reluctant to refer patients to other health professionals; it is the rare physician who routinely refers patients with stress-related or other behavioral disorders for behavioral treatment. In a recently reported study (Anda, Remington, Sienko, & Davis, 1987) researchers in the Michigan Department of Public Health Promotion and Education found that of 5,875 adults who smoked, only 44 percent had been told by their physician to stop smoking. Although physicians know the health risks of smoking, they are pessimistic about the patients' ability to make a lifestyle change. They also lack time, they are not always reimbursed by insurance companies for smoking-cessation counseling, and as noted, they hesitate to refer patients to non-physicians. A study conducted in 1982 (Bowen & Sammons, 1988) found that of 70 problem drinkers, less than half had been asked by their physicians about their drinking habits, and only 3 percent had been referred to a treatment program.

As medicine became scientific in this century and as specialization within medicine increased, two processes began: the tendency to treat the disease as an entity separate from the person (the result of specialization), and the acceptance of the biomedical model of disease. This combination has led to many spectacular treatments and to the ability to diagnosis disease regardless of the ability to treat it. However, the advances in medicine have created a "fix it" rather than a "prevent it" mentality, which has been accepted by medical professionals and patients. The emphasis on fixing the physical disease rather than preventing the disease at its psychosocial roots has permeated the society, from the individual who is concerned about health only when sick, to the government agencies that fund medical research on diagnosing and treating disease and fail to adequately fund social programs that prevent disease and illness.

The great achievements of scientific medicine have also fostered an unrealistic cultural belief in medicine and in physicians as conquerors of disease and guardians of health, with unquestioned authority (Starr, 1982). Patients expect an instant diagnosis, an instant cure, an instant relief, an instant quick fix. Patients are unhappy when they leave the physician's office without a diagnosis and without treatment of some sort, not realizing that the mysteries of physical disease and mind-body interaction far exceed the limits of the biomedical model and the ability of medicine to treat a problem.

Intentionally or not, physicians have perpetuated this belief by gaining power over all health-care delivery, through licensing laws that define "medicine" very broadly and make physicians the sole legitimate practitioners of medicine.

The medical industry has promoted worseness by not promoting wellness and by promoting dependency on medical treatment and complete trust in the medical system, rather than promoting self-responsibility for health and trust in oneself. This mentality is described by Lewis Thomas, a physician, cell biologist, previous director of the National Cancer Institute, and essayist:

> Nothing has changed so much in the health-care system over the past twenty-five years as the public's perception of its own health. The change amounts to a loss of confidence in the human form. The general belief these days seems to be that the body is fundamentally flawed, subject to disintegration at any moment, always on the verge of mortal disease, always in need of continual monitoring and support by health-care professionals. This is a new phenomenon in our society.
>
> We are really a quite healthy society, and we should be spending more time and energy in acknowledging this, and perhaps trying to understand more clearly why it is so. We are in some danger of becoming a nation of healthy hypochondriacs.
>
> (Thomas, 1977, pp. 43–44)

In an article titled "The Paradox of Health," Barsky (1988) says that although the nation's health status is improving, indicated by decreasing infant mortality and increased longevity, the experience of health is decreasing, as indicated by surveys over the past decades, with both men and women reporting more ill health in 1976 than in 1957, a trend that has continued. (Please read Box 20.2 now.) Barsky attributes this to several factors, including (1) increased health consciousness and decreased tolerance for minor symptoms, leading to increased use of medical services; (2) the commercialization of health—"Every producer tries to convince the public that something is dangerously wrong, or about to go wrong, and that immediate steps must be

BOX 20.2

SELF-ASSESSMENT OF HEALTH

The National Health Interview Survey asked respondents in different income brackets to rate their health as "excellent," "very good," "good," or "fair to poor." Here are the percentages of responses for "excellent" and "fair to poor":

Family Income	Excellent		Fair to Poor	
	1983	1986	1983	1986
Less than $10,000	28.9	27.7	21.1	20.4
$10,000–$14,999	34.0	31.9	13.7	14.3
$15,000–$19,999	36.9	34.4	10.4	11.4
$20,000–$34,999	43.7	42.7	6.9	7.0
$35,000 or more	52.8	50.1	4.6	4.3

Indeed, the experience of excellent health may be decreasing. In 1986, only 50 percent of the wealthiest individuals felt that their health was excellent, and only 27.7 of near-poverty responders had excellent health.

Note: There is a strong direct relationship between socioeconomic status as indicated by family income and self-assessment of health. As income drops to the poverty level, health status also drops; as the figures indicate, the poor are five times more likely to have poor health than the wealthy. These data are relevant to the discussion of poverty in Section Four.

Source: National Center for Health Statistics, *Health, United States (1987)*

taken to remedy the situation"; and (3) the fact that people now survive long enough to suffer the chronic diseases of modern life—"Thus, we live longer, but a greater proportion of our life is spent in ill health" (Barsky, 1988, p. 415). This gloomy finding highlights the importance of assuming self-responsibility for health early in life and abandoning the expectation that medicine is the guardian of health.

To some extent physicians have fostered the failure to trust in the natural healing power of the body and homeostasis by promoting the belief that the "doctor knows best" and by failing to promote self-responsibility and self-care. Physicians, however, are not solely responsible for this. The pharmaceutical industry contributes, the health insurance industry that reimburses sickness but not wellness contributes, and the patient contributes by lacking knowledge and by failing to take self-responsibility.

Several of these ingredients are epitomized in an insurance company flier included with some Visa credit card bills. The flier advertises a $400,000 cancer plan. In eye-catching print, the ad says, "Cancer Strikes Anywhere, At Any Age, Make Sure You Have the Protection You Need." Think for a moment of the meaning of this message. This fear-arousing statement suggests that cancer is something that "just happens," without cause—a disaster that strikes like lightning, unpredictable, inescapable—an external power that strikes us down. This message relies on ignorance and fear of cancer, and it fosters the belief that getting cancer is a matter of chance and that the ability to pay for medical treatment is the only protection. The brochure mentions nothing about prevention as protection.

People and institutions that profit from the treatment of illness and disease would seem to have a conflict of interest. Medicine is interested in health and is referred to as "health care." We cannot ignore the fact however, that because medical care is a for-profit enterprise in the United States, there is a conflict between keeping people out of the system and keeping people in the system, and between the professional value of treating all people and the unwillingness to treat people who cannot pay.

Countries such as Great Britain and Sweden have established nationalized health care in an attempt to solve the conflict of interest by reducing the profits that in this country go to physicians and institutions, including corporations that manage hospitals. National health care is also an attempt to solve the inequality in delivery of medical services that medicine as business cannot avoid. Ideally, national health care guarantees medical services for all and controls costs. In fact, nationalized health care is not without problems and in this country would require higher taxes or a fundamental shift in budget priorities. These conditions, and the opposition of medical groups, make nationalized medical care in this country unlikely in the near future.

Until recently the prevention of disease was not the concern of the physician working in a hospital or private office. Prevention was in the domain of public health departments and sanitation departments with the primary task of immunization and other forms of disease control. Today physicians understand the risk factors for chronic diseases and could play an important role in promoting health behaviors by using their "authority" to help people change.

In summary, if the scenario of "no medical services" came true, the medical industry, with its emphasis on the diagnosis and treatment of disease and illness, would not have prepared you for total responsibility for your health. In fact, this might be appropriate. The practice of medicine cannot be expected to have the total responsibility of teaching patients the principles and practice of health and wellness. We include the medical industry as a societal force that promotes worseness, however, because it has not promoted patient health. It has not encouraged nonmedical therapies and programs that do teach self regulation, self-responsibility, or prevention.

SECTION FOUR: VIOLENCE AND POVERTY

In this section we examine two societal conditions that seem to us to be, by definition, antihealth—conditions that destroy physical and psychological well-being of the victims, and that destroy and disgrace a healthy society—violence and the acceptance of poverty.

Violence

We do not have to argue that violence is bad for the victim, the aggressor, the family, business, society, or the planet. As we said in Chapter 12, Lifestyle and Health, violence destroys, damages, perpetuates fear and anxiety, alienates, prevents normal psychological development, and begets more violence.

And yet violence is big business—commercial, military, entertainment, sports. Flip through the latest *TV Guide*. About half of the photos show people with guns or depict violence or someone in terror, usually a woman. Now read the theme descriptions of the films and episodes; many focus on violence and revenge, including crime shows. This is entertainment for most Americans, adults and children.

We could write an entire chapter on the obvious connections of sex and violence in "entertainment." When our college showed *The Living Daylights* at the student center, a big-as-life poster advertising the film was hung in the lobby of our building. In the foreground was a sexy, barely dressed woman, holding a revolver loosely in one hand. In the background was handsome James Bond, pointing a revolver at her. Violence against women is increasing in movies, on television, and in life. Is there a connection? Is this destructive entertainment, or is this healthy entertainment? Is this just innocent fun, which entertains but never influences?

Knowing what you know about role models and imagery rehearsal, do you think that the extensive exposure to violence as entertainment and as news lowers a person's threshold for committing violence, raises it, or neither? Do you think that people become jaded, so that violence seems commonplace and therefore acceptable? Does watching violence teach violence? As the number of hours watching television goes up in this country, so does the violence. Is there a connection?

Recently we wondered why the entire nation needed to know that a woman went crazy in a small town in a southern state, walked into a grade school and shot several children, and later shot herself. What makes such an event national news? Are we better off for knowing about this insane, violent event; are we encouraged to take action against violence and against the social conditions that lead to it? And what news was not reported so that this event could be?

Here are some facts:

Family Violence

Every 18 seconds in the United States a woman is beaten by her husband, partner, or ex-husband. A married woman is six times more likely to be attacked by her partner in her own home than by a stranger on the street. Thousands of little girls are sexually molested by male relatives, repeatedly, each year. Police spend one-third to one-half of their time responding to domestic violence calls, which result in 40 percent of the injuries and 22 percent of the deaths of on-duty police officers. There are 800 shelters and safe-home networks for abused women and their children in the United States. New York City shelters were forced to turn away 85 percent of the women seeking shelter. Nationwide, shelters receive 50 percent more requests for help than they can accommodate (Midgley, 1987).

Child Maltreatment

Child abuse increased from 669,000 cases in 1976 to 1,928,000 cases in 1986. To what extent these data reflect an actual increase in child abuse is not clear, new reporting laws for professionals have clearly increased the frequency of reporting of suspected or actual abuse (National Center for Health Statistics, 1987). It is estimated that between 100,000 and 500,000 children are sexually molested each year (Fuller, 1987) and that less than 6 percent of the child molestations are reported (Lanyon, 1987).

Violence among Adolescents

In a 1987 survey of 11,419 eighth- and tenth-graders in 20 states, 77 percent of all respondents reported being in a fight in the previous year, and 14 percent had been robbed. Nineteen percent of the girls reported that in the past year someone had tried to force them to have sex. Twenty-nine percent of the respondents reported attempting suicide at least once (Centers for Disease Control, 1989).

Homicide

Homicides increased from 16,689 in 1984 to 19,527 in 1986. Homicides are the second-leading cause of death for teenagers in the United States and the leading cause of death for black males between the ages of 15 to 24. The homicide rate for black males is 500 percent higher than the national average of 72.5 per 100,000 (Blum, 1987; Rosenberg, Gelles, Holinger, Zahn, Stark, Conn, Fajman, & Karlson, 1987).

Rape

Rapes have increased from 37,990 in 1970 to 90,430 in 1986. Rape is an epidemic—one out of every three women living in the United States today will be raped and most experts agree that only half of all rapes are reported (Riesenberg, 1987). A rape occurs every six minutes in the United States. Fifty percent of all rapes are committed by acquaintances of the victims.

The long-term consequences of rape are well-known—frightening flashbacks of the attack, difficulty with sexual functioning, fear, physical injury, and pregnancy (Riesenberg, 1987).

Prisons

Prisons are overcrowded. Imprisonment rates have been escalating (see Figure 20.4). States are running out of money to pay for the prisons that are desperately needed to house the increasing number of criminals. Some states must turn baseball and football fields into prisons. Other states must crowd eight prisoners into a small cell. Many states release inmates prematurely to make room for new prisoners.

Yale professor John Archer and researcher Rosemary Gartner (1984), who conducted a 10-year international study of criminal violence, found that the United States is the most violent of the developed democratic countries in the world. From 1966–1970 homicide rates per 100,000 population for developed democratic

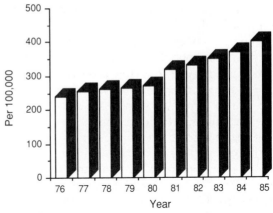

Figure 20.4. Increasing Male Imprisonment Rates, 1976–1985.
Source: Bureau of Justice Statistics.

countries are seen in Figure 20.5 and for cities in 20.6.

In the period 1966–1970, both Paris and New York City had more than 7 million inhabitants, but the crime rate in New York City was 10 times that in Paris. Philadelphia had the same number of homicides as the countries of England, Scotland, and Wales combined, a city of 2 million compared to three countries totaling 40 million inhabitants.

To understand the U.S. propensity for violence, Archer and Gartner (1984) examined the evidence for seven hypotheses about violence, using data from their study of 110 nations and 44 cities.

1. Economic hypothesis: Violence is caused by unemployment and poverty.
2. Catharsis hypothesis: Violence provides an outlet for aggressive instincts. Therefore societies whose wartime experience had been the most violent would show the greatest postwar decline in violent crimes.
3. Social disorganization hypothesis: Rapid industrialization, the breakup of families, property losses, changes in the labor force, and population migrations from country to city increase violence.

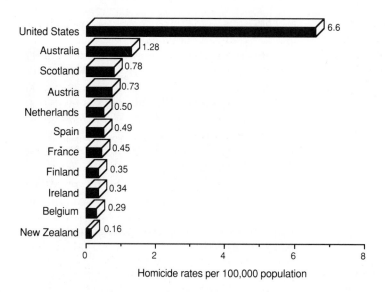

Figure 20.5. Homicide Rates for Developed Democratic Countries, Per 100,000 Population.
From Archer and Gartner (1984). *Violence and Crime in Cross-National Perspective.* **Adapted with Permission of Yale University Press.**

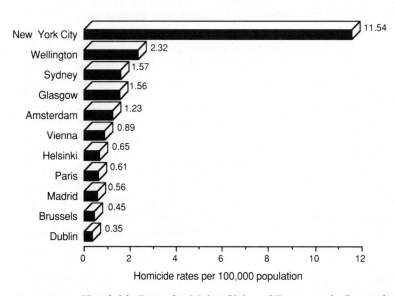

Figure 20.6. Homicide Rates for Major Cities of Democratic Countries, Per 100,000 Population. From Archer and Gartner (1984). *Violence and Crime in Cross-National Perspective.* **Adapted with Permission of Yale University Press.**

4. Artifacts hypothesis: Unusual demographic patterns such as the "baby boom" of the U.S. post-World War II period will increase the crime rate, and the reduction of the male population during war will decrease crime rate.
5. Social solidarity hypothesis: In less patriotic countries, people are less loyal to each other and to their country and therefore more homicides will occur than in "patriotic" countries.
6. Violent veteran hypothesis: War veterans are more likely to commit crimes, and thus countries with many veterans will have higher crime rates.
7. Legitimation of violence hypothesis:A country legitimatizes violence by honoring violence through military and espionage activity in the name of preserving the national interests; that is, government is a model for using violence to accomplish goals and settle disputes.

Based on crime rates, demographic data, and political history, Archer and Gartner found that the first six hypotheses of violence could not be substantiated. They found, however, that homicide rates and crime increased in all groups after a country had been in war. They state, "The legitimation model is the only one of the seven hypotheses presented here that is completely consistent with our finding of frequent and pervasive postwar homicide increases in combatant nations" (Archer & Gartner, 1984, p. 92). Archer and Gartner argue that the highest officials of the state legitimatize violence during war, and killing becomes praiseworthy and heroic. They speculate that the use of violence by a state to achieve its goals influences civilians to use violence as a means of settling conflict and accomplishing goals. Archer and Gartner cite Justice Louis Brandeis, who wrote in 1928: "Our government is the potent, the omnipresent teacher. For good or ill, it teaches the whole people by its example. Crime

is contagious. If the government becomes a lawbreaker, it breeds contempt for the law."

The extent to which the legitimization and use of violence by government "trickles down" to city streets and homes across the country is uncertain. However, the hypothesis that the government models violence is in agreement with the most widely accepted theory of violence, the social learning theory of Bandura (1973). Bandura suggests that violence is learned through modeling. Longitudinal studies of aggressive children (Eron, 1987), the effect of television viewing on aggressive behavior (Belson, 1978; National Institute of Mental Health, 1982), and experimental studies (Stuer, Applefield, & Smith, 1971) lend credence to the social-learning theory of violence.

When we think of "violence," we usually think of physical violence—physical injury that one person does to another. There is another form of violence that perpetuates physical injury on innocent victims from afar—corporate violence. In *Corporate Crime and Violence*, lawyer Russell Mokhiber (1988) states, "A man in a three-piece suit atop a Manhattan office building has the potential to inflict more violence on society than all the street thugs in New York City combined." Decisions about the safety of a medication, a car, or an insulating material such as asbestos can affect the health of thousands of people. For example, executives at the Johns Manville Company continued to market asbestos even though early company studies had determined that asbestos is harmful. In 1982 Manville Corporation paid $2.5 billion to victims of asbestos. Estimates are that 240,000 more Americans will die from asbestos-related cancer within the next 30 years. No mass reckless-homicide charges were ever brought against the executives who made the decision to conceal the information about the deadly effects of asbestos and to continue marketing asbestos (Mokhiber, 1988).

Psychologists Bandura (1973) and Monahan and Novaco (1978) believe that corporate violence results from the corporate decison-making process in which no single individual feels responsible for what is eventually done. Bandura calls this "rule by nobody." "Through division of labor, division of decision-making, and collective action, people can be contributors to cruel practices and bloodshed without feeling personally responsible or self-contemptuous for their part in it" (Bandura, 1973, p. 213).

Corporate violence is also legitimatized by the justice system. According to Mokhiber (1988), corporate officials who commit corporate crimes are rarely prosecuted or convicted. And if convicted, they receive light sentences and are sent to "country club" prisons. Present laws, such as the Consumer Product Safety Act, impose penalties of not more than $50,000 in fines and not more than one year in prison.

Violence as a way of life on the streets, in homes, and in offices is worthy of the attention of every health professional, indeed, of every

citizen. The roots of violence must be pulled up so that this particular tree cannot grow. This is an enormous task involving every level of society and aspect of culture, including values that directly or indirectly support or foster violence, conditions such as poverty that support and foster violence, and institutions that support and foster violence.

Poverty

Poverty is a health risk of enormous proportions. The poor in this country have higher sickness, disability, and death rates than any other group; infant mortality is higher and life span is shorter among the poor than any other group. More violence, more child abuse, and more alcoholism and substance abuse occur among the poor. Families with incomes below $7,000 are 10 times more likely to abuse their children than families with incomes over $25,000. And

---

BOX 20.3

POVERTY STATISTICS

1. Total poor increased from 8 million in 1979 to 22 million in 1985.
2. 6.8 percent of the population were poor in 1979, compared with 15.2 percent in 1987.
3. In 1985, 4 million workers received less than $7,500 annually. There were 30 percent fewer full-time jobs than in the 1970s. Forty-five percent of the jobs created in the 1980s were for part-time work.
4. In 1984, after-tax income increased 42.3 percent for the wealthiest one-fifth of the American families. After-tax income decreased for all other families.
5. One-fifth of all children now live in poverty.
6. Today, 37 percent of the low-income families do not have health insurance.
7. The homeless increased from 300,000 in 1976 to 2 million in 1984.
8. Teen pregnancy increased from 300,000 in 1979 to 2 million in 1984.
9. The largest group among the poor is single women with children.

The 1980s witnessed the first sharp increase in poverty in America since 1950.

Children's Defense Fund, 1988

poverty is increasing in the United States. In a study of poverty in six industrial nations, the wealthiest nation—the United States—had the highest poverty rate among children (Smeeding & Torry, 1988). Please read Box 20.3 now.

Of the poor, children suffer the most and are the least capable of changing their circumstances. The Children's Defense Fund, a private organization, is dedicated to providing "a strong and effective voice for the children of America who cannot vote, lobby, or speak for themselves." The goal of the fund is to "educate the nation about the needs of children and encourage preventive investment in children before they get sick, drop out of school, or get into trouble." The fund focuses on the state and

national level, on key issues that effect children in poverty: health, education, welfare, mental health, adolescent pregnancy prevention, and youth employment. In her book on the issues, *Families in Peril: An Agenda for Social Change*, Marian Edelman, president of the Children's Defense Fund, writes:

> The tide of misery that poverty breeds and that blacks have borne disproportionately throughout history has now spread to a critical mass of white American families and children. Thirty-three million—one-seventh of all Americans, including 13 million children—are now poor as a result of economic recession, structural changes in the economy, stagnated wages, federal tax and budget policies that favor the rich at the expense

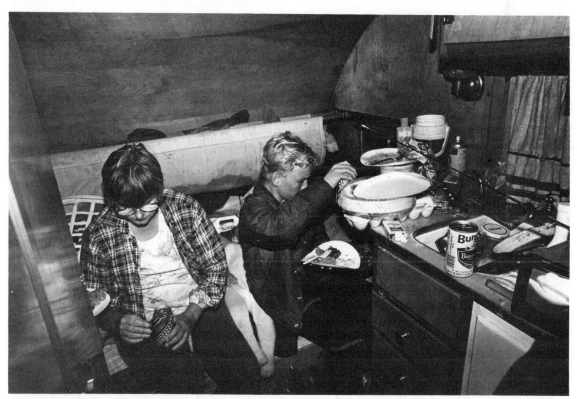

Today One-Fifth of All Children in the United States Live in Poverty. This Homeless Family Lives in a Tiny Trailer in a State Park.
Source: Stephen Shames, Visions Photo Inc., NY. © 1985.

of the poor, and changing family demographics that result in one in every five American children living in a female-headed household, and one in four being dependent upon welfare at some point in his or her lifetime.

The resultant rise in hunger, child and wife abuse, and homelessness has become a daily reality that has touched our lives either directly, through our neighbors or churches or synagogues, or indirectly, through our television screens.

(Edelman, 1987, pp. ix–x)

Blaming the poor for being poor has been a successful political dodge for many who argue against state and federal programs for helping those in poverty. The adage "If they wanted to work they would work" ignores the fact that there are more poor in this country than there are jobs for the poor, and the fact that today, at minimum wage, a full-time employee is unable to bring a family of three out of poverty. In 1979, 2.8 million workers could not pull their families out of poverty; in 1984 the number was more than 11.4 million (Edelman, 1987). The poor are getting poorer. Imagine that the family of three is a single mother and two children. If she earns just enough, she becomes ineligible for state and federal support, including medical services through Medicaid. The cycle of poverty continues.

Sociologists, psychologists, politicians, and others who study the dynamics of poverty know that the cycle of poverty is vastly more complex than simple statements such as "If they wanted to work they would work" suggest. In an extensive analysis of poverty and programs for the poor, Lisbeth Schorr, a lecturer in social medicine and health policy at Harvard Medical School, and broadcast journalist Daniel Schorr conclude:

The close association between poverty and risk holds for every component of risk—from premature birth to poor health and nutrition, from failure to develop warm, secure, trusting relationships early in life to child abuse, from family stress and chaos to failure to master school skills. Persistent and concentrated poverty virtually guarantee the presence of a vast collection of risk factors and their continuing destructive impact over time.

(Within Our Reach: Breaking the Cycle of Disadvantage, Schorr & Schorr, 1988, pp. 29–30).

The inverse relationship between health and social class has become stronger with the modernization of society. Many studies of social class have demonstrated that the middle and upper classes are not just wealthier than the lower class, they are also healthier (Kaplan, Haan, Syme, Minkler & Winkleby, 1987; Mechanic, 1983; Sagan, 1987). The physical disorders and conditions that are concentrated among the poor are listed in Box 20.4.

The poor do not receive the quantity or quality of medical care that the affluent and insured receive, and environmental factors undoubtedly contribute to the propensity of disease and illness among the poor. Nonetheless, epidemiologist Leonard Sagan argues that the biomedical model limits appreciation of psychosocial factors that predispose the poor to poor health, namely chronic stress, lack of social support, and authoritarian child-rearing that leads to a sense of helplessness and external locus of control. Sagan cites evidence, as we have in this text, that these psychosocial factors can impede immune resistance, and he argues that it is this decreased resistance to disease, not increased exposure to pathogens, that predisposes the poor to disease.

Sagan and others argue that increased medical services will not make poor people healthier and that the problem must be solved at the level of the source and not at the level of the symptom. Schorr and Schorr (1988) describe a "biomedical straight-jacket" in medical practice that, for example, permits a physician to treat an ear infection in a poverty-stricken child by treating the symptom while failing to realize that the symptoms will simply recur,

---

BOX 20.4

HEALTH PROBLEMS THAT ARE MORE FREQUENT AT LOWER SOCIOECONOMIC LEVELS IN THE UNITED STATES

Total mortality
Heart disease
Arthritis
Diabetes
Hypertension
Angina
Epilepsy
Rheumatic fever
Respiratory infections
Anemia
Lung cancer
Esophageal cancer

Sino-nasal cancer
Infant and child mortality
Neural tube defects
Tuberculosis
Unintentional injury
Low birth weight
Decreased survival from cancer
Decreased survival from heart attack
Restricted activity and bed days
Days in short-term hospitals
Number of hospital charges

Amler & Dull, 1987, *Closing the Gap: The Burden of Unnecessary Illness*

---

and may eventually cause deafness, because the treatment does not change the conditions in which the child lives.

To support his position that poor health among the poor in this country is not related to inadequate medical services, Sagan (1987) notes that in Britain, where the National Health Service provides care to all, the relationship between class and health persists; in spite of medical services, the poor suffer more disease and disability than the other classes. Sagan concludes:

> In addition, if this social class gradient of illness and mortality were the result of economic differences among social classes, one would anticipate that the effects would be limited to infectious diseases as a result of crowding, differences in food quality and quantity, and other environmental factors associated

with social class. The truth, however, is that all causes of death are influenced by social class—an observation that suggests a more generalized phenomenon. A more likely explanation is that social class membership reflects cultural or psychosocial differences in lifestyle, particularly those related to the family, reproduction, and parenting behavior.

(Sagan, 1987, p. 158)

Lifestyle habits relating to family and parenting affect children directly. Other lifestyle habits of adults do not explain the greater incidence of disease among poor children compared to other people, except as the habits of adults—such as smoking, drug use, and violence—impinge upon the child before and after birth. Poor lifestyle habits among the adult poor do contribute to sickness directly.

Compared to the general population, the poor tend to smoke more, have more alcohol and drug problems, more obesity (particularly in women), more accidents of all types, and more homicides and suicides (Kaplan, et al., 1987; Sagan, 1987).

Poverty, health, and education are also intricately connected. Many studies have shown an inverse relationship between level of education and sickness (Sagan, 1987). Education brings many blessings and seems to be a route out of poverty. The irony is that people in poverty are less educated than others, and the trend is increasing as teenage pregnancy and high school drop-out rates increase. Enhancing the educational advantage of poor children through Head Start programs is one element in the War on Poverty.

Poverty is a risk for illness, disease, and disability, and the causes are many: environmental conditions such as poor nutrition and inadequate housing, poor lifestyle habits including alcohol and drug abuse, psychological and physical abuse and the pervasiveness of violence, teenage pregnancy, poor education and illiteracy, unemployment and employment without adequate income, hazardous working conditions, demoralization and hopelessness, dysfunctional family life, single parenting, inadequate medical and psychological services. None of these conditions is limited to the poor, but they are concentrated among the poor. And while none of these alone (except perhaps violence) could cause the devastating effects of poverty, the poor in this country suffer many or all of these conditions. We cannot be surprised that the poor suffer more physical and mental illness and more disability than others in this country.

If you were raised in poverty, our scenario of no more medical services would have little impact on you. You would be so disadvantaged and so locked into a pattern of life that makes illness and disease likely that the chance of being able to change your circumstance for the sake of health would be slight.

SECTION FIVE: THE GOVERNMENT

Jesse Jackson used a compelling metaphor in his 1988 presidential campaign. He described a patchwork quilt of human needs, and he likened each patch to a particular group—women, the poor, children—struggling to meet its needs. He said, "They are right, but their patch is not big enough." A few groups have the power to get their needs met, but most groups do not have a big enough patch. The patch of the federal government is big enough. The federal government has the power to establish and finance policies for human and environmental health. The threads of the government's patch—the humans and regulations that are the government—could create a pattern, an emblem, so to speak, that would signify a united front in promoting health and wellness for all—but it does not. The current pattern is scattered, with support for some areas, such as medical research, and less support for other areas, such as health education and prevention. To some extent, the priorities of government are determined by the particular goals and social-economic philosophies of the administration in power and by special interests that have large patches.

In this section of the chapter, we focus on three interwoven aspects of the role of government in worseness: failure of government agencies to regulate business on behalf of human and environmental health, special interest groups that have the power to influence Congress, and the allocation of funds.

Regulatory Agencies

Government has always played a role in protecting citizens as need arises. The earliest health department, for example, was established in the mid-19th century as a response to an outbreak of cholera in New York City; the board established regulations to ensure proper sanitation. The history of government regulation is reflected in this example as a response to a problem rather than prevention of a problem.

Today regulatory agencies are created in response to man-made problems arising primarily from business and industry. After-the-fact regulation, however, is extremely difficult but has been the rule because of the fundamental separation of business and government and because business aggressively fights regulation.

From the point of view of consumers and environmentalists, regulatory agencies rarely do enough to ensure human and environmental health; from the business point of view, the agencies should be weakened because they hinder growth, development, and free trade. In the 1980s the Reagan administration agreed with business and initiated an anti-regulation trend. President Reagan and his first chairman of the Council of Economic Advisers, Murray Weidenbaum, argued that regulatory costs are too high and that budgets for regulatory agencies should be significantly reduced (Reagan, 1981; Weidenbaum, 1978).

Food and Drug Administration

At the turn of the century, the food industry was freewheeling. There was fraud in labeling, unsanitary conditions in meat processing, and hazardous chemicals in foods. Pharmaceutical companies were free to create all manner of suspicious concoctions, and fraudulent advertising was common. In 1906 Congress responded with the Food and Drug Act, which imposed regulations prohibiting the manufacture and interstate commerce in adulterated or mislabeled foods and drugs. In 1908 the Food and Drug Administration (FDA) was created to enforce the act.

Today the FDA sets standards for the safety and effectiveness of drugs, for foods and food additives, and for manufacturing practices of the food and cosmetics industries. In addition, the FDA sets standards for electronic product radiation and has the same regulatory functions for medical devices. The FDA also has the task of ensuring the accuracy of labeling of all products in its jurisdiction. It must carry out surveillance activities to ensure compliance with standards, and it is charged with monitoring the safety of imported foods and drugs.

The FDA ensures the safety of both prescription and the over-the-counter drugs. In the early 1960s it was the only regulatory agency in more than 46 countries that said "no" to thalidomide, believing that the pharmaceutical company that had created thalidomide had not demonstrated the drug's safety. This action prevented the tragedy that occurred in Europe—thousands of children were born without arms or legs or eyes. Please read Box 20.5 now. On the other hand, the FDA has approved drugs that are harmful or have not been adequately tested. For example, two arthritis drugs, Oraflex and Suprol, and an antihypertensive medication, Selacryn, caused death and disorders of many people before being banned. The history of Oraflex illustrates the danger of power and politics in drug regulation.

Oraflex was manufactured by Eli Lilly & Company and was sold in Great Britain two years before gaining approval by the FDA. During this time several deaths and other adverse reactions occurred. It was later proven that Lilly knew of the deaths but had failed to report these data to the FDA, as required by law. An FDA investigator discovered the problem and recommended that Oraflex not be approved. Nonetheless, Lilly received approval to market the drug in April 1982 and launched a $12 million advertisement and media campaign, including 6,100 press kits. By August, 62 deaths had occurred in Britain, and the drug was banned in that country on August 4, 1982. That afternoon Lilly suspended sales of Oraflex worldwide, having made $14 million in 14 weeks (Mokhiber, 1988; Negin, 1985).

The hesitancy and errors in FDA regulation of the pharmaceutical industry are paralleled in the food industry. For example, in the 1970s

---

BOX 20.5

THALIDOMIDE AND FRANCES KELSEY

Jim Jones is barely 2 feet tall and has no arms or legs and only one eye. Tom Smith has short flippers for arms and no legs. There are thousands of people such as Jim and Tom throughout the world whose mothers took an over-the-counter sedative drug for nausea during pregnancies in the 1960s. A German pharmaceutical company developed and aggressively marketed the drug in countries around the world. Frances Kelsey, M.D., had recently arrived at the FDA from a private medical practice in South Dakota. She was assigned the task of evaluating the safety of thalidomide. Dr. Kelsey found that the evidence presented for the safety of thalidomide lacked quality and, in fact, she found evidence that the drug might be unsafe for the fetus and recommended rejection of the drug in the United States. The pharmaceutical company that wanted to market the drug in the United States tried to pressure Dr. Kelsey's superiors into approving the drug. The FDA and Dr. Kelsey did not back down, and the drug was not approved. Years later when the tragedy of thalidomide became known throughout the world, President Kennedy awarded Dr. Kelsey a gold medal for her work at the FDA.

(Knightley, Evans, Potter, & Wallace, 1979).

---

it was known that 10 dyes caused cancer in animals. In spite of the prohibition against the use of additives that are found to cause cancer in animals, the FDA did not ban the use of these dyes, saying that more research was needed. In 1987, 4 of the 10 were approved. A citizens group sued the FDA in October 1987, and the U.S. Court of Appeals indicted the FDA for failing to prohibit chemicals that cause cancer. Finally, in July 1988, the FDA prohibited the sale of the four dyes (Wolfe, 1988a).

The FDA is plagued with problems, hindered by the enormity of the task and by an administration that favors deregulation. Some of these problems are: The allocation of money to the FDA has not kept pace with the plethora of domestic and imported products that it must regulate; the number of staff for carrying out FDA activities has been reduced; and the number of inspectors needed for surveillance is insufficient. The FDA cannot enforce regulations and must rely on other agencies, particularly the Justice Department to do so; it takes about 65 days to get contaminated food off the market from the time of discovery. The FDA relies primarily on food and drug companies to provide data on product safety; and FDA regulations can be ignored because fines for breaking the law are minuscule compared to the budgets of multimillion-dollar corporations.

In short, a lack of funds, personnel, and clout, as well as political pressure, can prevent the FDA from fulfilling its responsibility to protect the consumer. This is a repeating theme in other regulatory agencies.

Occupational Safety and Health Administration

The Occupational Safety and Health Administration (OSHA), created in 1970, is charged with protecting American workers in the workplace by setting and enforcing occupational safety and health standards. It has the task of identifying chemicals that are hazardous to workers' health. With more than

2,000 chemicals suspected of causing cancer, this is a difficult task (*Congressional Quarterly*, 1982). The difficulty is compounded when data on the safety of a chemical provided by the manufacturer conflicts with data that OSHA gathers. When data on a chemical conflict, OSHA may decide on the safety of the chemicals on a basis of the political climate. An unwise decision may cause the death of hundreds of workers. For example, asbestos was known to cause lung and gastrointestinal cancers for over 15 years before strict regulations were passed governing the use of asbestos in industry (*Congressional Quarterly*, 1982).

Although hundreds of chemicals including benzene, cadmium, ethylene oxide, formaldehyde, and vinyl chloride have been known to be hazardous for many years, OSHA did not require employers to inform employees of the presence of dangerous chemicals in the workplace until 1984. Philip Landrigan, director of Mount Sinai School of Medicine's Division of Environmental and Occupational Medicine in New York, reported before a Senate subcommittee that "by ignoring evidence on the dangers of formaldehyde for eight years, OSHA allowed more than 10,000 workers to get skin diseases in each of those years and between 7 and 48 workers to develop cancer" (cited in Wolfe, 1988b, p. 12). Landrigan also estimates that 65 workers may die from leukemia because of OSHA's nine-year delay in issuing a strong benzene standard.

Budget limitations prevent OSHA from investigating and enforcing health and safety regulations in the workplace. The number of inspectors was reduced from 1,038 to 655 in 1987. In 1980, OSHA conducted 16,000 inspections; in 1987, only 9,700 inspections were made (Wolfe, 1988b). Even when a company is found violating federal laws, punishment is seldom administered. For example, one company was charged with 40 violations of federal regulations in March 1987, and the only consequence for the company was a warning. According to the National Safety Workplace

Institute, injuries and illnesses increased by 20 percent between 1981 and 1987 in high-risk occupations such as mining. The National Institute for Occupational Safety and Health, a federal organization that promotes research on health and safety in the workplace, recommended that OSHA establish safety standards for 400 hazardous chemicals. By 1987 OSHA had issued regulations that decrease exposure to 24 chemicals such as lead, asbestos, and benzene. Other chemicals, such as bischloromethylether, that are highly carcinogenic continue to be used in industry (Wolfe, 1988b).

Like the FDA, OSHA has the task of regulating American business practices and is hindered by the same problems and pressures.

Environmental Protection Agency

Environmental Protection Agency (EPA) was created in 1970. As the term suggests, it is charged with the protection of the environment from industrial pollutants that endanger the environment and its inhabitants. The word "protection" is descriptive of the adversarial stance that is necessary. Naturally the EPA has enemies—the environmentalists who want stricter controls, and the industrialists who want fewer. As with other government regulatory agencies, the EPA is slow to create regulations, it fails to enforce existing regulations, and it often compromises in favor of industry.

Clean water, clean air, and a clean earth are essential for health and prevention of disease. Advancements in technology and industry have outpaced the ability of the EPA to protect Americans from hazardous wastes and chemicals, and industry is not required to disclose the risks of hazardous wastes to communities.

Like many other agencies, the EPA takes action only after a problem has developed. In two noteworthy cases—Love Canal in New York, and Woburn, Massachusetts—the citizens carried the burden of proving that the unusually high incidence of childhood disease, birth defects, and miscarriages had been caused by industrial contamination of the land and the water supply. In Woburn, residents discovered cancer-causing chemicals, benzene and chloroform, in two of the town wells used for drinking water. No action was taken by the EPA until researchers at Harvard University's School of Public Health clearly documented that the incidence of childhood leukemia in Woburn was twice that of the national average and concluded that exposure to the chemicals in the drinking water was the cause.

The Love Canal incident made national headlines in 1978, when 789 families had to be relocated because of water contamination by benzene, dioxin, methylene chloride, carbon tetrachloride, and 20,000 tons of other chemicals that were dumped into a nearby toxic waste site by Hooker Chemical Company. Citizens, headed by Lois Gibbs, who later founded Citizens Clearing House for Hazardous Waste, battled the chemical company and city, county, state, and federal health officials for many years before action was taken against the chemical company and the residents were moved (Levine, 1982; Mokhiber, 1988).

These are not isolated incidents. Countless other communities have had drinking water contaminated with pesticides, chemical solvents, and nuclear wastes. A 1980 EPA survey found that 350 waste disposal sites caused 168 cases of drinking-water contamination in 23 states. A more recent survey in Florida found that more than 700 wells were contaminated with pesticides. The Office of Technology Assessment (1986) reported that up to 35,000 sanitary landfills and trash dumps across the country may eventually pollute groundwater. Recently, the Pentagon announced that $10 billion would be needed to clean up the poisoned groundwater from the Rocky Mountain Arsenal near Denver, Colorado. The chemicals have poisoned a 30-square-mile area.

In May 1987, the prestigious National Academy of Sciences reported that one-third of all fruits and vegetables are sprayed with pesticides that may cause cancer. Each year,

2.6 billion pounds of pesticides are sprayed on fruits and vegetables. Most of the active ingredients in 1,000 pesticide products have not been fully tested. The EPA began testing the safety of farm chemicals in 1972; by 1986 it had completed its analysis on only 100, and only 30 had been tested for their toxic effects on humans (Mindell, 1987). The National Academy of Sciences stated that 28 pesticides currently used on food may cause 5.8 cases of cancer per 1,000 people exposed over a lifetime, or 1.46 million cancer cases in the United States over a 70-year period (Isaac & Gold, 1988).

Current government policy allows chemical companies to produce and sell chemicals with little restriction. Once on the market, regulation of a hazardous product is extremely difficult. In some instances the chemical company has been allowed to sell its stock of a hazardous chemical rather than suffer a financial loss by withdrawing the product from the market. For example, Alar, the substance used to make apples redder and firmer and to lengthen shelf life, is highly carcinogenic to humans, yet it continued to be used until 1990.

One of the most fascinating compromises that government has made on behalf of business is this provision: When the EPA bans a pesticide, the government, not the producer, must pay for the recall and disposal of the product. When the EPA suspended the weed killer Dinoseb, it estimated that $60 million to $120 million would be needed to reimburse the manufacturer for the unsold stock, to haul it away, and to dispose of it. This regulation decreases the likelihood that the EPA will ban hazardous pesticides.

Why do governmental regulatory agencies fail to carry out their mandates? The simple answer is: Congress has not allocated enough money. The complex answer involves priorities and the influence of special interest groups, described below. In the 1980s the EPA's budget was decreased each year; the 1988 budget was

11 percent less than the 1987 budget. The EPA's total budget for 1988 had less purchasing power than the 1976 budget, and yet new challenges face the EPA as industry supplies the world with energy and products, and as the by-products of production threaten the environment.

Acid rain, for example, is a major problem throughout North America. In the atmosphere, sulfur dioxide and nitrous oxides from power plants that burn coal and oil, and from motor vehicles, are converted into sulfuric and nitric acids. These acids are washed to earth in rain. As a result, groundwater is contaminated, buildings corrode, coastal waters deteriorate, forests and lakes are destroyed, and freshwater fish die (Mohnen, 1988). In spite of environmental damage, no policy has been established for dealing with the problem, and no money has been allocated to the EPA for implementing a policy. In fact, policies that could reduce the problem, such as the increased use of solar and wind energy, have been weakened. Tax deductions for solar and renewable energy have been eliminated, and budget allocations for research and development of alternative energies were decreased by $24 million in 1988 (Migdley, 1987).

Although the regulatory mechanisms were available for protecting the environment and human health, the 1980s was an antiregulation era. The antiregulation attitude is also fueled by the financial and political power of businesses that promote special interest at the expense of the human and environmental health. In the next section we describe the primary mechanisms through which special interest groups gain political influence and thereby, directly or indirectly, influence health in America.

Special Interest Groups

John Gardner, a secretary of Health, Education, and Welfare under President Nixon, believes that the impact of special interest groups on government policy is the major obstacle to health and wellness in this country (Common Cause, 1980). These groups represent the special interests of particular organizations such as the American Medical Association, the National Rifle Association, the Tobacco Institute, the American Dairymen's Association, and the National Beer Institute, to name a few. Special interest groups pay full-time lobbyists hundreds of thousands of dollars each year to promote their interests on Capitol Hill. There were 4,157 special interest groups registered in the United States in 1986 (Stern, 1988).

Special interest groups influence Congress by paying honoraria to senators and representatives. In 1987, members of Congress earned more than $9.5 million in this way. Senators receive $2,000 an hour, and representatives $1,000 an hour, for visiting an organization. In 1985 the Distilled Spirits Council paid $50,000 in honoraria to members of the tax-writing committee. Members of the House Appropriations Defense Subcommittee who are responsible for allocating money for defense, received more than $182,000 in honoraria from defense contractors in 1985. The 1987 chairman of the House Armed Services subcommittee on procurement earned $22,000 in honoraria from defense firms such as General Electric Company, General Dynamics Corporation, and Lockheed Corporation.

Special interest groups also target representatives who sit on the committees that regulate the activities that the special interest group represents. A member of the 1987 tax-writing committee received $40,000 from individuals connected with a major beer wholesaler. A senator on the Senate Finance Committee received $52,925 from individuals associated with the alcohol industry. A congressman on the 1987 tax-writing committee who received thousands of dollars from Anheuser-Busch, Inc., co-sponsored a House resolution opposing higher excise taxes on beer. In 1985–1986, individuals and political action committees representing the food industry gave $6,533,937 to congressional candidates.

Of this, $1,077,472 went to members of the agriculture committees (the agricultural committees consider legislation concerning farm and food industries). The chemical companies that make pesticides and herbicides gave $2,411,294 to congressional candidates in 1985 and 1986—$284,034 of that to members of agriculture committees. The Grocery Manufacturer's Association gave $3,252,589 to 1985–1986 congressional candidates, of which $499,719 went to members of agricultural committees. Members of the agriculture committees also received more than $109,500 in speaking fees from companies in the Grocery Manufacturer's Association. From 1979 to 1984, 13 defense contractors who have contracts with the Defense Department for building the MX missiles gave $4,519,141 to members of Congress, primarily to members of the Defense Appropriations Committee (Stern, 1988).

Special interest groups and individual companies also hire full-time lobbyists to represent their interests on Capitol Hill. For example, General Electric, the largest defense contractor, has 14 people in its lobbying office. Many of these lobbyists are former congressmen who served on defense appropriations committees or are former Pentagon officials. The Pharmaceutical Manufacturers Association paid a lobbying firm $3 million for one month's work (Stern, 1988).

Special interest groups can exert tremendous pressure on Congress. Wine and beer are taxed at the same rate as 37 years ago, 3 cents per bottle of wine and 3 cents per bottle of beer. Doubling the tax would bring $12 billion that could be used for prohealth programs. Another billion would come into the treasury if the tax deduction for paying excise taxes on wine and beer were eliminated, a deduction now claimed by large purchasers of alcohol products. When the Senate Finance Committee chairman proposed a tax increase on alcohol, he was overwhelmed by the alcohol industry. Dozens of lobbyists from the alcohol industry met with senators and representatives, particularly legislators who serve on tax committees. The National Beer Institute bought full-page ads criticizing the proposed increase in taxes in the hometown newspapers of legislators on tax committees. An extensive letter-writing campaign was instituted by the Beer Institute—50,000 cards went to legislators. The tax proposal did not get out of committee (Novak, 1988).

In addition to lobbying and other activities, special interest groups make large donations to political campaigns for the sole purpose of buying influence in governmental policy. Campaign contributions are made through a political action committee (PAC). In the next section we describe the activities of PACs with this question in mind: Can a legislator make prohealth decisions on behalf of all people while receiving donations for campaigning, and other benefits, from financially powerful

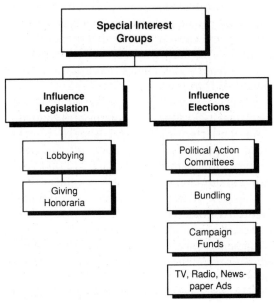

Figure 20.7. Special Interest Groups Influence Legislation and Elections.

groups with special interests that are not pro-health?

Political Action Committees

In 1986, $130 million was donated to congressional candidates by political action committees (PACs). Each senator running for re-election received more than $1 million. Eighty-eight percent of all PAC money goes to incumbents, giving them a significant financial edge. In 1986, 98 percent of the incumbents in the House of Representatives were re-elected. Of the top 15 PAC recipients in the House, 11 have been members of the Defense Appropriations subcommittee or the Armed Services Committee (Stern, 1988).

PAC money comes with strings attached. As Senator Thomas Eagleton of Missouri stated, "When you receive that money you know those folks have an expectation. You're not blind" (cited in Stern, 1988). Unless a candidate is independently wealthy, however, contributions from special interests groups are essential. The average cost of a winning campaign for the Senate in 1986 was $3,099,554. Robert F. Kennedy warned, "We are in danger of creating a situation in which our candidates must be chosen from among the rich . . . or from among those willing to be beholden to others" (cited in Stern, 1988).

In an attempt to prevent obvious bribery and to promote financial fairness in campaigns, federal campaign law places a $5,000 limit on direct donations to a candidate from a political action committee. In reality, however, there is no limit. The law states that a PAC can spend money freely on behalf of a candidate as long as there is no cooperation or collusion between the spender and the candidate's campaign. For example, the American Medical Association spent $100,000 on commercials and direct mailing for a candidate in Colorado who supported the association's proposal to limit the amount of malpractice awards against physicians. The

candidate won by a small margin. This activity was legal because the AMA had acted independently of the candidate's knowledge and cooperation.

PACs also "bundle." Contributions are collected from individuals and given to a candidate in a "bundle." in 1986, one PAC collected 168 individual contributions of $1,000 each and gave the chairman of the tax-writing committee the $168,000 in a bundle. Not surprisingly, the tax deduction that the PAC wanted to maintain was not eliminated (Stern, 1988).

There can be no doubt that money talks, and it talks politics. Through financial support, corporations and special interests gain the allegiance of candidates running for office who must receive money to manage a winning campaign. It is obvious that democracy and health issues are endangered by the current system of electing senators and representatives. Effective health policy-making, unbiased by special interest groups, is unlikely when an election is won with PAC money.

There seems to be no way out. Attempts to reduce PAC influence in politics by limiting campaign funding is voted on by a Congress that is elected with the campaign funds from PACs. "You get what you pay for" is true in government and in business. Because the American public does not contribute the millions of dollars necessary for campaigning for public office, the public does not command the loyalties of the senators and representatives who make decisions that affect the health and welfare of the American people.

The point here is that the largest "patch" that Americans have, the federal government—being no more than the people who run it—is vulnerable to pressure from special interest groups who do not have the health of people and the environment in mind, unless health is profitable.

In this subsection we focused on the primary method through which special interest groups win political favor and influence policy. This influence is evidenced in the allocation of funds in the national budget; in other words, in priorities.

Priorities and the Federal Budget

Funds follow power and priorities and are the bottom line of government. We can determine the priorities of government by examining the allocation of funds.

Figure 20.8 tells the story of priorities from 1982 to 1986. The military budget increased by 38 percent while allocations for health and human services decreased by 8 percent. The total military budget for the period 1981–1986 was $1.5 trillion, increasing by an average of $36 billion each year. During the same period, nonmilitary spending decreased by an average of $56 billion a year.

Poverty was not a priority for the U.S.

government in the 1980s. From 1980 to 1988, spending for the poor decreased by 21 percent (Conger, 1988). From 1982 to 1988, government spending for poor children decreased by $10 billion a year. Funds for the school lunch program, the breakfast program, and the child immunization program were cut. From 1982 to 1985, 3 million children were forced to drop out of the school lunch program, and 500,000 children were dropped from the breakfast program. Since 1981, the food stamp program has been cut by $6.8 billion, eliminating 1 million people from food stamps, and benefits have been reduced for another 20 million people. Food stamp benefits average 48 cents per person per meal.

Housing for the poor was not a priority. The 1988 budget reduced housing assistance from $6.9 billion to $4.1 billion. The Seattle Emergency Housing Service turned away 12,521 people in 1984; 58 percent of them

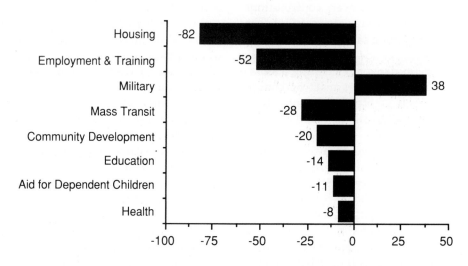

Percentage Increase/Decrease

Figure 20.8. Percent Increase and Decrease in Federal Spending, Adjusted for Inflation, from 1982–1986. (Military Figures Are Based on Department of Defense Data, December 1986; Housing Data Are from the Low Income Housing Information Service Based on Budget Authority Data Contained in the FY 1987 Budget of the United States Government; Other Domestic Program Estimates Are from the American Federation of State County and Municipal Employees Fiscal Planning Services, September, 1986. Adapted with Permission from Jobs with Peace Educational Fund Inc., Boston, MA.).

were children. The number of homeless families in New York City doubled in 1986. The Philadelphia Housing Authority has a waiting list of 23,000 families for public housing units. The number of families needing low-cost housing increased by 40 percent from 1981 to 1986 (Schwarz, 1988).

Job training and education were not a priority in the 1980s. From 1981 to 1986, job-training programs were cut by $9 billion. In 1983 funds for job training were cut by 70 percent, although unemployment rates increased to 10 percent. Investment in education shrunk from 9.8 percent of total spending in 1979 to 6.5 percent in 1983. Funds for the education of handicapped children were reduced in 1986 and 1987 (Schwarz, 1988).

Community projects were not a priority in the 1980s. Funds for wastewater treatment, public transportation, and bridge and road repair were cut by 50 percent.

Priorities of the federal government are also demonstrated in tax policies—who is taxed and who is not. In 1983, a mother with three children who earned $11,456 paid $1,384 in federal income taxes—more taxes than General Electric, Boeing Company, Dow Chemical Company, E.I. du Pont de Nemours & Co., Mobil Corp., Texaco, Inc., or American Telephone & Telegraph Co.; combined, these corporations earned $137 billion in profits. In the 1960s, corporate income taxes supplied one-quarter of all federal government revenues; in 1983, corporate income taxes contributed only 6.2 percent of all revenues. During this same period, defense contractors such as General Electric had profits of $6.5 billion, received $283 million in defense contracts from the government, and paid no income taxes. From 1981 to 1983, Boeing had profits of $1.5 billion and received $267 in tax refunds.

The situation in the 1980s was clear. Defense contracts consumed the lion's share of the budget; defense spending was the priority. Social programs, the development of new sources of energy, regulatory agencies, national health insurance, and protection of the environment were not priorities. In 1988 the federal budget was $1.2 trillion, and that was not enough, it was said, for health and education programs. Box 20.6 tells a different story. As the data in Box 20.6 indicate, the problem is one of priorities, not funds. If health for all—the World Health Organization definition of health—were a priority, the funds would be there.

Summary

We have given you a brief tour of ways in which the government promotes worseness and fails to promote health and well-being. We chose three areas that are interrelated: the failure of regulatory agencies, the power of special interest groups, and priorities. This was not a lesson in politics or economics, nor do we mean to suggest that the issues are simple. Changing budget priorities, for example, is a complex problem because the defense industry is entrenched in the economy. Our intent is to bring to your attention facts and concerns that you might not ordinarily associate with health issues and yet are related to health and wellness.

You may have noted that funding is a repeating theme. The allocation of funds is a tool that government has to express priorities; whoever controls the purse strings controls priorities. We have looked at ways in which priorities have not been prohealth and have been promilitary in the 1980s. In the 1980s the regulatory agencies that were meant to protect health were weakened, while special interest groups gained power to control policy.

To a great extent, the government represents society. But at the same time, it has the power to shape society, through its enormous financial resources and regulatory power, or through passivity, or withdrawal of funds. For this reason government cannot be ignored. We cannot remain aloof and never look into the muddy waters. In fact, there is a place for health professionals in all branches of government, and private citizens can influence government

| BOX 20.6 |

PRIORITIES?

Ten Pershing missiles out of a planned 380	could provide	$60 million for funding the school dropout prevention and recovery program
Ten B-1 bombers out of a planned 100	could provide	$5 billion for restoring cuts to school lunch, breakfast, and summer child-care food programs
Do not reactivate two World War II battleships	could provide	$1 billion emergency help for the homeless
One nuclear submarine out of 15 new subs	could provide	$2 billion for funding the youth training and employment act
$5 billion for removing tax deductions for alcohol-related entertainment	could provide	195,000 new jobs for production of alcohol fuel from renewable resources
$7 billion by increasing excise tax on beer and wine	could provide	430,000 new jobs in education by increasing student-teacher ratios from kindergarten through college
$8 billion by eliminating tobacco subsidies and tax deductions for advertising for tobacco and alcohol	could provide	268,000 new jobs to produce and install solar power systems
$10 billion by reducing waste and abuse in the Pentagon	could provide	265,000 new jobs in mass transit by producing streetcars, trains, and subways for all parts of the country

Source: Adapted from *Neither Jobs Nor Security* © by Employment Research Associates (1987)

through the united effort of citizens groups and through informed voting.

IIII➡

CONCLUSION

Worseness in this society has many sources: the food industry, the alcohol and tobacco industries, the violence industry, the medical industry, and the pharmaceutical industry; the government's failure to play more than a cursory role in primary prevention, its failure to support social programs, and its failure to regulate business on behalf of human and environmental health; and organized crime, drug trafficking, and the penal system. These "institutionalized" purveyors of worseness interact with societal and cultural factors including poverty, prejudice, violence, an ethos that places profit above public well-being, paranoia, greed, chronic stress that cuts across social classes, materialism, competitiveness, uncritical acceptance of authority, political disinterest and helplessness, and lack of spiritual values. To this conundrum can be added our society's steadfast belief that science and technology will prevail against disease and illness and the failure of individuals to take responsibility for personal, community, and world health.

We have described two interacting factors that underlie worseness. The quick-fix mentality, shared by consumers, medicine, business, and government, a mentality that prevents long-term solutions to long-term problems, and an economy that makes profit, not health or social responsibility, the motivating force.

Worseness occurs on many levels—personal, communal, industrial, governmental and global. It comes in personal choices about lifestyle, personal choice to "play the odds," personal choice to be a passive consumer of goods and services including medical services. It comes in community choices: to engage in or tolerate violence, alcoholism, or pollution. It comes in industrial choices: to pollute the water, soil, air, and food and endanger human and environmental health in the process of making a profit, to ignore government standards, and aggressively fight regulation, to seek short-term profit at the expense of long-term waste, and to commit corporate violence. It comes in societal choices manifested in government: the failure to regulate industry, to address the needs of the poor; and in the choice to make human health the highest priority, to be influenced by special interest groups, to seek quick-fix solutions to complex problems. It comes in global choices: the exploitation of Third World peoples by multinational corporations and the federal government, by exporting worseness and by controlling the Third World food supply and by increasing Third World dependency (Lappe & Collins, 1977). Worseness occurs in the failure to perceive the interconnectedness of our small world.

How sick are we? Are we a drugged, chemicalized, powerless, mesmerized people who cannot manage our own health? Substantial worseness is indicated by the data on nicotine use, alcoholism, violence on the streets, in homes and in corporations, the number of prescriptions given annually, the skyrocketing medical costs and costs of rehabilitation, the fact that America has the largest medical bill in the world, the increasing incidence of cancer and AIDS, increasing poverty, and increasing pollution.

Worseness, disease, and illness are not inevitable, but they are tenacious. We seem to eliminate one problem and create another. Infectious diseases have decreased, but chronic diseases have increased; we have a cornucopia of goods and services and energy, yet pollution of all types has increased; we have abundant birth control methods, yet teenage pregnancy is increasing; the wealthy are wealthier, yet the poor are poorer; communication systems are increasing, but the illiteracy rate is high; cigarette consumption among males is decreasing, yet, illicit drug use and associated violence increases; medical technology is the best in the world, but the overall health of the population is not increasing, and so on.

There is much to be distressed about, and much that every person can be challenged by and make a commitment to change.

Throughout this text we have emphasized self-responsibility, as did Knowles in his eloquent essay, saying it is the moral responsibility of each individual to take responsibility for health. Now we look beyond self-responsibility to social responsibility. We must look beyond self-responsibility because self-responsibility will not guarantee health in a sick society. When the air is polluted and the water is poisoned,

when there is violence on the streets and in homes, when drugs substitute for self regulation, when the federal budget committees cut health spending and regulatory agencies are weakened, when worseness industries and special interest groups can influence government policy, then both social responsibility and self-responsibility are needed.

Now you are ready for Chapter 21, Societal and Cultural Forces for Health and Wellness. We remind you that as in the classic fairy tales of good and evil, societal forces for health and against health are often found in the same domain.

Societal Forces for Health and Wellness

"Health for all by the year 2000."
—World Health Organization

A fresh wind is in the air—clean, wholesome, and energizing—it spreads across the land from state to state, affecting all areas of life. It heals and brings a zest for living—it is the fresh air of the "wellness movement."

Millions of people are exercising, eating good food, caring about their neighbors, cleaning up the environment, and feeling good. Health has become the number one value for thousands of people (Rubinstein, 1982). Businesses, schools, and colleges are developing health and wellness programs. Businesses are creating healthy work environments. Increasingly, the medical profession promotes a healthy lifestyle and public awareness of health hazards, and many hospitals have wellness programs. Health programs and health products are profitable. Companies that manufacture running shoes and sports equipment are profitable. Every day 60,000 pairs of running shoes are sold. Cereal companies advertise the importance of fiber, and margarine and peanut butter are advertised as "no cholesterol." Health spas have proliferated. Fun runs and bicycle races are popular, television and radio talk shows discuss health issues, and results of health and disease research are newsworthy. Self-help books of all types are popular, sales of video exercise and diet programs are up, and popular health magazines have large circulations. Aerobic classes and health programs are popular on public television; recreation and play

are on the increase. All over the country self-help and support groups flourish.

If our scenario from Chapter 20, "no medical services available," came true, these societal/cultural forces would help you maintain good health for the rest of life. Many of these ingredients of health were described in previous chapters; we do not elaborate on them here. In this chapter, we introduce a variety of model programs that point the way for health professionals and for society.

In Chapter 1, we described the concept of high-level wellness as developed by physician Halbert Dunn. High-level wellness includes five elements: zest for life, maximizing potential, purposeful direction, adapting to challenge, and social responsibility. Dunn emphasized that social wellness and social responsibility are essential to individual high-level wellness and that individual wellness means "social wellness on a world basis" (1961, p. 199). "All of us have our own particular spheres of interest and influence. It is our responsibility to take part in promoting social wellness within these spheres of daily activity. The well-being of society depends upon the you's and me's who make it up" (1961, p. 200). In this chapter we take up the fifth component in Dunn's concept of wellness, social responsibility. We examine societal forces that promote health and wellness.

In Section One, we describe wellness programs in business and industry and discuss a key issue in the success of these programs, cost-effectiveness. A program that is "cost-effective" saves money. As medical costs increase, businesses (which pay part of the employee's health insurance premium) and health insurance companies (which pay a large portion of medical costs) have jumped on the wellness bandwagon, because health and wellness save money. We also describe a growing trend in American industry, a trend that we became aware of while writing this chapter— protection of the environment and environmental consciousness. In Chapter 20, we emphasized the interaction of human health and environmental health and described the worsening of the environment. Here we describe efforts to enhance environmental health.

In Section Two, we examine health programs in colleges, universities, communities, and prisons. We also highlight model programs for preventing violence and the neglect and abuse of children. In Section Three, we discuss social policy, the promotion of health and wellness by state and federal governments. We highlight the Smoking Prevention Program in Minnesota and the U.S. Department of Health and Human Services. We include an important force for health and wellness in this culture— citizens groups. Common Cause, the Health Research Group, and Citizen's Clearing House for Hazardous Waste are examples of citizens groups that affect state and federal governments. Section Four widens the focus from our society to the global society. We highlight the World Health Organization's efforts to promote health throughout the world and describe a model community program that brings social responsibility and health to communities in Third World countries.

||||➡

SECTION ONE: WELLNESS IN BUSINESS

For the first time in the history of free enterprise, business has an incentive for promoting the health of the worker. A healthy worker saves the company money. Corporations know that the best way to lower medical costs is to keep people healthy. With medical costs increasing faster than inflation, business has an incentive for promoting wellness. By 1986, two-thirds of the Fortune 500 companies and half of all major corporations had in-house wellness programs (Orlandi, 1986).

> "Corporate health costs are rising so fast that if unchecked, within 8 years they will eliminate all profit for the average 500 company and for the 250 largest nonindustrial companies in this country."
>
> —John Creedon, chief of Metropolitan Life Insurance Company (cited in Goldsmith, 1986)

Wellness Programs

If you were an executive in a large corporation faced with increasing health insurance costs for employees, and you had to cope with loss of highly competent executives from heart attack, what would you do?

Live for Life

Faced with these problems, the Johnson & Johnson company took action. Beginning in 1979, Johnson & Johnson began the Live for Life (LFL) program for 28,000 employees in 50 plants. The goals of the program are "to provide the means for Johnson & Johnson employees to become the healthiest in the world and to control the increasing illness and accident costs of the corporation (Bly, Jones, & Richardson, 1986, p. 3236). The program is free for employees at company sites. Live for Life is a prototype of effective in-house wellness programs that reduce company costs by increasing employee health. If you were a corporate manager, you would study this program in detail.

The Live for Life program incorporates the basic elements of a wellness program:

1. Lifestyle assessment and health screening.

2. A lifestyle seminar that introduces employees to the basic concepts of wellness and the LFL program.
3. Classes for smoking cessation, weight control, good nutrition, and stress management. The program also includes yoga classes, alcohol education, physical fitness classes, and assertiveness training.
4. Alteration of the work environment; that is, nutritious food in the cafeteria, rewards for nonsmokers, exercise facilities, car pools, flexible scheduling of work time, and training programs to improve employee-manager relations.
5. Feedback and follow-up. Each employee receives a summary of lifestyle points earned during a three-month period for lifestyle improvement and fitness achievement. Participants are contacted by letter or telephone for their reactions and progress in the program.

Several studies have assessed the effectiveness of Johnson & Johnson's Live for Life Program. Bly and co-workers (1986) compared employees (N = 1,272) at four LFL plants who had participated in the program for two years with employees at four non-LFL plants (N = 751). Both groups of employees received health screenings in 1979 and 1981. Before and after comparisons were made between the two groups (Bly, et al., 1986). The results were:

A second study compared medical costs of three groups of employees after four years, 1979–1983:

1. employees who participated in the Live for Life program for more than 30 months (n = 5,192).
2. employees who participated in the Live for Life program from 18 to 30 months (n = 3,259).
3. employees who did not participate in the program (n = 2,955).

Employees in all three groups were similar in age, sex, stress levels, and health levels at the beginning of the study (Bly, et al., 1986).

The main saving was in hospitalization cost, which in 1983 was two times higher for the control group employees than the employees in the Live for Life program. Overall, the employees in the Live for Life programs saved Johnson & Johnson $980,316 in the four-year period.

Several other companies have reported reductions in medical costs from wellness programs. New York Telephone reported an annual savings of $2.7 million from its wellness program for 80,000 employees (Bruhn & Cordova, 1987). Blue Cross/Blue Shield of Indiana estimated a savings of $1.65 million over a four-year period from a wellness program for 2,400 employees (Goldsmith, 1986). Other companies report savings varying from $84.50 to $324.00 per employee (Bowne, Russell, & Morgan, 1984; Shephard, 1989).

	Live For Life Employees	Non-Live For Life Employees
Smoking cessation	23 percent	17 percent
High risk of coronary heart disease	13 percent	32 percent
Exercise improvement (men)	29 percent	19 percent
Exercise improvement (women)	20 percent	7 percent
Fitness	significant improvement	minimal or no improvement
Stress	significant decrease	minimal or the same
Work satisfaction	significant improvement	minimal or the same

Employees feel positive about wellness programs. In a survey of AT&T's 340,000 employees, 99 percent believed that the wellness program is valuable and should be made available to all employees. Employees also felt the wellness program showed that the company was interested in their well-being. Ninety-five percent of the employees rated the wellness program as "terrific" or "good" (Spilman, Goetz, Schultz, Bellingham, & Johnson, 1987).

Critics of corporate America point out that while corporations emphasize the individual's responsibility for sickness and health, the corporations may fail to take responsibility for the workplace environment (Sloan, 1987; Warner, 1987). Work overload, incompetent and abrasive managers, unclear job expectations, monotonous assembly-line work,

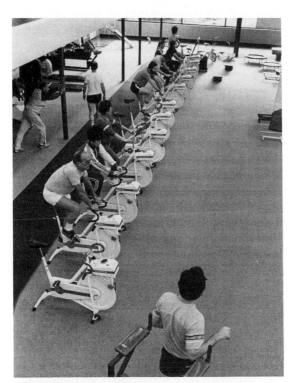

This Looks Like a Health Spa but in Fact Is a Room in a Large Plant. Worksite Wellness Programs Are a Positive Force for Health.
Source: Coors Wellness Center, Golden, CO.

piece work, shift work, and lack of control over working conditions are major factors in illness and stress in employees.

The critics are partially right. Health is not simply an individual matter; health also involves a healthy work environment. Many companies, however, make an effort to create a humane environment. Saab and Volvo eliminated the infamous assembly lines and now use units of workers who build the automobile as a team (Bruhn & Cordova, 1987). Flextime, popular in Europe, is gaining acceptance in American business. Fifteen million employees are under flextime, in which the time of arrival at work is flexible. In addition, American business is concerned with positive human relations at the worksite. Most corporations have training programs to enhance manager and employee relations (Goldsmith, 1986).

Today, the images of the ugly, noisy, unhealthy workplace and the angry, aggressive manager that were born with the Industrial Revolution are gone. Corporate America is becoming health conscious, providing wellness programs for employees and cleaning up the work environment. These are important contributions to health and wellness, but they are not enough. Because human health and environmental health are intimately related, corporate America has another obligation and contribution to health—protecting the natural environment by eliminating the by-products of production that pollute air, soil, and water and that threaten the health of all living creatures. We now describe several corporations that are environmentally conscious and are taking steps to reduce harm to the environment.

Business and a Healthy Environment

The image of business as a protector of the environment has captivated the management and workers of several large companies—the H. B. Fuller Company, Minnesota Mining & Mfg., Dow Chemical Co., Polaroid Corp.,

Digital Equipment Corp., Cleo Wrap Corporation, Safety Queen Corporation, and Wellman Plastics Corporation. A pioneer in this new field, Paul Pankratz, vice president of operations at Dow Chemical, promotes an "ecological" mentality in manufacturing that he calls "WRAP," for "Waste Reduction Always Pays." Pankratz has persuaded Dow Chemical that waste reduction is "the essence of good technology, and it's the right thing to do" (*Dow Today*, 1988). Pankratz began working on this concept in 1984, believing that ecological manufacturing could protect the environment and save money. This idea generated excitement at Dow Chemical, and early in the development, when the key people were discussing various waste-management ideas, Pankratz commented that it was important to wrap-up existing programs into one, and the acronym WRAP was born. WRAP conceptualizes the ecological perspective in manufacturing, saving the environment and saving money.

The creative excitement generated by Pankratz and his partners, Jerry Martin, director of environmental quality, and Ryan Delcombre, a chemical engineer, spread throughout Dow. In the following years, all segments of the Dow work force were challenged to generate ideas for effective waste management. In 1988 a computer control operator of a chemical reactor came up with the idea for recycling ethylene gas that would normally be released into the environment. This could save 10.5 million pounds of gas with a cost saving of $800,000 per year. Many other creative ideas for reducing waste and costs emerged:

1. From 1984 to 1987, Dow's Louisiana Division reduced total waste by 250 million pounds and saved $5.25 million through recycling methods such as re-routing waste stream and using materials in the water for production (Delcambre, 1987).
2. In 1987, another Louisiana plant began converting ethylene glycol (used in antifreeze) into an industrial-grade ethylene glycol, recycling 6 million pounds per year and reducing waste in the atmosphere.
3. In 1987, a plant in Michigan reduced total waste by 40 percent by making a series of small changes such as recycling solvents and improving equipment.
4. In 1987, a plant making latex in California developed a process that reuses wastewater, which formerly went to evaporation ponds. This reduced wastewater by 90 percent and eliminated the need for a landfill to store coagulated latex.

From 1986 to 1987, more than 25 waste reduction projects were developed in Dow plants. Each plant has established waste reduction goals and closely monitors all waste losses to air, water, and land. Dow has taken the leadership in waste management, and has encouraged more than 200,000 small companies to recycle chemical solvents such as trichlorethylene, which is used in dry cleaning.

Other companies have developed effective waste reduction programs. 3M, a worldwide company in 35 countries with a total net sales of $9.4 billion and the manufacturer of products such as Scotch Brand Tape, is a pioneer with its Pollution Prevention Program, called 3–P. From 1975 to 1988, 3M has cut air pollutants by 120,260 tons, sludge and solid waste by 314,000 tons, wastewater by 1.6 billion gallons, and water pollutants by 14,550 tons. The reduction in waste has saved 3M $420 million (Environmental Engineering and Pollution Control Department, 1988).

Wellman Plastic in Massachusetts has developed a technology for recycling 87 percent of all plastic products. Wellman recycles millions of pounds of plastic each year. For example, Wellman recycles the plastic bottles used by soft drink companies into plastics for products such as the felt on tennis balls and for polyester carpet (a third of the plastic used for polyester carpet comes from the Wellman plant).

In 1986, Cleo Wrap, the largest manufacturer of gift wrapping paper, switched from the solvent-based inks to water-based printing inks in all of its operations. This eliminated hazardous waste and the need for underground storage tanks, eliminated all above-ground solvent storage, reduced fire hazards and fire insurance premiums, and reduced the health risk associated with solvents (Office of Technology Assessment, 1986).

For years, solvents used in automotive garages went down the drain into disposal systems. Spotting an opportunity to make money and save the environment, Safety Queen of Elgin, Illinois, entered the business of recycling. Safety Queen gives drums to automotive garages for catching the solvents; the drums are picked up by the company, and the solvents are processed and sold back to the garages at a lower price than new solvents. Safety Queen recycles 99 percent of the used cleaning solvents collected. Safety Queen recycling has been so successful that it has, experienced record-breaking growth and profits 19 years in a row. Safety Queen has expanded to recycling of engine oil. Unfortunately, few states require recycling or the safe disposal of engine oil, but the technology is available.

Imagine the president of the Sierra Club, an active environmentalist group, acting as a consultant to a worldwide chemical company that makes over 10,000 products with 53 plants in 30 different cities and operations in 28 countries. When the H. B. Fuller Company of St. Paul, Minnesota, bought 200 acres for new research and development facilities, the president of the Sierra Club was hired to help the company design a work environment that would complement the ecology of the area. The result—a beautiful passive solar building, so efficient that in the cold Minnesota winters no fossil fuels are needed, surrounded by trees and wildlife—is a perfect example of Dunn's sense of environmental wellness in which beauty is integrated with function, for inspiration and joy.

H. B. Fuller is an adhesives company chaired by Elmer L. Andersen, an active environmentalist. From 1960 to 1962, Andersen was governor of Minnesota and spearheaded the establishment of Voyageurs National Park in the state's lake region. Andersen's concern for the preservation of the natural environment and for safety in the work environment is reflected in many company policies. The company has made a commitment to stop using solvent-based adhesives because of associated environmental and human safety issues, both in production and end use. Water-based and hot-melt adhesives are effective and safer alternatives, and those are the products the company emphasizes in its product development and marketing programs. The H. B. Fuller Company established a Worldwide Environment and Safety Committee led by its regulatory services director, Joe Pellish, to establish environmental policies and guidelines for Fuller plants around the world, even though many countries do not have pollution or safety regulations. "The programs will be consistent with standard worldwide requirements that will be established by and maintained by the Worldwide Environment and Safety Committee" (from the Worldwide Environment and Safety Policy statement adopted by the H. B. Fuller board of directors, October 17, 1986). The committee takes an active stance on all environmental issues, from the safety of the work environment to the safety of the chemicals used in the manufacturing process.

The Franklin Research and Development Corporation is an investment management company for institutions and individuals, created in 1982. The corporation specializes in ethical firms—firms that are socially and environmentally responsible—and evaluates companies according to their record of environmental and social responsibility. The

Atco Properties and Management Company pays its employees $500 to quit smoking. Bonnie Bell Incorporated pays employees 50 cents for each mile they run during the winter. Schere Brothers Lumber Company pays $300 to any employee who is sick fewer than three days a year. It pays to stay healthy!

demand for the Franklin Corporation's services became so great that in six years it accumulated assets of over $160 million. Franklin Corporation has become a major leader in promoting investments in ethical companies.

Corporate America is beginning to promote wellness and health across the business spectra and across the country. Wellness programs for employees enhance health and reduce medical costs, worksite safety programs reduce injuries and disease, and waste reduction and recycling processes save the environment. In business as in government, health promotion is a matter of priorities; the technology could undoubtedly be developed to ensure environmental health, and the behavioral techniques and knowledge of healthy lifestyle are already available to ensure employee health.

Summary

The proliferation of wellness programs in business is a positive trend for health and wellness. Business is also changing its attitude—from polluting the environment as a necessary cost of doing business, to preserving the environment—as a necessary part of doing good business. Many companies demonstrate that waste reduction saves money and the environment. As Paul Pankratz of Dow Chemical said, waste reduction is "the essence of good technology,

and it's the right thing to do" (*Dow Today*, 1988). These new forces for health in business are exciting and innovative, and they have the potential to enhance the health and wellness of millions of people in our society.

||||➡

SECTION TWO: PROGRAMS IN COLLEGES, HOSPITALS, COMMUNITIES, AND PRISONS

Forces for health and wellness are at work throughout society. Colleges, hospitals, and communities around the country have adopted wellness programs. We begin this section with a look at several exemplary programs in colleges, universities, and hospitals, and end with model programs in communities and prisons that prevent violence and promote health.

Wellness Programs in Colleges, Universities, and Hospitals

Compared to medical costs, health education is a bargain, and it reaches many people. From kindergarten to graduate school, educational institutions provide both the setting and the atmosphere for health and wellness education. We use our college as an example. Over the last 15 years, the Behavioral and Social Sciences Division of Aims Community College has developed wellness classes covering the entire lifespan, from the prenatal period to death. The programs are free to people 60 and over, and they cost $18 per credit for county residents. For people who cannot afford $18 per credit, tuition waivers are available. Thousands of people have taken these classes.

Biofeedback and Stress Management is one of the most popular classes. Participants learn a variety of behavioral skills, practice EMG feedback training in a biofeedback learning center, and practice thermal feedback training at home. Lectures include many topics in this textbook, such as the physiology of stress, identifying personal stressors, enhancing coping skills, positive goal-setting, positive self-talk, visualization, and cognitive restructuring.

Does a one-quarter class on stress management make a difference? Is health improved? To answer these questions, we obtained funds from the Colorado Board of Higher Education to evaluate the health status of students who took the class; the stress-profiling described in Chapter 5 was part of this study.

The study (Shellenberger, Turner, Green, & Cooney, 1986) included a control group of 200 subjects who received the 30-minute stress profile and completed the Minnesota Multiphasic Personality Inventory (MMPI) and the Cornell Medical Index, an inventory of 195 questions on medical symptoms. Three months after the profile, control subjects were given feedback on the stress profile and on the MMPI and CMI scores. The experimental group was students who completed the 10-week biofeedback and stress-management class. The students received the 30-minute stress profile and completed the MMPI and the CMI.

Follow-up health questionnaires were mailed to both groups two years later. The questionnaire covered current psychological and physiological health, including medication use, number of physician visits two years before taking the stress profile or class and two years after the profile or class, life changes, symptom history, and current satisfaction with life at work and at home. Completed questionnaires were returned by 78 people in the control group and by 50 students.

In comparison to the control group, students in the class significantly lowered physician visits, improved their mental and physical health, and reduced migraine headache, tension headache, heart palpitations, smoking, worrying, performance anxiety, general anxiety, insomnia, rage, bruxism, low-back pain, hay fever, ulcers, and high blood pressure.

We were pleased with the results. The biofeedback and stress-management class helped people develop coping skills, improve health, and reduce symptoms. The class was inexpensive and effective in reducing medical costs.

The University of Wisconsin at Stevens Point has pioneered in a comprehensive wellness program for faculty, staff, and students. The main components of the program are:

1. Lifestyle assessment.
2. Workshops and classes on assertiveness training, smoking cessation, weight control, nutrition, responsible use of alcohol, stress management, and physical fitness.
3. Alteration of the environment, such as adding nutritious food in the cafeteria and declaring no-smoking areas.
4. Use of a portable testing module for measuring lung capacity, blood pressure, resting pulse, muscle strength, and flexibility. The module is placed in dormitories, classrooms, and administrative buildings for use by everyone.
5. Lifestyle-improvement classes that can be taken for credit through the physical education department.
6. An annual national wellness-promotion conference for educators.

The Stevens Point program began in 1971. Although there are no long-term follow-up studies on students so far, the program provides a model for a large university.

Through its annual conference and programs, the University of Wisconsin at Stevens Point provides leadership for businesses, schools, hospitals, and government. Most of the participants at the wellness conference at Stevens Point are from hospitals. Many hospitals have wellness programs. The Michigan Hospital Association has promoted wellness programs in hospitals throughout the state. The American Hospital Association established the Center for Health Promotion in 1978 to help hospitals develop wellness programs. The center provides telephone consultations and audiovisual materials and publishes a health-promotion newsletter. Each year the center sponsors the Innovator's Conference. A select group of physicians, administrators, and health planners are invited to a three-day conference to share knowledge and plan new programs.

In the 1970s, the Swedish Medical Center in Englewood, Colorado, pioneered in a hospital-based wellness program. The tasks of the wellness program are:

1. To catalyze, coordinate, and provide high-quality wellness programs for improvement of health and realization of human potential.
2. To provide national leadership in the development of wellness and health promotion efforts.
3. To create supportive environments in hospitals, schools, churches, corporations, physicians' offices, government, and other community groups that help people initiate and maintain healthy lifestyles.
4. To explore the innovative role of the hospital in promoting the health of its community.

To accomplish these tasks, the Swedish Medical Center's program focuses on stress management, exercise, diet, smoking cessation, fitness testing, and substance-abuse prevention. The hospital has its own fitness and recreational facilities and coordinates recreational programs such as softball, fun runs, golf, ten-

nis, basketball, and skiing. The Swedish Medical Center also coordinates a hospital network for health promotion programs throughout the country.

The effectiveness of hospital-based wellness programs has not been determined. However, the change in identity of hospitals from "disease care centers" to "wellness centers" is bound to have significant implications for patients and staff and for the practice of medicine.

Prevention of Violence and Community Programs

The cycle of neglect, abuse, and violence begins early in life for many people. Programs for the prevention of violence and promotion of health have targeted populations at risk for violence and have initiated early intervention programs.

Prenatal/Early Infancy Project

Elmira, New York, at the northern end of Appalachia, in 1980 had the highest incidence of child abuse and neglect in New York state. It was also the most economically devastated part of the state and was described by *The New York Times* as a community "of lost jobs, broken families and fading hope" (Schorr & Schorr, 1987, p. 169). Pediatric psychologist David Olds, fresh from graduate school, had a plan that he thought might work with poor dysfunctional families in Elmira. His plan had trained nurses, skilled in providing social support and nursing care, visit the homes of families expecting a baby. The nurses would make visits during the prenatal period and continue to function as a resource after the baby was born.

An initial project was conducted with 400 poor families. Special effort was made to find families with pregnant teenagers and women who were unmarried, unemployed, or on welfare. A team of registered nurses was trained for 2 1/2 months and then began the home

---

At Sacred Heart Hospital in Yankton, South Dakota, an employee who feels great and wants to take a day off can call in and say, "I feel too great to go to work today." Employees are allowed three wellness days a year.

visits. The families were randomly assigned to one of the following groups: (1) health screening only; (2) health screening plus assistance in transportation to clinics; (3) screening, transportation, and home visits during pregnancy only; and (4) health screening, assistance in transportation, home visits during pregnancy, and home visits until the child was 2 years old.

The home visits by the nurses provided valuable health care, varying from family to family. One young couple expecting a baby in three months had not eaten for two days. The nurse helped them find emergency food and income, and then helped them find work. The nurses provided emotional support and also helped young mothers and fathers develop problem-solving skills for coping with the many stressors encountered day to day. In addition, the young mothers and fathers learned how to provide a healthy diet for themselves, and how to meet the emotional and physical needs of the newborn.

The families in the two treatment groups that received home visits from nurses had one-fifth the incidence of child abuse and neglect as other families, heavier and fewer premature babies, more parents returning to school, more parents finding employment, and fewer pregnancies over the next four years (Olds, Henderson, Tatelbaum, & Chamberlin, 1986a, 1986b). Replications of the nurse home-visit program have similar results. Child abuse and neglect declined significantly, and families became more functional.

Homebuilders

To prevent the spiral of family dissolution, neglect of children, and eventual placement of children of dysfunctional families in foster homes, the staff at the Catholic Children's Services in Tacoma, Washington, created a home-based program to help dysfunctional families.

In 1974, with a grant from the National Institute of Mental Health, Catholic Children's Services assembled a team of psychologists, social workers, and counselors to create a program for dysfunctional families; they called themselves Homebuilders. Homebuilders provide intensive care to families in distress, in the home. They describe themselves as a family intensive-care unit. Each team member is responsible for no more than three families; this gives team members the time to help the family resolve immediate crises and to teach coping skills. A family is referred to Homebuilders by social services when it is considered so dysfunctional that the children may have to be placed in a foster home. Often a family crisis is occurring when the referral is made, such as child abuse, a child running away, a suicide attempt, or an arrest. The staff works closely with teachers, juvenile court, employers, and social services.

Dysfunctional families are difficult to help; these families seem to be in continual crisis and they are suspicious of professionals. Homebuilders staff are able to break through the suspiciousness of dysfunctional families by providing intensive social support. For example, a mother with a history of abuse and neglect of her four children was referred to Homebuilders after she had been involved with many agencies and her children had been in a foster home for a short period of time. When the Homebuilder therapist visited the home, the mother did not want any advice on "raising kids." Instead she wanted help on getting her house together. The house was a mess and the children were unkempt and would not go to school because they were ridiculed by other students. The Homebuilder therapist focused on the immediate needs and helped the family get clothes, a refrigerator, blankets, and mattresses. Then she helped the mother scrub the walls and floors, an unusual therapeutic approach to dysfunctional families. As they worked together, the mother began to trust the therapist. The therapist also spent considerable time with the children, helping them with homework and visiting their teachers. During this time the therapist taught the basics of communication and coping skills. After several months, the family was functional. The mother was seeing a therapist at a local mental health center for ongoing support, the children were attending school regularly, and the two oldest children had obtained jobs. The Homebuilders' therapist was no longer needed. At the one-year follow-up the family was still functional. They had a sense of pride and closeness. The 16-year-old had decided to continue in school.

The Homebuilders program is very successful. Follow-up at six years showed a 92 percent success rate of rehabilitating families, preventing 849 children from being placed in foster care. By preventing long-term foster care, group care, or psychiatric hospitalization, Homebuilders estimates that for every dollar spent, six are saved (Kinney, Madsen, Fleming, & Haapakla, 1977).

Five states have instituted programs based on Homebuilders, most recently New York. Homebuilders is a model program. It demonstrates an effective approach for helping dysfunctional families.

Anger Control and Battering Couples

Violence in marriage cuts across socioeconomic levels. The Graduate School of Social Work at the University of Texas at Arlington has developed an intensive 10-week anger control program for violent couples that includes weekly group meetings and individual weekly therapy sessions. The couples learn "time out," relaxation, communication, empathy, cognitive restructuring, and assertiveness skills.

Participants experienced episodes of violence in their present family life. One-third of the participants was middle- or upper-class and two-thirds were lower-class. Participants voluntarily came to the sessions after reading about the program in the newspaper or hearing about it from a friend.

Professors Deschner and McNeill (1986) conducted a one-year follow-up study on 82 participants; complete preprogram and postprogram data were obtained from 69. Interviews, daily diaries, and questionnaires were used to assess the effectiveness of the program. Episodes of anger had significantly decreased, and participants perceived themselves and their partners as less angry. Eighty-five percent of the participants reported using anger control skills for at least eight months after the program. Incidents of abuse declined by 50 percent. Participants ranked the time-out skill as the most valuable and the one used most frequently. Using the time-out skill, one partner signals for time-out and the other partner acknowledges the need for a time-out. During time-out, couples relax or dispute angry self-talk. When they resume the dispute, each partner admits to the other that his or her fighting style was not perfect. Couples reported that reconciliation occurred quite rapidly after the time-out skill was used.

Clearly, couples can replace maladaptive and dysfunctional behaviors with new adaptive behaviors.

Intensive programs work. They prevent child abuse and neglect and family violence; in summary, they foster healthy families and the conditions for healthy development. These model programs are cost-effective and save society millions of dollars in social services cost. This work is primary prevention because it focuses on the cause of these problems.

Now we turn to an area that might be called secondary prevention, or changing a condition after it has occurred in an effort to prevent recurrence—the rehabilitation of criminals. Although generalizations can be inaccurate, experts know that people who find themselves in jail or in prison for serious or repeated offenses are likely to have come from abusive and dysfunctional families and have few occupational, social, and self regulation skills. For some, violence and crime are a way of life that is maintained in spite of the prison system, and, some would argue, because of it. Yet the situation is not hopeless; in this subsection we describe changes within the penal system that may change forever the institution that seems at times to foster criminal behavior rather than decrease it. These changes facilitate the development of the characteristics of the healthy person and break the cycle of crime and punishment.

Prisons and the Prevention of Violence

Currently, one in 350 Americans is serving time in prison (U.S. Bureau of the Census, 1987). Prisons and jails are breeding grounds for violence, and they perpetuate criminality. Assaults and homosexual rape are daily occurrences. In many prisons, inmates have no opportunity to learn skills for physical and psychological health that could free them from crime—job skills, self regulation skills, and fundamental academic skills. When prisoners are released they may be no better off than when they were incarcerated, and they may be angrier and more violent. Many criminals have no family or friends to return to, and their only social group is previous partners in crime. Prisoners lose their jobs, and many cannot pay for education and training. Jails and prisons may reinforce criminal behavior and provide all the ingredients for becoming an unhealthy person—a lack of self-esteem, a lack of positive human interaction, a lack of social support, a lack of a sense of control, and a lack of self regulation.

The traditional approach to treating criminals has been destructive to both inmates and the public, as indicated by a single statistic: The average recidivism rate is 80 percent (U.S. Bureau of the Census, 1987). This means that 80 percent of the people released from prison commit a second crime and are imprisoned again.

To compound the problem, on the average, prisoners now serve only one-fourth of the length of their sentence (U.S. Bureau of the Census, 1987). In 1987, the prison population reached a record of 546,659 inmates, and the FBI reported that violent crimes rose by 12 percent, the largest jump in two decades. At the same time, states are running out of money and room for prisoners. Overcrowding makes early release necessary. Warren Burger, chief justice of the United States in 1984, said, "Our system is too costly, too painful, too destructive, too inefficient for a truly civilized people."

But if you have been raped, or lost a loved one or a friend by homicide, or had a child molested, or been victimized in some other way, your attitude toward prisoners might be similar to that of many Americans: "Lock them up and throw away the key." Rehabilitating criminals is not a popular policy with the American public or with politicians. Public opinion regarding prisoners is so strong that in the 1988 presidential campaign, George Bush was able to make Michael Dukakis's prison reforms in Massachusetts a national issue that created negative feelings against prison reform. And as a society, we have been unwilling to provide sufficient money for rehabilitating criminals. The data indicate, however, that this attitude, and the current prison system, are failing. Most criminals are neither locked up forever nor rehabilitated. In the remainder of this section we introduce several new approaches to rehabilitation that foster psychosocial, moral, and spiritual development.

A variety of new rehabilitation programs teach psychological and practical skills needed for living successfully "on the outside." Skills range from reading maps and bus schedules to holding a job. The state of Virginia requires prisoners to be able to read above the sixth-grade level before receiving parole. Seven states require inmates to attend school if they read below the fifth-grade level.

Job-training programs help prisoners acquire vocational skills and are cost-effective. In Iowa, $7 million in annual sales from on-the-job training programs more than pays for prison and education expenses. "We're training people who won't come back to prison, and it costs taxpayers nothing," says Harry Cannon, director of prison industries. Florida recently contracted with a nonprofit firm, PRIDE (Prison Rehabilitation Industries and Diversified Enterprises), to create prison industries and provide training for prisoners, In 1987, prisoners earned $44 million dollars to pay for room and board and to repay crime victims. PRIDE is one of the most successful prison industries programs. It has established more than 30 different types of factories and shops within Florida prisons, including design and drafting, automobile renovation, printing, and manufacturing. To work in a factory or shop, prisoners must fill out applications and be interviewed for the job, which is important training for getting a job when released from prison. Prisoners who are accepted receive on-the-job training and wages. PRIDE also has a job-placement program for prisoners who are released.

Practical skills are not enough for inmates who lack self regulation skills such as goal-setting, delay of gratification, and self-discipline. In Mississippi inmates are taught self regulation skills in classes, and they learn self-discipline through rigorous physical exercises.

The long-term success of these rehabilitation programs is not known. Nevertheless, in contrast to the "talk" psychotherapy of the 1950s, which was ineffective in preventing recidivism (Lipton & Martinson, 1975), the new programs are likely to be successful because they focus on practical, occupational, and self regulation skills. It is clear, however, that these skills are not enough for many prisoners; social skills are also needed. Teaching social skills in a prison is not impossible and has far reaching benefits. We describe a recent innovation that dramatically changes the social environment in prisons—direct supervision.

Direct Supervision

Direct supervision is an innovative approach to prison management that has been adopted at more than 50 jails and prisons in the United States. "Direct supervision" refers to the environment shown in Figure 21.1. In direct supervision prisons, a central living room is surrounded by individual rooms, and guards are in direct contact with inmates, rather than in a guard room. Inmates have access to the living area, and the guards function as human-relations specialists with skills in communication, conflict resolution, and crisis intervention. Discipline by logical consequences is the rule. The guards head off conflicts before they develop, and they have the power to administer logical consequences immediately, according to the severity of the misbehaviors. The logical consequence of fighting is being locked in one's room; other consequences are extra cleanup duty, loss of television or telephone privileges, and loss of recreational facilities. In direct supervision facilities for men, 40 percent of the guards are women. This may be a significant factor in the success of direct supervision programs, although we have no data on the influence of women in prison.

The consequences of direct supervision are positive for both staff and prisoners (Krauth & Clem, 1987; Nelson, O'Toole, Krauth, & Whitmore, 1984; Sigurdson, 1985, 1987). Incidents of violence are reduced by 50 percent. In the first two years after the New York City Jail adopted direct supervision, there were no incidents of vandalism, no homicides, no suicides, and no sexual assaults. The number of fights in two years were comparable to the monthly rate in other jails. In the first 18 months of direct supervision at the Contra Costa County jail in California, there were no incidents of homosexual rape. In another large jail in an adjacent county, homosexual rapes averaged five a night. Vandalism is almost nonexistent in direct supervision jails. Ninety-five percent of all inmates function very well under direct supervision. The remaining 5 percent are either mentally ill or extremely violent and are placed in highly restricted environments (Sigurdson, 1985, 1987).

Direct supervision enhances the well-being

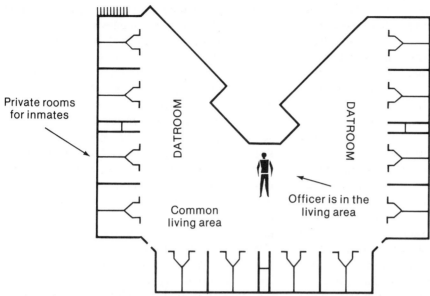

Figure 21.1. Direct Supervision Prison Design. Adapted from *Direct Supervision Jails: Interview with Administrators,* National Institute of Corrections Information Center, Boulder, CO.

of both guards and prisoners. Prisoners are treated with dignity, and guards are treated as professionals and are challenged by the job. Life satisfaction is high, and absenteeism for guards is decreased by 70 percent compared with rates in traditional prison environments.

The positive results of direct supervision prisons are no mystery. Study Figure 21.1 from a social engineering perspective. You can see that a social unit is created in which people communicate freely, do not feel isolated, and above all, are trusted.

A classic problem remains—the social environment outside the prison that the prisoner returns to when released. Typically, prisoners return to the same environment that fostered the criminal behavior. The gains made in prison may be undermined by the old environment. Prisoners need a supportive group to associate with after release, in which noncriminal behavior is reinforced. Several volunteer groups are dedicated to this problem such as Koinonia, Road to Emmaeus, Prisoners' Fellowship, Institute for Alternatives to Violence, and Kairos.

Forces for health and wellness are at work for people even in prisons and jails, places where violence and degradation are common: direct-supervision prisons, educational programs, job-training programs such as PRIDE, and self regulation training programs. Direct-supervision prisons find that 95 percent of criminals respond positively to humane treatment. Prisoners are not immune to the dynamics of health and wellness—love, self regulation skills, positive expectations, enhancing self-esteem, and discipline based on logical consequences.

Summary

The cycle of disadvantaged and dysfunctional families can be broken by intensive intervention programs such as Homebuilders in Washington and the pediatric nurse program in Appalachia. Educational programs in colleges and hospitals help families and individuals learn skills for healthy living. Even hardened criminals are capable of transformation through programs that teach practical and psychosocial skills, through social support, and through a meaningful purpose in life. Direct-supervision programs bring wellness to staff and prisoners. Violence and tension are reduced, prisoners are treated with dignity, and staff members feel a new sense of pride as professionals in conflict resolution. These exciting new programs demonstrate that people can overcome difficult problems when they are given the resources and encouragement.

Society has the experience, the knowledge, and the resources to reach for the goal of "wellness for all by the year 2000", to which this text is dedicated. The major issue is priorities: Will the government allocate resources and establish policy for enhancing the health of all people, and will people respond with responsibility?

IIII▶

SECTION THREE: THE POLITICS OF HEALTH —SOCIAL ENGINEERING

This chapter focuses on forces outside the individual—social forces—that promote personal health and wellness. The previous sections described private and public programs designed specifically to foster behavior change in individuals and examined several of these programs in detail. In this section we shift perspective from the specific program and its effect on behavior to the level at which programs and health policies are initiated, the level of social policy. "Social policy" refers to laws, regulations, guidelines, and programs that are created by government to affect the health of citizens, either by promoting health behavior or by discouraging or preventing worseness behavior. Personal health and social policy are intertwined.

Social policy is in the political domain in the sense that creating social policy is a function of local, state, and federal governments. "Social engineering" refers to changing individual behavior through social policy, and it bridges a conceptual gap between political process and social policy and psychology. When we talk about the effect of social policy on health, we are talking about social engineering.

We have many examples of the effects of social policy on health behavior: the ban on smoking in public places, raising the drinking age to 21, requiring the use of seat belts in cars, bans on alcohol and tobacco advertising, requiring bicyclists and motorcyclists to wear helmets, and stiff driving-under-the-influence penalties. These policies may have a greater effect on preventing disease and injury than attempts to change individual behavior by working directly with individuals. For example, raising the legal drinking age from 18 to 21 has been more successful in reducing alcohol-related auto fatalities than programs designed to help the drunk driver. Forty percent of all deaths in people age 15–24 are caused by car accidents, and half of these deaths involve a drunk driver. To counter this, in 1982, Tennessee increased the penalties for driving under the influence, and in 1984 raised the drinking age to 21 years. These policies were accompanied by high-profile programs in high schools against driving under the influence. Alcohol-related deaths declined by 33 percent in the 15–18 year group, and by 38 percent in the 19–20 year group (Decker, Graitcer, & Schaffner, 1988). In 1987, the National Highway Traffic Safety Administration reported a 13 percent drop in fatal accidents and 1,000 lives saved in states that raised the drinking age to 21.

Health professionals in many fields—public health, community health, health education, and health psychology—study the dynamics of social policy and its effects on health. Health professionals can play an important role in determining and implementing social policy.

We begin this section by describing the process through which one state, Minnesota, developed a social policy and legislation to achieve a particular health goal.

The State of Minnesota

In 1981, the Minnesota Department of Health established the goal of a smoke-free society by the year 2000 (Minnesota had already banned smoking in public places outside of designated areas in 1975 with passage of the Minnesota Clean Air Act). To accomplish this goal, the Minnesota Department of Health established the Center for Nonsmoking and Health in the summer of 1983. The center had two researchers, a health educator, and the state epidemiologist. It provided research evidence on the beneficial

effects of nonsmoking on health and acted as coordinator of statewide nonsmoking programs (see Figure 21.2). Also in 1983, the Minnesota commissioner of health appointed a technical advisory committee to develop a statewide plan for actively promoting nonsmoking. Members of the advisory committee represented medicine, labor, wholesale/retail sales, education, insurance, nursing, advertising, community action, hotel/restaurant management, and local and state government.

The Technical Advisory Committee produced a report in September 1984 titled, *The Minnesota Plan for Nonsmoking and Health.* The report made 39 recommendations for five target areas through which nonsmoking would be promoted: (1) school and youth education,

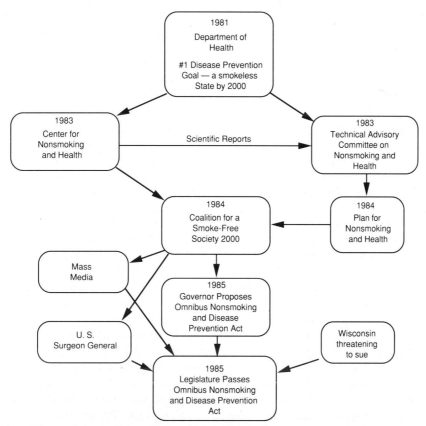

Figure 21.2. Flow Chart of the Political Process for Passage of the Nonsmoking Bill in Minnesota.

(2) public education and communications, (3) regulatory measures, (4) economic incentives and disincentives, and (5) information and program evaluation (Schultz, Onoen, Pechecek, Harty, Skubic, Gust, & Dean, 1986). The report proposed the following legislation:

1. Increase the state cigarette excise tax by 7 cents per pack.
2. Prohibit the free distribution of cigarettes.
3. Provide worksite nonsmoking programs.
4. Develop tobacco-use prevention programs for adolescents.
5. Provide statewide and community grants for nonsmoking programs.
6. Provide funds for technical assistance and program evaluations.
7. Promote public education through media campaigns.

The report created considerable discussion. More than 2,000 copies were distributed to legislators, public health professionals, and reporters.

To implement the plan, representatives from the American Cancer Society, American Lung Association, American Heart Association, the Minnesota Public Health Association, the Minnesota Department of Health, health insurance companies, and health maintenance organizations formed the Minnesota Coalition for a Smoke-Free Society 2000. The coalition actively promoted the plan through the mass media and through invited speakers including Surgeon General Everett Koop. The coalition influenced the governor to introduce a legislative bill, the Omnibus Nonsmoking and Disease Prevention Act. Revenues from the increased excise tax on cigarettes would pay for the antismoking programs.

The tobacco industry immediately lobbied against the bill. Nine lobbyists were hired to represent Philip Morris, Cos. Inc., R. J. Reynolds, Inc., Brown and Williams Inc., the Tobacco Institute, and state candy and tobacco groups. Nationally known economists, researchers, and lawyers provided "expert witness" testimony against the bill. Ads opposing the bill appeared in newspapers throughout the state. The R. J. Reynolds company sent preaddressed postcards to smokers throughout the state for mailing to state senators.

The Minnesota Legislature was committed to reducing taxes in 1985. Many legislators believed that the Omnibus Nonsmoking and Disease Prevention Act conflicted with a mandate from citizens to reduce taxes. On the other hand, money for sewer construction projects was badly needed, and it could be acquired through the cigarette excise tax increase. The state of Wisconsin was threatening to sue Minnesota for dumping sewage into the Mississippi River.

After much debate, the omnibus bill was attached to a larger bill that included a $1 billion cut in personal income tax. The proposed excise tax was reduced from 7 cents to 5 cents, and distribution of free cigarettes was not banned.

The political process by which the Omnibus Nonsmoking and Disease Prevention Act became law (Figure 21.2) is an example of the various factors involved in promoting health legislation and creating social policy. The widespread support by the citizens of Minnesota, the support of influential corporations and businesses, and the lobbying efforts of the Minnesota Coalition for a Smoke-Free Society 2000 effectively countered the tremendous pressure exerted by the tobacco industry (Schultz, Onoen, Pechacek, Harty, Skubic, Gust, & Dean, 1986).

Other states are actively promoting health legislation. In 1988, Massachusetts was the first state to pass a universal health insurance law that requires all employers to provide health insurance. Small employers with five or fewer employees will not have to provide insurance, but their workers will be able to obtain insurance through the state group insurance plan (Bule, 1988). North Carolina has developed a model pollution-prevention program called Pollution Prevention Pays Program (Office of Technology Assessment, 1986). The state provides information, technical assistance, and grants to businesses and educational institutions for developing recycling and waste-reduction programs. The program has received support from all segments of the state, including business and citizens groups.

Achieving legislation for health programs in the United States involves a struggle between the forces for and against health. Even at the state level the political process is often arduous and complicated, and it requires advocates who have persistence, patience, and the ability to cooperate with diverse groups of people and cope with the paradoxical forces in our society.

The Federal Government, Health Promotion, and Protection

With its immense financial resources and bureaucracy, the government can play a central role in promoting health and well-being in this country. Many government programs fund health research and public information services. Reports from the Office of the Surgeon General are influential directives that guide research and funding. The 1964 surgeon general's report on the association of cigarette smoking and lung cancer is credited with increasing public awareness of the hazards of tobacco use and stimulating the surge of programs for prevention of smoking. The Office of Technology and Assessment is an agency of Congress whose function is to update Congress on technological developments that affect human health. The director of the agency is appointed by a bipartisan committee of Congress. The agency has taken a leadership role in uniting business and citizens groups to promote waste reduction, and it provides industry with the latest information on technology for recycling waste. The Office of Technology and Assessment also evaluates the

effectiveness of government agencies involved in health protection, such as the Environmental Protection Agency.

The federal government spends more money on health promotion and health protection than any other organization in the United States. In 1987, $50 million was spent on health, education, and social services, and another $23 million went to research and development. Many innovative community, school, and family programs are financed by federal agencies within the Department of Health and Human Services. For example, the School Health Education Evaluation program that evaluated health education in schools described in Chapter 13 was funded and developed by the Center for Health Promotion and Education, a division of the Centers for Disease Control, which is part of the Public Health branch. Most of the health-promotion programs in communities are funded by the various institutes that are divisions within the National Institutes of Health. The Minnesota Healthy Heart Program is funded by the Heart, Lung, and Blood Institute. Many drug and alcohol prevention programs are funded by the Alcohol, Drug Abuse, and Mental Health Institute. Some of the research in behavioral medicine discussed in Chapter 15 was funded by the various institutes within the Department of Health and Human Services.

Many agencies within the Department of Health and Human Services are designed to protect the health and safety of the public. As discussed in Chapter 20, the mandate of the Food and Drug Administration is to protect the public from harmful medications and from carcinogens in food. One function of the National Institute for Occupational Safety and Health is protection of workers from harmful exposure to toxic chemicals. The Centers for Disease Control conducts extensive research on disease and prevention of disease, and is now strenuously working to help curb the AIDS epidemic.

An entire book could be written on the

federal programs that promote the health of the American people. When adequate funding and personnel are available, governmental agencies are powerful forces for health and wellness. University of Arizona professor John Schwarz argues in his book, *America's Hidden Success* (1988), that many government programs are more efficient than businesses and are effective in improving the health of the American people. "Hidden success" refers to successful health and education programs such as Head Start, job training, job creation, and Aid to Families with Dependent Children. In one decade, poverty was reduced by 60 percent and infant mortality by 50 percent. Head Start helped thousands of children improve their intellectual and social abilities (Conger, 1988).

Schwarz argues that only federal programs can solve the problems of poverty, infant mortality, and child neglect, as well as the health problems of thousands of elderly, disabled, and disadvantaged people in the United States. Nonprofit groups such as United Way can help, but such groups lack the resources, money, and organization to coordinate a national program to deal with national problems. Even in the best of economic times, the circumstances of disabled and disadvantaged people are not improved. When federal health and education programs were cut back in the 1980s, the effects were significant: infant mortality increased in 1985, unemployment reached higher levels than in the 1970s, and homelessness and poverty significantly increased. As we know from the 1970s, a strong government that vigorously promotes health and education can be a blessing for millions of people, and it can promote a healthy nation.

In spite of this potential, it is a fact that the government may fail to foresee problems that will eventually endanger human and environmental health, and the government may fail to enforce existing regulations, particularly when the violator is corporate America. And it is a fact that corporate America is reluctant to regulate itself on behalf of human and environmental

health when doing so threatens profits. It might seem then that the average citizen is at the mercy of government and business, having little power to affect either. This is not so. We next discuss what is, in our estimation, one of the most important societal forces for health, citizens groups, which, to use the previous metaphor, join the small patch of the individual to a large patch that represents common goals for the common good, a patch that is far greater in power than the individual patches.

Citizens Groups and Health Promotion

A citizens group is a response to a need that individuals alone cannot pursue, lacking knowledge, time, money, legal support, political influence, or even a voice. The Children's Defense Fund, for example, was created to fight for the well-being of children, who have no voice of their own. Groups such as the Sierra Club and Greenpeace fight to protect the environment and all of its inhabitants, the majority of which have no voice at all.

We highlight three citizens groups that are diverse in history and focus but that have a common need to pursue—the health and well-being of citizens everywhere.

Ralph Nader and the Health Research Group

A 32-year-old lawyer from Connecticut took on General Motors. In 1965, Ralph Nader had just written a book, *Unsafe at Any Speed*, criticizing the automobile industry for failing to include safety features in cars and for failing to ensure the mechanical safety of new cars. In particular, Nader criticized the design of the Chevrolet Corvair, which caused it to flip over at speeds of 35–60 mph. The U.S. Senate brought Nader and GM together in a hearing that became high drama as Nader fought the auto giant. When it was discovered that GM had played foul by trying to slander Nader, the senators and the public were outraged.

Nader emerged as a public hero, the underdog fighting the giants on behalf of the common people. It was an appropriate image.

Nader's persistence and publicity from the hearing hastened the passage of the first Federal Auto Safety Law in 1966. By recalling unsafe cars (more than 1 million have been recalled) and by requiring safety features on cars, the law has helped save more than 85,000 lives and has protected more than 1 million people involved in accidents from serious injury (Claybrook, 1985).

Knowing that it is impossible to fight corporate giants alone and without money, Nader helped create more than 15 citizens groups, including Public Citizen, an organization composed of six research groups (Figure 21.3). One of the most important groups, the Health Research Group (HRG), was founded in 1971 by Nader and physician Sidney Wolfe. The HRG investigates health topics and lobbies Congress, and in conjunction with the Litigation Group (also founded by Nader), sues governmental agencies that fail to enforce regulations designed to protect the American people. Some of the topics that the Health Research Group has pursued are:

> *Smokeless tobacco:* In the last few years, thousands of teenage boys started using chewing tobacco and snuff. In 1984 the Health Research Group petitioned the Federal Trade Commission to require warning labels on smokeless tobacco products and advertising. It also urged minor and major league baseball clubs to curtail the use of smokeless tobacco, believing that the habit among ballplayers encourages younger boys to chew. Director Wolfe says, "Much of

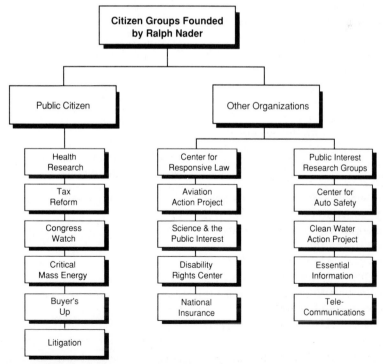

Figure 21.3.   Citizen Groups that Ralph Nader Helped to Establish.

the phenomenal growth in the use of smokeless tobacco among teenage boys is certainly due to the use of these products by professional athletes" (Negin, 1985, October).

Drugs: The Health Research Group studies the scientific research on hundreds of drugs to evaluate their safety and effectiveness. When the Health Research Group finds that a drug is not safe, it petitions the Food and Drug Administration to ban the drug. For example,

the Health Research Group found that a painkilling drug, Suprol, had caused more than 300 cases of kidney damage and petitioned the FDA to prohibit sale of Suprol. Suprol was finally taken off the market in May 1987, after the drug had been banned by all the European countries.

Food products: The Health Research Group evaluates research on a variety of food additives. It advocates fast-food labeling, including processing information,

---

CAMPAIGN RECOGNIZES SAFE FOOD TRAILBLAZERS

"Clean your plate" Mom always chided—but then she probably didn't think about the additives, pesticides, and contaminants that riddle the modern food supply. Making supper healthful again is the objective of a coalition called Americans for Safe Food, which bestowed the 1988 "Safe Food Trailblazer" awards on several companies, states, and individuals for their innovative efforts to provide a clean food supply to the nation. The recipients include:

Texas and Washington, for establishing programs for certifying organic farms to ensure that production methods conform to state standards.

Purity Supreme, whose 65 New England supermarkets carry natural beef that is virtually free of drug and pesticide residues.

Farmers Wholesale Cooperative, a distributorship owned by Washington State organic farmers, which has expanded the market for their certified organic produce to a dozen supermarkets in Seattle and Olympia.

Rep. Ted Weiss, a New York Democrat,

for exposing gross dereliction of duty by the Food and Drug Administration with regard to regulating food dyes and animal drugs.

Minnesota, Wisconsin, and California, for funding research and training in sustainable agriculture, including helping farmers reduce chemical inputs.

Iowa, for its innovative tax on pesticides and nitrogen fertilizer that will help fund a $64.5 million, five-year program to promote sustainable agriculture, combat chemical contamination of drinking water, and study toxic chemicals' impact on health.

Community Supported Agriculture of South Egremont, Massachusetts, for its project in which 75 households bought shares in an organic farm and share in its production.

Rep. George Brown, a California Democrat, and Sen. Patrick Leahy, a Vermont Democrat, for their leadership in appropriating $3.9 million for alternative agricultural research.

Source: Public Citizen, (1988, July/August)

so that customers know what they are eating: for example, what type of fat the fast-food processor uses in making french fries.

Hazardous Chemicals: Thousands of chemicals are produced each year. Many, such as asbestos, cause cancer, lung disease, heart disease, or other problems. Workers who handle these chemicals may be at risk for disease and injury. For many years the Health Research Group advocated that all workers have the right to know what toxic substances are present in the workplace, and finally it sued the Occupational Safety and Health Administration for failing to issue regulations. The U.S. Court of Appeals agreed with the Health Research Group and required OSHA to issue stringent "right to know" regulations.

The Health Research Group serves as a watchdog for health issues. It monitors the societal forces that jeopardize health, it does the homework and research, and it takes action not possible by the individual citizen. The Health Research Group also publishes a newsletter, *Health Letter.* Like all other citizens groups, the Health Research Group helps the private citizen be an informed consumer and encourages individual action. For example, Americans for Safe Food, a branch of the Center for Science in the Public Interest, provides a packet of instructions on how to organize a local group for pressuring supermarkets to provide safe food. It also publishes a newsletter, *Nutrition Action,* that informs the consumer about the food industry and food and promotes wise decision-making, in action and in eating.

The vast network of citizens organizations that began with the frustration and dedication of one person, Ralph Nader, is a repeating story in the development of citizens groups; the next group that we highlight is another example.

Citizen's Clearinghouse for Hazardous Waste

After Lois Gibbs' family moved to Niagara Falls, New York, her 6-year-old son was always sick. He had asthma, convulsions, blood disorders, and urinary tract problems that required two operations. Lois knew that their house was near an old dump, Love Canal, that had been covered up, and she was aware that many residents were worried about chemicals seeping into basements and yards, but she did not make the connection with her son until June 1978, when an article in the local paper described the chemicals in the dump and their effects— lung disease and neurological disorders. The school that her son attended was built on the dump site.

Lois was convinced that her son's problems had been caused by the Love Canal dump site and wanted to transfer him to another school. The school board refused, saying ". . . we'll have to recognize there's a risk to the other children as well. We'd have to close the school and we're not about to do that to please one overemotional mother" (Citizen's Clearinghouse for Hazardous Waste, 1986, p. 8). Not to be put off so easily, Lois began to take action, a difficult step for someone who was neither bold nor outspoken. She began by going door-to-door, talking to residents about their concerns and asking for support in organizing a community homeowners association for the purpose of pressuring local and state officials to close the school, pay restitution for property loss, and clean up the dump site. With help from several people, Lois learned about the chemicals in the dump and the risks to health, how to get her message to the press, and how to confront government officials; she also learned that many adults were sick and that many had children with birth defects. In August the state health commissioner announced a plan for Love Canal: The school was closed, a cleanup was proposed, and families with pregnant women or children under 2 years were told to move immediately, with no assistance from the state, federal government, or the chemical company that had created the dump but claimed no responsibility. For Lois Gibbs and her partners at Love Canal, that was just the beginning of dealing with citizens' needs and local, state, and federal bureaucracy, and of learning to organize and fight for rights. Four years later, the Love Canal homeowners were finally moved from their homes through a federal grant and remuneration from the chemical company (Levine, 1982).

Through the experience of Love Canal, Lois Gibbs became an informed leader. She learned that many toxic dump sites throughout the country are endangering the health of citizens, while county, state, and federal officials attempt to hide the facts, as they did at Love Canal. In time, Gibbs became well known and received calls from around the country. She realized that to continue the work, she would

need to create a clearinghouse for information in the best location, Washington, D.C. In 1981 Lois formed the Citizen's Clearinghouse for Hazardous Waste (CCHW). People called the clearinghouse saying, "We think we have a Love Canal in our back yard. What should we do?" Soon, hundreds of citizens and groups joined the CCHW. As of June 1988, there were 3,650 CCHW groups across the United States, with 1,600 affiliate groups such as local chapters of the Sierra Club. A heterogeneous membership includes all economic, racial, and political groups; poisoned groundwater knows no boundaries. The function of the CCHW is to protect citizens from toxic wastes. Many state laws ban the dumping of toxic wastes, but the laws were rarely enforced before the CCHW became influential. According to the U.S. Office of Technology Assessment, the CCHW has been more effective than any other group in

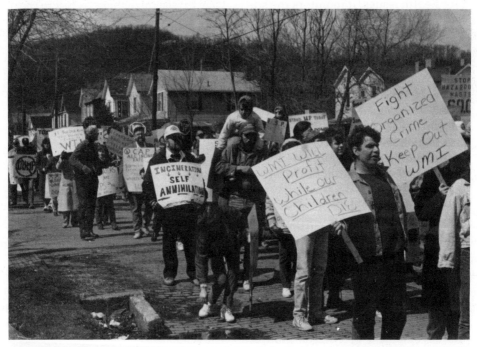

Citizens Can Play an Active and Powerful Role in Safeguarding Health by Protesting and Changing Unhealthy Conditions.
Source: Citizens Clearinghouse on Waste.

enforcing state laws against dumping of toxic wastes.

The CCHW is an "old-fashioned" American movement that expresses American values of neighbor helping neighbor and people accepting social responsibility for the health promotion for all. Many other citizens groups could be described, with histories similar to the CCHW's. Mothers Against Drunk Drivers (MADD) is a case in point: A national organization with branches in many cities (and a student organization, Students Against Drunk Drivers), started by one parent with a grievance against society and laws that permit the killing of thousands by drunken drivers, with little consequence to the driver. It is a similar story of overcoming resistance with citizens' support, of organizing, and of gaining power through organization and cooperation. Like the CCHW and many other citizens groups, MADD is also the story of persistence toward the goal of improving the quality of life for all.

The organization that we next describe works at another level, changing the process of government itself.

Legislative Decision-Making and Common Cause

> Dear Friend, I would like to ask you to join me in forming a new independent, non-partisan organization to help in rebuilding the nation. It will be known as Common Cause . . . . a citizen's lobby concerned not with the advancement of special interests but with the well-being of the nation.

So began John Gardner's letter to the American people in August 1970. The media called Gardner's program the "Lost Cause." Yet, within six months 100,000 Americans had joined Common Cause. By 1986 Common Cause had 290,000 members.

Gardner founded Common Cause because, after spending five years as Secretary of Health, Education, and Welfare under Nixon, he was convinced that certain fundamental

characteristics of the legislative process hindered the development of social and health programs and made it possible for special interests to gain power over the legislative process. We briefly describe three challenges that Common Cause tackled on behalf of all citizens.

Government in the Sunshine. The first change that Common Cause sought was a ruling that congressional committees must meet and vote in open sessions, except in cases of national security. This procedure became known as the sunshine rule. By 1973, committees in the House of Representatives agreed to open meetings, and by 1975 the Senate adopted the sunshine rule for its committees and for 50 executive branch agencies. In addition, by 1975, 48 state legislatures had adopted the sunshine rule for all their committee meetings. The significance of the sunshine rule to the legislative process is clear. Legislators are more accountable for their decisions when those decisions are public. There are no more "closed doors"; the public can be informed and can hold legislators accountable. This gives power to the public and forces legislators to be more public-minded.

Public Funding of Presidential and Congressional Campaigns.

For Sale
The United States Government
All bids will be handled in secrecy.

So read a letter in 1970 that Common Cause sent to its members. Common Cause was convinced that elected officials cannot represent the public fairly when they depend on special interest groups for campaign funds, an issue discussed in Chapter 20. Common Cause took up a common need, public financing of political campaigns. Common Cause first targeted public financing of presidential campaigns and was successful. In 1974, President Ford signed into law the public financing of presidential elections. Presidential elections are now financed in part by millions of citizens who designate $1 of their taxes, on the tax return form, for the presidential election fund. Candidates may still receive donations from citizens and groups, but they do not have to depend solely on those gifts. While this does not eliminate the inequity in funding, it is an important attempt to make political campaigns a matter of issues, not money. While not yet successful in getting Congress to support public financing of congressional campaigns, Common Cause persists in working toward that goal.

Ethics in Government.   For years, Common Cause worked for a strong bill on ethics in government. The result: In 1978, President Carter signed the Ethics in Government Act. Now, all members of the House and Senate, federal judges, and high-ranking officers of the executive branch, must reveal their financial holdings and sources of income. This law exposes conflicts of interest by government leaders, such as the hypothetical case of a congressman who holds shares in a weapons manufacturing company and sits on a congressional committee that allocates funds for defense contracts.

Common Cause has been instrumental in bringing many other important changes in legislative procedure. Two examples are the elimination of the seniority system in Congress and replacing it with the democratic election of committee members, and the sunset law, which requires periodic review of regulatory agencies (McFarland, 1984).

Summary

Citizens groups serve an essential function in society. They give the individual a voice and help the individual in need. There are dozens of citizens groups in the United States; we could include groups such as Easter Seals, United Way, the Red Cross, Goodwill Industries, and many others. The citizens groups that are of interest to us in this section are those that are organized to safeguard human and environmental health by influencing government and social policy. These groups perform a task that the ordinary citizen cannot accomplish. They continually monitor government and business activities; they do the homework that the average person cannot do. Having done this work, these groups take action in two ways—they pressure government to make prohealth decisions, occasionally through court action, and they make their findings and research available to the public through publications and newsletters. The latter function of citizens groups is invaluable; only the informed citizen can be socially responsible.

Health is a political issue because, directly or indirectly, activities at all levels of government influence health, from prenatal care programs and the immunization of children to medical care for the elderly, from seat-belt laws to punishing drunken drivers, from workplace safety standards to standards for pesticide use and drug efficacy, from funding health research to funding health programs in schools, from establishing national health goals to taking the steps to reach those goals.

Social policy and individual health are intimately connected. When social policy is designed to influence a specific health hazard or promote a specific health behavior, it is called social engineering. In this section we discussed the steps that Minnesota took toward "a smoke-free society by the year 2000," an example of social engineering through social policy. The federal government has both the organizational structure and the sources for creating and implementing nationwide social policies that both dramatically and subtly improve the health of the nation.

The politics of health and the development of social policy are not solely in the hands of the government, nor is the individual powerless to influence social policy. Through common goals, cooperation, and persistence, citizens groups play an important role in safeguarding and promoting the health and well-being of all citizens.

The politics of health and wellness are not separate from the dynamics of health and wellness.

IIII➡

SECTION FOUR: INTERNATIONAL FOCUS

We can think of the individual as a circle within the larger circle of the family within the larger circle of the community, within the larger circle of society, within the larger circle of the planet. We can think of one dynamic of health and wellness as the interaction of these many circles. Now we broaden the focus to the global level. As the nations of the world interact politically and economically, and as the world grows "smaller," the need for global consciousness and global solutions to health problems increases. The forces against health and wellness are not confined to national boundaries, nor are the forces for health and wellness.

In this section we describe two such forces, an international organization devoted to "health for all by the year 2000," the World Health Organization, and a model program for villagers in Third World countries.

The World Health Organization

The United Nations, founded in 1946, is dedicated to preventing war and to improving the well-being of all peoples. Several organizations within the United Nations focus on health issues: the World Food Program, the Children's Fund (UNICEF), Earthwatch (an environmentalist organization), and the World Health Organization (WHO). We concentrate on the World Health Organization.

The World Health Organization was established in 1948, as an agency responsible for directing and coordinating international activities for health promotion. More than 165 countries are members. At the 1977 WHO Conference, 156 countries agreed on the goal of "Health for all by the year 2000." That vision challenged the government representatives, who carried the message home. Dr. Halfdan Mahler, director-general of WHO, stated, "Few could have foreseen then to what extent this move would fire the imagination of people throughout the world. That it did, showed how timely the call was to bring about a social revolution in community health" (Mahler, 1981). The next year, the WHO conference at Alma-Ata, in the Soviet Union, devised a strategy, primary health care, for achieving the goal. The strategy of primary health care focuses on "community involvement in the spirit of self-reliance and self-determination to achieve essential health." It was agreed that communities would share with government the responsibility of health for all. The essential ingredients for health were outlined:

Safe drinking water and sanitation.
Adequate nutrition.
Immunization against the major infectious diseases of childhood.
Reduction of communicable diseases in the developing countries in the year 2000 to the 1980 levels in developed countries.
Prevention of noncommunicable diseases through healthy lifestyles and controlling the physical and psychosocial environments.
Maternal and child health care, including family planning.
Health education for preventing and controlling health problems.
Availability of essential drugs.
Access to medical treatment.

The strategy of primary health care gives priority to the role of nurses and health workers. Health workers are chosen by the local community to receive medical training. The health worker helps the community establish prevention programs such as immunization, improved diet, and improved sanitation. The health worker also visits sick people in their homes and prescribes medications and gives inoculations when necessary.

In May 1986, the World Health Organization evaluated its progress toward achieving health for all by the year 2000 (*World Health,* 1988 January/February). Some examples are:

1. Through an expanded program of immunization, smallpox was eliminated throughout the world in 1979. The goal of WHO is to immunize all children by 1990 against communicable diseases such as measles, polio, diptheria, tetanus, whooping cough, and tuberculosis.
2. About 370,000 people have been trained to administer immunizations.
3. A rational policy on medication distribution and a list of 36 essential medications, such as penicillin, were agreed upon.
4. Standards were established for breast milk substitutes.
5. An international program on oral rehydration therapy for diarrhea illnesses was created.
6. Crisis-intervention and emergency-preparation programs were created.
7. Sanitation and water programs for underdeveloped countries were developed through the Community Water Supply and Sanitation Program.
8. The Global Program on AIDS has disseminated information on AIDS prevention throughout the world.
9. A 10-year-old program, Tropical Diseases Research, has resulted in a worldwide network of scientists sharing technology and information.
10. A worldwide antismoking campaign was initiated.

The World Health Organization provides leadership and education to all nations through its journals, committees, projects, and conferences. It is a model of cooperation and action among nations.

The World Health Organization also emphasizes the importance of community self-responsibility and self-determination in developing countries. In Third World countries, where it is common to have insufficient means of transportation, scarce energy and food, scarce medical services, and inadequate "public" services, each village must become a unified and self-sufficient community. In the next section we describe a model program for villages that began in Sri Lanka.

Sarvodaya Self-Help Movement

Sri Lanka, previously Ceylon, is an island nation the size of West Virginia off the southern tip of India. Sri Lanka is one of the oldest democracies in the Third World, and its 14.5 million citizens are proud of their role in self-governance. Sri Lanka has several religious groups, Hindus, Buddhists, Moslems, and Christians. Conflicts between the wealthy Hindus and the poor Buddhists, and between westernized English-speaking city-dwellers and Sinhalese-speaking rural people, continually disrupt the social life and natural beauty of this island paradise. Sri Lanka is one of the poorest nations in the world. In 1984, the annual per capita income was $340.

The Sarvodaya movement was introduced into this setting of poverty and social and religious conflict by a student of the philosophy and practical teachings of Mahatma Gandhi. *Sarvodaya* means the awakening to social consciousness of one and all, manifested through social action for the good of all. "May all beings be well and happy" is the slogan of the Sarvodaya movement.

In 1958 a high school science teacher, A. T. Ariyaratna, went to India to study the Gandhian movement. The Gandhian ideals of truth, nonviolence, and self-reliance expressed his own deeply felt beliefs. After many years of study, Ariyaratna returned to Sri Lanka to develop a program for implementing the Gandhian techniques in poor villages. Like Gandhi, Ariyaratna had a vision of the self-sufficient village (Macy, 1985).

Ariyaratna began the Sarvodaya program by training 16- and 17-year-old students to work in villages through work camps, a program that we might call work/study. During the training, the students lived in villages and worked side by side with the villagers, digging a latrine, building a road, or clearing a canal. Through this work experience the student learned the fundamental teaching—the interdependence of all aspects of life—social, economic, political, moral, cultural, and spiritual. This teaching reflects an understanding of life that is common to Eastern philosophies: One's work and livelihood and social activity are not separate from one's spiritual life. The awareness of the interdependence comes through working with others to bring all people to their highest level of well-being.

Today, many villagers become Sarvodaya workers and are trained through the same work camp process. After completing the work camp, and having learned the principles of Sarvodaya, the worker is prepared to work in a village when invited to do so. The villagers decide on the work project to be carried out in their village; often this is the first time that the villagers have joined together to discuss and make decisions. It is the birth of community consciousness and self-determination, the goals of the Sarvodaya movement. The Sarvodayan worker learns to listen, to be patient, and to respect each villager.

Through the villagers' working together and preparing meals together, through meeting to discuss the work project, through song and dance, and through prayer and meditation, a sense of unity and cohesion emerges. "We build the road and the road builds us" and "the road we build may wash away, but the attitudes we build do not" are common sayings of Sarvodayan participants.

The work in the villages honors local spiritual traditions and rituals. The priest is present at all times, and the meetings and celebrations are held in the local temple or church. The priests say, "Don't sit in your temple like a rich monk waiting for *dana* (nirvana). Go to the people, go to the poorest, work with them." The principles of love and nonviolence, truth, and being of service are taught in all of the religions of Sri Lanka. These principles unite Christians, Buddhists, Moslems, and Hindus, who can work together for the common good when they live by these principles.

Organizing from the grass roots up and not from the top down is a central idea in the Sarvodayan movement, arising from the dedication to self-determination. Many of the most active workers in the villages are children and teenagers. The idealism and energy of these young people are contagious in the community. The young people are trusted, and they participate in the village council with the elders. They are encouraged to contribute their views and to share responsibility for community development. It is no surprise that young people are attracted to the Sarvodayan movement, and many of the Sarvodayan workers who work in the villages are 16 and 17 years old. After visiting Sri Lanka, a World Bank official said, "What strikes me most is that Sarvodaya does not regard unemployed youth as a liability—as most societies do, where they are a drain on the economy and can be volatile and destructive. Somehow Sarvodaya has been able to turn them into an asset" (Macy, 1985, p. 96).

Sarvodayan communities have lasted through civil conflict and guerrilla war during the 1980s in Sri Lanka. They have maintained their spiritual values and traditions of nonviolence, truth, and self-sufficiency in spite of intense pressures for modernization and technology by government. Most Sarvodayan workers maintain their independence from the government and work on their own with little pay, helping new communities begin a path of social responsibility and self-sufficiency.

The Sarvodayan emphasis on awakening to the interdependence of all aspects of life has helped extremely poor people gain a sense of community spirit, social responsibility, and community power. This is the natural result of villagers working together on projects for the good of all and of rekindling the villagers' religious heritage. The religious pluralism, the nonpartisan stance in politics, and the nonviolent approach to human conflict and human development enables the Sarvodayan movement to survive fluctuations in government and civil conflicts. Sarvodayan workers say:

> Your village may boast of having a post office, telephones, electricity . . . but that is not what constitutes being developed. Development is in your head, your mind.

> Right Mindfulness—that means stay open and alert to the needs of the village. Look to see what is needed—latrines, water, road. Try to enter the minds of the people, to listen behind their words. Practice mindfulness in the *shramandana* (community work project) camp: Is the food enough? Are people getting wet? Are the tools in order? Is anyone being exploited?"

> In Sarvodaya we act now. We make shramadanas, training programs, preschools. We don't divide people; we show them how they can change (Macy, 1985).

The success of the Sarvodaya movement is measured in the 4,000 villages in Sri Lanka that have become self-determining communities, attending to the needs of all and working together to fulfill the slogan "May all beings be well and happy."

In 1970 the Sarvodaya Institute was founded in Sri Lanka as a training center. By 1985, 100,000 workers had been trained and were working in Africa, India, and Thailand. The spread of the Sarvodayan movement is perhaps a sign that the principles of community and unity for the good of all are truly international.

CONCLUSION

The wind of wellness is blowing in many directions: down the corridors of corporate America, through the classroom doors, into the jungle villages of Third World countries. It rustles papers on the desks of Capitol Hill, it raises dust in citizens groups, and it whispers in the trees of city parks. It makes waves on the American shores, and it ripples lifestyles. Someday it will turn the corner and blow down the streets of ghettos everywhere.

Today we have more knowledge about the dynamics of health and wellness than ever before. We know the basic steps to high-level wellness. We know how to prevent illness and disease and how to promote health and wellness, and we understand the importance of both. Prevention of chronic disease and illness motivates thousands of people to lose weight, exercise, eat a low-fat diet, and manage stress.

We have also learned that health pays and sickness costs. As medical costs have soared, the financial incentive to stay well gains power. Financial incentives are the key to wellness programs in business and the motivator in stay-well insurance, and they make sense to the average citizen. Health professionals know that incentives are essential to motivating behavioral change. Yet, although the goal of health is widely espoused, the incentives are not in keeping with this goal. We have not yet found a way to motivate our entire population to live today for the long-term gains of tomorrow.

Managing social incentives for health and wellness is an aspect of social engineering, and it is achieved through public policy. We can imagine a significant change in health behavior if, for example, it became the policy to give everyone who reached 65 at ideal weight a substantial tax refund. We could expect a significant cost reduction in Medicare coverage, knowing that one-fourth of middle-age Americans are obese and that obesity is a major health risk. Regulations established by public policy—regulations that govern business and the behavior of individuals—profoundly affect health. Lowering the speed limit and enforcing it saves lives and injury; increasing the drinking age and enforcing it saves lives and injury; requiring the use of seat belts in automobiles and enforcing it saves lives and injury.

Public policy at the state and federal levels can be influenced by special interest groups, but the emergence of citizens groups is changing the balance of power. Safe cars, safe foods, safe drugs, and safe water are actively pursued by these groups. The work of citizens groups is invaluable to American health. It provides a vehicle for social responsibility, which, we believe, must be part of the dynamics of health and wellness, as is self-responsibility. Public policy affects everyone, just as social conditions affect everyone, and

social responsibility expressed through political action is important to everyone.

Social responsibility implies action, and it also implies an attitude. The perceptual and behavioral shift from self-responsibility to social responsibility is important because personal health and well-being are intimately connected to the greater social sphere and are influenced by societal forces. Social responsibility also implies a consciousness of the connectedness of all things, environmental and human, and it implies a sense of community, worldwide community and local community. Worldwide community is the message of the World Health Organization that brings people from many countries together to cooperatively solve problems that affect everyone.

It is clear that we have enough knowledge of the dynamics of health and wellness, enough research, enough financial and human resources, and enough organizational structure in government, citizens groups, and schools to strive for "health for all by the year 2000."

References

Abrams, D., Monti, P., Pinto, R., Elder, J., Brown, R., & Jacobus, S. (1987). Psychosocial stress and coping in smokers who relapse or quit. *Health Psychology, 6,* 289–303.

Achterberg, J. (1985). *Imagery and healing: Shamanism and modern medicine.* Boulder, CO: New Science Library.

Achterberg, J., & Lawlis, G. F. (1978). *Image of cancer.* Champaign, IL: Institute for Personality and Ability Testing.

Achterberg, J., & Lawlis, G. F. (1980). *Bridges of the body mind: Behavioral approaches to health care.* Champaign, IL: Institute for Personality and Ability Testing.

Achterberg, J., Lawlis, G. F., Simonton, C., & Simonton, S. (1977). Psychological factors and blood chemistries as disease outcome predictors for cancer patients. *Multivariate Clinical Experimental Research,* December.

Achterberg, J., Matthews-Simonton, S., & Simonton, C. (1977). Psychology of the exceptional cancer patient: A description of patients who outlive life expectancies. *Psychotherapy: Theory, Research and Practice, 41,* 416–422.

Adams, E., Blanken, A., Gfroerer, J., & Ferguson, L. (1988). *Overview of selected drug trends.* Washington, DC: National Institute on Drug Abuse.

Ader, R., & Cohen, N. (1984). Behavior and the immune system. In D. W. Gentry (Ed.), *Handbook of behavioral medicine,* (pp. 117–173). New York: Guilford Press.

Adler, C., & Adler, S. (1983). Physiologic feedback and psychotherapeutic intervention for migraine: A 10-year follow-up. In V. Pfafenrath, P. Lundberg, & O. Sjaastad (Eds.), *Updating in headache,* (pp. 217–223). Berlin: Springer-Verlag Press.

Adolescent Pregnancy Prevention Clearinghouse (1986). *Model programs: Preventing adolescent pregnancy and building self-sufficiency.* Washington DC: Children's Defense Fund.

Ajzen, I., & Fishbein, M. (1980). *Understanding attitudes and predicting behavior.* Englewood Cliffs, NJ: Prentice-Hall.

Alberti, R., and Emmons, M. (1970). *Your perfect right.* San Luis Obispo, CA: Impact Publishers.

Albrecht, K. (1979). *Stress and the manager: Making it work for you.* Englewood Cliffs, NJ: Prentice-Hall.

Alcoholics Anonymous (1980). *Do you think you're different?* New York: Alcoholics Anonymous World Services, Inc.

Alcoholics Anonymous (1981). *Young people and AA.* New York: Alcoholics Anonymous World Services, Inc.

American Cancer Society (1984). *Cancer facts & figures.* New York.

American College of Sports Medicine (1980). *Guidelines for graded exercise testing and exercise prescription.* Philadelphia: Lea & Febiger.

American Heart Assocation (1985). *Heart facts.* Dallas.

American Humane Association (1981). Child Protection Division. Denver: National Study of Child Neglect and Abuse Reporting.

American Psychiatric Association. *Diagnostic and statistical manual of mental disorders: Third edition.* (1980). Washington, DC.

American Psychological Association, American Educational Research Association, and National Council on Measurements Used in Education (1954). Technical recommendations for psychological tests and diagnostic techniques. *Psychological Bulletin* (Supplement), 51, (2), Part 2.

American Psychologist (1982). Awards for distinguished scientific contributions: 1981. Volume 37, No. 1, 32–51.

Amler, R., & Dull, H. (1987). *Closing the gap: The burden of unnecessary illness.* New York: Oxford University Press.

Anda, R., Remington, P., Sienko, D., & Davis, R. (1987). Are physicians advising smokers to quit? *Journal of the American Medical Association, 257,* 1916–1918.

Anderson, G. E. (1972). *College schedule of recent experience.* Unpublished master's thesis, Department of Guidance and Counseling, North Dakota State University, Fargo, North Dakota.

Andrasik, F., & Blanchard, E. (1987). The biofeedback treatment of tension headache. In J. Hatch, J. Fisher, & J. Rugh, *Biofeedback: Studies in clinical efficacy,* (pp. 281–320). New York: Plenum Press.

Andrasik, F., & Holroyd, K. (1983). Specific and nonspecific effects in the biofeedback treatment of tension headache: 3-year follow-up. *Journal of Consulting and Clinical Psychology, 51,* 634–636.

Andrasik, F., Blanchard, E., Neff, E., & Rodichok, L. (1984). Biofeedback and relaxation training for chronic headache: A controlled comparison of booster treatments and regular contacts for long-term maintenance. *Journal of Consulting and Clinical Psychology, 52,* 609–615.

Anthony, J. E. (1987). Children at high risk for psychosis growing up successfully. In J. Anthony & B. Cohler (Eds.), *The invulnerable child* (pp. 147–184). New York: Guilford Press.

Anthony, J. E., (1974). The syndrome of the psychologically invulnerable child. In E. J. Anthony & C. Koupernik (Eds.), *The child in his family 3: Children at psychiatric risk.* New York: Wiley.

Anthony, J. E., & Cohler, B. (Eds.) (1987). *The invulnerable child.* New York: Guilford Press.

Antonovsky, A. (1987). *Unraveling the mystery of health: How people manage stress and stay well.* San Francisco: Jossey-Bass.

Archer, D., & Gartner, R. (1984). *Violence and crime in cross-national perspective.* New Haven, CT: Yale University Press.

Ardell, D. (1977). *High level wellness.* New York: Bantam Books.

Arena, J., Blanchard, E., Andrasik, F., Cotch, P., & Myers, P. (1983). Reliability of psychophysiological assessment. *Behavior Research and Therapy, 21,* 447–460.

Arnold, C. (1985). Health and life. *Journal of the American Medical Association, 25,* 2897.

Assagioli, R. (1965). *Psychosynthesis.* New York; Viking Press.

Bacon, M., Child, I., & Barry, H. (1963). A cross-cultural study of some correlates of crime. *Journal of Abnormal Social Psychology, 66,* 291–300.

Bacon, S. (1987). *The evolution of the Outward Bound process.* Greenwich, CT: Outward Bound Press.

Bahnson, C. B. (1969). Psychophysiological complementarity in malignancies: Past work and future vistas. *Annals of the New York Academy of Sciences, 164,* 319–333.

Banderia, M., Bouchard, M., & Granger, L., (1982). Voluntary Control of Autonomic Responses: A Case for a Dialogue Between Individual and Group Experimental Methodologies. *Biofeedback and Self-Regulation, 7,* 317–329.

Bandura, A. (1973). *Aggression: A social learning analysis.* Englewood Cliffs, NJ: Prentice-Hall.

Bandura, Albert (1977). Self-efficacy: Toward a unifying theory of behavioral change. *Psychological Review, 84,* 191–215.

Bandura, Albert (1986). *The social foundations of thought & action.* Englewood Cliffs, NJ: Prentice-Hall.

Bandura, A., & Adams, N. E. (1977). Analysis of self-efficacy theory of behavioral change. *Cognitive Therapy and Research, 1,* 287–308.

Bandura, A., & Mischel, A. (1965). Modification of self-imposed delay of reward through exposure to live and symbolic models. *Journal of Personality and Social Psychology, 2,* 698–705.

Barefoot, J., Dahlstrom, G., & Williams, R. (1983). Hostility, CHD incidence, and total mortality: A 24-year follow-up study of 255 physicians. *Psychosomatic Medicine, 45,* 5963.

Barefoot, J., Dodge, K., Peterson, B., Dahlstrom, W., & Williams, R. (1989). The Cook-Medley Hostility Scale: Item content and ability to predict survival. *Psychosomatic Medicine, 54,* 46–57.

Barkley, R. (1981). *Hyperactive children: A handbook for diagnosis and treatment.* New York: Guilford Press.

Barnard, J. (1987). Introduction in M. Rose and R. Thomas (Eds.), *Children with chronic conditions: Nursing in a family and community context.* Orlando, FL: Grune & Stratton.

Barsky, A. (1988). The paradox of health. *The New England Journal of Medicine, 318,* 414–418.

Bartrop, R., Lockhurst, E., Lazarus, L., Kiloh, L., & Penny, R. (1977). Depressed lymphocyte function after bereavement. *Lancet, 1,* 834–836.

Basmajian, J. (1963). Control and training of individual motor units. *Science, 141,* 440–441.

Basmajian, J. (1974). *Muscles alive.* Baltimore: Williams & Wilkins.

Baumrind, D. (1971). Current patterns of parental authority. *Developmental Psychology Monograph, 4* (1, Part 2).

Baumrind, D. (1973). The development of instrumental competence through socialization. In A. D. Pick (Ed.), Minnesota symposia on child psychology (Vol. 7). Minneapolis: University of Minnesota Press.

Beck, A., & Katcher, A. (1983). *Between pets and people.* New York: G. P. Putnam.

Beck, Aaron (1979). *Cognitive therapy and emotional disorders.* New York: New American Library.

Belson, W. (1978). *Television violence and the adolescent boy.* London: Teakfield.

Benjamin, L. (1963). Statistical treatment of the law of initial values (LIV) in autonomic research: A review and recommendation. *Psychosomatic Medicine, XXV,* 556–566.

Benson, H. (1975). *The relaxation response.* New York: William Morrow.

Benson, H., & McCallie, Jr., D. (1979). Angina pectoris and the placebo effect. *New England Journal of Medicine, 300,* 1424–1429.

Benson, H., & Proctor, W. (1985). *Beyond the relaxation response.* New York: Berkeley Publishing.

Bergman, L., & Magnusson, D. (1986). Type A behavior: A longitudinal study from childhood to adulthood. *Psychosomatic Medicine, 48,* 134–142.

Berkman, L., & Syme, S. (1979). Social networks, host resistance, and mortality: A nine-year follow-up study of Alameda County residents. *American Journal of Epidemiology, 109,* 186–204.

Berkman, L., and Breslow, L. (1983). *Health and ways of living: The Alameda County study.* New York: Oxford University Press.

Berman, Philip (Ed.) (1986). *The courage of conviction.* New York: Ballantine Books.

Bertalanffy, L., von (1968). *General systems theory.* New York: Brazilier.

Beyer, J., DeGood, D., Ashley, L., & Russell, G. (1983). Patterns of postoperative analgesic use with adults and children following cardiac surgery. *Pain, 17,* 71–81.

Birk, L. (Ed.) (1973). *Biofeedback: Behavioral medicine,* (pp. 147–165). New York: Grune & Stratton.

Black, S., Humphrey, J. H., and Niven, J. (1963). Inhibition of mantoux reaction by direct suggestion under hypnosis. *British Medical Journal,* Vol. 6, 925–929.

Blanchard, E., Andrasik, F., Ahles, T., Teders, S., & O'Keefe, D. (1980). Migraine and tension headache: A meta-analytic review. *Behavior Therapy, 11,* 613–631.

Blanchard, E., Andrasik, F., Guarnieri, P., Neff, D., & Rodichok, L. (1987). Two-, three-, and four-year follow-up on the self-regulatory treatment of chronic headache. *Journal of Consulting & Clinical Psychology, 55,* 257–259.

Blanchard, E., Appelbaum, K., Guarnieri, P., Neff, D., Andrasik, F., Jaccard, J., & Barron, K. (1988). Two studies of the long-term follow-up of minimal therapist contact treatments of vascular and tension headache. *Journal of Consulting and Clinical Psychology, 56,* 427–432.

Blanchard, E., McCoy, G., Musso, A., Gerardi, M., Pallmeyer, T., Gerardi, R., Cotch, P., Siracusa, K., & Andrasik, F. (1986). A controlled comparison of thermal biofeedback and relaxation training in the treatment of essential hypertension: I. Short-term and long-term outcome. *Behavior Therapy, 17,* 563–579.

Blanchard, E., & Schwarz, S. (1987). Adaptation of a multicomponent treatment for irritable bowel syndrome to a small-group format. *Biofeedback & Self-Regulation, 12,* 63–69.

Blanchard, E., Schwarz, S., & Neff, D. (1988). Two-year follow-up of behavioral treatment of irritable bowel syndrome. *Behavior-Therapy, 19,* 67–73.

Blanchard, E., Schwarz, S., & Radnitz C. (1987). Psychological assessment and treatment of irritable bowel syndrome. *Behavior Modification, 11,* 348–372.

Blue-Cross/Blue-Shield (1978). *Stress.* Chicago: Blue-Cross/Blue-Shield.

Blum, R. (1987). Contemporary threats to adolescent health in the United States. *Journal of the American Medical Association, 257,* 3390–3395.

Blumberg, E. M., West, P., & Ellis, F. (1954). A possible relationship between psychological factors and human cancer. *Psychosomatic Medicine, 16,* 277–286.

Bly, J., Jones, R., & Richardson, J. (1986). Impact of worksite health promotion on health care costs and utilization. *Journal of the American Medical Association, 256,* No. 23, 3235–3240.

Bopp, M. (1985). *Developing healthy communities: Fundamental strategies for health promotion.* Lathbridge, Alberta: Four Worlds Development Press.

Borysenko, Joan (1985). Healing motives: An interview with David C. McClelland. *Advances, 2,* 29–41.

Botvin, G., & Dusenbury, L. (1988). Substance abuse prevention and the promotion of competence. Unpublished manuscript. Cornell University Medical College.

Botvin, G., & Eng, A. (1982). Efficacy of a multicomponent approach to the prevention of cigarette smoking. *Preventive Medicine, 11,* 199–211.

Botvin, G., & Eng, A. (1980). A comprehensive school based smoking prevention program. *Journal of School Health, 50,* 209–213.

Botvin, G., & Wills, T. (1985). Personal and social skills training: Cognitive-behavioral approaches to substance abuse prevention. In C. Bell & R. Battjes (Eds.), *Prevention research: Deterring drug abuse among children and adolescents.* Washington, DC: NIDA Research Monograph.

Botvin, G., Baker, E., Renick, N., Filazzola, A., & Botvin, E. (1984). A cognitive-behavioral approach to substance abuse prevention. *Addictive Behaviors, 9,* 137–147.

Botvin, G., Renick, N., & Baker, E. (1983). The effects of scheduling format and booster sessions on a broad-spectrum psychosocial approach to smoking prevention. *Journal of Behavioral Medicine, 6,* 359–379.

Boulding, K. (1978). *Ecodynamics.* Beverly Hills, CA: Sage.

Bowen, O., & Sammons, J. (1988). The alcohol-abusing patient: A challenge to the profession. *Journal of the American Medical Association, 260,* 2267–2270.

Bowne, D., Russell, M., Morgan, J., et al., (1984). Reduced disability and health care costs in an industrial fitness program. *Journal of Occupational Medicine, 26,* 809–816.

Bradshaw, J. (1988). *The family.* Pompano Beach, FL: Health Communications.

Braud, L. (1978). The effects of frontal EMG biofeedback and progressive relaxation upon hyperactivity and its behavioral concomitants. *Biofeedback & Self-Regulation, 3,* 69–89.

Braud, L., Lupin, M., & Braud, W. (1975). The use of electromyographic biofeedback in the control of hyperactivity. *Journal of Learning Disabilities, 8,* 21–26.

Brody, J., & Shafer, D. (1982). Contributions of parents and peers to children's moral socialization. *Developmental Review, 2,* 31–75.

Brody, J. (1981). *Jane Brody's nutrition book.* New York: Bantam Books.

Brown, A., Palincsar, A., & Purcell, L. (1984). Poor readers: Teach don't label. In U. Neisser (Ed.), *The academic performance of minority children: A new perspective.* Hillsdale, NJ: Erlbaum.

Brown, B. (1977). *New mind, new body.* New York: Harper & Row.

Brown, D. P., and Fromm, E. (1987). *Hypnosis and Behavioral Medicine.* Hillsdale, NJ: Erlbaum.

Brownell, K., Colletti, G., Ersner-Hershfield, R., Hershfield, S., & Wilson, G. (1977). Self control in school children: Stringency and leniency in self determined and externally imposed performance standards. *Behavior Therapy, 8,* 442–455.

Brownell, K., & Foreyt, J. (1985). Obesity. In D. Barlow (Ed.), *Clinical handbook of psychological disorders.* Hillsdale, NJ: Erlbaum.

Brownell, K., & Kaye, F. (1982). A school-based behavior modification, nutrition education, and physical activity program for obese children. *American Journal of Clinical Nutrition, 35,* 277–283.

Brownell, K., & Wadden, T. (1986). Behavior therapy for obesity: Modern approaches and better results. In K. Brownell & J. Foreyt (Eds.), *Handbook of eating disorders,* (pp. 180–197). New York: Basic Books.

Brownell, K., Marlatt, G., Lichtenstein, E., & Wilson, G. (1986). Understanding and preventing relapse. *American Psychologist, 41,* 765–782.

Brudny, J., Grynbaum, B., & Korein, J. (1974). Spasmodic torticollis: Treatment by feedback display of the EMG. *Archives of Physical Medicine and Rehabilitation, 55,* 49–53.

Brudny, J., Korein, J., Grynbaum, B., Belandres, P., & Gianutsos, J. (1979). Helping hemiparetics to help themselves. *Journal of the American Medical Association, 241,* 814–820.

Bruhn, J., & Cordova, F. (1987). Promoting healthy behavior in the workplace. *Health Values, 11,* 39–48.

Bruhn, J., & Wolf, S. (1978). Update on Roseto, Pa.: Testing a prediction. *Psychosomatic Medicine, 40,* 86.

Bruhn, J., & Wolf, S. (1979). *The Roseto story.* Norman, OK: University of Oklahoma Press.

Bruhn, J. (1965). An epidemiological study of myocardial infarctions in an Italian-American community. *Journal of Chronic Disease, 18,* 353–365.

Bruhn, J., Chandler, B., Miller, C., Wolf, S., & Lynn, T. (1966). Social aspects of coronary heart disease in two adjacent, ethnically different communities. *American Journal of Public Health, 56,* 2493–2506.

Brunton, P. (1972). *A search in secret India.* New York: Weiser.

Bry, A. (1976). *Directing the movies of your mind.* New York: Harper & Row.

Buckalew, M. W., and McDonagh, C. (1987). Self-regulation in an undergraduate psychology course: Results from a performance examination. *Biofeedback and Self-Regulation, 11,* 321–328.

Budzynski, T. (1973). Biofeedback procedures in the clinic. *Seminars in Psychiatry, 4,* 537–547.

Budzynski, T. (1977). Systematic desensitization. Dual Cassette Tape Recording, catalogue No. T–35, New York: BioMonitoring Applications.

Budzynski, T. (1979). Strategies in headache treatment. In J. Basmajian (Ed.), *Biofeedback—principles and practice for clinicians,* (pp. 132–151). Baltimore: Williams & Wilkins.

Budzynski, T. H., & Stoyva, J. M. (1969). An instrument for producing deep muscle relaxation by means of analog information feedback. *Journal of Applied Behavioral Analysis, 2,* 231–237.

Budzynski, T. H., Stoyva, J. M., Adler, C. S., & Mullaney, D. J. (1973). EMG biofeedback and tension headache: A controlled outcome study. In L. Birk (Ed.), *Biofeedback: Behavioral medicine,* New York: Grune & Stratton.

Budzynski, T. H., Stoyva, J. M., & Adler, C. S. (1970). Feedback-induced relaxation: Application to tension headache. *Journal of Behavior Therapy and Experimental Psychiatry, 1,* 205–211.

Budzynski, T., & Stoyva, J. (1972). Biofeedback techniques in behavior therapy. In D. Shapiro (Ed.), *Biofeedback and Self-Control,* (pp. 437–457). Chicago: Aldine Publishing.

Bule, J. (1988, July). MA: Victory in worker bill, *APA Monitor,* p. 26.

Bulloch, K. (1985). Neuroanatomy of lymphoid tissue: A review, in R. Guillemin (Ed.), *Neuromodulation of immunity,* (pp. 111-135). New York: Raven Press.

Burg, M., Blumenthal, J., Barefoot, J., Williams, R., & Haney, T. (1986). Social support as a buffer against the development of coronary artery disease. Paper presented at the Society of Behavioral Medicine Meeting, San Francisco.

Burns, David (1985). *Intimate connections.* New York: Morrow.

Burns, David (1980). *Feeling good.* New York: New American Library.

Burton, D. (1988). Do anxious swimmers swim slower? Reexamining the elusive anxiety-performance relationship. *Journal of Sport & Exercise Psychology, 10,* 45–61.

Burton, L. (1981). A critical analysis and review of the research on Outward Bound and related programs (Doctoral dissertation, Rutgers

University), *Dissertation Abstracts International, 42,* 1581B.

Bush, H. S., Thompson, M., and Van Tubergen, N. (1985). Personal assessment of stress factors for college students. *Journal of School Health, 55,* No. 9, 370–375.

Bush, J., & Holmbeck, G. (1987). Pain in children: A review of the literature from a developmental perspective, *Psychology and Health, 1,* 215–236.

Caffrey, B. (1968). Reliability and validity of personality and behavioral measures in a study of coronary heart disease, *Journal of Chronic Diseases, 21,* 191–204.

Caffrey, B. (1970). A multivariate analysis of sociopsychological factors in monks with myocardial infarctions. *American Journal of Public Health, 60,* 452–458.

Caffrey, B. (1978). Psychometric procedures applied to the assessment of the coronary-prone behavior pattern. In Dembroski, T. M., Weis, S. M., Shield, J. L., Haynes, S. G., and Feinleib, M. (Eds.), *Coronary-Prone Behavior,* (pp. 89–93). New York: Springer-Verlag.

Cairns, D., Thomas, L., Mooney, V., & Pace, J. B. (1975). A comprehensive treatment approach to chronic low back pain. *Pain, 2,* 301–308.

Cairns, J. (1985, November). The treatment of diseases and the war against cancer. *Scientific American, 253,* 51–59.

California Department of Mental Health (1982). *Friends can be good medicine.*

Campos, J., Barrett, K., Lamb, M., Goldsmith, H., & Stenberg, C. (1983). Socioemotional development. In M. Haith & J. Campos (Eds.), *Handbook of child psychology.* New York: Wiley.

Cannon, Walter B. (1932). *The wisdom of the body.* New York: W. W. Norton.

Carkhuff, R., & Berenson, B. (1976). *Teaching as treatment,* Amherst, MA: Human Resource Development.

Carmelli, D., Rosenman, R., & Chesney, M. (1987). Stability of the Type A structured interview and related questionnaires in a 10-year follow-up of an adult cohort of twins. *Journal of Behavioral Medicine, 10,* 513–525.

Carter, J., & Russell, H. (1984a). Use of biofeedback relaxation procedures with learning disabled children. In J. Humphrey (Ed.), *Stress in childhood,* (pp. 277–300). New York: AMS Press.

Carter, J., & Russell, H. (1984b). Results of a long-term federally funded program on biofeedback and learning disabilities. In J. Lubar (Chairman), *The use of EEG for diagnosis and treatment of minimal brain dysfunction syndrome and attention deficit disorders in children.* Symposium presented at Biofeedback Society of America, Albuquerque, NM.

Cautela, J. R. (1967). Covert sensitization. *Psychological Reports, 20,* 459–468.

Center for Attitudinal Healing (1978). *There is a rainbow behind every dark cloud.* Millbrae, CA: Celestial Arts.

Centers for Disease Control (1989). Smoking-attributable mortality, morbidity, and economic costs—California. *Journal of the American Medical Association, 261,* 2942–2945.

Centers for Disease Control (1989). Results from the national adolescent student health survey. *Journal of the American Medical Association, 261,* 2025–2031.

Centers for Disease Control (1989). Update: Acquired immunodeficiency syndrome—United States, 1981–1988. *Journal of the American Medical Association, 261,* 2609–2617.

Cerulli, M., Nikoomanesh, P., & Schuster, M. (1979). Progress in biofeedback conditioning for fecal incontinence. *Gastroenterology, 76,* 742–749.

Chaves, J., & Barber, T. (1974). Cognitive strategies, experimenter modelling, and expectation in the attenuation of pain. *Journal of Abnormal Psychology, 83,* 356–363.

Chesney, M., Black, G., Chadwick, J., & Rosenman, R. (1981). Psychological correlates of the Type A behavior pattern, *Journal of Behavioral Medicine, 4,* 217–229.

Chilcote, R., & Baehner, R. (1980). Atypical bleeding in hemophilia: Application of the conversion model to the case study of a child. *Psychosomatic Medicine, 42,* 221–230.

Children's Defense Fund (1988). *A children's defense budget.* Washington, DC.

Chodoff, Paul (1986). Survivors of the Nazi holocaust, in Rudolf H. Moos (Ed.), *Coping with life crises,* (pp. 407–414). New York: Plenum Press.

Churchland, P. M. (1984). *Matter and consciousness: A contemporary introduction to the philosophy of mind.* Cambridge, MA: Bradford.

Citizen's Clearinghouse for Hazardous Waste (1986). *Five Years of Progress 1981-1986.* Arlington, Virginia: CCHW.

Clarke, J., Morris, G., & Cooney, J. (1987). Assessment of the physiological stress response associated with migraine and tension headaches. *Clinical Biofeedback & Health, 10,* 58–67.

Clarke-Stewart, K. A., & Fein, G. G. (1983). Early childhood programs. In M. M. Haith & J. J. Campos (Eds.), *Handbook of child psychology: Infancy and developmental psychology.* New York: Wiley.

Claybrook, J. (1985, October). Unsafe at any speed. *Public Opinion,* p. 5.

Cluss, P., & Fireman, P. (1985). Recent trends in asthma research. *Annals of Behavior Medicine, 7,* 11–16.

Cohen, I. R. (1988, April). The self, the world, and autoimmunity. *Scientific American, 258,* 52–60.

Cohen, J. J. (1985). Stress and the human immune response. *Journal of Burn Care and Rehabilitation, 6,* 167–173.

Cohen, J., Syme, S., Jenkins, C., Kagan, A., & Zyzanski, S. (1979). Cultural context of Type A behavior and risk for CHD: A study of Japanese-American males. *Journal of Behavioral Medicine, 2,* 375–384.

Cohen, R., Blanchard, E., Ruckdeschel, J., & Smolen, R. (1986). Prevalence and correlates of post-treatment and anticipatory nausea and vomiting in cancer chemotherapy. *Journal of Psychosomatic Research, 30,* 643–654.

Cohen, S. (1988). Psychosocial models of the role of social support in the etiology of physical disease. *Health Psychology, 7,* 269–297.

Colten, M., & Janis, I. (1982). Effects of moderate self-disclosure and the balance-sheet procedure. In I. Janis (Ed.), *Counseling on personal decisions: Theory and research on short-term helping relationships.* New Haven, CT: Yale University Press.

Common Cause (1980). *A decade of citizen action.* Washington, DC: Common Cause.

Conger, John (1988). Hostages to fortune: Youth, values and the public interest. *American Psychologist, 43,* 291–300.

Congressional Quarterly (1982). Food: Is it safe to eat? Washington, DC.

Connell, D., Turner, R., & Mason, E. (1985). Summary of findings of the school health education evaluation: Health promotion effectiveness, implementation, and costs. *Journal of School Health, 55,* 316–321.

Consortium for Longitudinal Studies (1983). *As the twig is bent . . . lasting effects of preschool programs.* Hillsdale, NJ: Erlbaum.

Consumer Reports (1987, September). Ban cigarette advertising? 565–569.

Cooper, C. R., Grotevant, H. D., & Condon, S. M. (1982). Individuality and connectedness in the family as a context for adolescent identity formation and role-taking skill (pp. 54–55). In H. D. Grotevant & C. R. Cooper (Eds.), *Adolescent development in the family,* San Francisco: Jossey-Bass.

Cooper, K. (1982). *The aerobics program for total well-being.* New York: M. Evans and Co.

Coppotelli, H., & Orleans, C. (1985). Partner support and other determinants of smoking cessation maintenance among women. *Journal of Consulting and Clinical Psychology, 53,* 455-460.

Cormier, W., & Cormier, L. (1979). Interviewing strategies for helpers: A guide to assessment, treatment ¡ and evaluation. Monterey, CA: Brooks/Cole.

Cornwall, M. (1987). The social bases of religion: A study of factors influencing religious belief and commitment, *Review of Religious Research, 29,* 44–56.

Corr, C. A., & Corr, D. M. (Eds.), (1985). *Hospice approaches to pediatric care.* New York: Springer.

Costa, P., Zonderman, A., McCrae, R., & Williams, R. (1986). Cynicism and paranoid alienation in the Cook and Medley HO Scale. *Psychosomatic Medicine, 48,* 283–285.

Cousins, Norman (1979). *The anatomy of an illness as perceived by the patient.* New York: W. W. Norton.

Cousins, Norman (1983). *The healing heart.* New York: W. W. Norton.

Cousins, Norman. (1976). Anatomy of an illness as perceived by the patient, *New England Journal of Medicine, 295,* 1458–1463.

Cousins, Norman (1981). *Anatomy of an illness as perceived by the patient: Reflections on healing and regeneration.* New York: Bantam.

Crumbaugh, James., & Maholick, L. T. (1976). *Purpose-in-Life Test.* Munster, IN: Psychometric Affiliates.

Cummings, M., Iannotti, R., & Zahn-Waxler, C. (1985). Influence of conflict between adults on the emotions and aggression of young children. *Developmental Psychology, 21,* 495–507.

Curtis, R. L. (1975). Adolescent orientations toward parents and peers. *Adolescence, 10,* 483–494.

Cutrona, E. (1982). Transition to college: Loneliness and the process of social adjustment. In L. A. Peplau and D. Perlman (Eds.), *Loneliness: A sourcebook of current theory, research, and therapy.* New York: Wiley-Interscience.

D'Zurilla, T., & Goldfried, M. (1971). Problem solving and behavior modification. *Journal of Abnormal Psychology, 78,* 107–126.

Danskin, D. G., & Danskin, D. V. (1988). *Quick-mini stress management strategies for you a person with a disability.* Manhattan, KS: Guild Hall Publications.

Dash, J. (1980). Hypnosis for symptom amelioration. In J. Kellerman (Ed.), *Psychological aspects of childhood cancer.* Springfield, IL: Charles C Thomas.

David, O., Clark, J., & Voeller, K. (1972). Lead and hyperactivity. *Lancet, 2,* 900–903.

David-Neel, A. (1971). *Magic and mystery in Tibet.* New York: Dover Publication.

Davis, J., & Glaros, A. (1986). Relapse prevention and smoking cessation. *Addictive Behaviors, 11,* 105–114.

DeBacker, G., Dramaix, M., Kittel, F., & Kornitzer, M. (1983). Behavior, stress, and psychosocial traits as risk factors. *Preventive Medicine, 12,* 32–36.

Decker, M., Graitcer, P., & Schaffner, W. (1988). Reduction in motor vehicle fatalities associated with an increase in the minimum drinking age. *Journal of American Medical Association, 260,* 3604–3610.

Decker, P., & Nathan, B. (1985). *Behavior modeling training.* New York: Praeger.

Deffenbacher, J., & Shelton, J. (1978). A comparison of anxiety management training and desensitization in reducing test and other anxieties. *Journal of Counseling Psychology, 26,* 120–127.

Deffenbacher, J. (1986). Cognitive and physiological components of test anxiety in real-life exams. *Cognitive Therapy and Research, 10,* 635–644.

Deffenbacher, J., Zwemer, M., Whisman, R., & Sloan, R. (1986). Irrational beliefs and anxiety. *Cognitive Therapy and Research, 10,* 281–292.

Defore, F. (1983). *The life of a child.* New York: Viking Press.

Delcambre, P. (1987, September 2). Waste reduction—Bring back gumbo. *Dow Today.* Midland, MI: Dow Chemical News & Information Services.

Dembroski, T., MacDougall, J., Williams, R., Haney, T., & Blumenthal, J. (1985). Components of Type A hostility, and anger-in: Relationship to angiographic findings. *Psychosomatic Medicine, 47,* 219–233.

Dembroski, T. M. (1978). Reliability and validity of methods used to assess coronary-prone behavior. In Dembroski, T. M., Weiss, S. M., Shields, J. L., Haynes, S. G., and Feinleib, M. (Eds.), *Coronary-prone behavior,* (pp. 95–106). New York: Springer-Verlag.

Dement, W. (1976). Dreams. Public address at the University of Northern Colorado, Greeley, CO.

Demone, H. (1973). The nonuse and abuse of alcohol by male adolescents. In M. Chafetz (Ed.), *Proceedings on the Second Annual Alcoholism conference.* DHEW Publication (HSM) 73–9083.

Denkowski, K., Denkowski, G., & Omizo, M. (1983). The effects of EMG-assisted relaxation training on the academic performance, locus of control, and self-esteem of hyperactive boys. *Biofeedback & Self-Regulation, 8,* 363–375.

Department of Health and Human Services (1987). *National household survey on drug abuse: Population estimates 1985.* Rockville, MD: National Institute of Drug Abuse.

Deschner, J., & McNeil, J. (1986). Results of anger control training for battering couples. *Journal of Family Violence, 1,* 111–120.

Desoille, R. (1965). *The directed daydream.* Psychosynthesis Research Foundation, issue 18, 1–33.

Deubner, D. (1977). An epidemiologic study of migraine and headache in 10–12 year olds. *Headache 17,* 173–180.

Devine, E., & Cook, T. (1983). A meta-analytic analysis of effects of psychoeducational interventions on length of postsurgical hospital stay. *Nursing Research, 32,* 267–274.

Dewey, J. (1933). *How we think: A restatement of the relation of reflective thinking to the educative process* (rev. ed.). New York: D. C. Heath.

Diagnostic and Therapeutic Technology Assessment. (1989). Gastric restrictive surgery, *Journal of the American Medical Association, 261,* 1491–1494.

Diamond, S. (1976). Biofeedback: Treatment of choice in childhood migraine. Biofeedback Research Society Annual meeting, Colorado Springs, CO.

Diamond, S., & Franklin, M. (1975). Autogenic training with biofeedback in the treatment of children with migraine. *Therapy in Psychosomatic Medicine,* 190–192.

DiCara, L. V. (1972). Learning of cardiovascular responses: A review and a description of physiological and biochemical consequences. In J. Stoyva, T. X. Barber, L. DiCara, J. Kamiya, N. Miller, & D. Shapiro (Eds.), *Biofeedback and self-control,* Chicago: Aldine Publishing.

DiClemente, C., & Prochaska, J. (1982). Self-change and therapy change of smoking behavior: A comparison of processes of change in cessation and maintenance. *Addictive Behaviors, 7,* 133–142.

Diesendorf, M. (1976). *The magic bullet.* Canberra, England: Society for Social Responsibility in Science.

Dillon, K., Minchoff, B., & Baker, K. (1985–1986). Positive emotional states and enhancement of the immune system. *International Journal of Psychiatry in Medicine, 15,* 13–18.

DiMatteo, M., & DiNicola, D. (1982). *Achieving patient compliance: The psychology of the medical practitioner's role.* New York: Pergamon Press.

Disorbio, J. (1984). The effects of the kiddie quieting response on stress and anxiety of elementary school children. (Doctoral dissertation, University of Northern Colorado, 1983). *Dissertation Abstracts International, 44,* (11), 3523.

Dobson, K. (Ed.). (1988). *Handbook of cognitive-behavioral therapies.* New York: Guilford Press.

Dotevall, G. (1985). *Stress and common gastrointestinal disorders,* New York: Praeger.

Dow Today (1988, May). Dow USA units are presented awards for showing that "Waste Reduction Always Pays," No. 47.

Dreikurs, R., & Stoltz, V. (1964). *Children the challenge.* New York: Hawthorn Books.

Drossman, D. A., Powell, D. W., & Sessions, J. T. (1977). The irritable bowel syndrome. *Gastroenterology, 73,* 811–822.

Drotman, D. P. (1985). Chemicals, health and the environment. In Daniel S. Blumenthal (Ed.), *Introduction to environmental health,* New York: Springer.

Drug Topics (1988, April 4). Big money in anxiolytics.

Drug Utilization in the U.S.—1986 (1987). Rockville, MD: Office of Epidemiology and Biostatistics, Food and Drug Administration.

Dubow, E., Huesmann, L., & Eron, L. (1987). Mitigating aggression and promoting prosocial behavior in aggressive elementary schoolboys. *Behaviour Research and Therapy, 25,* 527–532.

Dunbar, Flanders (1939). Editorial, *Psychosomatic Medicine, 1,* p. 3.

Dunkel-Schetter, C. (1984). Social support and cancer: Findings based on patient interviews and their implications. *Journal of Social Issues, 40,* 77–98.

Dunn, H. (1961). *High-level wellness.* Arlington, VA: Beatty Press.

Dweck, C. (1986). Motivational processes affecting learning. *American Psychologist, 41,* 1040–1048.

Edelman, M. (1987). *Families in peril: An agenda for social change.* Cambridge, MA: Harvard University Press.

Eland, J., & Anderson, J. (1977). The experience of pain in children. In A. Jacox (Ed.), *Pain—A source book for nurses and other health professionals.* Boston: Little Brown.

Elder, S., & Eustis, N. (1975). Instrumental blood pressure conditioning in out-patient hypertensives. *Behaviour Research and Therapy, 13,* 185–188.

Eliot, R., & Breo, D. (1984). *Is it worth dying for?* New York: Bantam Books.

Ellis, A. (1975). *A new guide to rational living.* North Hollywood, CA: Wilshire Books.

Employment Research Associates (1987). *Neither jobs nor security.* Lansing, Michigan: ERA.

Engel, G. L. (1977). The need for a new medical model: A challenge for biomedicine. *Science, 196,* 129–136.

Englehardt, L. (1976). The application of biofeedback techniques within a public school setting. Presentation at the Biofeedback Research Society Seventh Annual Meeting, March 1976, Colorado Springs, CO.

Environmental Engineering and Pollution Control Department (1988). Pollution Prevention Pays. St. Paul, Minnesota: 3M.

Epilepsy Foundation of America (1975). *Epilepsy.* Washington DC.

Epstein, L., Figueroa, J., Farkas, G., & Beck, S. (1981). The short-term effects of feedback on accuracy of urine glucose determinants in insulin-dependent diabetic children. *Behavior Therapy, 12,* 560–564.

Erikson, Erik (1980). *Identity and the life cycle.* New York: W. W. Norton.

Eron, L. (1987). The development of aggressive behavior from the perspective of a developing behaviorism. *American Psychologist, 42,* 435–442.

Eron, L., & Huesmann, L. (1984). The relation of pro-social behavior to the development of aggression and psychopathology. *Aggressive Behaivor, 10,* 243–253.

Evans, F. J. (1985). Expectancy, therapeutic instructions, and the placebo response. In L. White, B. Tursky, & G. Schwartz (Eds.), *Placebo: Theory, research, and mechanisms,* (pp. 215–226). New York: Guilford Press.

Evans, R. (1976). Smoking children: Developing a social-psychological strategy of deterrence. *Journal of Preventive Medicine, 5,* 122–127.

Evans, R. (1988). How can health life-styles in adolescents be modified? Some implications from a smoking prevention program. In D. Routh (Ed.), *Handbook of Pediatric Psychology,* (pp. 321–331). New York: Guilford Press.

Evans, R., Rozelle, R., Mittelmark, M., Hansen, W., Bane, A., & Havis, J. (1978). Deterring the onset of smoking in children: Knowledge of immediate physiological effects and coping with peer pressure, media pressure, and parent modeling. *Journal of Applied Social Psychology, 8,* 126–135.

Eysenck, H. J. (1987). Anxiety, learned helplessness, and cancer: A causal theory. *Journal of Anxiety Disorders, 1,* 87–104.

Eysenck, H. J. (1988). Personality, stress, and cancer: Prediction and prophylaxis. *British Journal of Medical Psychology, 61,* 57–75.

Fahrion, S. (1978). Autogenic biofeedback treatment for migraine. In M. E. Granger (Ed.), *Research and clinical studies in headache,* (pp. 47–71).

Fahrion, S., Mills, S., Parks, P., Nichols, J., Bremer, S., & Norris, P. (1987). Self-regulation of blood pressure in patients with borderline essential hypertension and those at "intermediate risk." *Biofeedback & Self-Regulation, 12,* 142, 143.

Fahrion, S., Norris, P., Green, A., Green, E., & Snarr, C. (1987). Biobehavioral treatment of essential hypertension: A group outcome study. *Biofeedback & Self-Regulation, 11,* 257–278.

Farley, G. (1981). Cognitive development. In R. Simons & H. Pardes (Eds.), *Understanding human behavior in health and illness.* Philadelphia: Williams & Wilkins Co.

Farquhar, J, Maccoby, N., & Solomon, D. (1984). Community applications of behavioral medicine. In W. Gentry (Ed.), *Handbook of behavioral medicine,* (pp. 437–478). New York: Guilford Press.

Farquhar, J. (1978). *The American way of life need not be hazardous to your health.* New York: W. W. Norton.

Farquhar, J., Maccoby, N., & Solomon, D. (1984). Community applications of behavioral medicine. In W. Gentry (Ed.), *Handbook of Behavioral Medicine,* (pp. 437–478). New York: Guilford Press.

Feist, J., & Brannon, L. (1988). *Health psychology.* Belmont, CA: Wadsworth.

Fenly, Leigh. (1977, August 28). "Welfare Workers' Stress Takes Toll." *San Diego Union,* San Diego, CA.

Fentress, D., Masek, J., Mehegan, J., & Benson, H. (1986). Biofeedback and relaxation response training in the treatment of pediatric migraine. *Developmental Medicine and Child Neurology, 28,* 139–146.

Feshbach, N. (1984). Empathy, empathy training, and the regulation of aggression in elementary school children. In R. M. Kaplan, V. Konecni, & R. Novaco (Eds.), *Aggression in children and youth,* (pp. 192–208). The Hague: Martinus Nijhoff.

Feuerstein, M., & Gainer, J. (1982). Chronic headache: Etiology and management. In D. Doleys, R. Meredith, & A. Ciminero (Eds.), *Behavioral medicine: Assessment and treatment strategies.* New York: Plenum Press.

Feuerstein, M., Bush, C., & Corbisiero, T. (1982). Stress and chronic headache: A psychophysiological analysis of mechanisms. *Journal of Psychosomatic Research, 26,* 167–182.

Fields, M. O. (1978). Wife beating: Facts and figures. *Victimology, 2,* 643–647.

Finley, W. (1977). Operant conditioning of the EEG in two patients with epilepsy: Methodologic and clinical considerations. *Pavlovian Journal, 12,* 93–111.

Fischer-Williams, M., Nigl, A., & Sovine, D. (1981). *A textbook of biological biofeedback.* New York: Human Services Press.

Fischman, L. (1987). Type A on trial. *Psychology Today,* February, 42–50.

Fisher, C. L., Gill, C., Daniels, J. C., Cobb, E. K., Berry, C. A., and Ritzman, S. E. (1972). Effects of space flight environment on man's immune system. *Aerospace Medicine 43,* 856–859.

Fletcher, B. (1970). *Students of Outward Bound Schools in Great Britain.* Unpublished manuscript, University of Bristol School of Education, England.

Cited in Bacon, S. (1987), *The evolution of the Outward Bound process.* Greenwich, CT: Outward Bound Press.

Fletcher, Sally, (1986). *The challenge of epilepsy.* Santa Rosa, CA: Aura Press.

Flor, H., Haag, G., & Turk, D. (1986). Long-term efficacy of EMG biofeedback for chronic rheumatic back pain. *Pain, 27,* 195–202.

Foa, E., Blau, J., Prout, M., & Latimer, P. (1977). Is horror a necessary component of flooding (implosion)? *Behaviour Research and Therapy, 15,* 397–402.

Fontana, A., Rosenberg, R., Kerns, R., & Marcus, J. (1986). Social insecurity, the Type A behavior pattern, and sympathetic arousal. *Journal of Behavioral Medicine, 9,* 79–88.

Forbes (1980, September 1). No wonder, *126,* 14–15.

Fordyce, W. E. (1976). *Behavioral methods for chronic pain and illness.* St. Louis, MO: Mosby.

Forman, S. (1982). Stress management for teachers: A cognitive-behavioral program. *Journal of School Psychology, 20,* 180–187.

Foster, W., & Seltzer, A. (1986). A portrayal of individual excellence in the urban ghetto. *Journal of Counseling and Development, 64,* 579–582.

Fowler, J., Budzynski, T., & VandenBergh, R. (1976). Effects of an EMG biofeedback relaxation program on the control of diabetes: A case study. *Biofeedback & Self-Regulation, 1,* 105–112.

Francis, S., (1988, February 15). U. S. Industrial Outlook—1988, *Medical Benefits,* (pp. 1–2). Charlottesville, VA: Kelly Communications.

Frankenhauser, M. (1977). Job demands, health and wellbeing. *Psychosomatic Research, 21,* 313–321.

Frankenhauser, M. (1980). Psychological aspects of life stress. In S. Levine & H. Ursin (Eds.), *Coping and health.* New York: Plenum Press.

Frankenhauser, M., & Rissler, A. (1970). Effects of punishment on catecholamine release and efficiency of performance. *Psychopharmacologia 17,* 378–390.

Frankl, Viktor, E. (1963). *Man's search for meaning.* New York: Pocket Books.

Free, N., Green, B., Grace, M., Chernus, L., & Whitman, R. (1985). Empathy and outcome in brief focal-dynamic therapy. *American Journal of Psychiatry, 142,* 917–921.

Freedman, R., Ianni, P., & Wenig, P. (1983). Behavioral treatment of Raynaud's disease. *Journal of Consulting and Clinical Psychology, 51,* 539–549.

Freedman, R., Ianni, P., & Wenig, P. (1985). Behavioral treatment of Raynaud's disease: long-term follow-up. *Journal of Consulting and Clinical Psychology, 53,* 136.

French, J. R. P., & Caplan, R. D. (1972). Organizational stress and individual strain. In A. J. Marrow (Ed.), *The failure of success,* pp. 30–66.

French-Belgian Collaborative Group (1982). Ischemic heart disease and psychological patterns: Prevalence and incidence studies in Belgium and France. *Advances in Cardiology, 29,* 25–31.

Freud, S. (1955). *The interpretation of dreams.* New York: Basic Books.

Friedman, E. (1980). Animal companions and one-year survival of patients after discharge from a coronary care unit. *Public Health Reports, 95,* 307–312.

Friedman, E. (1983). Social interaction and blood pressure: Influence of animal companions. *The Journal of Nervous and Mental Disease, 171,* 461–65.

Friedman, M., & Rosenman, R. H. (1974). *Type A behavior and your heart.* Greenwich, CT: Fawcett Publications.

Friedman, M., and Ulmer, D. (1984). *Treating type A behavior.* New York: Random House.

Friedman, M., Thoresen, C., Gill, J., Ulmer, D., Powell, L., Price, V., Brown, B., Thompson, L., Rabin, D., Breall, W., Bourg, E., Levy, R., & Dixon, T. (1986). Alteration of type A behavior and its effect on cardiac recurrences in post myocardial infarction patients: Summary results of the recurrent coronary prevention project. *American Heart Journal, 112,* 653–675.

Frieze, I. (1979). Perceptions of battered wives. In I. Frieze, D. Bar-Tal, & J. Carrol (Eds.), *New approaches to social problems,* (pp. 79–108). San Francisco: Jossey-Bass.

Frontiers of Psychiatry (December, 1973). *Roche Report, 3,* pp. 1–2.

Frymoyer, J. (1988). Back pain and sciatica. *New England Journal of Medicine, 318,* 291–300.

Fuller, A. (1989). Child molestation and pedophilia. *Journal of the American Medical Association, 261,* 602–606.

Funk, S., & Houston, B. K. (1987). A critical analysis of the hardiness scale's validity and utility. *Journal of Personality and Social Psychology, 53,* 572–578.

Furedy, J. (1985). Specific vs. placebo effects in biofeedback: Science-based vs. snake-oil behavioral medicine. *Clinical Biofeedback & Health, 8,* 155–162.

Ganellen, R. J., & Blaney, P. H. (1984). Hardiness and social support as moderators of the effects of life stress. *Journal of Personality and Social Psychology, 47,* 156–163.

Gardner, G. G., and Olness, K. (1981). *Hypnosis and hypnotherapy with children.* New York: Grune & Stratton.

Garmezy, N., & Tellegren, A. (1984). Studies of stress-resistant children: Methods, variables and preliminary findings. In F. Morrison, C. Lord, and D. Keating (Eds.), *Advances in applied developmental psychology,* (pp. 231–287). New York: Academic Press.

Garmezy, N. (1983). Stressors of childhood. In N. Garmezy and M. Rutter (Eds.), *Stress, coping and development in children,* (pp. 43–83). New York: McGraw Hill.

Garmezy, N. (1986). Stress resistant children: The search for protective factors. In J. E. Stevenson (Ed.), *Aspects of current child psychiatry research.* Oxford, England: Pergamon.

Gartner, A., & Riessman, F. (Eds.), (1984). *The self-help revolution.* New York: Human Sciences Press.

Gatchel, R. J., and Baum, A. (1983). *An introduction to health psychology.* New York: Random House.

Gentry, W. (1984). Behavioral medicine: A new research paradigm. In W. Gentry (Ed.), *Handbook of Behavioral Medicine,* 1–12. New York: Guilford Press.

Getchell, B. (1987). *The fitness book.* Indianapolis: Benchmark Press.

Giles, S. (1978). Separate and combined effects of biofeedback training and brief individual psychotherapy in the treatment of gastrointestinal disorders. Doctoral dissertation, University of Colorado, Boulder.

Giles-Sims, J. (1983). *Wife battering: A systems theory approach.* New York: Guilford Press.

Giovacchini, P. L., & Muslin, H. (1965). Ego equilibrium and cancer of the breast. *Psychosomatic Medicine, 27,* 524–532.

Gjerde, P. F. (1985). Adolescent depression and parental socialization patterns: A prospective study. Paper presented at the biennial meeting of the Society for Research in Child Development. Toronto, Ontario.

Glassman, Judith (1983). *The cancer survivors and how they did it.* New York: The Dial Press.

Goebel, M., Viol, G., Lorenz, G., & Clemente, J. (1980). Relaxation and biofeedback in essential hypertension: A preliminary report of a six-year project. *American Journal of Clinical Biofeedback, 3,* 20–29.

Gold, A., Goodwin, F., and Chvouzos, G. (1988). Clinical and biochemical manifestations of depression. *New England Journal of Medicine, 319,* 348–353.

Gold, M., & Yanof, D. S. (1985). Mothers, daughters, and girlfriends. *Journal of Personality and Social Psychology, 49,* 645–659.

Gold, P., Goodwin, F., & Chvousos, G. (1988). Clinical and biochemical manifestations of depression. *New England Journal of Medicine, 319,* 348–353.

Goldfried, M. R. (1971). Systematic desensitization as training in self-control. *Journal of Consulting and Clinical Psychology, 37,* 228–234.

Goldfried, M. R. (1977). The use of relaxation and cognitive relabeling as coping skills. In R. B. Stuart (Ed.), *Behavioral self-management: Strategies, techniques and outcomes,* (pp. 71–116). New York: Brunner/Mazel.

Goldner, V. (1984). Overeaters anonymous. In A. Gartner & F. Riessman (Eds.), *The self-help revolution,* (pp. 65–72). New York: Human Sciences Press.

Goldsmith, M. (1986). Worksite wellness programs: Latest wrinkle to smooth health care costs. *Journal of the American Medical Association, 256,* 1089–1095.

Golins, G. (1980). *Outward Bound and troubled youth.* Greenwich, CT: Outward Bound USA.

Good, T., & Weinstein, R. (1986). Schools make a difference: Evidence, criticisms, and new directions. *American Psychologist, 41,* 1090–1097.

Goodkin, Karl. (1986). *Journal of Psychosomatic Research, 30,* No. 1.

Gortmaker, S., et al. (1988). Increasing pediatric obesity in the United States. *American Journal of Disorders of Children, 141,* 535–540.

Gottlieb, S. (1988). Why study PAC's. *Law and Society Review, 21,* 907–909.

Graham, L., et al. (1983). Five-year follow-up of a behavioral weight loss program. *Journal of Consulting and Clinical Psychology, 51,* 322–323.

Green, E., & Green, A. (1977). *Beyond biofeedback.* New York: W. W. Norton.

Green, E., Green, A., & Norris, P. (1980). Self-regulation training for control of hypertension. *Primary Cardiology, 6,* 126–137.

Green, E. E., Green, A. M., and Walters, E. D. (1969). Feedback technique for deep relaxation. *Psychophysiology, 6,* 371–377.

Green, J., & Shellenberger, R. (1986a). Biofeedback research and the ghost in the box: A reply to Roberts. *American Psychologist, 41,* 1003–1005.

Green, J., & Shellenberger, R. (1986b). Clinical biofeedback training and the ghost in the box: A reply to Furedy. *Clinical Biofeedback and Health, 9,* 96–105.

Green, J. (1983). Biofeedback therapy with children. In W. Rickles, J. Sandweiss, D. Jacobs, R. Grove, & E. Criswell (Eds.), *Biofeedback and family practice medicine,* (pp. 121–144). New York: Plenum Press.

Greene, W. A., & Miller, G. (1958). Psychological factors and reticuloendothelial disease. *Psychosomatic Medicine, 20,* 124–144.

Greer, S., & Morris, T. (1975). Psychological attributes of women who develop breast cancer: A controlled study. *Journal of Psychosomatic Research, 19,* 147–153.

Greer, S., Morris, T., & Pettingale, K. (1979). Psychological response to breast cancer: Effect on outcome. *Lancet, 2,* 785–788.

Grevert, P., & Goldstein, A. (1985). Placebo, analgesia, naloxone, and the role of endogenous opiods. In L. White, B. Tursky, & G. Schwartz (Eds.), *Placebo: Theory, research and mechanisms,* (pp. 332–350). New York: Guilford Press.

Griswold-Ezekoye, Stephanie (1985). The multicultural model in chemical abuse prevention and intervention. *Journal of Children in Contemporary Society, 18,* 203–230.

Gross, S., & Gardner, G. (1980). Child pain: Treatment approaches. In W. Smith, H. Merskey, & S. Gross (Eds.), *Pain: Meaning and management,* (pp. 127–142). New York: Spectrum.

Grossarth-Matticek, R., Bastiaans, J., and Kanazir, D. T. (1985). Psychosocial factors as strong predictors of mortality from cancer, ischaemic heart disease and stroke: The Yugoslav prospective study, *Journal of Psychosomatic Research, 29,* 167–176.

Grossarth-Matticek, R., Eysenck, H., Vetter, H., & Frentzl-Beyme, R. (1986). The Heidelberg prospective intervention study. Paper presented at the First International Symposium on Primary Prevention and Cancer, March 1986, Antwerp.

Contents of the paper are discussed in H. Eysenck, (1987), Anxiety, learned helplessness, and cancer: A causal theory, *Journal of Anxiety Disorders, 1,* 87–104.

Grossarth-Matticek, R., Kanazir, D., Schmidt, P., & Veter, H. (1982). Psychosomatic factors in the process of carcenogenesis. *Psychotherapy and Psychosomatics, 28,* 284–302.

Grossarth-Matticek, R., Kanazir, D., Vetter, H., & Jankovic, M. (1983). Smoking as a risk factor for lung cancer and cardiac infarct as mediated by psychosocial variables: A prospective investigation. *Psychotherapy and Psychosomatics, 39,* 94–105.

Gruber, B., Hall, N., Hersh, S., & Dubois, P. (1988). Immune system and psychologic changes in metastatic cancer patients while using ritualized relaxation and guided imagery. *Scandanavian Journal of Behavior Therapy, 17* (1), 25–46.

Guarnieri, P., Blanchard, E., Andrasik, F., & Neff, D. (1986). Two-, three-, and four-year prospective follow-up on the behavioral treatment of chronic headache. *Biofeedback & Self-Regulation, 11,* 59–60.

Guglielmi, R., Roberts, A., & Patterson, R. (1982). Skin temperature biofeedback for Raynaud's disease: A double-blind study. *Biofeedback & Self-Regulation, 7, 99–119.*

Guidano, V. F. (1988). A systems, process-oriented approach to cognitive therapy. In *Handbook of cognitive-behavioral therapies,* Keith S. Dobson, (Ed.), New York: Guilford Press.

Gunby, P. (1988a). Tobacco row. *Journal of the American Medical Association, 260,* 1835.

Gunby, P. (1988b). Something really new this television season: Coordinated campaign against drunk driving. *Journal of the American Medical Association, 260,* 1830–1831.

Guyton, A. (1977). *Textbook of medical physiology.* Philadelphia: W. B. Saunders.

Haan, N. (1985). Processes of moral development: Cognitive or social disequilibrium? *Developmental Psychology, 21,* 996–1006.

Hadley, J., & Staudacher, C. (1985). *Hypnosis for change.* Oakland, CA: New Harbinger Publications.

Hahn, M. (1966). *California Life Goals Evaluation Schedule.* Palo Alto, CA: Western Psychological Services.

Hall, H. (1983). Hypnosis and the immune system: A review with implications for cancer and the psychology of healing. *American Journal of Clinical Hypnosis, 25,* Nos. 2–3; 92–103.

Hall, N., & Goldstein, A. (1985). Neurotransmitters and host defense. In R. Guillemin (Ed.), *Neuromodulation of immunity,* (pp. 143–153). New York: Raven Press.

Hamburg, D., Elliott, G., & Parron D. (Eds.), (1982). *Health and behavior: Frontiers of research in the biobehavioral sciences.* Washington, DC: National Academy Press.

Harlow, L., Newcomb, M., & Bentler, P. (1986). Depression, self-derogation, substance use, and suicide ideation: Lack of purpose in life as a mediational factor. *Journal of Clinical Psychology, 42,* 5–19.

Harrington, D., Block, J., & Block, J. (1987). Testing aspects of Carl Roger's theory of creative environments: Child-rearing antecedents of creative potential in young adolescents. *Journal of Personality and Social Psychology, 52,* 851–856.

Harrington, G. (1987). *Real food, fake food, and everything in between.* New York: Macmillan.

Haugen, G. B., Dixon, H. H., and Dickel, H. A. (1963). *A therapy for anxiety tension reduction.* New York: Macmillan.

Hawkins, J., Lishner, D., Catalano, Jr., R., & Howard, M. (1985). Childhood predictors of adolescent substance abuse: Toward an empirically grounded theory. *Journal of Children in Contemporary Society, 18,* 11–47.

Hawkins, N., Davies, R., & Holmes, T. H. (1957). Evidence of psychosocial factors in the development of pulmonary tuberculosis. *American Review of Tuberculosis & Pulmonary Disorders, 75,* 768–780.

Hawton, K. (1986). *Suicide and attempted suicide among children and adolescents.* London: Sage Publications.

Haynes, R. B. (1982). Patient compliance with antihypertensive treatment: An introduction. In R. B. Haynes, M. E. Mattson, & T. O. Engebretson, Jr. (Eds.), *Patient compliance to prescribed antihypertensive medication regimens: A report to the National Heart, Lung, and Blood Institute,* xiii–xiv. Bethesda, MD: NIH Publications.

Haynes, S., & Matthews, K. (1988). Coronary-prone behavior: Continuing evolution of the concept. *Annals of Behavior Medicine, 10,* 47–59.

Haynes, S. G., Feinleib, M., and Kannel, W. B. (1980). The relationship of psychosocial factors to coronary heart disease in the Framingham Study III. Eight-year incidence of coronary heart disease. *American Journal of Epidemiology, 3,* 37–58.

Health Care Financing Administration (1989). *Medicare data.* Baltimore: U.S. Department of Health and Human Services.

Hecker, M., Chesney, M., Black, G., & Frautschi, N. (1988). Coronary-prone behaviors in the Western Collaborative Group Study. *Psychosomatic Medicine, 1,* 153–164.

Henry, J., & Stephens, P. (1977). *Stress, health, and the social environment: A sociobiologic approach to medicine.* New York: Springer-Verlag.

Herman, R. (1973). Augmented sensory feedback in the control of limb movement. In *Neural organization and its relevance to prosthetics,* (pp. 197–215). Orlando, FL: Symposia Specialists.

Heyward, W. L., and Curran, J. W. (1988). The epidemiology of AIDS. *Scientific American, 259,* 72–81.

Higgins, A., Power, C., & Kohlberg, L. (1984). The relationship of moral atmosphere to judgments of responsibility. In W. M. Kurtines & J. Gewirtz (Eds.), *Morality, moral behavior, and moral development.* New York: Wiley-Interscience.

Higgins, C., & Whitley, K. (1982). Health policy and the tobacco subsidy. *Health Values, 6,* 25–29.

Hilgard, E., & Hilgard, J. (1983). Hypnosis in the relief of pain. Los Altos, CA: Kaufman.

Hillman, L. C., Stace, N. H., & Pomare, E. W. (1984). Irritable bowel patients and their long-term response to a higher fiber diet. *The American Journal of Gastroenterology, 79,* 107.

Hinkle, L., & Plummer, N. (1952). Life stress and industrial absenteeism. *Industrial Medicine and Surgery, 21,* 363–375.

Hinkle, L. E. (1974). The effect of exposure to cultural change, social change, and changes in interpersonal relationships on health. In B. S. Dohrenwend & B. P. Dohrenwend (Eds.), *Stressful life events: Their nature and effects.* New York: Wiley.

Hobbs, N., Perrin, J., & Ireys, H. (1985). *Chronically ill children and their families.* San Francisco: Jossey-Bass.

Hockey, R. (Ed.), (1983). *Stress and fatigue in human performance.* New York: Wiley.

Hoffman, M. L. (1982). Development of prosocial motivation. In N. Eisenberg (Ed.), *The development of prosocial behavior.* New York: Academic Press.

Hoffman, M. L. (1977). *Empathy, its development and prosocial implications.* In C. B. Keasey (Ed.),

Nebraska symposium on motivation, Vol. 25. Lincoln: University of Nebraska Press.

Hogan, R., & Nicholson, R. (1988). The meaning of personality test scores. *American Psychologist, 43,* 621–626.

Holahan, C., & Moos, R. (1985). Life stress and health: Personality, coping and family support in stress resistance. *Journal of Personality and Social Psychology, 49,* 739–747.

Holmes, T. H., & Rahe, R. H. (1967). The social adjustment rating scale. *Journal of Psychosomatic Research, 11,* 213–218.

Holt, R. (1964). Imagery: The return of the ostracized. *American Psychologist, 19,* 254–264.

House, J., Robbins, C., & Metzner, H. (1982). The association of social relationships and activities with mortality: Prospective evidence from the Tecumseh Community Health Study. *American Journal of Epidemiology, 116,* 123–140.

Houston, B., & Kelly, K. (1987). Type A behavior in housewives: Relation to work, marital adjustment, stress, tension, health, fear-of-failure and self esteem. *Journal of Psychosomatic Research, 31,* 55–61.

Hoyt, M., & Janis, I. (1975). Increasing adherence to a stressful decision via a motivational balance-sheet procedure: A field experiment. *Journal of Personality and Social Psychology, 31,* 833–839.

Hubert, N., & Wachs, T. (1985). Parental perceptions of the behavioral components of infant easiness/difficultness. *Child Development, 56,* 1525–1537.

Hudzinski, L. (1983). Neck musculature and EMG biofeedback in treatment of muscle contraction headache. *Headache, 23,* 86–90.

Hughes, J. F., Gust, S. W., Keenan, R. M., Fenwick, J. W., & Healey, M. L. (1989). Nicotine vs. placebo gum in general medical practice. *Journal of the American Medical Association, 261,* 1300–1305.

Hull, J., Van Treuren, R., & Virnelli, S. (1987). Hardiness and health: A critique and alternative approach. *Journal of Personality and Social Psychology, 53,* 518–530.

Hunsley, J. (1987). Internal dialogue during academic examinations. *Cognitive Therapy & Research, 11,* 653–664.

Hunter, Beatrice (1971). *Consumer beware!* New York: Bantam Books.

Hutschnecker, A. A. (1951). *The will to live.* New York: Prentice-Hall.

Igoe, J. (1980). Project health PACT in action. *American Journal of Nursing, 80,* 2016–2021.

Illich, Ivan. (1975). *Medical nemesis: The expropriation of health.* New York: Pantheon.

Ince, L., Zaretsky, H., Lee, M., Kerman-Lerner, P., & Adler, J. (1987). Utilization of EMG biofeedback for restoration of function in stroke patients. *Biofeedback & Self-Regulation, 12,* 148.

Irwin, M., Daniels, M., Smith, T. L., Bloom, E., and Weiner, H. (1987). Impaired natural killer cell activity during bereavement. *Brain, Behavior and Immunity, 1,* 98–104.

Isaac, K., & Gold, S. (Eds.), (1988). *Eating clean: Overcoming food hazards.* Washington, DC: Center for the Study of Responsive Law.

Jacobson, E. (1929). *Progressive relaxation.* Chicago: University of Chicago Press.

Jacobson, E. (1934). *You must relax.* New York: McGraw Hill.

James, W. (1890). *The principles of psychology.* New York: Henry Holt & Co.

James, W. (1912). *Lectures to teachers.* New York: Henry Holt & Co.

Jampolsky, G. (1983). *Teach only love: The seven principles of attitudinal healing.* New York: Bantam Books.

Jampolsky, J. (1983). *Teach only love.* New York: Bantam Books.

Janis, I. (1958). *Psychological stress.* New York: Wiley.

Janis, I. (1982). *Stress, attitudes, and decisions.* New York: Praeger.

Janis, I. (1983a). *Short-term counseling.* New Haven, CT: Yale University Press.

Janis, I. (1983b). The role of social support in adherence to stressful decisions. *American Psychologist, 38,* 143–160.

Janis, I. (1984). The patient as decision maker. In W. Gentry (Ed.), *Handbook of behavioral medicine.* New York: Guilford Press.

Janis, I., & Hoffman, D. (1982). Effective partnerships in a clinic for smokers. In I. L. Janis (Ed.), *Counseling on personal decisions: Theory and research on short-term helping relationships.* New Haven, CT: Yale University Press.

Janis, I., & Mann, L. (1977). *Decision making. A psychological analysis of conflict, choice and commitment.* New York: Macmillan.

Janis, I., & Mann, L. (1965). Effectiveness of emotional role-playing in modifying smoking habits and attitudes. *Journal of Experimental Research in Personality, 1,* 89–90.

Janz, N. K., & Becker, M. H. (1984). The health belief model: A decade later. *Health Education Quarterly, 11* (1), 1–47.

Jay, S., Elliott, C., & Varni, J. (1986). Acute and chronic pain in adults and children with cancer. *Journal of Consulting and Clinical Psychology, 54,* 601–607.

Jay, S., Elliott, C., Ozolins, M., Olson, R., & Pruitt, S. (1985). Behavioral management of children's distress during painful medical procedures. *Behaviour Research and Therapy, 23,* 513–520.

Jay, S., Katz, E., Elliott, C., & Siegel, S. (1987). Cognitive-behavioral and pharmacologaic interventions for children's distress during painful medical procedures. *Journal of Consulting and Clinical Psychology, 55,* 860–865.

Jayasuriya, D. (1981). Regulating the drug trade in the Third World, *World Health Forum, 2,* 423–426.

Jemmott, J. B., III., Borysenko, J., Borysenko, M., McClelland, D., Chapman, R., Meyer, D., & Benson, H. (1983). Academic stress, power motivation, and decrease in salivary secretory immunoglobulin A secretion rate. *Lancet, 1,* 1400–1402.

Jenkins, C. D. (1971). Psychologic and social precursors of coronary disease. *New England Journal of Medicine, 284,* 307–317.

Jenkins, C. D., Rosenman, R. H., and Friedman, M. (1968). Replicability of rating the coronary-prone behavior pattern. *British Journal of Preventive Society of Medicine, 22,* 16–22.

Jessor, R., & Jessor, S. (1977). *Problem behavior and psychosocial development: A longitudinal study of youth.* New York: Academic Press.

Johnson, J. H., & Sarason, I. G. (1979). Moderator variables in life stress research. In I. G. Sarason & C. D. Spielberger (Eds.), *Stress and anxiety.* Washington, DC: Hemisphere Publishing.

Johnston, L., O'Malley, P., & Bachman, J. (1988). *Illicit drug use, smoking, and drinking by America's high school students, college students, and young adults, 1975–1987.* Washington, DC: National Institute of Drug Abuse.

Jones, E., Forrest, J., Goldman, N., Henshaw, S., Lincoln, R., Rosoff, J., Westoff, C., & Wulf, D. (1985). Teenage pregnancy in developed countries: Determinants and policy implications. *Family Planning Perspectives, 17,* 53–63.

Jones, D. R. (1986). What repatriated prisoners of war wrote about themselves. In Rudolf Moos (Ed.), *Coping with life crises: An integrated approach.* New York: Plenum Press.

Jones, W., Hobbs, S., & Hockenbury, D. (1982). Loneliness and social skill deficits. *Journal of Personality and Social Psychology, 42,* 682–689.

Jung, C. G. (1963). *Memories, dreams, reflections.* New York: Vintage Books.

Jurish, S., Blanchard, E., Andrasik, F., Teders, S., Neff, D., & Arena, J. (1983). Home- versus clinic-based treatment of vascular headache. *Journal of Consulting and Clinical Psychology, 51,* 741–751.

Justice, B. (1987). *Who gets sick.* Houston, TX: Peak Press.

Kagan, J., Kearsley, R., & Zelazo, P. (1978). *Infancy: Its place in human development.* Cambridge, MA: Harvard University Press.

Kamiya, J. (1971). Conditioned discrimination of the EEG alpha rhythm in humans. In T. X. Barber, L. DiCara, J. Kamiya, N. Miller, D. Shapiro & J. Stoyva (Eds.), *Biofeedback and self-control,* (pp. 279–290). Chicago: Aldine Publishing.

Kamiya, J. (1979). Autoregulation of the EEG alpha rhythm: A program for the study of consciousness. In E. Peper, S. Ancoli, M. Quinn (Eds.), *Mind-body integration: Essential readings in biofeedback.* New York: Plenum Press.

Kanfer, F. H. (1970). Self-regulation: Research, issues and speculations. In C. Neuringer and J. L. Michael (Eds.), *Behavior modification in clinical psychology.* New York: Appleton-Century-Crofts.

Kanfer, F. H., & Hagerman, S. (1980). The role of self-regulation. In L. P. Rehm (Ed.), *Behavior therapy for depression: Present status and future directions.* New York: Academic Press.

Kaplan, G., & Reynolds, P. (1987). Depression and cancer mortality and morbidity: Prospective evidence from the Alameda County study. *Journal of Behavioral Medicine, 11,* 1–13.

Kaplan, G. A., Haan, M. N., Syme, S. L., Minkler, M., & Winkleby, M. (1987). Socioeconomic status and health. In Robert Amler and H. Dull (Eds.), *Closing the gap: The burden of unnecessary illness* (pp. 125–129). New York: Oxford University Press.

Kaplan, H. (1975). Increases in self-rejection as an antecedent of deviant responses. *Journal of Youth and Adolescence, 4,* 281–292.

Kaplan, J., Powell, K., Sikes, R., Shirley, R., & Campbell, C. (1982). An epidemiologic study of the benefits and risks of running. *Journal of the American Medical Association*, 248, 3118–3121.

Karasek, R., Theorell, T., Schwartz, J., Pieper, C., & Alfredsson, L. (1982). Job, psychological factors and coronary heart disease: Swedish prospective findings and U.S. prevalence findings using a new occupational inference method. *Advances in Cardiology*, 29, 62–67.

Katz, R., & Singh, N. (1986). Reflections on the ex-smoker: Some findings on successful quitters. *Journal of Behavioral Medicine*, 9, 191–202.

Kazdin, A., & Wilcoxon, L. (1976). Systematic desensitization and nonspecific treatment effects: A methodological evaluation. *Psychological Bulletin*, 83, 729–758.

Keefe, F., & Hoelscher, T. (1987). Biofeedback in the management of chronic pain syndromes. In J. Hatch, J. Fisher, & J. Rugh (Eds.), *Biofeedback: Studies in clinical efficacy*, (pp. 211–253). New York: Plenum Press.

Keller, M., & Baumann, L. (1986). Further comments on psychology and nursing. *American Psychologist*, 41, 1169–1170.

Kellerman, J. (1980). *The psychological aspects of childhood cancer*. Springfield, IL: Charles C. Thomas.

Kendall, P. C., & Hollon, S. D. (1981). Assessing self-referent speech: Methods in the measurement of self-statements. In P. C. Kendall & S. D. Hollon (Eds.), *Assessment strategies for cognitive-behavioral interventions*. New York: Academic Press.

Kendall, P. C., Williams, L., Pechacek, T. F., Graham, L. E., Shisslack, C., & Herzoff, N. (1979). Cognitive-behavioral and patient education interventions in cardiac catheterization procedures: The Palo Alto Medical psychology project. *Journal of Consulting and Clinical Psychology*, 47, 49–58.

Kewman, D., & Roberts, A. (1980). Skin temperature biofeedback and migraine headaches. *Biofeedback & Self-Regulation*, 5, 327–345.

Kiecolt-Glaser, J., and Glaser, R. (1988). Psychological influences on immunity. *American Psychologist*, 43, 892–898.

Kiecolt-Glaser, J., Fisher, L., Ogrocki, P., Stout, J., Speicher, C., & Glaser, R. (1987). Marital quality, marital disruption, and immune function. *Psychosomatic Medicine*, 49, 13–34.

Kiecolt-Glaser, J., Garner, W., Speicher, C., Penn, D. Holliday, J., & Glaser, R. (1984). Psychosocial modifiers of immunocompetence in medical students. *Psychosomatic Medicine*, 46, 7–14.

Kiecolt-Glaser, J., Glaser, R., Strain, E., Stout, J., Tarr, K., Holliday, J., & Speicher, C. (1986). Modulation of cellular immunity in medical students, *Journal of Behavioral Medicine*, 5, 5–21.

Kiecolt-Glaser, J., Speicher, C., Holliday, J., & Glaser, R. (1984). Stess and the transformation of lymphocytes by Epstein-Barr virus. *Journal of Behavioral Medicine*, 7, 1–12.

Kiecolt-Glaser, J., Stephens, R., Lipetz, P., Speicher, C., & Glaser, R. (1985). Distress and DNA repair in human lymphocytes. *Journal of Behavioral Medicine*, 3, 311–320.

Kiecolt-Glaser, J. K., Glaser, R., Willinger, D., Stout, J., Messick, G., and Sheppard, S. (1985). Psychosocial enhancement of immunocompetence in a geriatric population. *Health Psychology*, Vol 4, 25–41.

Kiecolt-Glaser, J. K., & Glaser, R. (1987). Psychosocial moderators of immune function. *Annals of Behavioral Medicine*, 9 (2), 16–20.

Kiecolt-Glaser, J. K., Kennedy, S., Malkolf, S., Fisher, L., Speicher, C. E., and Glaser, R. (1988). Marital discord and immunity in males. *Psychosomatic Medicine*, 50, 213–229.

Kierkegaard, S. (1954). *Fear and trembling and the sickness unto death*. New York: Doubleday.

Kiesler, C. A. (Ed.), (1971). *The psychology of commitment*. New York: Academic Press.

King, A., & Arena, J. (1984). Behavioral treatment of chronic cluster headache in a geriatric patient. *Biofeedback and Self-Regulation*, 9, 201–208.

Kinney, J., Madsen, B., Fleming, T., & Haapala, D. (1977). Homebuilders: Keeping families together. *Journal of Consulting and Clinical Psychology*, 45, 667–673.

Kipnis, D., & Schmidt, S. (1984). Patterns of managerial influence: Shotgun managers, tacticians, and bystanders. *Organizational Dynamics*, 12, 58–67.

Kissen, D. M., & Eysenck, H. J. (1962). Personality in male lung cancer patients. *Journal of Psychosomatic Research*, 6, 123–127.

Kissen, D. M., Brown, R. I. (1969). A further report on personality and psychosocial factors in lung cancer, *Annals of the New York Academy of Sciences*, 164, 535–544.

Kissen, D. M. (1963). Personality characteristics in males conducive to lung cancer. *British Journal of Medical Psychology, 36,* 27–36.

Kissen, D. M. (1967). Psychosocial factors, personality and lung cancer in men aged 55–64. *British Journal of Medical Psychology, 40,* 29–43.

Kissen, D. M. (1968). Some methodological problems in clinical psychosomatic research with special reference to chest disease. *Psychosomatic Medicine, 30,* 324–325.

Kissen, D. M. (1964). Relationship between lung cancer, cigarette smoking, inhalation, and personality. *British Journal of Medical Psychology, 37,* 203–216.

Kleinmuntz, B. (1987). The predictive power of the polygraph: The lies lie detectors tell. *Journal of the American Medical Association, 257* (2), 189–190.

Klopfer, B. (1957). Psychological variables in human cancer, *Journal of Projective Techniques, 31,* 331–340.

Knightley, P., Evans, H., Potter, E., & Wallace, M. (1979). *Suffer the children: The story of Thalidomide.* New York: Viking Press.

Knowles, John (Ed.), (1977). *Doing better and feeling worse: Health in the United States.* New York: W. W. Norton.

Kobasa, S., & Puccetti, M. (1983). Personality and social resources in stress resistance. *Journal of Personality and Social Psychology, 45* (4), 839–850.

Kobasa, S. (1979). Stressful life events, personality and health: An inquiry into hardiness. *Journal of Personality and Social Psychology, 37,* 1–11.

Kobasa, S. (1982a). Commitment and coping in stress resistance among lawyers. *Journal of Personality and Social Psychology, 42,* 707–717.

Kobasa, S. (1982b). The hardy personality: Towards a social psychology of stress and health. In J. Suls & G. Sanders (Eds.), *Social psychology of health and illness.* Hillsdale, NJ: Erlbaum.

Kobasa, S. (1984a). Barriers to work stress: II. The "hardy" personality. In W. D. Gentry, H. Benson, & C. J. de Wolff (Eds.), *Behavioral medicine, work, stress and health.* The Hague: Martinus Nihoff.

Kobasa, S. (1984b). How much stress can you survive? *American Health Magazine,* September, 64–77.

Kobasa, Suzanne (1979). Stressful life events, personality and health: An inquiry into hardiness. *Journal of Personality and Social Psychology, 37,* 1–11.

Kobasa, S., Maddi, S., Kahn, S. (1982). Hardiness and health: A prospective study. *Journal of Personality and Social Psychology, 42,* 168–177.

Koestler, A. (1964). *The act of creation.* New York: Macmillan.

Kohen, D. P., Olness, K. N., Colwell, S. O., and Heimel, A. (1984). The use of relaxation-mental imagery (self-hypnosis) in the management of 505 pediatric behavioral encounters. *Developmental and Behavioral Pediatrics, 5,* 21–25.

Kohlberg, L. (1969). Stage and sequence: The cognitive developmental approach to socialization. In D. A. Goslin (Ed.), *Handbook of socialization theory and research.* Chicago: Rand McNally.

Kohlberg, L. (1981). *The philosophy of moral development: Moral stages and the idea of justice.* New York: Harper & Row.

Kohn, M., & Schooler, C. (1983). *Work and personality.* Norwood, NJ: Ablex.

Kohn, M. (1959). Social class and parental values. *American Journal of Sociology, 64,* 337–351.

Koocher, G. P., and O'Malley, J. E. (1981). *The Damocles Syndrome: Psychosocial consequences of surviving childhood cancer.* New York: McGraw-Hill.

Korein, J., Brudny, J., Grynbaum, B., Sachs-Frankl, G., Weisinger, M., & Levidow, L. (1976). Sensory feedback therapy of spasmodic toricollis and dystonia: Results in treatment of 55 patients. In R. Eldrige & S. Fahn (Eds.), *Advances in Neurology (Vol. 40).* New York: Raven Press.

Krauth, B., & Clem, C. (1987). *Direct supervision jails: Interviews with administrators.* Boulder CO: National Institute of Corrections Information Center.

Krueger, R. B., Levy, E. M., Cathcart, E. S., Fox, B. H., & Black, P. H. (1984). Lymphocyte subsets in patients with major depression: Preliminary findings. *Advances, 1* (1), 5–9.

Kuczynski, L. (1983). Reasoning, prohibitions, and motivations for compliance. *Developmental Psychology, 19,* 126–134.

Labbe, E., & Williamson, D. (1983). Temperature biofeedback in the treatment of children with migraine headaches. *Journal of Pediatric Psychology, 8,* 317–326.

Lacey, J., & Lacey, B. (1962). The law of initial value in the longitudinal study of autonomic constitution: Reproducibility of autonomic responses and response patterns over a four-year interval. *Annals of the New York Academy of Science, 98,* 1257.

Lalonde, M. (1974). *A new perspective on the health of Canadians.* Montreal: Government of Canada.

Lambert, N., Sandoval, J., & Sassone, D. (1979). Prevalence of treatment regimens for children considered to be hyperactive. *American Journal of Orthopsychiatry, 49,* 482–490.

Landy, F. (1986). Stamp collecting versus science: Validation as hypothesis testing. *American Psychologist, 41,* 1183–1192.

Lang, P. (1977). Research on the specificity of feedback training: Implications for the use of biofeedback in the treatment of anxiety and fear. In J. Beatty and H. Legewie (Eds.), *Biofeedback & behavior,* (pp. 323–330). New York: Plenum Press.

Lang, P. J. (1979). A bio-informational theory of emotional imagery. *Psychophysiology, 16,* 495–512.

Lanyon, R. (1986). Theory and treatment in child molestation. *Journal of Clinical and Consulting Psychology, 45,* 176–182.

Lappe, F. M., and Collins, J. (1977). *Food first: Beyond the myth of scarcity.* New York: Ballantine Books.

Larsson, B., & Melin, L. (1986). Chronic headaches in adolescents: Treatment in a school setting with relaxation training as compared with information-contact and self-registration. *Pain, 25,* 325–336.

Lazar, I., & Darlington, R. (1982). Lasting effects of early education: A report from the consortium for longitudinal studies. *Monographs of the Society for Research in Child Development, 47* (Whole No. 195).

Lazarus, R., & Folkman, S. (1984). *Stress, appraisal, and coping.* New York: Springer.

Lazarus, R. (1981, July). Little hassles can be hazardous to health. *Psychology Today,* 58–62.

Lazarus, R. S., and Folkman S. (1984a). *Stress, appraisal, and coping.* New York: Springer.

Lazarus, R. S., and Folkman, S. (1984b). Coping and adaptation. In W. Doyle Gentry, (Ed.), *Handbook of behavioral medicine.* New York: Guilford Press.

Lazarus, R., & DeLongis, A. (1981). Psychological stress and coping in aging. *American Psychologist, 38,* 245–254.

Leach, B., & Norris, J. (1977). Factors in the development of Alcoholics Anonymous (A.A.). In B. Kissin & H. Begleiter (Eds.), *The biology of alcoholism* (Vol. 5, *Treatment and rehabilitation of the chronic alcoholic).* New York: Plenum Press.

Lehman, D., Ellard, J., Wortman, B. (1986). Social support for the bereaved: Recipients' and providers' perspectives on what is helpful. *Journal of Consulting and Clinical Psychology, 54,* 438–446.

Lepper, M. (1983). Social control processes, attributions of motivation, and the internalization of social values. In E. Higgins, D. Ruble, & W. Hartup (Eds.), *Social Cognition and Social Behavior.* New York: Cambridge University Press.

LeShan, E., (1975). Can your emotions help you resist cancer? cited in *Women's Day.* Greenwich, CT: Fawcett Publications.

LeShan, L. (1959). Psychological states as factors in the development of malignant disease: A critical review. *Journal of the National Cancer Institute, 22,* 1–18.

LeShan, L. (1966). An emotional life history pattern associated with neoplastic disease. *Annals of the New York Academy of Sciences, 125,* 780–793.

LeShan, L. (1977). *You can fight for your life.* New York: Harcourt Brace Jovanovich.

Leuner, H. (1978). Basic principles and therapeutic efficacy of guided affective imagery. In J. Singer (Ed.), *The power of human imagination.* New York: Plenum Press.

Levenkron, J., & Moore, G. (1988). The Type A behavior pattern: Issues for intervention research. *Annals of Behavior Medicine, 10,* 78–83.

Leventhal, H., & Watts, J. (1966). Sources of resistance to fear-arousing communications on smoke and lung cancer. *Journal of Personality, 34,* 313–321.

Leventhal, H. (1968). Experimental studies of anti-smoking communications. In L. Berkowitz (Ed.), *Recent advances in social psychology, Vol. 5,* (pp. 95–121). New York: Academic Press.

Leventhal, H. (1970). Findings and theory in the study of fear communications. In L. Berkowitz (Ed.), *Recent advances in social psychology, Vol. 5,* (pp. 119–186). New York: Academic Press.

Leventhal, H., & Everhart, D. (1979). Emotion, pain, and physical illness. In C. Izard (Ed.), *Emotions and psychopathology.* New York: Plenum Press.

Leventhal, H., Meyer, D., Nerenz, D. (1980). The common sense representation of illness danger. In S. Rachman (Ed.), *Medical psychology, 2.* New York: Pergamon Press.

Leventhal, H., Meyer, D., & Gutmann, M. (1980). The role of theory in the study of compliance to high blood pressure regimens. In R. Haynes, M. Mattson, & T. Engebretson, Jr., (Eds.), Patient compliance to prescribed antihypertensive medication regimens: A report to the National Heart, Lung, and Blood Institute. Bethedsa, MD: NIH publication No. 81-2102.

Leventhal, H., Singer, R., & Jones, S. (1965). Effects of fear and specificity of recommendations upon attitudes and behavior. *Journal of Personality and Social Psychology, 2,* 20–29.

Leventhal, H., Zimmerman, R., & Gutmann, M. (1984). Compliance: A self-regulation perspective. In W. Gentry (Ed.), *Handbook of behavioral medicine.* New York: Guilford Press.

Levine, Adeline (1982). *Love Canal: Science, politics, and people.* Lexington, MA: Lexington Books.

Levine, D., Green, J., Deeds, S., Chalox, J., Rusell, R., & Finlay, S. (1979). Health education for hypertensive patients. *Journal of the American Medical Association, 241,* 1700–1703.

Levine, S. (1987). Stress, pressure, and peak performance, *Ms.* magazine, 37.

Levy, S. M., and Wise, B. (1988). Psychosocial risk factors and cancer progression. In C. Cooper (Ed.), *Stress and breast cancer.* New York: Wiley.

Levy, S. M., Herberman, R. B., Maluish, A. M., Schlien, B., & Lippman, M. (1985). Prognostic risk assessment in primary breast cancer by behavioral and immunological parameters. *Health Psychology, 4* (2), 99–113.

Libo, L., & Arnold, G. (1983a). Relaxation practice after biofeedback therapy: A long-term follow-up study of utilization and effectiveness. *Biofeedback & Self-Regulation, 8,* 217–227.

Libo, L., & Arnold, G. (1983b). Does training to criterion influence improvement? A follow-up study of EMG and thermal biofeedback. *Journal of Behavioural Medicine, 6,* 397–404.

Lipton, D., & Martinson, R. (1975). *The effectiveness of correctional treatment: A summary of evaluation studies.* New York: Holt, Rinehart and Winston.

Locke, S. (1986). *The healer within.* New York: Dutton.

London, P., & Engstrom, D. (1982). Mind over pain. *American Health, 1,* 62–67.

London, P. (1970). The rescuers. In J. Macaulay & L. Berkowitz (Eds.), *Altruism and helping behavior.* New York: Academic Press.

Longabaugh, R., McCrady, B., Fink, E., Stout, R., McAuley, T., Doyle, C., & McNeill, D. (1983). Cost-effectiveness of alcoholism treatment in partial vs. inpatient settings: Six month outcomes. *Journal of Studies on Alcohol, 44,* 1049–1071.

Lopez, F., & Thurman, C. (1986). A cognitive-behavioral investigation of anger among college students. *Cognitive Therapy & Research, 10,* 245–256.

Lovin, R. (1988). The school and the articulation of values. *American Journal of Education, 96,* 143–161.

Lubar, J., & Bahler, W. (1976). Behavioral management of epileptic seizures following EEG biofeedback training of the sensorimotor rhythm. *Biofeedback & Self-Regulation, 1,* 77–104.

Lucas, G. (Dir.). *Star Wars* (film). Hollywood, CA: Twentieth-Century Fox Film Corporation.

Lupin, M., Braud, L., Braud, W., & Duer, W. (1976). Children, parents, and relaxation tapes. *Academic Therapy, 12,* 105–113.

Lyles, J., Burish, T., Krozely, M., & Oldham, R. (1982). Efficacy of relaxation training and guided imagery in reducing the adversiveness of cancer chemotherapy. *Journal of Consulting and Clinical Psychology, 40,* 509–529.

Lynch, J. J. (1985). *The language of the heart.* New York: Basic Books.

MacDougall, J. M., Dembroski, T. M., Dimsdale, J. E., & Hackett, T. (1985). Components of Type A, hostility, and anger-in: Further relationships to angiographic findings. *Health Psychology, 4,* 137–152.

MacKay, Judith (1989). Battlefield for the tobacco war. *Journal of the American Medical Association, 261,* 28–29.

MacLeod, J. (1983). Biofeedback in the management of partial anal incontinence. *Diseases of the Colon and Rectum, 26,* 244–246.

Macklin, E., & Rubin, R. (1983). *Contemporary families and alternate lifestyles.* Beverly Hills, CA: Sage.

Macy, J. (1985). *Dharma and development: Religion as resource in the Sarvodaya self-help movement.* West Hartford, CT: Kumarian Press.

Maddi, S., & Kobasa, S. (1984). *The hardy executive.* Homewood, IL: Dow Jones-Irwin.

Maddi, S., Kobasa, S., & Hoover, M. (1979). An alienation test. *Journal of Humanistic Psychology, 19,* 73–76.

Magos, A. L., et al., (1986). Treatment of premenstrual syndrome by subcutaneous oestradiol implants and cyclical oral norethisterone: Placebo controlled study. *British Medical Journal, 292,* 1629–1633.

Mahler, H. (1981). "World Health Day 1981" *WHO Chronicle, 35,* 79–85.

Mahoney, M. (1974). *Cognitive and behavior modification.* Cambridge, MA: Ballinger.

Mahoney, M. (1977). Personal science: A cognitive learning therapy. In A. Ellis & A. Grieger (Eds.), *Handbook of rational emotive therapy.* New York: Springer.

Mahoney, M., & Avener, M. (1977). Psychology of the elite athlete: An exploratory study. *Cognitive Therapy & Research, 1,* 135–141.

Mahoney, M. J. (1988). The cognitive sciences and psychotherapy: Patterns in a developing relationship. In *Handbook of cognitive-behavioral therapies,* K. S. Dobson, (Ed.), New York: Guilford Press.

Mann, J., & Chin, J. (1988). AIDS: A global perspective. *New England Journal of Medicine, 319,* 302–303.

Marks, I. (1975). Behavioral treatments of phobic and obsessive-compulsive disorders: A critical appraisal. In R. Hersen, R. M. Eisler, & P. M. Miller (Eds.), *Progress in behavior modification. Vol. 1.* New York: Academic Press.

Marlatt, G., & Gordon, J. (1980). Determinants of relapse: Implications for the maintenance of behavior change. In P. O. Davidson & S. M. Davidson (Eds.), *Behavioral medicine: Changing health life-styles,* (pp. 410–452). Elmsford, NY: Pergamon.

Marlatt, G., & Gordon, J. (Eds.), (1985). *Relapse prevention: Maintenance strategies in addictive behavior change.* New York: Guilford Press.

Marlatt, G. A. (1983). The controlled-drinking controversy: A commentary. *American Psychologist, 38,* 1097–1110.

Martelli, M., Auerback, S., & Alexander, J. (1987). Stress management in the health care setting: Matched interventions with patient coping styles. *Journal of Consulting and Clinical Psychology, 55,* 201–207.

Martin, R., & Lefcourt, H. (1983). Sense of humor as a moderator of the relation between stressors and moods. *Journal of Personality and Social Psychology, 45,* 1313–1324.

Marx, M., Garrity, T., & Bowers, F. (1975). The influence of recent life experience on the health of college freshmen. *Journal of Psychosomatic Research, 19,* 87–98.

Maslach, C. (1982). *Burnout: The cost of caring.* Englewood Cliffs, NJ: Prentice-Hall.

Maslow, A. (1968). *Toward a psychology of being.* New York: Van Nostrand Reinhold.

Maslow, A. (1970). *Motivation and personality.* New York: Harper & Row.

Masters, J., Burish, T., Hollon, S., & Rimm, D. (1987). *Behavior therapy.* New York: Harcourt Brace Jovanovich.

Matarazzo, J. D. (1980). Behavioral health and behavioral medicine: Frontiers for a new health psychology. *American Psychologist, 35,* 807–817.

Matarazzo, J. D. (1984). Behavioral health: A 1990 challenge for the health sciences professions. In J. D. Matarazzo, S. Weiss, J. Herd, N. Miller, & S. M. Weiss (Eds.), *Behavioral health: A Handbook of health enhancement and disease prevention.* New York: Wiley.

Mather, L., & Mackie, J. (1983). The incidence of postoperative pain in children. *Pain, 15,* 271–282.

Matheson, D., Bruce, R., & Beauchamp, K. (1974). *Introduction to experimental psychology.* New York: Holt, Rinehart & Winston.

Matthews, D. B. (1984). A study of psychosocial effects of relaxation training on rural preadolescents. (Research Bulletin No. 34). Orangeburg, SC: South Carolina State College. (ERIC Document Reproduction Service No. ED 252 801).

Matthews, K. (1982). Psychological perspectives on the Type A behavior pattern. *Psychological Bulletin, 92,* 293–323.

Matthews, K., Glass, D., Rosenman, R., & Bortner, R. (D1977). Competitive drive, Pattern A, and coronary heart disease: A further analysis of some data from the Western Collaborative Group Study. *Journal of Chronic Diseases, 30,* 489–498.

Matthews, K., & Krantz, D. (1976). Resemblances of twins and their parents in pattern A behavior. *Psychosomatic Medicine, 28,* 140–144.

Matthews, K., & Woodall, K. (1988). Childhood origins of overt Type A behaviors and cardiovascular reactivity to behavioral stressors. *Annals of Behavioral Medicine, 10,* 71–77.

Matthews, K., Rosenman, R., Dembroski, T., McDougall, J., & Harris, E. (1984). Familial resemblance in components of the Type A behavior pattern: A reanalysis of the California Type A twin study. *Psychosomatic Medicine, 46,* 512–522.

Mayron, J., Mayron, E., Ott, J., & Nations, R. (1976). Light, radiation, and academic achievement: Second year data. *Academic Therapy, 11,* 397–407.

McCartney, K. (1985). Day care. Paper presented at the annual meeting of the American Association for the Advancement of Science, Los Angeles.

McClelland, D. C. (1979). Inhibited power motivation and high blood pressure in men. *Journal of Abnormal Psychology, 88,* 182–190.

McClelland, D. C. (1985). *Human motivation.* Glenview, IL: Scott, Foresman.

McClelland, D. C. (1989). Motivational factors in health and disease. *American Psychologist, 44,* 675–683.

McClelland, D. C., & Kirshnit, D. (1982). Effects of motivational arousal on immune functions. Unpublished manuscript, Harvard University, Department of Psychology and Social Relations, discussed in D. C. McClelland (1985), *Human motivation.* Glenview, IL: Scott, Foresman.

McClelland, D., Constantin, C., Regalado, D., & Stone, C. (1982). Effects of child-rearing practices on adult maturity. In D. C. McClelland (Ed.), *The development of social maturity,* (pp. 209–248). New York: Academic Press.

McCrady, B., Dean, L., Dubreuil, D., & Swanson, S. (1985). The problem drinkers' project: A programmatic application of social-learning-based treatment. In G. Marlatt & J. Gordon (Eds.), *Relapse prevention: Maintenance strategies in addictive behavior change.* New York: Guilford Press.

McFall, R., & Hammen, L. (1971). Motivation, structure, and self-monitoring: Role of nonspecific factors in smoking reduction. *Journal of Consulting and Clinical Psychology, 37,* 80–86.

McFall, R., & Lillesand, D. (1971). Behavioral rehearsal with modeling and coaching in assertion training. *Journal of Abnormal Psychology, 77,* 313–323.

McFarland, A. (1984). *Common Cause.* Chatham, NJ: Chatham House Publishers.

McGoldrick, M., & Pearce, J. (1981). Family therapy with Irish Americans. *Family Process, 20,* 223–241.

McGrady, A., Woerner, M., Bernal, G., & Higgins, J. (1987). Effect of biofeedback-assisted relaxation on blood pressure and cortisol levels in normotensives and hypertensives. *Journal of Behavioral Medicine, 10,* 301–310.

McKay, M., Davis, M., & Fanning, P. (1981). *Thoughts & feelings.* Richmond, CA: New Harbinger Publications.

Mechanic, D. (1983). *Handbook of health, health care and the health professions.* New York: Free Press.

Medalie, J. H., & Goldbourt, U. (1976). Angina pectoris among 10,000 men, II: Psychosocial and other risk factors. *American Journal of Medicine, 60,* 910–921.

Medical World News (1973, March 9). "Biofeedback in Action," 47–60.

Meer, J. (1985, July). Loneliness. *Psychology Today,* 28–33.

Meichenbaum, D. (1977). *Cognitive-behavior modification: An integrative approach.* New York: Plenum Press.

Meichenbaum, D. (1985). *Stress inoculation training.* New York: Pergamon Press.

Melamed, B., & Bush, J. (1985). Family factors in children with acute illness. In D. Turk, & R. Kerns (Eds.), *Health, illness, and families: A life-span perspective,* (pp. 183–219). New York: Wiley.

Menninger, Karl (1963). *The vital balance.* New York: Viking Press.

Middaugh, S., Kee, W., & Barchiesi, F. (1987). Biofeedback and chronic pain rehabilitation treatment outcome in geriatric patients. *Biofeedback and Self-Regulation, 12,* 156–157.

Midgley, J. (1987). *The new women's budget.* Philadelphia: Women's International League for Peace and Freedom.

Miller, L., & Bizzel, R. (1984). Long-term effects of four preschool programs: Ninth- and tenth-grade results. *Child Development, 55,* 1570–1587.

Miller, A. (1981). *Prisoners of childhood.* New York: New American Library.

Miller, A. (1984). *Thou shalt not be aware: Society's betrayal of the child.* New York: New American Library.

Miller, A. (1984). *For your own good: Hidden cruelty in child-rearing and the roots of violence.* New York: New American Library.

Miller, F., & Jones, H. (1948). The possibility of precipitating the leukemia state by emotional factors, *Blood, 8,* 880–885.

Miller, N. (1975/76). Clinical applications of biofeedback: Voluntary control of heart rate, rhythm, and blood pressure. In T. Barber (Ed.),

Biofeedback and Self-Control, (pp. 367–377). Chicago: Aldine Publishing.

Miller, N. E. (1971). Learning of visceral and glandular responses. In J. Kamiya, T.X. Barber, L. DiCara, N. Miller, D. Shapiro, J Stoyva (Eds.), *Biofeedback and self-control,* Chicago: Aldine-Atherton.

Miller, O. B. (Ed.), (1925). Shingebiss: A Chippewa Indian tale. In *My bookhouse: In the nursery.* Chicago, IL: The Bookhouse for Children.

Milner, M. (1983). Technology to aid and abet biofeedback approaches. In P. Firestone & P. Mc-Grath (Eds.), *Advances in behavioral medicine for children and adolescents,* (pp. 131–160). London: Erlbaum Associates.

Mindell, E. (1987). *Unsafe at any meal.* New York: Warner Books.

Minuchin, S., & Fishman, H. (1979). The psychosomatic family in child psychiatry. *Annals of the American Academy of Child Psychiatry, 18,* 76–90.

Mischel, W. (1968). *Personality and assessment.* New York: Wiley.

Mischel, W. (1976). *Introduction to personality.* New York: Holt, Rinehart & Winston.

Mischel, W., Shoda, Y., & Peake, P. (1988). The nature of adolescent competencies predicted by preschool delay of gratification. *Journal of Personality and Social Psychology, 54,* 686–696.

Mischel, W., & Leibert, R. M. (1966). Effects of discrepancies between observed and imposed reward criteria on their acquisition and transmission. *Journal of Personality and Social Psychology, 3,* 45–53.

Mischel, W. (1961). Preference for delayed reinforcement and social responsibility. *Journal of Abnormal and Social Psychology, 62,* 1–7.

Mischel, W. (1974). Processes in delay of gratification, In L. Berkowitz (Ed.), *Advances in experimental social psychology, Vol. 7.* New York: Academic Press.

Mischel, W. (1984). Convergences and challenges in the search for consistency. *American Psychologist, 39,* 355.

Mischel, W. (1976). *Introduction to personality.* New York: Holt, Rinehart and Winston.

Mohnen, V. (1988). The challenge of acid rain. *Scientific American, 259,* 30–38.

Mokhiber, R. (1988). *Corporate crime and violence.* San Francisco: Sierra Books.

Monahan, J., & Novaco, R. (1978). Corporate violence: A psychological analysis. In P. Lipsitt & B. Sales (Eds.), *New directions in psychological research,* New York: Van Nostrand Reinhold.

Morales, B. (1981, June). Eyesight: A barometer of health. *Let's Live,* 63–67.

Moreno, J. (1947). *The theatre of spontaneity,* New York: Beacon House.

Morris, D., Nathan, R., Goebel, R., and Blass, N. H. (1985). Hypoanesthesia in the morbidly obese. *Journal of the American Medical Association, 253,* 3292–3295.

Morrow, Gary (1986). Effect of the cognitive hierarchy in the systematic desensitization treatment of anticipatory nausea in cancer patients: A component comparison with relaxation only, counseling, and no treatment. *Cognitive Therapy and Research, 10,* 421–446.

Moskovitz, S. (1983). *Love despite hate: Child survivors of the holocaust and their adult lives.* New York: Schocken Books.

Mostofsky, D. I., & Balaschak, B. A. (1977). Psychobiological control of seizures. *Psychological Bulletin,* Vol. 84, 723–750.

MRFIT Study Group (1979), The MRFIT behavior pattern study I: Study design, procedures, and reproducibility of behavior pattern judgments. *Journal of Chronic Disease, 32,* 293–305.

MRFIT Study Group (1982). Multiple Risk Factor Intervention Trial: Risk factor changes and mortality results. *Journal of the American Medical Association, 248,* 1465–1477.

Murphy, P., Darwin, J., & Murphy, D. (1977). EEG feedback training for cerebral dysfunction: A research program with learning disabled adolescents. *Biofeedback & Self-Regulation, 2,* 288.

Murphy, T., Pagano, R., & Marlatt, G. (1986). Lifestyle modification with heavy alcohol drinkers: Effects of aerobic exercise and meditation. *Addictive Behaviors, 11,* 1751–186.

Najjar, M., & Rowland, M. (1987). Anthropometric reference data and prevalence of overweight—United States, 1976–1980. DHHS publication No. (PHS) 87–1688. Hyattsville, MD: U.S. Department of Health and Human Services.

Nakagawa-Kogan, H., Betrus, P., Beaton, R., Burr, R., Larson, L., Mitchell, P., & Wolf-Wilets, V. (1984). Management of stress response clinic: Perspective of five years of biofeedback and stress management treatment of stress-related disorders by nurses. *Biofeedback Society of America Proceedings,* Alburquerque, NM.

National Advisory Committee on Handicapped Children (1968). *Special education for handicapped children, first annual report.* Washington, DC: U.S. Department of Health, Education, and Welfare.

National Center for Health Statistics (1986). *Health, United States,* DHHS Pub. No. (PHS) 88–1232. Washington, DC: U.S. Government Printing Office.

National Center for Health Statistics (1987). *Health, United States,* DHHS Pub. No. (PHS) 88–1232. Washington, DC: U.S. Government Printing Office.

National Center for Health Statistics (1986). *Vital and Health Statistics,* Series 10, No. 156. Department of Health and Human Services publication (PHS) 86–1584. Washington, DC: U.S. Government Printing Office.

National Institute of Mental Health (1982). *Television and behavior: Ten years of scientific progress and implications for the eighties: I. Summary report.* Washington, DC: U.S. Department of Health and Human Services.

National Institute on Drug Abuse (1987). *National trends in drug use and related factors among American high school students and young adults, 1975–1986.* Washington, DC: U.S. Government Printing Office.

National Institute on Drug Abuse (1988). Data from the drug abuse warning network (DAWN), July–December, 1987. DHHS Publication No. (ADM) 88–1582. Washington, DC: U.S. Government Printing Office.

Neff, D., & Blanchard, E. (1987). A multi-component treatment for irritable bowel syndrome. *Behavior Therapy, 18,* 70–83.

Negin, E. (1985, December). Eli Lilly guilty in Oraflex case. *Public Opinion,* pp. 6–7.

Negin, E. (1985, October). The big chew. *Public Opinion,* p. 4.

Nelson, R. W., O'Toole, M., Krauth, B., & Whitmore, C. (1984). *Direct supervision models.* Boulder, CO: National Institute of Corrections Center.

Neugebauer, R. (1984). The reliability of life-event reports. In B. S. Dohrenwend & B. P. Dohrenwend (Eds.), *Stressful life events and their contexts,* 108–130, New Brunswick, NJ: Rutgers University Press.

New Realities. (1987, November/December). Attitudinal healing centers, Volume 8, pp. 54–55.

Newman, R., Seres, J., Yospe, L., & Garlington, B. (1978). Multidisciplinary treatment of chronic pain: Long-term follow-up of low-back pain patients. *Pain, 4,* 283–292.

Nichols, P., & Chen, T. (1981). *Minimal brain dysfunction: A prospective study.* Hillsdale, NJ: Erlbaum.

Nielsen, D., & Holmes, D. (1980). Effectiveness of EMG biofeedback training for controlling arousal in subsequent stressful situations. *Biofeedback & Self-Regulation, 5,* 235–245.

Nielsen Television Index (1982). *National Audience Demographic Report.* Northbrook, Ill: A.C. Nielsen.

Niles, W. (1986). Effects of a moral development discussion group on delinquent and predelinquent boys. *Journal of Counseling Psychology, 33,* 45–51.

Noel, J., Forsyth, D., & Kelley, K. (1987). Improving the performance of failing students by overcoming their self-serving attributional biases. *Basic & Applied Social Psychology, 8.* 151–162.

Nomellini, S., & Katz, R. (1983). Effects of anger control training on abusive parents. *Cognitive Therapy and Research, 7,* 57–68.

Norris, P. A., and Porter, G. (1987). *I choose life.* Walpole, NH: Stillpoint Publishing.

Novaco, R. (1975). *Anger control: The development and evaluation of an experimental treatment.* Lexington, MA: D. C. Heath.

Novaco, R. W. (1977). A stress inoculation approach to anger management in the training of law enforcement offices. *American Journal of Community Psychology, 5,* 327–346.

Novaco, R. W. (1980). Training of probation counselors for anger problems. *Journal of Counseling Psychology, 27,* 385–390.

Novak, V. (1988, May/June). Under the influence. *Common Cause Magazine,* 19–23.

Nowell, C., & Janis, I. (1982). Effective and ineffective partnerships in a weight-reduction clinic. In I. Janis (Ed.), *Counseling on personal decisions: Theory and research on short-term helping relationships.* New Haven, CT: Yale University Press.

Nuckolls, K., Cassel, J., & Kaplan, B. (1972). Psychosocial assets, life crises and the prognosis of pregnancy. *American Journal of Epidemiology, 95,* 431–441.

O'Connell, K. A. (1988). Nursing perspectives on behavioral medicine training: A rose by some other name would be better. *Annals of Behavioral Medicine, 10,* 1988, 11–14.

O'Leary, A. (1985). Self-efficacy and health. *Behaviour Research and Therapy, 233,* 437–451.

Office of Technology Assessment (1986). *Serious reduction of hazardous waste.* OTA–ITE–317. Washington, DC: U.S. Government Printing Office.

Olds, D., Henderson, C., Chamberlin, R., & Tatelbaum, R. (1986a). Improving the delivery of prenatal care and outcomes of pregnancy: A randomized trial of nurse home visitation. *Pediatrics, 77,* 16–28.

Olds, D., Henderson, C., Chamberlin, R., & Tatelbaum, R. (1986b). Preventing child abuse and neglect: A randomized trial of nurse home visitation. *Pediatrics, 78,* 65–78.

Olness, K. (1986). Hypnotherapy in children: New approach to solving common pediatric problems. *Postgraduate Medicine, 79,* 95–105.

Olness, K. (1977). Hypnosis in-service education in a children's hospital. *American Journal of Clinical Hypnosis, 20,* 80–83.

Olness, K., MacDonald, J., & Uden, D. (1987). Comparison of self-hypnosis and propranolol in the treatment of juvenile classic migraine. *Pediatrics, 79,* 593–597.

Omizo, M. (1980a). The effects of biofeedback-induced relaxation training in hyperactive adolescent boys. *Journal of Psychology, 105,* 131–138.

Omizo, M. (1980b). The effects of relaxation and relaxation training on dimension of self concept (DOSC) among hyperactive male children. *Educational Research Quarterly, 5,* 22–30.

Orlandi, M. (1986). The diffusion and adoption of worksite health promotion innovations: An analysis of barriers, *Preventive Medicine, 15,* 522–536.

Orme-Johnson, D. W., and Farrow, J. T. (Eds.), (1977). *Scientific research on the transcendental meditation program, Volume I.* New York: Maharishi European Research University Press.

Osler, William (1921). *The evolution of modern medicine.* New Haven, CT: Yale University Press.

Outward Bound, (1988). Outward Bound and troubled youth: The treatment outcome literature. Greenwich, CT: Outward Bound Press.

Overeaters Anonymous (1981). *To the man who wants to stop compulsive overeating, welcome.* Torrance, CA: Overeaters Anonymous Inc.

Owan, T., Palmer, I., & Quintana, M. (1987). *School/community-based alcoholism/substance abuse prevention survey.* Washington, DC: Indian Health Service.

Ownby, R. (1983). The neuropsychology of attention deficit disorders in children. *Journal of Psychiatric Treatment and Evaluation, 5,* 229–236.

Oxendine, J. (1980). Emotional arousal and motor performance. In R. Suinn (Ed.), *Psychology in sports,* 103–111. Minneapolis: Burgess Publishing.

Palmblad, J., Cantell, K., Strander, H., Froberg, J., Karlsson, C. G., Levi, L., Gronstrom, M., and Unger, P. (1976). *Journal of Psychosomatic Research, 20,* 193–199.

Parcel, Guy (1985). Comments from the field. *Journal of School Health, 55,* 345–347.

Parke, R., & Slaby, R. (1983). The development of aggression. In E. Hetherington (Ed.), *Handbook of child psychology.* New York: Wiley.

Parry, Glenys. (1986). Paid employment, life events, social support, and mental health in working-class mothers. *Journal of Health and Social Behavior, 27,* 193–208.

Patel, C., & North, W. (1975). Randomized controlled trial of yoga and biofeedback in management of hypertension. *Lancet, 2,* 93–95.

Patel, C. (1973). Yoga and biofeedback in the management of hypertension. *Lancet, 2,* 1053–1055.

Patel, C. (1975a). Yoga and biofeedback in the management of "stress" in hypertensive patients. *Clinical Science and Molecular Medicine, 48,* 171–174.

Patel, C. (1975b). 12-month follow-up of yoga and biofeedback in the management of hypertension, *Lancet, 1,* 62–64.

Patel, C. (1984). A holistic approach to cardiovascular diseases. *The British Journal of Holistic Medicine, 1,* 30–41.

Patel, C., Marmot, M., Terry, D., Carruthers, M., Hunt, B., & Patel, M. (1985). Trial of relaxation in reducing coronary risk: Four year follow up. *British Medical Journal, 13,* 1103–1106.

Paternite, C., & Loney, J. (1980). Childhood hyperkinesis: Relationship between symptomatology and home environment. In C. Whalen & B. Henker (Eds.), *Hyperactive children: The social ecology of identification and treatment,* (pp. 105–141). New York: Academic Press.

Patterson, G., & Stouthamer-Loeber, M. (1984). The correlation of family management practices and delinquency. *Child Development, 55,* 1299–1307.

Peavey, B., Lawlis, F., and Goven, A. (1985) Biofeedback-assisted relaxation: Effects on phagocytic capacity. *Biofeedback & Self-Regulation, 10,* 33–47.

Peele, A. (1985). *The meaning of addiction: Compulsive experience and its interpretation.* Lexington, MA: Lexington Books.

Pelletier, K. (1977). *Mind as healer, mind as slayer.* New York: Delta.

Penfield, W. (1950). The cerebral cortex and the mind of man. In P. Laslett (Ed.), The physical basis of mind. Oxford, England: Blackwell.

Penfield, W. (1975). *The mystery of the mind.* Trenton, NJ: Princeton University Press.

Peper, E., & Grossman, E. (1979). Thermal biofeedback training in children with headache. In E. Peper, S. Ancoli, & M. Quinn (Eds.), *Mind/body integration.* New York: Plenum Press.

Peper, E., Smith, K., & Waddell, D. (1987). Voluntary wheezing versus diaphragmatic breathing with inhalation (Voldyne) feedback: A clinical intervention in the treatment of asthma. *Clinical Biofeedback and Health, 10,* 83–89.

Peplau, L., & Goldston, S. (1984). Preventing the harmful consequences of severe and persistent loneliness. DHHS Publication No. (ADM) 84–1312. Washington, DC: U.S. Government Printing Office.

Perls, F. (1969). *Gestalt therapy verbatim.* Moab, UT: Real People Press.

Perry, C., Klepp, K., & Shultz, J. (1988). Primary prevention of cardiovascular disease: Communitywide strategies for youth, *Journal of Consulting and Clinical Psychology, 56,* 358–364.

Perry, C., & Jessor, R. (1985). The concept of health promotion and the prevention of adolescent drug abuse. *Health Education Quarterly, 12,* 169–184.

Perry, C., Klepp, K., & Sillers, C. (1989). Communitywide strategies for cardiovascular health: The Minnesota heart health program youth program. *Health Education Research, 4,* 87–101.

Perry, C., Luepker, R., Murray, D., Kurth, C., Mullis, R., Crockett, S., & Jacobs, D. (1988b). Parent involvement with children's health promotion: The Minnesota Home Team. *American Journal of Public Health, 78,* 1156–1160.

Perry, D., Maccoby, N., & McAlister, A. (1980). Adolescent smoking prevention: A third-year follow-up. *World Smoking and Health, 1,* 40–45.

Perry, S., & Heidrich, G. (1982). Management of pain during débridement: A survey of U.S. burn units. *Pain, 13,* 267–280.

Persky, V. W., Kempthorne-Rawson, J., & Shekelle, G. (1987). Personality and risk of cancer: 20-Year follow-up of the Western Electric study. *Psychosomatic Medicine, 49,* 435–449.

Peterson, C., & Seligman, M. (1984). Causal explanations as a risk factor for depression: Theory and evidence. *Psychological Review, 91,* 347–374.

Peterson, C., & Seligman, M. (1987). Explanatory style and illness. *Journal of Personality, 55,* 237–265.

Peterson, L., & Ridley-Johnson, R. (1980). Pediatric hospital response to a survey on prehospitalization preparation for children. *Journal of Pediatric Psychology, 5,* 1–7.

Petosa, R., & Oldfield, D. (1985). A pilot study of the impact of stress management techniques on the classroom behavior of elementary school students. *Journal of School Health, 55,* 69–71.

Petty, R. E., Ostrom, T. M., & Brock (Eds.), (1981). *Cognitive responses in persuasion.* Hillsdale, NJ: Erlbaum.

Phares, E. (1976). *Locus of control in personality.* Morristown, NJ: General Learning Press.

Phillips, D., & Feldman, K. (1973). A dip in deaths before ceremonial occasions: Some new relationships between social integration and mortality. *American Sociological Review, 38,* 678–696.

Pickering, T., James, G., Boddie, C., Harshfield, G., Blank, S., & Laragh, J. (1988). How common is white coat hypertension? *Journal of the American Medical Association, 259,* 225–228.

Pierce, J., Fiore, M., Novotny, T., Hatziandreu, E., & Davis, R. (1989). Trends in cigarette smoking in the United States. *Journal of the American Medical Association, 261,* 61–65.

Pines, M. (1979). Superkids, *Psychology Today,* January, 53–63.

Pines, M. (1984, March). Psychology Today conversation: Michael Rutter: Resilient children. *Psychology Today, 18,* 60–65.

Pomerleau, O., & Brady, J. (1979). Introduction: The scope and promise of behavioral medicine. *Behavioral medicine: Theory and practice,* xi–xxvi. Baltimore: Williams & Wilkins.

Porter, G., & Norris, P. (1985). *Why me?* Walpole, NH: Stillpoint Publishing.

Powell, L., & Thoresen, C. (1987). Modifying the Type A behavior pattern: A small group treatment approach. In J. Blumenthal & D. Mc-Kee (Eds.), *Applications in behavioral medicine and health psychology: A clinician's source book,* (pp. 171–207). Sarasota, FL: Professional Resource Exchange.

Price, V. (1984). *Type A behavior pattern.* New York: Academic Press.

Pritikin, N. (1979). *The Pritikin program for diet and exercise.* New York: Grosset & Dunlap.

Project Peacock (1982). *Donahue with Kids,* CBS Broadcasting.

Public Citizen, (1988, July/August). Campaign recognizes safe food trailblazers. Washington, DC.

Radil-Weiss, T. (1983). Men in extreme conditions: Some medical and psychological aspects of the Auschwitz Concentration Camp. *Psychiatry, 46,* 259–269.

Radke-Yarrow, M., & Zahn-Waxler, C. (1984). Roots, motives, and patternings in children's prosocial behavior. In E. Staub, D. Bar-Tal, J. Karylowski, & J. Reykowski (Eds.), *Handbook of child psychology: Vol. 4, Socialization, personality, and social development,* (pp. 775–911). New York: Wiley.

Rahe, R., Hervig, L., & Rosenman, R. (1978). Heritability of Type A behavior. *Psychosomatic Medicine, 40,* 478–486.

Random House Dictionary (1979). New York: Random House.

Reagan, R. (1981, February 5). *Report to the Nation on the Economy,* radio broadcast reported in Sandoz & Crabb, Jr., (Eds.), *A Tide of Discontent,* p. 217.

Redd, W., & Andrykowski, M. (1982). Behavioral intervention in cancer treatment: Controlling aversion reactions to chemotherapy. *Journal of Consulting and Clinical Psychology, 50,* 1018–1029.

Redd, W. (1984). Control of nausea and vomiting in chemotherapy patients. *Postgraduate Medicine, 75,* 104–113.

Redfield, R. R., and Burke, D. S. (1988). HIV infection: The clinical picture. *Scientific American, 259,* 90–99.

Reed, H., & Janis, I. (1974). Effects of a new type of psychological treatment on smokers' resistance to warnings about health hazards. *Journal of Consulting and Clinical Psychology, 42,* 748.

Regenstein, L. (1986). *How to survive in America the poisoned.* Washington, DC: Acropolis Books.

Reich, B. (1989). Non-invasive treatment of vascular and muscle contraction headache: A comparative longitudinal clinical study. *Headache, 29,* 34–41.

Reiter, J., Andrews, D., & Janis, C. (1987). *Taking control of your epilepsy.* Santa Rosa, CA: Basics Publishing.

Renneker, R., Cutler, R., Hora, J., Bacon, C., Bradley, G., Kearney, J., & Cutler (1963). Psychoanalytic explorations of emotional correlates of cancer of the breast. *Psychosomatic Medicine, 25,* 96–108.

Reynolds, P., & Kaplan, G. (1986). Social connections and cancer: A prospective study of Alameda County residents. Paper presented at the Society of Behavioral Medicine Meeting, March 5–7, San Francisco.

Rhodewalt, F., & Zone, J. (1989). Appraisal of life change, depression, and illness in hardy and nonhardy women. *Journal of Personality and Social Psychology, 56,* 81–88.

Rice, P. L. (1987). *Stress and health: Principles and practice for coping and wellness.* Pacific Grove, CA: Brooks/Cole Publishing.

Riesenberg, D. (1987). Treating a societal malignancy—Rape. *Journal of the American Medical Association, 257,* 726–727.

Rivera, E., & Omizo, M. (1980). The effects of relaxation and biofeedback on attention to task and impulsivity among male hyperactive children. *The exceptional child, 27,* 41–51.

Robins, L. (1974). The Vietnam drug user returns. *Special Action Office Monograph,* May 1974 (Series A, No. 2).

Robins, L., Helzer, J., Heselbrock, M., & Wish, E. (1980). Vietnam veterans three years after Vietnam. In L. Brill & C. Winick (Eds.), *The yearbook of substance use and abuse (Vol. 11).* New York: Human Sciences Press.

Robinson, D. (1979). *Talking out of alcoholism: The self-help process of Alcoholics Anonymous.* London: Croom, Helm.

Rodin, J. (1984). Interview with Faye Abdellah, U.S. deputy surgeon general, *American Psychologist, 1,* 68–69.

Rose, M. H., and Thomas, R. B. (1987). *Children with chronic conditions: Nursing in a family and community context.* Orlando, FL: Grune & Stratton.

Rosen, T., Terry, N., & Leventhal, H. (1982). The role of esteem and coping in response to a threat communication. *Journal of Research in Personality, 16*, 90–107.

Rosenbaum, L. (1986). Biofeedback with family therapy for diabetes mellitus. In J. Humphrey (Ed.), *Human stress: Current selected research.* New York: AMS Press.

Rosenbaum, L. (1988). *Biofeedback frontiers: Self-regulation of stress reactivity.* New York: AMS Press.

Rosenbaum, L., Tanenberg, R., & Eastman, R. (1986). Insulin/dextrose infusion system confirms biofeedback effect: IDDM case study. *Diabetes, 35, Supplement 1,* Abstract No. 44.

Rosenbaum, M. (1980a). Schedule for assessing self-control behaviors: Preliminary findings. *Behavior Therapy, 11,* 109–121.

Rosenbaum, M. (1980b). Individual differences in self-control behaviors and tolerance of painful stimulation. *Journal of Abnormal Psychology, 89,* 581–590.

Rosenbaum, M. (1983). Learned resourcefulness as a behavioral repertoire for the self-regulation of internal events: Issues and speculations. In M. Rosenbaum, C. M. Franks, and Y. Jaffe (Eds.), *Perspectives on behavior therapy in the eighties.* New York: Springer.

Rosenbaum, M., & Smira, K. B. (1986). Cognitive and personality factors in the delay of gratification of hemodialysis patients. *Journal of Personality and Social Psychology, 51,* 357–364.

Rosenberg, M., Gelles, R., Holinger, P., Zahn, M., Stark, E., Conn, J., Fajman, N., & Karlson, T. (1987). Violence: Homicide, assault, & suicide. In Amler & Dull (1987). *Closing the gap: The burden of unnecessary illness* (pp. 164–180). New York: Oxford University Press.

Rosenberg, R., & Beck, S. (1986). Preferred assessment methods and treatment modalities for hyperactive children among clinical child and school psychologists. *Journal of Clinical Child Psychology, 15,* 142–147.

Rosenhan, D. (1970). The natural socialization of altruistic autonomy. In J. Macaulay & L. Berkowitz (Eds.), *Altruism and helping behavior.* New York: Academic Press.

Rosenman, R. H., Brand, R. J., Sholtz, R. I., and Friedman, M. (1976). Multivariate prediction of coronary heart disease during 8.5 year follow-up in the Western Collaborative Group Study. *American Journal of Cardiology 37,* 93–910.

Rosenthal, R. (1971). Teacher expectations and their effects upon children. In G. Lesser (Ed.), *Psychology and educational practice.* Glenview, IL: Scott, Foresman.

Ross, M., & Ross, A. (1980). Commentary: Parents' experience of health care for the terminally ill child. In M. Jospe, J. Nieberding, & B. Cohen (Eds.), *Psychological factors in health care,* (pp. 409–425). Lexington, Mass: Lexington Books.

Rotter, J., Seeman, M., & Liverant, S. (1962). Internal vs. external locus of control: A major variable in behavior theory. In N. F. Washburne (Ed.), *Decisions, values and groups,* (pp. 473–516). London: Pergamon.

Rozensky, R., & Pasternak, J. (1985). Obi-Wan Kenobi, "The Force," and the art of biofeedback: A headache treatment for overachieving young boys. *Clinical Biofeedback & Health, 8,* 9–13.

Rubenstein, C. (1986). A consumer's guide to psychotherapy. In C. Tavris (Ed.), *Every woman's emotional well-being.* New York: Doubleday.

Russell, D., & Cutrona, C. (1985). Loneliness and physical health among the rural elderly. Paper presented at the annual meeting of the American Psychological Association, Los Angeles.

Russell, D. (1982). *Rape in marriage.* New York: Macmillan.

Rutter, M. (1983). Stress, coping and development. In N. Garmezy & M. Rutter (Eds.), *Stress, coping and development in children,* (pp. 1–42). New York: McGraw-Hill.

Safer, D., & Krager, J. (1985). Prevalence of medication treatment for hyperactive adolescents. *Psychopharmacology Bulletin, 21,* 212–215.

Sagan, L. (1987). *The health of nations.* New York: Basic Books.

Santrock, J. (1987). *Adolescence.* Dubuque, Iowa: Wm. C. Brown.

Sarason, I., & Sarason, B. (1981). Teaching cognitive and social skills to high school students. *Journal of Consulting and Clinical Psychology, 49,* 908–918.

Sarason, I. G. (1975a). Text anxiety, attention, and the general problem of anxiety. In C. D. Spielberger & I. G. Sarason *Stress and Anxiety, Volume 1,* (pp. 165–187). New York: Wiley.

Sarason, I. G. (1975b). Anxiety and self-preoccupation. In I. G. Sarason & C. D. Spielberger (Eds.),

Stress and Anxiety, Volume 2, (pp. 27–44). New York: Wiley.

Sarason, I., Johnson, J., Berberich, J., & Siegel, J. (1979). Helping police officers to cope with stress: A cognitive-behavioral approach. *American Journal of Community Psychology, 7,* 593–603.

Sarason, I. G., Johnson, J. H., Sarason, B. R. (1978). Assessing the impact of life changes: Development of the Life Experiences Survey. *Journal of Consulting and Clinical Psychology, 46,* 932–946.

Sarason, I. G., Sarason, B. R., & Johnson, J. H. (1985). Stressful life events: Measurement, moderators, and adaptation. In S. Burchfield (Ed.), *Stress: Psychological and physiological interactions.* Washington, DC: Hemisphere.

Sargent, J. D., Green, E. E., and Walters, E. D. (1972). The use of autogenic feedback training in a pilot study of migraine and tension headaches. *Headache, 12,* 120–124.

Scarr, S. (1984). *Mother care, other care.* New York: Basic Books.

Schachter, S. (1982). Recidivism and self-cure of smoking and obesity. *American Psychologist, 37,* 436–444.

Schaefli, A., Rest, J., & Thoma, S. (1985). Does moral education improve moral judgment? A meta-analysis of intervention studies using the Defining Issues Test. *Review of Educational Research, 55,* 319–352.

Schell, O. (1985). *Modern meat.* New York: Vintage Books.

Scherwitz, L., Graham II, L. E., Grandits, G., & Billings, J. (1987). Speech characteristics and behavior-type assessment in the multiple risk factor intervention trial (MRFIT) structured interviews, *Journal of Behavioral Medicine, 10,* 173–195.

Schleifer, S., Keller, S., Meyerson, A., Rasking, M., Davis, K., & Stein, M. (1984). Lymphocyte function in major depressive disorder. *Archives of General Psychiatry, 41,* 484–486.

Schleifer, S., Keller, S., McKegney, F., & Stein, M. (1979). The influence of stress and other psychosocial factors on human immunity. Paper presented at the 36th Annual Meeting of the Psychosomatic Society, Dallas.

Schleser, R., Meyers, A., & Montgomery, T. (1980). A cognitive behavioral intervention for improving basketball performance. Paper presented at the Association for the Advancement of Behavior Therapy, 18th Annual Convention, New York.

Schlesinger, Arthur (1976). *The American way of violence.*

Schlichter, K. J., & Horan, J. J. (1981). Effects of stress inoculation on the anger and aggression management of institutionalized juvenile delinquents. *Cognitive Therapy and Research, 5,* 359–365.

Schmale, A., & Iker, H. (1966). The psychological setting of uterine cervical cancer. *Annals of the New York Academy of Sciences, 125,* 807–813.

Schmidt, S., & Kipnis, D. (1987). The perils of persistence. *Psychology Today, 21,* 32–34.

Schmied, L., & Lawler, K. (1986). Hardiness, Type A behavior, and the stress-illness relation in working women. *Journal of Personality and Social Psychology, 51,* 1218–1223.

Schmieder, R., Friedrich, G., Neus, H., Rudel, H., & von Eiff, A. (1984). The influence of beta blockers on cardiovascular reactivity and Type A behavior pattern in hypertensives. *Psychosomatic Medicine, 45,* 417–423.

Schneider, C. (1983). Biofeedback treatment of irritable bowel syndrome. Paper presented at the annual meeting of the Biofeedback Society of America, Denver.

Schneider, J., Smith, C., Whitcher, S. (1988, June). The relationship of mental imagery to white blood cell (neutrophil) function: Experimental studies of normal subjects. Presentation at the Tenth Annual International Conference on Mental Imagery, New Haven, CT.

Schorr, L., & Schorr, D. (1988). *Within our reach: Breaking the Cycle of Disadvantage.* New York: Doubleday.

Schultz, J., & Luthe, Wolfgang (1959). *Autogenic training* New York & London: Grune & Stratton, 1965.

Schultz, J., Moen, M., Pechacek, T., Harty, K., Skubic, M., Gust, S., & Dean, A. (1986, Autumn). The Minnesota plan for nonsmoking and health: The legislative experience. *Journal of Public Health Policy,* pp. 300–313.

Schwartz, G., & Shapiro, D. (1973). Biofeedback and essential hypertension: Current findings and theoretical concerns. In L. Bird (Ed.), *Biofeedback: Behavioral medicine.* New York: Grune & Stratton.

Schwartz, G. E. (1984). *Psychobiology of health: A new synthesis.* In B. Hammonds & C. Scheirer

(Eds.), *Psychology and health,* (pp. 149–193). Washington, DC: American Psychological Association.

Schwartz, G. E., & Weiss, S. M. (1978). Behavioral medicine revisited: An amended definition. *Journal of Behavioral Medicine, 1,* 249–252.

Schwartz, G. E., & Weiss, S. M. (1977). What is behavioral medicine? *Psychosomatic Medicine, 39,* 377–381.

Schwartz, R. (1986). The internal dialogue: On the asymmetry between positive and negative coping thoughts. *Cognitive Therapy and Research, 10,* 591–605.

Schwarz, J. (1985). Child psychopathology. In S. Pfeiffer (Ed.), *Clinical child psychology: An introduction to theory, research, and practice,* (pp. 93–176). New York: Harcourt Brace Jovanovich.

Schwarz, John (1988). *American's hidden success: A reassessment of public policy from Kennedy to Reagan.* New York: Norton.

Science Digest (1981, May). How much of a brain do you need? Volume 89, p. 110.

Segal, N. (1985). Holocaust twins: Their special bond. *Psychology Today* (August), 52–58.

Seligman, M. (1975). *Helplessness.* San Francisco: Freeman.

Selye, H. (1976). *The stress of life.* New York: McGraw-Hill.

Selye, H. (1978). On the real benefits of eustress. *Psychology Today,* 12 (10), 60–64.

Senate Select Committee on Nutrition and Human Needs (1977). *Dietary goals for the United States, 2nd Edition.* Washington, DC: U.S. Senate.

Seres, J., & Newman, R. (1976). Results of treatment of chronic low back pain at the Portland Pain Center. *Journal of Neurosurgery, 455,* 32–36.

Setterlind, S. (1986). An experimental study of relaxation training in Swedish schools. Presentation at the Seventeenth Annual Biofeedback Meeting, New Orleans.

Shaffer, J. W., Graves, P. L., Swank, R. T., & Pearson, T. (1987). Clustering of personality traits in youth and the subsequent development of cancer among physicians. *Journal of Behavioral Medicine, 10,* 441–447.

Shaver, P., Furman, W., & Buhrmester, D. (1985). Transition to college: Network changes, social skills, and loneliness. In S. Duck and D. Perlman (Eds.), *Understanding personal relationships: An interdisciplinary approach.* London: Sage.

Sheehan, Kay. (1987). A psychotherapeutic model of power struggle resolution based on a synthesis of Gandhi's satyagraha and Adler's/Driekurs' theories and methods. Unpublished doctoral dissertation, University of Northern Colorado, Greeley.

Sheehy, G. (1985). *Pathfinders.* New York: Bantam Books.

Shekelle, R., Gayle, M., Ostfeld, A., & Paul, O. (1983). Hostility, risk of coronary heart disease & mortality, *Psychosomatic Medicine, 45,* 109–114.

Shekelle, R., Raynor, W. J., Ostfeld, A. M., Garron, D. C., Bieliauskas, L. A., Liu, S., Maliza, C., & Ogelsby, P. (1981). Psychological depression and 17 year risk of death from cancer, *Psychosomatic Medicine, 43,* 117–125.

Shekim, W., Dekirmenjian, H., & Chapel, J. (1977). Urinary catecholamine metabolites in hyperkinetic boys treated with d-amphetamine. *American Journal of Psychiatry, 134,* 1276–1279.

Shellenberger, R., & Green, J. (1986). *From the ghost in the box to successful biofeedback training.* Greeley, CO: Health Psychology Publications.

Shellenberger, R., & Green, J. (1987). Specific effects and biofeedback versus biofeedback-assisted self-regulation training. *Biofeedback and Self-Regulation, 12,* 185–209.

Shellenberger, R., & Lewis, M. (1986). Reliability of stress profiling, in *Biofeedback Society of America Proceedings,* San Francisco.

Shellenberger, R., Amar, P., Schneider, C., & Stewart, R. (1989). *Clinical efficacy and cost effectiveness of biofeedback therapy: Guidelines for third-party reimbursement.* Wheat Ridge, CO: Association for Applied Psychophysiology and Biofeedback.

Shellenberger, R., Turner, J., Green, J., & Cooney, J. (1986). Health changes in a biofeedback and stress management program, *Clinical Biofeedback & Health, 9,* 23–24.

Shephard, R. (1989). Exercise and employee-wellness initiatives. *Health Education Research, 4,* 233–243.

Sheridan, Charles (1980). Outline of a research strategy for biofeedback-based therapy. *American Journal of Clinical Biofeedback, 3,* 107–113.

Shiffman, S. (1982). Relapse following smoking cessation: A situational analysis. *Journal of Consulting and Clinical Psychology 50,* 71–86.

Shiffman, S. (1984). Coping with temptations to smoke. *Journal of Consulting and Clinical Psychology, 52,* 261–267.

Shiffman, S., Read, L., Maltese, J., Rapkin, D., & Jarvik, M. (1985). In G. Marlatt & J. Gordon (Eds.), *Relapse prevention: Maintenance strategies in addictive behavior change.* New York: Guilford Press.

Shultz, J., Moen, M., Pechacek, T., Harty, K., Skubaic, M., Gust, S., & Dean, A. (1986, Autumn). The Minnesota plan for nonsmoking and health: The legislative experience. *Journal of Public Health Policy,* 300–313.

Siegel, B. (1986). *Love, medicine, and miracles.* New York: Harper & Row.

Sigurdson, H. (1985). *The Manhattan House of Detention: A study of modular direct supervision.* Boulder, CO: National Institute of Corrections Center.

Sigurdson, H. (1987). *Pima County detention center: A study of modular direct supervision.* Boulder, CO: National Institute of Corrections Center.

Simon, S., Howe, L., & Kirschenbaum, H. (1972). *Values clarification: A handbook of practical strategies for teachers and students.* New York: Hart.

Simonton, C., Matthews-Simonton, S., & Creighton, J. (1978). *Getting well again.* Los Angeles: J. P. Tarcher.

Singer, Jerome (1974). *Imagery and daydream methods in psychotherapy and behavior modification.* New York: Academic Press.

Singer, Jerome (1976, July). Fantasy: The foundation of serenity. *Psychology Today.*

Sloan, R. (1987). Workplace health promotion: A commentary on the evolution of a paradigm. *Health Education Quarterly,* 14, 181–194.

Smeeding, T. M., & Torry, B. B. (1988). Poor children in rich countries. *Science,* 242, 873–877.

Smith, G., Jr., O'Rourke, D., Conger, C., Charlton, R., Steele, R., & Smith, S. (In press). Psychological modulation of antigen specific cell-mediated immunity. *Psychosomatic Medicine.*

Smith, G. R., and McDaniel, S. M. (1983). Psychologically mediated effects on the delayed hypersensitivity reaction to tuberculin in humans. *Psychosomatic Medicine,* 46, 65–70.

Smith, G. R., McKenzie, J. M., Marner, D. J., and Steele, R. W. (1985). *Archives of Internal Medicine,* 145, 2110–2112.

Smith, M., Collisan, M., & Hurrell, J. (1978). A review of NIOSH psychological stress research. In *Occupational Stress,* Washington, DC: DHEW (NIOSH) Publication No. 78–156.

Smoll, F., & Smith, R. (1984). Leadership research in youth sports. In J. Silva & R. Weinberg (Eds.), *Psychological foundations of sport,* (pp. 351–385). Champaign, IL: Human Kinetics.

Solano, C., Batten, P., & Parish, E. (1982). Loneliness and patterns of self-disclosure. *Journal of Personality and Social Psychology,* 43, 524–531.

Solomon, G., Kay, N., & Morley, J. (1983). Endorphins: A link between personality, stress, emotions, immunity, and disease? In N. Plotnikoff, R. Faith, A. Murgo, & R. Good (Eds.), *Enkephalins and endorphins, stress and the immune system,* (pp. 129–137). New York: Plenum Press.

Sosa, R., Kennell, J., Klaus, M., Robetson, S., & Urrutia, J. (1980). The effect of a supportive companion on perinatal problems, length of labor and mother-infant interaction. *New England Journal of Medicine,* 303, 597–600.

Spielberger, C. E., Edwards, C. D., Montuori, J., & Lushene, R. (1986). Children's State-Trait Anxiety Inventory. Palo Alto, CA: Consulting Psychologists Press.

Spielberger, C., & London, P. (1982, March-April,). Rage boomerangs. *American Health,* 52–56.

Spielberger, C., Jacobs, G., Russell, S., & Crane, R. (1983). Assessment of anger: The State-Trait Anger Scale. In J. Butcher, C. Spielberger (Eds.), *Advances in Personality Assessment,* Vol., 2. New York: Erlbaum.

Spilman, M., Goetz, A., Schultz, J., Bellingham, R., & Johnson, D. (1987). Effects of a corporate health promotion program. *Journal of Occupational Medicine,* 29, (4).

Spinetta, J., Elliot, E., Hennessey, J., Knapp, V., Sheposh, J., Sparta, S., & Sprigle, R. (1982). The pediatric psychologist's role in catastrophic illness. In J. Tuma (Ed.), *Handbook for the practice of pediatric psychology* (pp. 165–220). New York: Wiley.

Spirito, A., Russo, D., & Masek, B. (1984). Behavioral interventions and stress management training for hospitalized adolescents and young adults with cystic fibrosis. *General Hospital Psychiatry,* 6, 211–218.

Spivack, G., & Shure, M. B. (1974). *Social adjustment of young children.* San Francisco: Jossey-Bass.

Srole, L., & Fisher, A. K. (1984). The midtown Manhattan longitudinal study versus the mental paradise lost doctrine: A controversy joined. In Mednick, Harway, & Finello (Eds.), *Handbook of longitudinal research,* (pp. 225–255). New York: Praeger.

Srole, L., & Fisher, A. K. (1980). The midtown Manhattan longitudinal study versus "The Mental Paradise Lost" doctrine. *Archives of General Psychiatry, 37,* 209–221.

Stacy, B. (1987, July). Helping kids cope with terminal illness. *East-West Journal.*

Standards for Educational and Psychological Testing (1985). Prepared by the committee to develop standards for educational and psychological testing of the American Educational Research Association, The American Psychological Association, and the National Council on Measurement in Education. Washington DC: American Psychological Association.

Starr, Paul. (1982). *The social transformation of American medicine.* New York: Basic Books.

Steig, R. L., & Williams, R. C. (1983). Cost effectiveness study of multidisciplinary pain treatment of industrial-injured workers. *Seminars in Neurology, 3,* 370–376.

Steiner, S., & Dince, W. (1981). Biofeedback efficacy studies: A critique of critiques. *Biofeedback and Self-Regulation, 6,* 275–288.

Steiner, S., & Dince, W. (1983). A reply on the nature of biofeedback efficacy studies. *Biofeedback and Self-Regulation, 7,* 499–504.

Sterman, M. B. (1984). The role of sensorimotor rhythmic EEG activity in the etiology and treatment of generalized motor seizures. In T. Elbert et al., (Eds.), *Self Regulation of the Brain and Behavior,* Berlin: Springer-Verlag.

Sterman, M. B. (1986). Epilepsy and its treatment with EEG feedback therapy. *Annals of Behavioral Medicine, 8,* 21–25.

Sterman, M. B., & Friar, L. (1971). Suppression of seizures in an epileptic following sensorimotor EEG feedback training. *Electroencephalography and Clinical Neurophysiology, 33,* 89–95.

Sterman, M. B., & MacDonald, L. (1978). Effects of central cortical EEG feedback training on incidence of poorly controlled seizures. *Epilepsia, 19,* 207–222.

Sterman, M. B., & Wyrwicka, W. (1967). EEG correlates of sleep: Evidence for separate forebrain substrates. *Brain Research, 6,* 143–163.

Stern, A. (1981). Asthma and emotion. *Psychosomatic Medicine, Vol 43,* 365–372.

Stern, J., Brown, M., Ulett, G., & Sletten, I. (1977). A comparison of hypnosis, acupuncture, morphine, Valium, aspirin, and placebo in the management of experimentally induced pain. In W. Edmonston (Ed.), Conceptual and investigative approaches to hypnosis and hypnotic phenomena. *Annals of the New York Academy of Science, 296,* 175–193.

Stern, P. (1988). *The best Congress money can buy.* New York: Pantheon.

Steuer, F., Applefield, J., & Smith, R. (1971). Televised aggression and interpersonal aggression of preschool children. *Journal of Experimental Child Psychology, 11,* 442–447.

Stevenson, H. (1974). Reflections on the China Visit. *Society for Research in Child Development Newsletter,* Fall, 3.

Stitt, P. A. (1981). *Fighting the food giants.* Manitowoc, WI: Natural Press.

Stolbach, L. L., & Brandt, U. C. (1988). Psychosocial factors in the development and progression of breast cancer. In Cary L. Cooper (Ed.), *Stress and Breast Cancer.* New York: Wiley.

Stone, G., Hindz, W., & Schmidt, G. (1975). Teaching mental health behaviors to elementary school children. *Professional Psychology, 6,* 34–40.

Stout, C., Morrow, J., Brandt, E., & Wolf, S. (1964). Unusually low incidence of death from myocardial infarction: Study of an Italian American community in Pennsylvania. *Journal of American Medical Association, 188,* 845–849.

Stout, D., Thorton, B., & Russell, H. (1980). Effect of relaxation training on student persistence and academic performance. *Psychological Reports, 47,* 189–190.

Stoyva, J., & Budzynski, T. (1974). Cultivated low arousal—an antistress response? In L. DiCara (Ed.), *Biofeedback and Self-Control,* (pp. 265–290). Chicago: Aldine Publishing.

Straus, M. A., Gelles, R. J., & Steinmetz, S. K. (1980). *Behind closed doors: Violence in the American family.* Garden City, NY: Anchor Books.

Stroebel, Charles (1983). *OR: The quieting reflex.* New York: Berkley Books.

Stroebel, E., & Stroebel, C. (1980). *The Kiddie QR: A choice for children.* New Haven, CT: QR Institute.

Stroebel, L., & Stroebel, C. (1984). The quieting reflex: A psychophysiologic approach for helping children deal with healthy and unhealthy stress.

In James Humphrey (Ed.), *Stress in childhood*, (pp. 251–276). New York: AMS Press.

Strupp, H., & Binder, J. (1984). *Psychotherapy in a new key*. New York: Basic Books.

Stuart, R. B. (Ed.), (1977). *Behavioral self-management: Strategies, techniques and outcomes*. New York: Brunner/Mazel.

Stuart, R., & Mitchell, C. (1980). Self-help groups in the control of obesity. In A. J. Stunkard (Ed.), *Obesity*. Philadelphia: W. B. Saunders.

Stumphauzer, J. S. (1972). Increased delay of gratification in young prison inmates through imitation of high delay peer models. *Journal of Personality and Social Psychology, 21*, 10–17.

Suinn, R. (1976). Visual motor behavior rehearsal for adaptive behavior. In J. Krumboltz and C. Thoresen (Eds.), *Counseling methods*. New York: Holt, Rinehart and Winston.

Suinn, R. (1983). Imagery and sports. In A. Sheikh (Ed.), *Imagery: Current theory, research, and application*, (pp. 507–533). New York: Wiley.

Suinn, R. (1986). *Seven steps to peak performance*. Toronto: Hans Huber.

Suinn, R. M., & Richardson, F. (1971). Anxiety management training: A nonspecific behavior therapy for anxiety control. *Behavior Therapy, 2*, 493–510.

Suinn, R. M. (1980). Pattern A behaviors and heart disease: Intervention approaches. In J. M. Ferguson & C. B. Taylor (Eds.). *Advances in Behavioral Medicine*, (pp. 5–28). New York: Spectrum Publications.

Surwit, R., Shapiro, D., & Good, M. (1978). Comparison of cardiovascular biofeedback, neuromuscular biofeedback, and meditation in the treatment of borderline essential hypertension. *Journal of Consulting and Clinical Psychology, 45*, 252–262.

Swan, M., Stark, W., Hammerman, D., & Lesis, C. (1983). Research in outdoor education: Summaries of doctoral studies, Vol. III. Reston, VA: AAHPRD.

Swanson, M., & Kinsobourne, M. (1980). Food dyes impair performance of hyperactive children on a laboratory learning test. *Science, 207*, 1485–1487.

Swearingen, R. (1978). A humanistic approach to the management of fractures. *Today's Clinician*, February, 21–25.

Taber, C. W. (1970). *Taber's cyclopedic medical dictionary*. Phildadelphia: F. A. Davis.

Tanner, Ogden. (1976). *Stress*. New York: Time-Life Books.

Taub, E. (1977). Self-regulation of human tissue temperature. In G. E. Schwartz & J. Beatty (Eds.), *Biofeedback theory and research*, (pp. 265–300). New York: Academic Press.

Taylor, S. E. (1986). *Health psychology*. New York: Random House.

Temoshok, L., & Heller, B. (1981). Stress and Type C versus epidemiological risk factors in melanoma. Paper presented at the 89th Annual Convention of the American Psychological Association, Los Angeles.

Temoshok, Lydia (1985). Biopsychosocial studies on cutaneous malignant melanoma: Psychosocial factors associated with prognostic indicators, progression, psychophysiological and tumor-host response. *Social Science and Medicine, 20* (8) 833–840.

The American Nurse. (1974, May). Scope of Practice Statement for PNP's Issued, p. 5.

Thoits, Peggy, A. (1986). Social support as coping assistance. *Journal of Consulting and Clinical Psychology, 54*, 416–423.

Thomas, A. (1980). *The dynamics of psychological development*. New York: Brunner/Mazel.

Thomas, C. B. (1988). Cancer and the youthful mind: A forty-year perspective. *Advances, 5* (2), 42–58.

Thomas, C., Dusynski, K., & Shaffer, J. (1979). Family attitudes in youth as potential predictors of cancer. *Psychosomatic Medicine, 41*, 287–301.

Thomas, J., Koshy, M., Patterson, L., Dorn, L., & Thomas, K. (1984). Management of pain in sickle cell disease using biofeedback therapy: A preliminary study. *Biofeedback & Self Regulation*, 413–420.

Thomas, L. (1980). *The medusa and the snail*. New York: Bantam Books.

Thomas, L. (1977). On the science and technology of medicine. In J. H. Knowles (Ed.), *Doing better and feeling worse: Health in the United States*. New York: W. W. Norton.

Thompson, W. G., & Heaton, K. W. (1980). Functional bowel disorders in apparently healthy people. *Gastroenterology, 79*, 283–388.

Thoreson, C., & Mahoney, M. (1974). *Behavioral self-control*. New York: Holt, Rinehart & Winston.

Tiffany, S., Martin, E., & Baker, T. (1986). Treatments for cigarette smoking: An evaluation of the contributions of aversion and counseling procedures, *Behavior Research and Therapy, 24,* 437–452.

Tipton, R., & Riebsame, W. (1987). Beliefs about smoking and health: Their measurement and relationship to smoking behavior. *Addictive behaviors. 12,* 217–223.

Toomey, M. (1972). Conflict theory approach to decision making applied to alcoholics. *Journal of Personality and Social Psychology, 24,* 199–206.

Tsokos, G., & Balow, J. (1983). Regulation of human cellular immune responses by glucocorticosteroids. In N. Plotnikoff, R. Faith, A. Murgo, & R. Good (Eds.), *Enkephalins and endorphins, stress and the immune system,* (pp. 38–44). New York: Plenum Press.

Tuma, J. (1982). *Handbook for the practice of pediatric psychology.* New York: Wiley.

Turk, D., & Flor, H. (1984). Etiological theories and treatments for chronic back pain: Psychological models and intervention. *Pain, 19,* 209–234.

Turk, D., Meichenbaum, D., & Genest, M. (1983). *Pain and behavioral medicine: A cognitive-behavioral perspective.* New York: Guilford Press.

U.S. Bureau of the Census (1987). *Statistical abstract of the United States, 1987* (107th edition). Washington, DC: U.S. Government Printing Office.

U.S. Department of Education (1986). *High school and beyond.* Washington, DC: U.S. Government Printing Office.

U.S. Department of Health and Human Services (1984). *The 1984 report of the Joint National Committee on Detection, Evaluation, and Treatment of High Blood Pressure.* (DHHS Publication No. NIH 84–1088). Washington, DC: U.S. Government Printing Office.

U.S. Department of Health and Human Services (1979). *Healthy people: The surgeon general's report on health promotion and disease prevention, 1979.* Washington, DC: U.S. Government Printing Office.

U.S. Department of Agriculture (1985). *Dietary guidelines for Americans, second edition.* Washington, DC: U.S. Government Printing Office.

U.S. Department of Health and Human Services (1986). *The 1990 health objectives for the nation: A midcourse review.* Washington, DC: U.S. Government Printing Office.

U.S. Department of Health and Human Services (1988). Births, marriages, divorces, and deaths for September 1988, *Monthly Vital Statistics Report. 37,* 10–12.

U.S. Department of Health and Human Services (1988). *Health United States 1987.* Hyattsville, MD: National Center for Health Statistics.

U.S. Department of Labor (1984). Current labor statistics, *Monthly Labor Review, 107,* 1, 8.

Vaillant, George E. (1977). *Adaptation to life.* Boston: Little Brown.

Valdez, M. (1985). Effects of a biofeedback-assisted attention training in a college population, *Biofeedback and Self-Regulation, 10,* 315–324.

Van Nostrand, J., Zappolos, A., Hing, E., Bloom, B., Hirsch, B., & Foley, D. (1979). The national nursing home survey: 1977 summary for the United States. (DHEW publication No. PHS 79-1794). Washington, DC: U.S. Government Printing Office, Statistics Series, 13–43.

Varni, J. (1981). Self regulation techniques in the management of chronic arthritic pain in hemophilia. *Behavior Therapy, 12,* 185–194.

Varni, J., & Gilbert, A. (1982). Self regulation of chronic arthritic pain and long term analgesic dependence in a hemophiliac. *Rheumatology Rehabilitation, 22,* 171–174.

Varni, J., Gilbert, A., & Dietrich, S. (1981). Behavioral medicine in pain and analgesia management for the hemophilic child with factor VIII inhibitor. *Pain, 11,* 121-126.

Vartiainen, E., McAlister, A., Puska, P., Viri, L., Tossavainen, K., Niskanen, E., & Pallonen, U. (1986). *Short term effects of school and community-based programs to prevent smoking and alcohol abuse among adolescents.* Department of Epidemiology, National Public Health Institute, Finland.

Veninga, R., & Spradley, J. (1981). *The work/stress connection: How to cope with job burnout.* Boston: Little Brown.

Vincent, M., Clearie, A., & Schluchter, M. (1987). Reducing adolescent pregnancy through school and community-based education. *Journal of the American Medical Association, 257,* 3382–3386.

Vivekananda, Swami (1955). *Raja-Yoga.* New York: Ramakrishna-Vivekanda Center.

Vormbrock, J., & Grossberg, J. (1988). Cardiovascular effects of human-pet dog interactions. *Journal of Behavioral Medicine, 11,* 509–517.

Wald, A. (1981). Use of biofeedback in the treatment of fecal incontinence in patients with meningeomyelocele. *Pediatrics, 68*, 45–49.

Wald, A. (1983). Biofeedback for neurogenic fecal incontinence: Rectal sensation is a determinant of outcome. *Journal of Pediatric Gastroenterology & Nutrition, 2*, 302–306.

Walker, C., Milling, L., & Bonner, B. (1988). Incontinence disorders: Enuresis and encopresis, In D. Routh (Ed.), *Pediatric psychology*, (pp. 363–397). New York: Guilford Press.

Walker, L. E. (1980). Battered women. In A. M. Brodsky & R. T. Hare-Mustin (Eds.), *Women and psychotherapy*, (pp. 339–363). New York: Guilford Press.

Wallace, G., Goldstein, B., Nathan, P. (1985). *Introduction to psychology*. Dubuque, IA: William C. Brown.

Wankle, L., & Thompson, C. (1977). Motivating people to be physically active: Self-persuasion vs. balanced decision making. *Journal of Applied Social Psychology, 7*, 332–340.

Warner, K. (1987). Selling health promotion to corporate America: Uses and abuses of the economic argument. *Health Education Quarterly, 14*, 39–55.

Waters, W., Williamson, D., Bernard, B., Blouin, D., & Faulstich, M. (1987). Test-retest reliability of psychophysiological assessment. *Behaviour Research and Therapy, 25*, 213–221.

Watkins, P., & Eisler, R. (1988). The Type A behavior pattern, hostility, and interpersonal skill. *Behavior Modification, 12*, 315–334.

Watterson, K. (1988). *The safe medicine book*. New York: Ballantine Books.

Weidenbaum, M. (1978, April). The costs of government regulation of business, *Joint Economic Committee*, p. 16. Washington DC: United States Congress.

Weiner, I., (1982). *Children and adolescent psychopathology*. New York: Wiley.

Weinstein, K., Davison, G., DeQuattro, V., & Allen, J. (1987). Type A behavior and cognitions: Is hostility the bad actor? *Health Psychology, 6*, 55.

Weinstein, N. D. (1987). Introduction: studying self-protective behavior. In N. D. Weinstein (Ed.), *Taking Care: Understanding and encouraging self-protective behavior*. Cambridge: Cambridge University Press.

Weinstein, N. D. (1988). The precaution adoption process. *Health Psychology, 7* (4) 355–386.

Weissman, A. (1979). *The dysfunctional attitude scale: A validation study*. Unpublished dissertation. University of Pennsylvania.

Weissman, A., & Beck, A. (1978). *Development and validation of the Dysfunctional Attitude Scale: A preliminary investigation*. Paper presented at the Annual Meeting of the American Educational Research Association. Toronto.

Wenger, M. A., Bagchi, B. K., & Anand, B. K. (1961). Experiments in India on "voluntary" control of the heart and pulse. *Circulation, 24*, 1319–1325.

Werder, D., & Sargent, J. (1984). A study of childhood headache using biofeedback as a treatment alternative. *Headache, 24*, 122–126.

Werner, E., & Smith, R. (1982). *Vulnerable, but invincible: A longitudinal study of resilient children and youth*. New York: McGraw Hill.

Werner, E. (1984). Resilient children. In *Young Children*. Washington, DC: National Association for the Education of Young Children.

Werner, E. (1989). High risk children in young adulthood: A longitudinal study from birth to 32 years. *American Journal of Orthopsychiatry, 59*, 72–81.

West, L. J., & Stein, M. (Eds.), (1982). *Critical issues in behavioral medicine*. Philadelphia: J. B. Lippincott.

Wetmore, R. (1972). The influence of Outward Bound school experience on the self-concept of adolescence boys. University Microfilms, 72–25, 475.

White, Robert (1959). Motivation reconsidered. *Psychological Review, 66*, 297–333.

Whitehead, W., Burgio, K., & Engel, B. (1985). Biofeedback treatment of fecal incontinence in geriatric patients. *Journal of the American Geriatric Society, 33*, 320–324.

Whitehead, W., Parker, L., Basmajian, L., Morrill-Corbin, E., Middaugh, S., Garwood, M., Cataldo, M., & Freeman, J. (1986). Treatment of fecal incontinence in children with spina bifida: Comparison of biofeedback and behavior modification. *Archives of Physical Medicine and Rehabilitation, 67*, 218–224.

Whitehead, W., Parker, L., Masek, B., Cataldo, M., & Freeman, J. (1981). Biofeedback treatment for fecal incontinence in patients with meningomyelocele. *Developmental Medical Child Neurology, 23*, 313–322.

Wiebe, D., & McCallum, D. (1986). Health practices and hardiness as mediators in the stress-illness relationship. *Health Psychology, 5,* 425–438.

Williams, R., & Anderson, N. (1987). Hostility and coronary heart disease. In J. Elias & P. Marshall (Eds.), *Cardiovascular disease and behavior,* (pp. 17–37). New York: Harper & Row.

Williams, R., Haney, T., Lee, K., Kong, Y., Blumenthal, J., & Whalen, R. (1980). Type A behavior, hostility, and atherosclerosis. *Psychosomatic Medicine, 42,* 539–549.

Wilson, S. C., and Barber, T. X. (1983). The fantasy-prone personality: Implications for understanding imagery, hypnosis, and parapsychological phenomena. In *Imagery: Current theory, research, and applications,* Anees Sheikh (Ed.), New York: Wiley.

Wirsching, M., Stierlin, H., Hoffman, F., Weber, G., & Wirshing, B. (1982). Psychological identification of breast cancer patients before biopsy, *Journal of Psychosomatic Research, 26,* 1–10.

Wittkower, Eric (1977). Historical perspective of contemporary psychosomatic medicine, In Z. J. Lipowski, D. Lipsitt, & P. Whybrow (Eds.), *Psychosmatic Medicine,* (pp. 3–13). New York: Oxford University Press.

Wolf, S., & Fischer-Williams, M. (1987). The use of biofeedback in disorders of motor function. In J. Hatch, J. Fisher, & J. Rugh (Eds.), *Biofeedback: Studies in clinical efficacy,* (pp. 153–179). New York: Plenum Press.

Wolff, H. (1952). *Stress and disease.* Springfield, IL: Charles C Thomas.

Wolf, S., & Goodell, H. (1968). *Harold G. Wolff's stress and disease.* Springfield, IL: Charles C Thomas.

Wolfe, S. (Ed.), (1988a). Medical update, *Health Letter, 4,* 11.

Wolfe, S. (Ed.), (1988b). Reagan administration does not believe worker health is important, *Health Letter, 4,* 12.

Wolpe, J. (1958). *Psychotherapy by reciprocal inhibition.* Stanford, CA: Stanford University Press.

Wood, C. (1987). Buffer of hardiness: An interview with Suzanne C. Ouellette Kobasa. *Advances, 4,* 37–45.

World Health (1988, January/February). Health for all—all for health, pp. 16–20.

World Health Organization (1947). Constitution of the World Health Organization, *Chronicle of the World Health Organization, I,* 29–43.

World Health Organization (1987, March). Cigarettes smoked outstrip population growth, p. 30.

Worldwide Environmental and Safety Committee (1986, October 17). Worldwide environmental and safety policy statement. St. Paul, Minnesota: H.B. Fuller Company.

Wybran, J. (1985). Enkephalins, endorphins, substance P, and the immune system. In R. Guillemin (Ed.), *Neuromodulation of immunity,* (pp. 157–160). New York: Raven Press.

Yarrow, L. J., MacTurk, R. H., Vietze, P. M., McCarthy, M. E., Klein, R. P., & McQuiston, S. (1984). Developmental course of parental stimulation and its relationship to mastery motivation during infancy. *Developmental Psychology, 20,* 492–503.

Young, J. D., & Cohen, Z. A. (1988, January). How killer cells kill. *Scientific American, 258,* 38–44.

Yussen, S. (1977). Characteristics of moral dilemmas written by adolescents. *Developmental Psychology, 13,* 162–163.

Zahn-Waxler, C., & Radke-Yarrow, M. (1979). A developmental analysis of children's responses to emotions in others. Paper presented at the biennual meeting of the Society for Research in Child Development, San Francisco, March.

Zastowny, T., Kirschenbaum, D., & Meng, A. (1986). Coping skills training for children: Effects on distress before, during, and after hospitalization for surgery. *Health Psychology, 5,* 231–247.

Zeltzer, L., Dash, J., & Holland, J. (1979). Hypnotically induced pain control in sickle cell anemia. *Pediatrics, 64,* 533–536.

Ziegler, D., Hassanein, R., & Couch, J. (1977). Characteristics of life headache histories in a nonclinic population. *Neurology, 27,* 265–269.

Index